Animal Medicine: A Guide for Veterinary Practitioners

Animal Medicine: A Guide for Veterinary Practitioners

Edited by Herbert Dundas

SYRAWOOD
PUBLISHING HOUSE

New York

Published by Syrawood Publishing House,
750 Third Avenue, 9th Floor,
New York, NY 10017, USA
www.syrawoodpublishinghouse.com

Animal Medicine: A Guide for Veterinary Practitioners
Edited by Herbert Dundas

International Standard Book Number: 978-1-68286-553-8 (Hardback)

Cataloging-in-Publication Data

Animal medicine : a guide for veterinary practitioners / edited by Herbert Dundas.
     p. cm.
Includes bibliographical references and index.
ISBN 978-1-68286-553-8
1. Veterinary medicine. 2. Animals--Diseases. 3. Animal health. I. Dundas, Herbert.
SF745 .A55 2018
636.089--dc23

TABLE OF CONTENTS

PREFACE

Animal medicine or veterinary medicine deals with the treatment and care as well as prevention of diseases in animals. This book on animal medicine explores all the important aspects of the field in the present day scenario. Animal medicine is a vast field and has various branches that diverge according to the nature of the ailment and the treatment required. Veterinarians also seek to prevent contagious diseases that are prevalent among animals as well zoonotic diseases that pose a threat to human beings as well. While understanding the long-term perspectives of the topics, the book makes an effort in highlighting their impact as a modern tool for the growth of the discipline. This book will prove to be immensely beneficial to students and researchers in this field.

This book is the end result of constructive efforts and intensive research done by experts in this field. The aim of this book is to enlighten the readers with recent information in this area of research. The information provided in this profound book would serve as a valuable reference to students and researchers in this field.

At the end, I would like to thank all the authors for devoting their precious time and providing their valuable contribution to this book. I would also like to express my gratitude to my fellow colleagues who encouraged me throughout the process.

Editor

Human Induced Rotation and Reorganization of the Brain of Domestic Dogs

Taryn Roberts[1]*, Paul McGreevy[1], Michael Valenzuela[2,3]*

1 Faculty of Veterinary Science, University of Sydney, Sydney, New South Wales, Australia, **2** School of Psychiatry, University of New South Wales, Sydney, New South Wales, Australia, **3** Brain and Ageing Research Program, Faculty of Medicine, University of New South Wales, Sydney, New South Wales, Australia

Abstract

Domestic dogs exhibit an extraordinary degree of morphological diversity. Such breed-to-breed variability applies equally to the canine skull, however little is known about whether this translates to systematic differences in cerebral organization. By looking at the paramedian sagittal magnetic resonance image slice of canine brains across a range of animals with different skull shapes (N = 13), we found that the relative reduction in skull length compared to width (measured by Cephalic Index) was significantly correlated to a progressive ventral pitching of the primary longitudinal brain axis (r = 0.83), as well as with a ventral shift in the position of the olfactory lobe (r = 0.81). Furthermore, these findings were independent of estimated brain size or body weight. Since brachycephaly has arisen from generations of highly selective breeding, this study suggests that the remarkable diversity in domesticated dogs' body shape and size appears to also have led to human-induced adaptations in the organization of the canine brain.

Editor: Rafael Linden, Universidade Federal do Rio de Janeiro, Brazil

Funding: MV is supported by a University of New South Wales Vice Chancellor's Fellowship. TR was funded by a Postgraduate Scholarship from the Natural Sciences and Engineering Research Council of Canada. Funders had no role in study design, data collection and analysis, decision to publish, or preparation of the manuscript.

Competing Interests: The authors have declared that no competing interests exist.

* E-mail: taryn@bell.net (TR); michaelv@unsw.edu.au (MV)

Introduction

The domestic dog, *Canis familiaris*, exhibits more morphological variation than any other species. Through human selection, breeds have diverged significantly from the form of their closest ancestor, the grey wolf (*Canis lupus*), with the greatest variation evident in the size and shape of the skull [1], which range from 7 to 28 cm in length [2]. Wolves are dolichocephalic (long skulled) but not as extreme as some breeds of *Canis familiaris*, such as greyhounds and Russian wolfhounds (Borzois) [2]. Canine brachycephaly (short-skulledness) is found only in domestic dogs and is related to paedomorphosis in these animals [3]. Puppies of all breeds are born with short snouts, and so the longer skull of dolichocephalic animals emerges during post partum development [4]. Other morphological differences in head shape between brachycephalic and dolichocephalic dogs include changes in the craniofacial angle (angle between the basilar axis and hard palate) [5], morphology of the temporomandibular joint [6], and radiographic anatomy of the cribiform plate [7].

Little is known about breed-dependent changes in morphology of the domesticated dog brain. For example, the standard veterinary text, *Miller's Anatomy of the Dog*, notes skull differences between brachy- and dolichocephalic dogs but refers only in passing to the brain [1]. In the 1960s, Seiferle presented a comparison of the brains of brachy- and dolichocephalic dogs, and his diagrams depict brachycephalic brains that are rounded and shortened in the anterior-posterior plane, with a pronounced shift in the position of the olfactory lobe [8]. There has since been little attention to the neuromorphological changes in brachycephalic

dogs, or what effects these may have on canine behavior or health. At a behavioral level, brachycephaly may be associated with an increased ability to focus and respond to human pointing gestures [9], potentially due to differences in retinal ganglion cell distribution [2]. More generally, reduction in skull length in carnivores correlates with a reduction in olfactory lobe size, hypothetically due to restriction in the development of frontal brain regions [10].

Canine brain research has thus far focused on clinical reports of breed specific disorders, such as pug encephalitis [11], or syringohydromyelia in Cavalier King Charles spaniels [12], or of comparisons between two or three breeds on a given morphological metric, and often these studies have used only one breed to represent a skull type. While the comparison of skull extremes is informative, it would also be of value to investigate whether morphological differences in skull shape across a wide variety of breeds are accompanied by differences in brain organization. Cephalic index (CI) is a simple and useful method of characterizing skull morphology, calculated by dividing skull width by skull length [2,9,13,14], and its use allows an examination of brain organization across the full continuum of dog skull shapes.

In the current study, our aim therefore was to examine the effect of differences in the shape of the canine skull on spatial organization of the brain, focusing on the relationship between the olfactory lobe and supratentorial (above the cerebellum) brain mass, as well as changes of the long axis of the brain. We analyzed paramedian sagittal magnetic resonance image (MRI) slices taken from dogs across a wide range of cephalic indices and developed a number of mathematical measures for capturing these relationships.

Methods

Subjects

Eleven recently euthanized dogs of different breeds obtained from a local pound were used in this study. Euthanized dogs from local dog shelters are sometimes used for teaching veterinary anatomy at the University of Sydney as permissible under NSW law, and the university's Animal Ethics Committee confirmed in writing to MV that use of such dogs for the purpose of our study did not require specific committee approval. The investigators had no influence on the fate of these dogs, and conducted no ante-mortem selection or interaction with the individual animals. Deceased animals were MRI scanned within four hours *post mortem* prior to routine cremation. The age of these subjects was not known, and their dominant breed was determined by experienced veterinarians. Two live dogs (both English springer spaniels) were also scanned with owner consent, and were given clearance by the University of Sydney Animal Ethics Committee as part of a larger canine brain ageing study (Ethics approval N00-3-2007-6-4571), resulting in a total sample of N = 13 dogs. None of the dogs in this study were markedly under- or over-weight.

MR Imaging

Imaging was conducted at the University of Sydney Veterinary Teaching Hospital using a 0.25 Tesla Esaote Vet Grande MRI System (Software release 9.2) with a gradient strength of 20mt/meter and a resonance frequency (RF) strength of 900 watts. All dogs were positioned in sternal recumbency, using RF dual phase array C2 or C4 coils, with the exception of Dog 9 which was scanned in lateral recumbency with a RF linear C1 coil due to large cranial size.

Spin Echo TE Sagittal T1 images were obtained for all 13 dogs (TR 610/TE 18, 3/0.3 mm slice thickness, FOV/RFOV 250×250, 1 NEX and a 250×24 Matrix) with the brain positioned at the isocentre. If the tip of the nose was not visible on the first sagittal scan, dogs were repositioned in the coil with the hard palate at the isocentre and scanned with the same protocol to permit measurement of hard palate angulation.

Cephalic Measurements and Skull Type

Skull length and width were measured on intact dog heads using digital calipers. Skull width was measured at the widest point of the zygomatic arches, and skull length from the external occipital protuberance to the tip of the nose (Figure 1). Cephalic index (CI) was calculated as (skull width/skull length) ×100 [2]. Since the range of cephalic indices defining domestic dog skull types as *dolichocephalic*, *mesocephalic* or *brachycephalic* are not entirely consistent across the literature [1,15,16,17], high- vs low CI grouping was based on median split in our analyzes.

For the purpose of comparison, we were interested in any documented accounts of CI in the wolf (Canis lupus), but could find none. We were, however, able to estimate CI on the basis of two independent sources: 1) www.skullsite.co.uk – an amateur collection of various different animal skulls, including a wolf skull picture and corresponding morphological measurements, and 2) Multi-planar specimen pictures of a gray wolf skull archived by the University of Michigan's Museum of Zoology [18].

MR Image Analysis

Using Analyze (Biomedical Imaging Resource), each dog's brain was realigned to the hard palate, as per veterinary radiological convention [2]. A paramedian sagittal slice depicting the olfactory lobe at its most distinct was selected and the region of interest of the brain and olfactory lobe were manually traced. Only the

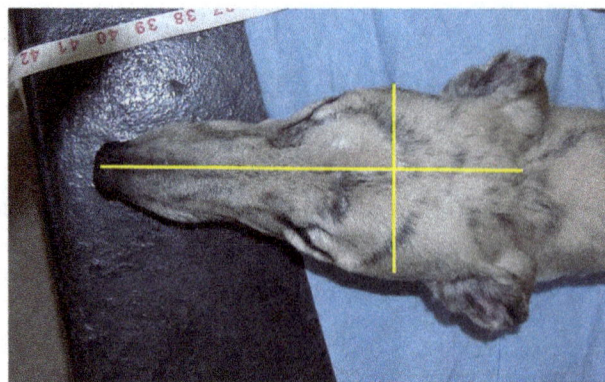

Figure 1. Cephalic Index Measurement. For measurement of the cephalic index, skull width was measured from one zygomatic arch to the other and skull length was measured from the nose to the occipital protuberance. Cephalic index (CI) was calculated as (skull width/skull length) ×100.

supratentorial cerebral hemisphere was traced due to ambiguities in demarcation of the brainstem on sagittal imaging. Planimetric 2D estimates of cerebral size and olfactory volume based on these traced images were calculated using Analyze. Traced images were then saved in Portable Networks Graphic (.png) format and imported into Matlab (MathWorks), for calculation of the centre of mass of the brain (CoM$_{brain}$) and olfactory lobe (CoM$_{OL}$).

We then established a longitudinal axis (LA), as the longest possible line drawn from the most rostral point of the frontal lobe to the furthest caudal point of the occipital lobe (Figure 2). The angle of deflection between the hard palate and LA was used to calculate *pitch*, in effect a measure of dorsal-ventral cerebral axis rotation.

To analyse the position of the olfactory lobe relative to the cerebral hemisphere, all brains were now realigned to the LA, in effect normalizing for any differences in brain pitch. We measured the angle of deflection of a line drawn between the CoM$_{OL}$ and the CoM$_{brain}$ *relative to the LA axis* (Figure 3b) using Microsoft Picture Manager and the program Universal Desktop Ruler (Version 3.3.3269, AVP Soft, www.AVPSoft.com).

The angle of deflection between the CoM of the brain and that of the olfactory lobe was then calculated. Because variation in brain shape was observed and may have biased deflection measurements, a second method of characterization was also used: a dorsal-ventral linear displacement ratio between CoM$_{OL}$ and the CoM$_{brain}$.

As MRI slices were 3 mm thick, only one suitable slice depicting a distinct olfactory lobe was available for most dogs. The area contained within manual traces of the olfactory bulb was multiplied by the slice thickness to estimate *olfactory bulb volume*. In those two dogs where two slices through the olfactory bulb were present, the average was used. Furthermore, in these two dogs, choice of slice had a negligible effect on calculation of CoM, leading to angle measurement differences of less than 2 degrees.

Statistical analyses

Analysis was performed using the Statistical Package for the Social Sciences (PASW 18.0 for Windows, SPSS inc, www.spss.com). Pearson correlations were calculated between skull shape, body weight and height, angle of the longitudinal axis and deviation of the olfactory lobe. Because of the small sample size of

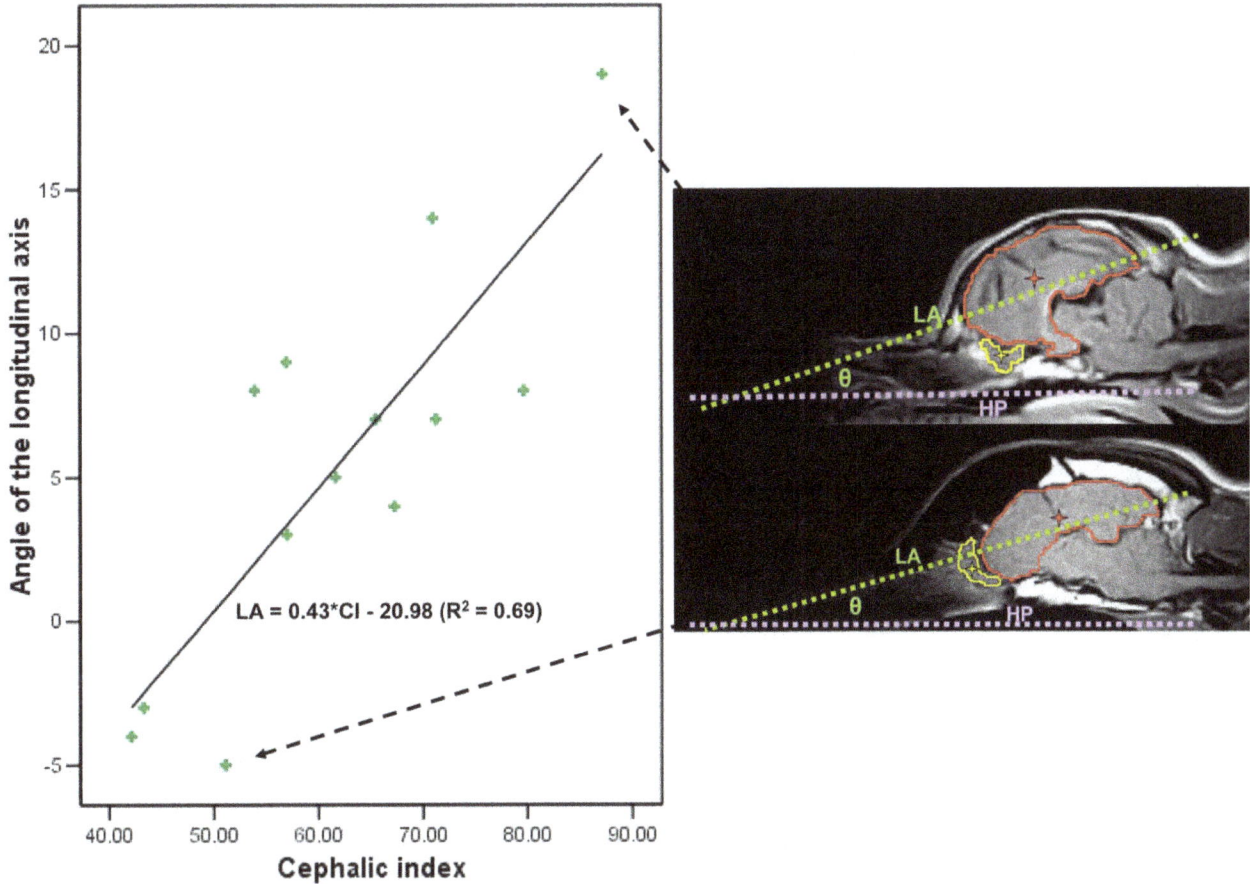

Figure 2. Pitching of the Primary Longitudinal Brain Axis. Cephalic index and longitudinal axis with respect to the hard palate. Individual sagittal scans for dogs at each extreme are shown with the brain outlined in red and centre of mass indicated by a red star. The olfactory bulb has also been outlined in yellow and centre of mass shown in yellow star. HP: Hard Palate reference line. LA: Longitudinal axis. θ = Angle of interest.

the brachycephalic and dolichocephalic groups, to test for effects of low or high CI we divided the CI range at the mid-point of CI scores present in this study ($CI_{mid} = 64.5$) and performed independent sample t-tests to look for differences in angle of the longitudinal axis and deflection of the olfactory lobe between low (CI 42.17–61.70, n = 7) and high (CI 65.48–87.23, n = 6) CI groups.

Results

Animals

The type of dogs in this study and their morphological and intracranial measurements are summarized in Table 1. Whilst dogs in the high CI group (i.e., brachycephalic end of spectrum) tended to be smaller and weigh less, none of these comparisons were significantly different.

Morphology

Cephalic index (CI) in domestic dogs ranged from 42.2 in a greyhound to 87.2 in a shih tzu cross. In general, body size and weight were closely related to CI in the domestic dogs studied in this sample (see inter-correlations in Table 2). Body weight was therefore used as a covariate in subsequent analyzes.

In the two wolf records we could find, CI varied between 50.9 (137 mm/269 mm *100 based on www.skullsite.co.uk measure-

ments) to 51.9 (8.3AU/16AU *100 based on University of Michigan figure).

Intracranial Volume Estimates

There were no significant differences between dogs in the high versus low CI groups in terms of estimated brain size or olfactory lobe volume (see Table 1).

Cerebral Axis Rotation

Upon observing the midsagittal images, it was apparent even to the naked eye that dogs with the most brachycephalic skulls had markedly rotated cerebral hemispheres, with the brain pitched ventrally at the anterior pole. This was confirmed quantitatively, as can be seen in Figure 2. There was a significant correlation between pitch rotation and CI (r = 0.828, p<0.001, N = 13). This relationship was not eliminated when either controlling for body weight (partial correlation = 0.69, p = 0.012, df = 10) or estimated brain size (partial correlation = 0.72, p = 0.009, df = 10).

This association appeared to be more specific to rostral-caudal skull length (r = −0.771, p<0.002, N = 13), rather than with skull width. For every mm of attenuated skull length relative to width, the canine brain pitched ventrally at the anterior pole by 0.43 degrees. The average angle of the LA Axis of the low CI group (mean: 1.86, SD = 5.84, n = 7) and the high CI group (mean: 9.83,

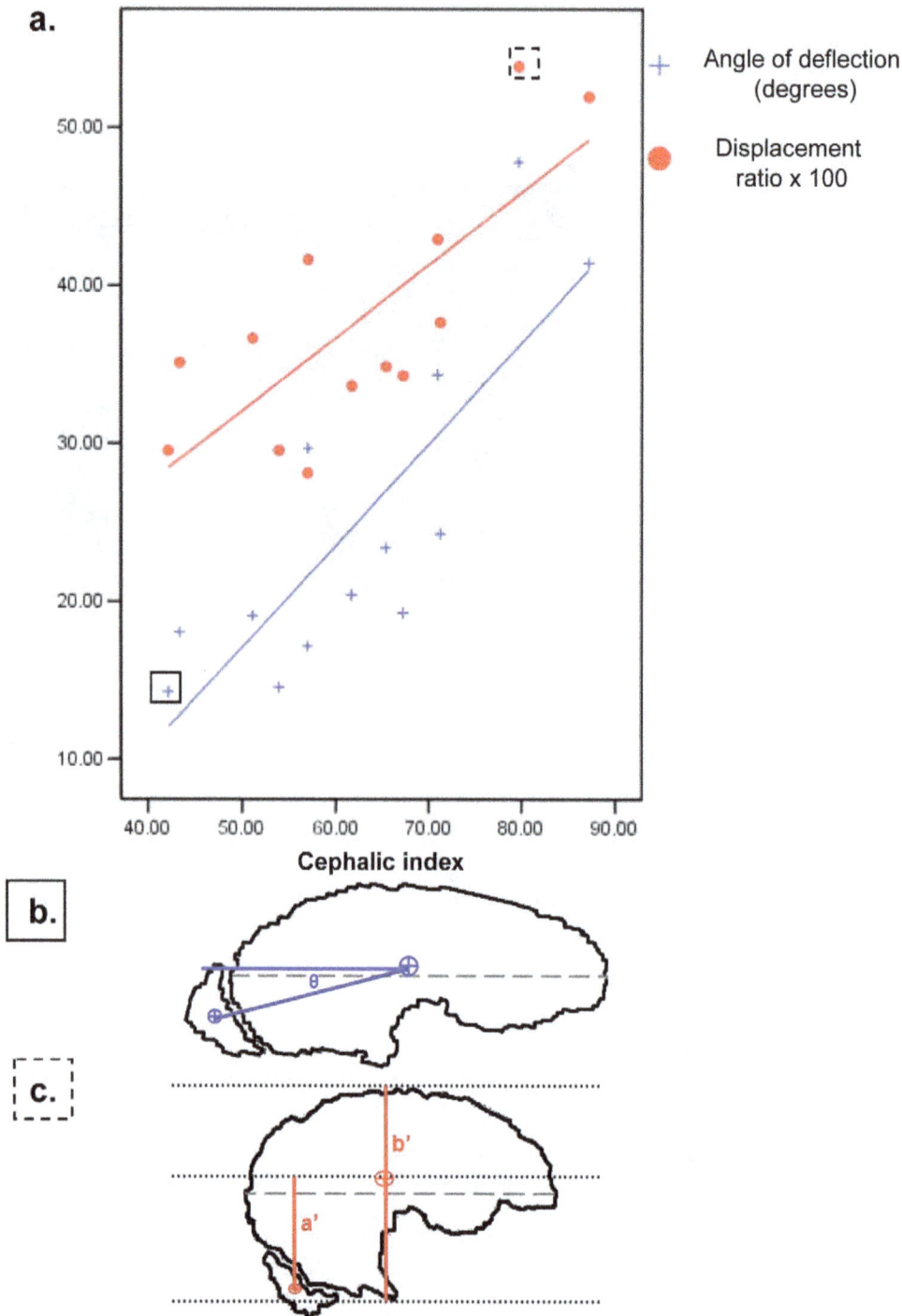

Figure 3. Deviation of the Olfactory Lobe. a) Cephalic index and deviation of the olfactory lobe using two different methods after normalization of cerebral axis to horizontal. Two exemplar dogs highlighted in boxes are illustrated in parts b) and c) below. b) Angle of deflection method: angle in degrees between centre of mass of brain (CoM$_{brain}$) and centre of mass of olfactory lobe (CoM$_{OL}$). c) Displacement method: Ratio of the ventral-dorsal distance from centre of mass of brain and centre of mass of olfactory lobe (a') to overall brain height (b').

SD = 5.57, n = 6) were significantly different (t = 2.507, 95%CI of mean difference: −14.98 – −0.97, p = 0.029).

Olfactory-Brain Deflection

Equally striking on the midsagittal images of the dogs scanned in this study was a repositioning of the olfactory lobe relative to the rest of the brain in dogs with reduced skull length. This deflection of the olfactory lobe from the longitudinal axis correlated significantly with CI when measured both in terms of angular deflection (r = 0.814, p = 0.001, N = 13 **Fig 3a,b**) and displacement ratio (r = 0.763, p = 0.002, N = 13, **Figure 3a,c**). The correlation between CI and angular deflection was not eliminated

Table 1. Characteristics of dogs in this study by cephalic index group (N = 13).

	High CI (brachycephalic)	Low CI (dolichocephalic)	T-test statistic	p-value
N	6	7	–	–
Male	50%	43%	–	–
Breeds	Akita cross, Mastiff cross, Maltese, Staffordshire bull terrier, Shih tzu cross	Greyhound, English springer spaniel, Australian cattle dog cross, Jack Russell terrier, Pit bull cross	–	–
Sagittal brain size (mm^2)	1475.21±369.4	1722.3±358.6	1.31	0.217
Olfactory lobe volume (mm^3)	255.9±114.3	334.2±110.4	1.26	0.234
Body weight (kg)	14.9±9.7	21.3±7.5	1.33	0.211
Height (cm)	40.8±13.9	55.3±12.9	1.95	0.78

CI: cephalic index. Mean values ± SD.

when controlling for either body weight (partial correlation = 0.64, p = 0.026, df = 10), estimated brain size (partial correlation = 0.66, p = 0.02, df = 10), or olfactory lobe volume (partial correlation = 0.73, p = 0.007, df = 10).

Both measures of deviation correlated negatively with skull length (angle r = −0.927, p = 0.000, n = 13; displacement r = −0.861, p = 0.000, n = 13) and the angle of deflection correlated negatively with skull width (angle r = −0.562, p = 0.046, n = 13). The low CI group (mean = 19.0, SD = 5.22, n = 7) and the high CI group (mean = 31.8, SD = 11.31, n = 6) displayed significantly different average olfactory angular deflection values (t = 2.677, 95%CI of mean difference: −23.18 – −2.26, p = 0.022). Individual animals' skull and cerebral morphology measurements are presented in Table 3.

Discussion

Our study introduces two new observations about the organization of the brain of the domestic dog. Approximately 69% of the variance in overall pitch of the brain, and 66% of the variance in the relative position of the olfactory lobe, was explained by skull shape as revealed by cephalic index. Increasingly brachycephalic dogs were found a have a more ventrally rotated cerebral axis and a more ventrally shifted olfactory bulb position. Interestingly, these relationships appear to be highly sensitive to CI because rather than appearing beyond a critical threshold, they were found across a wide range of skull shapes and were independent of body weight or brain size.

Canine brachycephaly is purely a human invention. For example, to the best of our knowledge the cephalic index of the wolf (*Canis lupus*) approximates 51 to 52, whilst in our sample of domesticated dogs, ranged from 42 to 87. A complex interplay of breed pressures since canines began human cohabitation about 12,000 years ago [19]– including selection for behavioral, functional, and more recently, aesthetic traits – has led to their amazing physical diversity [9,20]. Some have speculated as to whether this prepotent physical variation intimates a unique level of plasticity in the canine genome [21]. Added to this, no other animal has enjoyed the level of human affection and companionship as the dog, nor undergone such a systematic and deliberate intervention in its biology through selective breeding.

This diversity is no less prominent than in the wide variation in the shape and size of the canine skull. In this study, this variability was found to extend to the organization of the canine brain. We found a strong correlation between high CI and both cerebral axis rotation (ventrally at the anterior pole) and a 'ventralization' of

Table 2. Pearson Correlation Data for Skull Shape, Body Size, Body Weight, Angle of the Longitudinal Axis and Deflection of the Olfactory Lobe for N = 13 Dogs.

	Skull Length (mm)	Skull Width (mm)	Body weight (kg)	Body height (cm)	Angle of the Longitudinal axis	Deflection of the olfactory lobe (angle)	Deflection of the olfactory lobe (distance ratio)
Cephalic Index	−.839**	−.093	− .661*	−.762**	.020**	.814**	.763**
Skull Length (mm)		.591*	.945**	.953**	−.771**	−.927**	−.861**
Skull Width (mm)			.708**	.554*	−.196	−.562*	−.550
Body weight (kg)				.954**	−.665*	−.842**	−.765**
Body height (cm)					−.671*	−.846*	−.796**
Angle of the Longitudinal axis						.604*	.493
Deflection of the olfactory lobe (angle)							.971**

**: Correlation is significant at the 0.01 level (2-tailed).
*: Correlation is significant at the 0.05 level (2-tailed).

Table 3. Individual skull and brain measurements for dogs in this study (n = 13) in the current series.

	Breed	Sex	CI	CI group	Skull length (mm)	Skull width (mm)	Angle of the LA	Deviation of the Olfactory Lobe (Angle)	Deviation of the Olfactory Lobe (Displacement)
1	Greyhound	F	42.17	L	239.5	101	−4	14.26	29.56
2	Greyhound	M	43.36	L	260.6	113	−3	18.05	35.12
3	English springer spaniel	F	51.11	L	229.5	117	−5	19.09	36.67
4	English springer spaniel	F	53.93	L	214.0	115	8	14.54	29.57
5	Australian cattle dog cross	M	57.00	L	216.5	123	9	17.15	28.12
6	Jack Russell terrier	M	57.04	L	163.4	93.2	3	29.7	41.64
7	Pit bull cross	F	61.70	L	216.7	134	5	20.42	33.63
8	Akita cross	M	65.48	H	205.4	135	7	23.39	34.85
9	Mastiff cross	M	67.28	H	222.2	150	4	19.28	34.27
10	Maltese	F	70.94	H	120.1	85.2	14	34.33	42.92
11	Staffordshire bull terrier	F	71.24	H	186.7	133	7	24.27	37.67
12	Shih tzu cross	F	79.69	H	116.7	93	8	47.81	53.89
13	Shih tzu cross	M	87.23	H	113.6	99.1	19	41.42	51.98

Low (L) and High (H) Cephalic index (CI) group based on median split. LA: longitudinal axis.

olfactory lobe location. Our analysis suggested this was most strongly associated with skull shortening rather than loss of skull girth in increasingly brachycephalic dogs.

But how could skull shortening affect cerebral organization? Studies of human craniosynostosis [22,23] and immature head banding [23] suggest that the development of brain shape and size is closely interrelated to the configuration of dura matter as well as the co-developing cranial vault. Changes to any of one of these factors can lead to changes in the others [22]. Differences in canine skull length resulting from artificial human selection pressures may have led to alterations in cerebral development most evident in brachycephalic versus dolicocephalic dogs. Specifically, rostral intracranial volumetric restriction during development of short-skulled dogs may explain the combination of axis rotation and olfactory bulb repositioning. Regodon et al (1993) also noted that reduced skull length in brachycephalic dogs gives rise to a more perpendicular development of the cranium relative to the facial axis [5]. These anatomical adaptations could hence represent a biological solution to a 'space problem'. The olfactory bulb seems to have migrated to a potential space ventral to the orbital frontal cortex, thereby freeing the anterior pole for normal development of the frontal cortex. Alternatively, animals at the dolichocephalic end of the spectrum may have sufficient 'spare capacity' in the cranial vault to permit olfactory bulb development almost directly anterior to the frontal lobe. Either of these possible explanations relies on an evolutionary and developmental preference to preserve frontal lobe volume. Future studies could therefore directly compare frontal lobe morphology in brachy- and dolichocephalic dogs.

Because differences in cranial morphology across dog breeds were closely associated with major neuroanatomical changes, whether these also lead to differences in behavior is a major open question. We cannot yet infer whether the progressive cerebral reorganization found in more brachycephalic dogs have direct functional sequelae. Interestingly, brachycephalic breeds are not typically selected for scent work because of poor olfaction assumed due to crowding of ethmoturbinate bones. Our data suggests a second possible explanation related to anterior-posterior compression of the skull and repositioning of the olfactory lobe relative to

the rest of the brain. More broadly, dogs with different skull shapes may behave differently [9], but this is not entirely consistent [24]. Improved behavioral measurement of sensory, motor and cognitive function in domestic dogs is therefore a high priority.

Skull-shape dependent changes in the position of the olfactory bulb also predict a fascinating consequence for the adult rostral migratory stream (RMS). The RMS is a track of neural precursors that originates in the subependymal zone of the lateral ventricles and terminates in the olfactory bulb, contributing to neural turnover in this brain structure in both rodents and humans [25,26]. Whilst its functional significance remains unresolved, neurogenesis within the RMS is closely connected to olfaction [27,28]. Given the predictable nature of differences in the location of the canine olfactory lobe based on cranial shape, our findings also predict a rule-based change in the spatial course of the RMS within the brain of domestic dogs. Histological confirmation of this prediction, and any possible behavioral implications for olfaction, are of intense interest for future research.

Finally, a potential limitation on our conclusions is that larger dogs generally tend to have larger brains and manifest a more dolichocephalic cranial morphology, and smaller dogs the opposite. The effects of cranial morphology on brain organization may therefore be confused with those of body and brain size. There are, however, two main reasons why this was unlikely to have been a major confounder in our study. Firstly, there were no significant differences in body weight or estimated brain size between our comparison groups. Secondly, since our study may have been underpowered in this respect, we also took care to control for body weight and brain size in our correlational analyses. So even after accounting for brain size or body weight differences, there was strong evidence for a correlation between CI and both cerebral axis and olfactory lobe position. The effects of skull shape on cerebral axis and olfactory lobe position therefore appear to be independent of body or brain size.

To further disambiguate these competing influence on canine brain organization, future research may also profit by studying those interesting dog 'outliers' which break the usual body size-cephalic index norm. These include dolichocephalic breeds with low bodyweight (such as the Italian greyhound), and brachycephalic breeds of high bodyweight (such as the Neapolitan mastiff). Use of high resolution 3D MR imaging as often used in human brain studies would also allow more accurate calculation of whole brain volume, as well as possible changes in lobar organization or grey and white matter distribution.

Overall, our findings suggest that the remarkable variability evident in canine morphology is also apparent in the dog's cerebral organization. We found strong and independent correlations between cephalic index and pitching of the long brain axis, as well as ventral positioning of the olfactory lobe. Further investigation of the inter-relationships between skull shape, brain organization and behavior represent fascinating directions for future canine research.

Acknowledgments

The authors are grateful to G. Burland, D. Slade and J. van Ekris for their assistance in sourcing materials for this study, as well as to K. Hughes and H. Laurendet for support in acquiring magnetic resonance images, and for the collaboration of the University of Sydney Veterinary Teaching Hospital throughout the project. C. Suo is kindly thanked for technical assistance throughout the duration of the data analysis. K. Keay is thanked for constructive comments and assistance with the artwork presented in this manuscript. This manuscript reports on a study by TR towards her Masters in Veterinary Studies.

Author Contributions

Conceived and designed the experiments: PDM MJV. Performed the experiments: TR. Analyzed the data: TR MJV. Contributed reagents/materials/analysis tools: PDM MJV. Wrote the paper: TR PDM MJV.

References

1. Evans HE, Christensen GC, eds (1979) Miller's Anatomy of the Dog. 2nd ed. ed. Philadelphia: WB Saunders.
2. McGreevy P, Grassi T, Harman A (2003) A Strong Correlation Exists between the Distribution of Retinal Ganglion Cells and Nose Length in the Dog. Brain, Behavior and Evolution 63: 13.
3. Goodwin D, Bradshaw JWS, Wickens SM (1997) Paedomorphosis affects visual signals of domestic dogs. Animal Behaviour 53: 297–304.
4. Coppinger R, Schneider R (1995) Evolution of working dogs. In: Serpell J, ed. The Domestic Dog: its evolution, behaviour and interactions with people. Cambridge: Cambridge University Press. pp 21–47.
5. Regodon S, Vivo JM, Franco A, Guillen MT, Robina A (1993) Craniofacial angle in dolicho-, meso- an brachycephalic dogs: radiological determination and application. Annals of Anatomy 175: 361–363.
6. Dickie AM, Sullivan M (2001) The effect of obliquity on the radiographic appearance of the temporomandibular joint in dogs. Veterinary Radiology & Ultrasound 42: 205–217.
7. Schwarz T, Sullivan M, Hartung K (2000) Radiographic anatomy of the cribiform plate (Lamina cribosa). Veterinary Radiology & Ultrasound 41: 220–225.
8. Seiferle E (1966) Zur topographie des gehirns bei lang - und kurzkopfigen hunderassen. Acta Anatomica 63: 346–362.
9. Gacsi M, McGreevy P, Kara E, Miklosi A (2009) Effects of selection for cooperation and attention in dogs. Behavioural and Brain Functions 5: 31.
10. Gittleman JL (1991) Carnivore olfactory bulb size: allometry, phylogeny and ecology. Journal of Zoology 225: 253–272.
11. Flegel T, Henke D, Boettcher Irene C, Aupperle H, Oechtering G, et al. (2008) Magnetic resonance imaging findings in histologically confirmed pug dog encephalitis. Veterinary Radiology & Ultrasound 49: 419–424.
12. Cerda-Gonzalez S, Olby NJ, McCullough S, Pease AP, Broadstone R, et al. (2009) Morphology of the caudal fossa in cavalier king charles spaniels. Veterinary Radiology & Ultrasound 50: 37–46.
13. Evans KE, McGreevy PD (2006) The distribution of ganglion cells in the equine retina and its relationship to skull morphology. Anatomia, Histologia, Embryologia 35: 1–6.
14. Evans KE, McGreevy PD (2006) Conformation of the equine skull: A morphometric study. Anatomia, Histologia, Embryologia 35: 221–227.
15. Lignereux Y, Regodon S, Pavaux, CI (1991) Typologie cephalique canine. Revue de Medicine Veterinaire 142: 469–480.
16. Onar V, Pazvant S (2001) Skull Typology of Adult Male Kangal Dogs. Anatomia, Histologia, Embryologia 30: 41–48.
17. Stockard CR (1941) The genetic and endocrine basis for differences in form and behavior. New York: The Wistar Institute of Anatomy and Biology.
18. Myers P, Espinosa R, Parr CS, Jones T, Hammond GS, et al. (2008) The Animal Diversity Web (online).
19. Ostrander E (2007) Genetics and the Shape of Dogs. American Scientist Volume 95: 406.
20. Asher L, Diesel G, Summers JF, McGreevy PD, Collins LM (2009) Inherited defects in pedigree dogs. Part 1: Disorders related to breed standards. The Veterinary Journal 182: 402–411.
21. Hock C, Konietzko U, Streffer J, et al. (2003) Antibodies against beta-amyloid slow cognitive decline in Alzheimer's disease. Neuron 38: 554.
22. Aldridge K, Kane AA, Marsh JL, Panchal J, Boyadjiev SA, et al. (2005) Brain morphology in nonsyndromic unicoronal craniosynostosis. The Anatomical Record Part A: Discoveries in Molecular, Cellular, and Evolutionary Biology 285A: 690–698.
23. Cheverud J, Kohn L, Konigsberg L, Leigh S (1992) Effects of fronto-occipital artificial cranial vault modification on the cranial base and face. American Journal of Physical Anthropology 88: 323–345.
24. McGreevy PD, Brueckner A, Thomson PC, Branson NJ (2010) Motor laterality in four breeds of dog. Journal of Veterinary Behavior: Clinical Applications and Research Accepted.
25. Alvarez-Buylla A, Garcia-Verdugo JM, Tramontin AD (2001) A unified hypothesis on the lineage of neural stem cells. Nature Reviews Neuroscience 2: 287–293.
26. Curtis MA, Kam M, Nannmark U, Anderson MF, Axell MZ, et al. (2007) Human Neuroblasts Migrate to the Olfactory Bulb via a Lateral Ventricular Extension. Science 315: 1243–1249.
27. Curtis MA, Monzo HJ, Faull RLM (2009) The rostral migratory stream and olfactory system: smell, disease and slippery cells. In: Verhaagen J, ed. Progress in Brain Research: Elsevier. 548 Pages.
28. Martoncikova M, Lievajova K, Cova J, Blasko J, Racekova E (2010) Odor enrichment influences neurogenesis in the rostral migratory stream of young rats. Acta Histochem In Press

2

Discovery of Molecular Mechanisms of Traditional Chinese Medicinal Formula Si-Wu-Tang Using Gene Expression Microarray and Connectivity Map

Zhining Wen[1,2], **Zhijun Wang**[3], **Steven Wang**[3], **Ranadheer Ravula**[3], **Lun Yang**[1,4], **Jun Xu**[5], **Charles Wang**[6], **Zhong Zuo**[7], **Moses S. S. Chow**[3], **Leming Shi**[1,4]*, **Ying Huang**[3]*

1 National Center for Toxicological Research, U.S. Food and Drug Administration, Jefferson, Arkansas, United States of America, 2 College of Chemistry, Sichuan University, Chengdu, Sichuan, China, 3 Department of Pharmaceutical Sciences and Center for Advancement of Drug Research and Evaluation, College of Pharmacy, Western University of Health Sciences, Pomona, California, United States of America, 4 Department of Clinical Pharmacy and Center for Pharmacogenomics, School of Pharmacy, Fudan University, Shanghai, China, 5 Clinical Transcriptional Genomics Core, Medical Genetics Institute, Cedars-Sinai Medical Center, David Geffen School of Medicine at UCLA, Los Angeles, California, United States of America, 6 Functional Genomics Core, Beckman Research Institute, City of Hope Comprehensive Cancer Center, Duarte, California, United States of America, 7 School of Pharmacy, Faculty of Medicine, The Chinese University of Hong Kong, Hong Kong, China

Abstract

To pursue a systematic approach to discovery of mechanisms of action of traditional Chinese medicine (TCM), we used microarrays, bioinformatics and the "Connectivity Map" (CMAP) to examine TCM-induced changes in gene expression. We demonstrated that this approach can be used to elucidate new molecular targets using a model TCM herbal formula Si-Wu-Tang (SWT) which is widely used for women's health. The human breast cancer MCF-7 cells treated with 0.1 µM estradiol or 2.56 mg/ml of SWT showed dramatic gene expression changes, while no significant change was detected for ferulic acid, a known bioactive compound of SWT. Pathway analysis using differentially expressed genes related to the treatment effect identified that expression of genes in the nuclear factor erythroid 2-related factor 2 (Nrf2) cytoprotective pathway was most significantly affected by SWT, but not by estradiol or ferulic acid. The Nrf2-regulated genes *HMOX1*, *GCLC*, *GCLM*, *SLC7A11* and *NQO1* were upregulated by SWT in a dose-dependent manner, which was validated by real-time RT-PCR. Consistently, treatment with SWT and its four herbal ingredients resulted in an increased antioxidant response element (ARE)-luciferase reporter activity in MCF-7 and HEK293 cells. Furthermore, the gene expression profile of differentially expressed genes related to SWT treatment was used to compare with those of 1,309 compounds in the CMAP database. The CMAP profiles of estradiol-treated MCF-7 cells showed an excellent match with SWT treatment, consistent with SWT's widely claimed use for women's diseases and indicating a phytoestrogenic effect. The CMAP profiles of chemopreventive agents withaferin A and resveratrol also showed high similarity to the profiles of SWT. This study identified SWT as an Nrf2 activator and phytoestrogen, suggesting its use as a nontoxic chemopreventive agent, and demonstrated the feasibility of combining microarray gene expression profiling with CMAP mining to discover mechanisms of actions and to identify new health benefits of TCMs.

Editor: Matej Oresic, Governmental Technical Research Centre of Finland, Finland

Funding: This work was supported by the U.S. Food and Drug Administration. The preparation of Si-Wu-Tang product was supported by the Innovation and Technology Fund (ITS/112/07) from the Innovation and Technology Commission of the Hong Kong Special Administrative Region of the People's Republic of China. This study was partially supported by the Innovation and Technology Grant (ITS/446/09) from the Innovation and Technology Commission of the Hong Kong Special Administrative Region of the People's Republic of China. The funders had no role in study design, data collection and analysis, decision to publish, or preparation of the manuscript. The views presented in this article do not necessarily reflect those of the U.S. Food and Drug Administration.

Competing Interests: The authors have declared that no competing interests exist.

* E-mail: leming.shi@gmail.com (LS); yhuang@westernu.edu (YH)

Introduction

Traditional Chinese medicines (TCMs) have been used in China and other Asian countries for over 5,000 years for the prevention and treatment of a variety of diseases. In contrast to target-oriented Western medicine, TCM uses a holistic and synergistic approach to restore the balance of *Yin-Yang* of body energy so the body's normal function, or homeostasis, can be restored [1]. Traditional Chinese herbal medicines often consist of a combination of individual herbs to form specific formulae aimed to increase therapeutic efficacy and reduce adverse effects [2]. Theoretically, multiple active phytochemical components in the TCM formulae may simultaneously target multiple molecules/pathways and thus potentially achieve superior effect as compared to single compounds alone [3]. However, while about 100,000 herbal formulae have been recorded and there are many empiric examples of successful clinical use of TCM, relationship of the essential phytochemical components in each of the formulae to molecular targets/pathway has not been identified for most TCM due to lack of suitable methodology to tackle the complex mechanisms. Lack of molecular evidence for targets diminishes the scientific validity of the claimed usefulness of TCM, despite the availability of empiric clinical experience. Thus, new methods for molecular target/pathway identification are sorely needed to advance the modernization of TCM.

The microarray technology and associated bioinformatic data mining tools provide an opportunity to simultaneously analyze a large number of genes/targets associated with complex therapeutic effects of TCM [4]. The working principle for this genomic approach is that the phenotype of a cell, including the function and response to the environment, is ultimately determined by its gene expression profiles. Analyzing the changes of gene expression profiles after treatment by TCM in vitro or in vivo may help reveal their mechanisms of action [4,5]. In addition, because the use of medicinal herbs may mimic or oppose the effects of concurrently used drugs, gene expression profiling using microarrays can also be used for revealing the mechanism of herb-drug interactions [6].

A few studies have used microarray-based transcriptional profiling to evaluate TCMs or their components [5,7,8,9,10]. The identified genes modulated by the TCM provided insights into molecular understanding of activity [4,11]. However, the real challenge is to reliably detect differentially expressed genes and dissect the functional relevance of identified genes to pharmacological mechanisms from these microarray studies [12]. The improper study design and unsuitable data analysis may lead to unreliable and less accurate results derived from the microarray studies [13,14,15,16]. To compare and integrate data derived from multiple different array experiments even for a single TCM component represents another technical challenge [12]. Special quality control criteria for array processing and analysis need to be used to overcome previous problems associated with microarray technologies.

Recently, the Connectivity Map (CMAP) database containing microarray expression data from cultured cell lines (e.g., human breast cancer cell line MCF-7) treated with bioactive small molecules with known mechanism of action and disease application has been described [17]. The current version of CMAP contains more than 7,000 expression profiles representing treatments from 1,309 compounds (http://www.broadinstitute.org/cMAP/) and in several studies, the CMAP database has been used for discovery of functional connections between drugs, genes, and diseases through the common gene-expression changes on the same cell lines [17,18,19,20,21]. Using CMAP, drugs affecting common molecular pathways can be identified and putative mechanism of action of unknown drugs can be explored. It may provide a useful tool for TCM when combined with microarray analysis.

To demonstrate the potential application of this approach for discovery of molecular mechanisms of TCM, we studied a model TCM formula, Si-Wu-Tang (SWT, directly translated as Four Agents Decoction) [22]. SWT has been used in China and Japan for about 1,000 years for the relief of menstrual discomfort, climacteric syndrome, peri- or postmenopausal syndrome and other estrogen-related diseases [22,23,24,25,26]. It has been reported to have sedative, anti-coagulant and antibacterial activities as well as effects on vasodilatation and hematopoiesis [27]. SWT has also been shown to possess an inhibitory effect on radiation-induced bone marrow damage [27,28]. However, the mechanism of the pharmacological action of SWT has not yet been clarified. The SWT formula is composed of four herbs, Radix *Rehmanniae praeparata*, Radix *Angelicae Sinensis*, Rhizoma *Ligustici Chuanxiong* and Radix *Paeoniae Alba* [22]. At least nine bioactive phytochemicals have been reported for SWT: paeoniflorin, paeonol, gallic acid, ferulic acid, Z-ligustilide, ligustrazine, butylphthalide, senkyunolide A and catalpol [25]. Of these compounds, ferulic acid (FA) and paeoniflorin have been recommended as the chemical markers for quality assessment of SWT [29,30,31,32]. In view of wide empiric use of SWT and known chemical components already reported, in the present study, we profiled the gene expression of MCF-7 cells treated with SWT, its component FA as well as estradiol using Affymetrix microarray Human U133Plus2.0 (Figure 1). We demonstrated the

feasibility of applying the combined microarray and CMAP approach in identifying molecular mechanisms of SWT.

Results

Hierarchical clustering analysis for quality assessment of array data and identification of treatment effects

Hierarchical clustering analysis was used to assess the overall quality of the microarray data (**Figure 2a**). A high correlation coefficient (colored in red in the heatmap of correlation coefficients) means that the gene expression profiles from two microarrays are very similar. The three replicates in each treatment group showed high pair-wise correlation in terms of log2 gene expression. In addition, samples treated with estradiol and high concentration of SWT showed dramatically different expression profiles compared to that of the control group. The visual observation of the clustering results indicates satisfactory reproducibility of microarray experiments for the biological replicates in each treatment group and significant treatment effects of estradiol and SWT, warranting further analyses and interpretation of their treatment effects.

Three replicates of MCF-7 control and MCF-7 treated with ferulic acid at low, medium and high concentrations were used for hierarchical clustering analysis in **Figure 2b**. For every dose-treatment group, the three replicates in the same group did not cluster together, indicating that there was no clear treatment effect even at the high concentration of ferulic acid. It seems that the treatment effects of ferulic acid on MCF-7 are minimal at the doses tested in this study.

In inspecting the treatment effects of SWT at low, medium and high concentrations along with the three replicates of estradiol treatment, hierarchical clustering analysis (**Figure 2c**) clearly demonstrated the high reproducibility of the replicates in each treatment group and strong treatment effects for estradiol and SWT at high concentration. The figure also shows clustering of the three replicates in the medium or low concentration of SWT treatment, but the degree of the treatment effect was much smaller than that for high-concentration SWT treatment. The expression profiles for the three replicates in the estradiol treatment group also clustered tightly together and were dramatically different from those of the control group samples. The expression profiles of the estradiol group were also dramatically different from those of the high-concentration SWT treatment group.

Identification of differentially expressed genes

Because there are 54,675 probe sets on the Affymetrix Human U133Plus 2.0 microarray, 2,734 probe sets would be expected by chance to show a $p < 0.05$. By comparing the number of probe sets with a $p < 0.05$ for each treatment group (**Table 1**) with that expected by chance (2,734), we can roughly assess the degree of the treatment effect. By applying the same cutoffs of t-test p value < 0.05 and fold change > 1.5, the differentially expressed genes were selected separately from comparing each treatment group with the control group. The number of differentially expressed genes varied dramatically depending on the treatment group. The high-concentration SWT and estradiol treatments resulted in the highest numbers of genes differentially expressed, whereas the treatment effect of ferulic acid appeared to be minor for all concentrations, and there was no clear dose-response relationship. On the other hand, the numbers of genes differentially expressed as a result of SWT treatment showed a clear dose-response trend, with an increase from low dose (7 genes, corresponding to 10 probe sets) to medium dose (71 genes, corresponding to 90 probe sets) and a big jump from medium dose to high dose (1,911 genes,

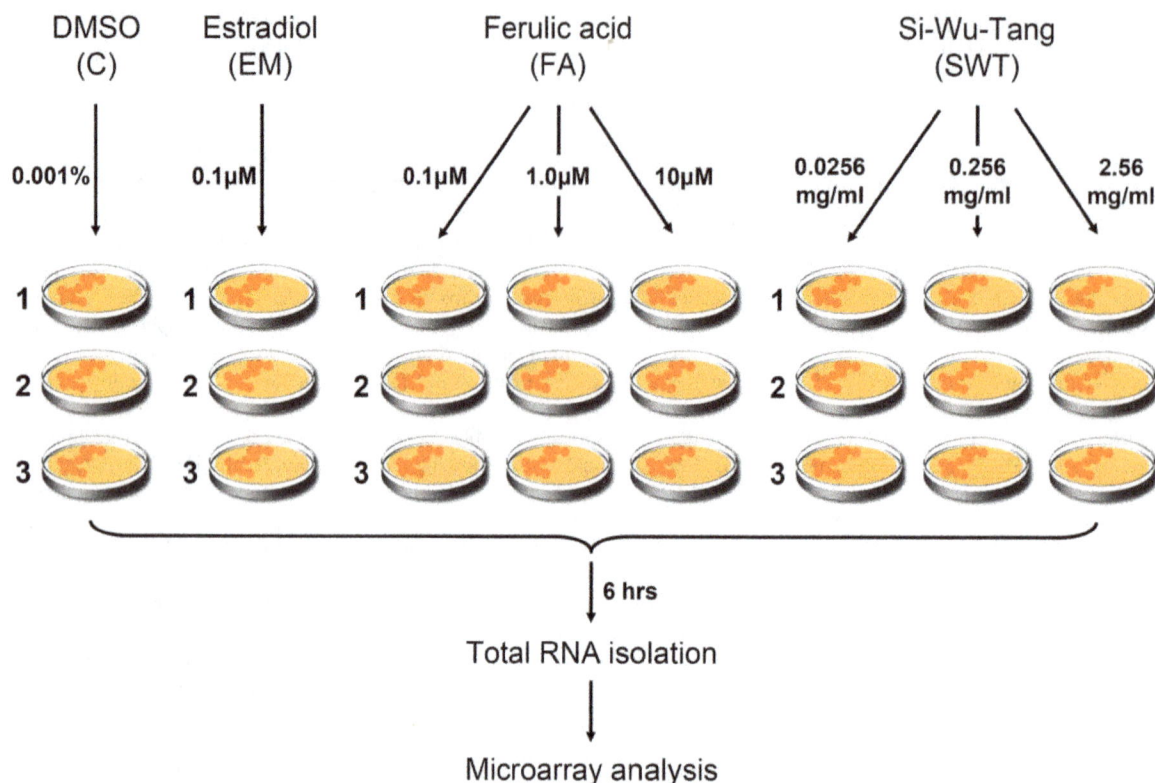

Figure 1. Experimental design of microarray gene expression profiling. The 24 samples were obtained from MCF-7 cells which were divided into eight treatment groups. 0.001% DMSO was used as the vehicle control (C). The cells were treated with 0.1 µM estradiol, FA at three concentrations (0.1, 1.0, and 10 µM) and SWT at three concentrations (0.0256, 0.256, and 2.56 mg/ml). For each treatment group, 3 biological replicates were included.

corresponding to 2,979 probe sets). The treatment with estradiol (0.1 µM) changed the expression of 830 unique genes (corresponding to 1,292 probe sets). However, only 337 genes were commonly regulated by both estradiol treatment and the high-concentration SWT treatment, indicating similarities and differences in the mechanisms of action between the two agents. Consistently, by controlling the false discovery rate (FDR) at the level of 0.05, only the high-concentration SWT and estradiol treatments resulted in genes differentially expressed (**Table 1**).

Canonical pathway analysis by IPA software: the Nrf2-mediated oxidative stress response pathway is most significantly impacted by high-concentration SWT treatment

The pathway names, Fisher's exact test p values, and the ratios of impacted genes for the top 10 IPA pathways most significantly enriched with genes differentially expressed from SWT and estradiol treatments are listed in **Table 2**. For the low-concentration SWT treatment, none of the IPA pathways was significantly enriched, mainly because of the very small number of differentially expressed genes (10 probe sets, corresponding to 7 genes). For medium-concentration SWT treatment, several IPA pathways related to the metabolism of xenobiotics by CYP450, C21-steroid hormone metabolism, cell cycle, and molecular mechanisms of cancer were highly enriched with differentially expressed genes. Genes differentially expressed from high-concentration SWT treatment group were most significantly enriched in several cancer signaling pathways. In particular, the Nrf2-mediated oxidative stress response pathway, which has

recently been found to play an important role in cancer prevention, was the most significantly impacted pathway ($p = 4.55 \times 10^{-9}$). About 23% (42/183) of the genes in the Nrf2 pathway were either up- or down-regulated by high-concentration SWT treatment (**Figure 3**).

We also used the expression profile of estradiol treatment as the query to search the IPA pathway database. The top 10 hits (**Table 2**) include pathways related to cell cycle, molecular mechanisms of cancer, and p53 signaling. These pathways are well-known to be associated with the biological functions of estradiol, validating the quality of microarray gene expression data in this study and the utility of the IPA pathway analysis approach. Notably, although the Nrf2-mediated oxidative stress response pathway was significantly impacted by high-concentration SWT treatment, it was not affected by estradiol treatment at the condition tested in this study.

Pathway analysis in KEGG database

None of the KEGG pathways was significantly enriched with the differentially expressed genes from low-concentration SWT treatment group and only 8 KEGG pathways were significantly enriched from medium-concentration SWT treatment. Instead, there were 25 and 19 KEGG pathways significantly enriched with differentially expressed genes from high-concentration SWT treatment and estradiol treatment, respectively. The top 10 significantly impacted KEGG pathways were listed in **Table 3**. Comparing the KEGG pathways listed in **Table 3** with the IPA pathways listed in **Table 2**, we can see that pathways related to signaling of cancer, cell cycle and metabolism were significantly

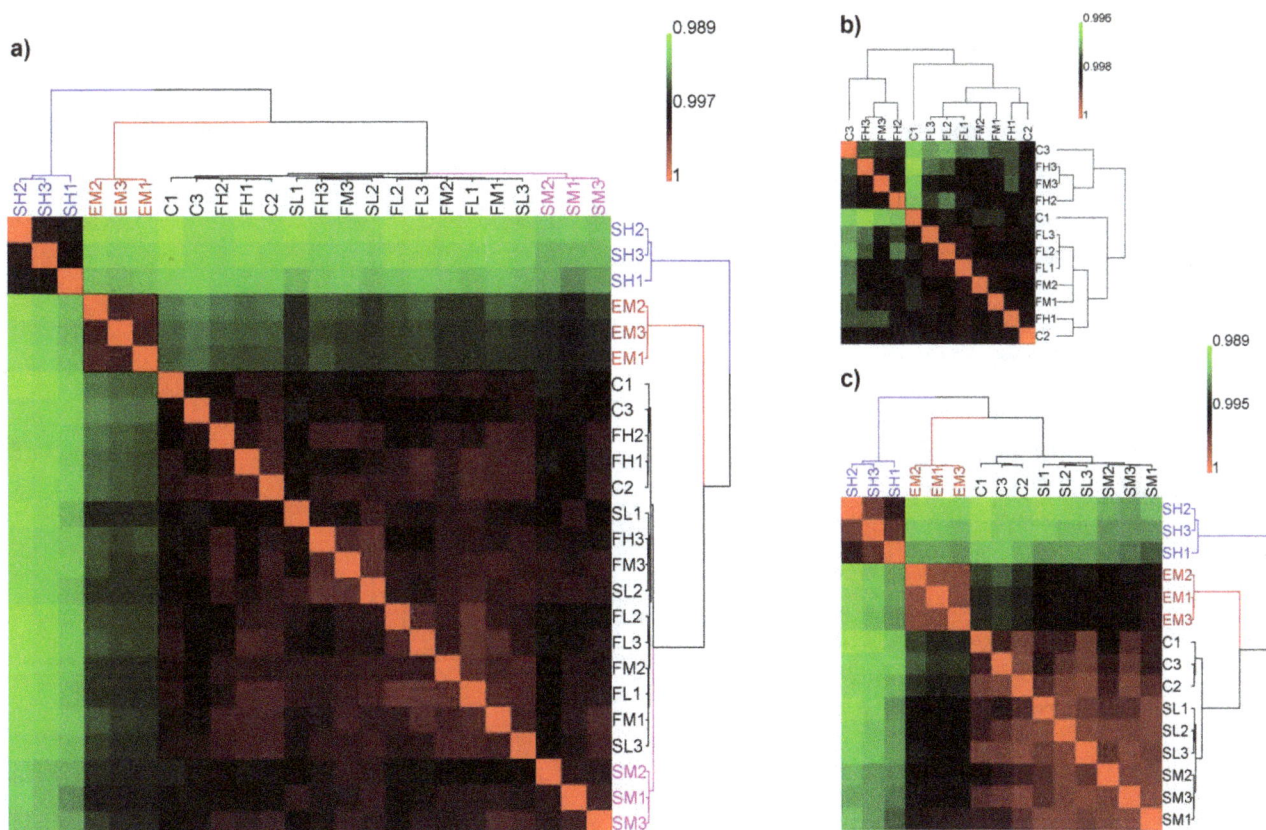

Figure 2. The hierarchical clustering analysis and heatmap of the correlation coefficients between gene expression profiles. (A) All 24 samples from the 8 treatment groups; (B) controls and ferulic acid treatments; and (C) controls and treatments by estradiol and SWT. There was good reproducibility between the three biological replicates in each treatment group. No clear treatment effect was observed for ferulic acid treatments. Low- and medium-concentration SWT treatments showed mild effects, while the strongest treatment effects were seen from estradiol and high-concentration SWT treatments.

impacted by estradiol treatment and by SWT treatments at medium- and high-concentrations, highlighting the commonalities between the pharmacological effects of estradiol and SWT.

Identification of dose-responsive genes and pathways

Since genes or pathways that show dose-dependent changes are most likely reflecting valid pharmacological action from a drug, we therefore created two lists of differentially expressed genes (probe sets, $p < 0.05$) from SWT treatments at medium and high concentrations in comparison to the controls and identified common genes by overlapping the two lists. From this list of common genes, we can determine dose-responsive genes for which the expression level increased or decreased and mapped these to unique gene symbols in the IPA software. In total, 1,240 unique

Table 1. Treatment information and the number of differentially expressed genes of each treatment group.

Treatment	Concentration	Hybridization name	No. of probe sets ($p<0.05$, FC>1.5)	No. of genes ($p<0.05$, FC>1.5)	No. of probe sets ($p<0.05$)*	No. of probe sets (FDR<0.05)
Control	-	C1, C2, C3	-	-	-	-
Estradiol	0.1 µM	EM1, EM2, EM3	1,292	830	11,595	3,598
Ferulic acid	0.1 µM	FL1, FL2, FL3	9	8	2,965	0
	1 µM	FM1, FM2, FM3	6	4	3,332	0
	10 µM	FH1, FH2, FH3	3	3	2,270	0
SWT	0.0256 mg/mL	SL1, SL2, SL3	10	7	3,578	0
	0.256 mg/mL	SM1, SM2, SM3	90	71	5,409	0
	2.56 mg/mL	SH1, SH2, SH3	2,979	1911	13,296	6,673

*For the U133Plus2 microarrays with 54,675 probe sets, 2,734 (54,675×0.05) probe sets are expected by chance to have a p value <0.05.
FDR: false discovery rate.

Table 2. Top IPA pathways enriched with differentially expressed genes and their corresponding Fisher's exact test p values.

Treatment	IPA pathway name	p-value	Total number of genes in the IPA pathway	Ratio[*]
SWT at high concentration	Nrf2-mediated Oxidative Stress Response	4.55e-09	183	0.230
	p53 Signaling	2.37e-07	92	0.283
	Molecular Mechanisms of Cancer	6.17e-07	372	0.164
	Glucocorticoid Receptor Signaling	3.68e-06	280	0.168
	CD40 Signaling	2.92e-05	67	0.254
	Pancreatic Adenocarcinoma Signaling	3.26e-05	116	0.207
	EGF Signaling	3.26e-05	49	0.286
	B Cell Receptor Signaling	7.57e-05	154	0.188
	TGF-β Signaling	8.81e-05	83	0.229
	HGF Signaling	1.22e-04	103	0.214
SWT at medium concentration	Cell Cycle: G1/S Checkpoint Regulation	4.28e-05	59	0.068
	Role of CHK Proteins in Cell Cycle Checkpoint Control	2.27e-04	35	0.086
	Aryl Hydrocarbon Receptor Signaling	1.18e-03	154	0.026
	Molecular Mechanisms of Cancer	1.21e-03	372	0.016
	C21-Steroid Hormone Metabolism	2.11e-03	71	0.028
	Metabolism of Xenobiotics by Cytochrome P450	3.47e-03	209	0.014
	TR/RXR Activation	3.71e-03	97	0.031
	p53 Signaling	4.22e-03	92	0.033
	Cell Cycle Regulation by BTG Family Proteins	7.06e-03	36	0.056
	ATM Signaling	1.46e-02	53	0.038
SWT at low concentration	None of the pathways was significantly enriched with differentially expressed genes.			
Estradiol	Role of BRCA1 in DNA Damage Response	5.10e-09	61	0.246
	Cell Cycle: G1/S Checkpoint Regulation	2.69e-07	59	0.220
	Role of CHK Proteins in Cell Cycle Checkpoint Control	6.22e-06	35	0.257
	Aryl Hydrocarbon Receptor Signaling	7.09e-06	154	0.117
	Hereditary Breast Cancer Signaling	1.85e-05	129	0.124
	Molecular Mechanisms of Cancer	2.80e-05	372	0.083
	Pyrimidine Metabolism	5.74e-05	231	0.078
	Glycosphingolipid Biosynthesis - Globoseries	3.86e-04	46	0.130
	p53 Signaling	3.87e-04	92	0.130
	Pancreatic Adenocarcinoma Signaling	1.21e-03	116	0.103

*The ratio is calculated by dividing the number of differentially expressed genes found in the pathway by the total number of genes involved in the pathway.

genes were identified as dose-responsive genes that are associated with the pathways in the IPA software. The intensity of these genes obviously increased or decreased when the concentration of SWT treatments increased from 0.0256 mg/mL (SL) to 2.56 mg/mL (SH). **Table 4** lists the names, Fisher's exact test p values, and the ratios of affected genes for the top 10 IPA pathways most significantly enriched with the dose-responsive genes to SWT. The Nrf2 pathway is again on the top of list. Among all the 1,240 genes showing dose-responsive changes, 24 upregulated and 7 down-regulated genes could be assigned to the Nrf2 pathway. **Figure 4** showed that 10 out of the 15 most upregulated genes (probe sets) are regulated by the Nrf2 pathway according to PubMed literature search. Because of recently reported cancer prevention role of the Nrf2 pathway, our data suggest that SWT may have an Nrf2-inducing activity and may possess cancer chemopreventive effects.

Mapping gene expression profiles to the CMAP reference database

Since the same cell line (MCF-7) and same treatment period (6 h) were used to generate the above dataset as the CMAP dataset, comparison analysis can be done between the two datasets. Estradiol is the common drug used in both datasets. Thus, to further evaluate the quality and usability of the gene expression data generated in this study, we first used the gene expression profile from estradiol treatment as a query to search the CMAP database. If our data are in good quality and the CMAP approach works, we should expect the gene expression profiles of MCF-7 cells treated with estradiol in CMAP to show up on the list of top hits. Indeed, when the top 200 (100 up-regulated and 100 down-regulated) differentially expressed genes were used as the query, the CMAP profile of estradiol treated MCF-7 cells surfaced

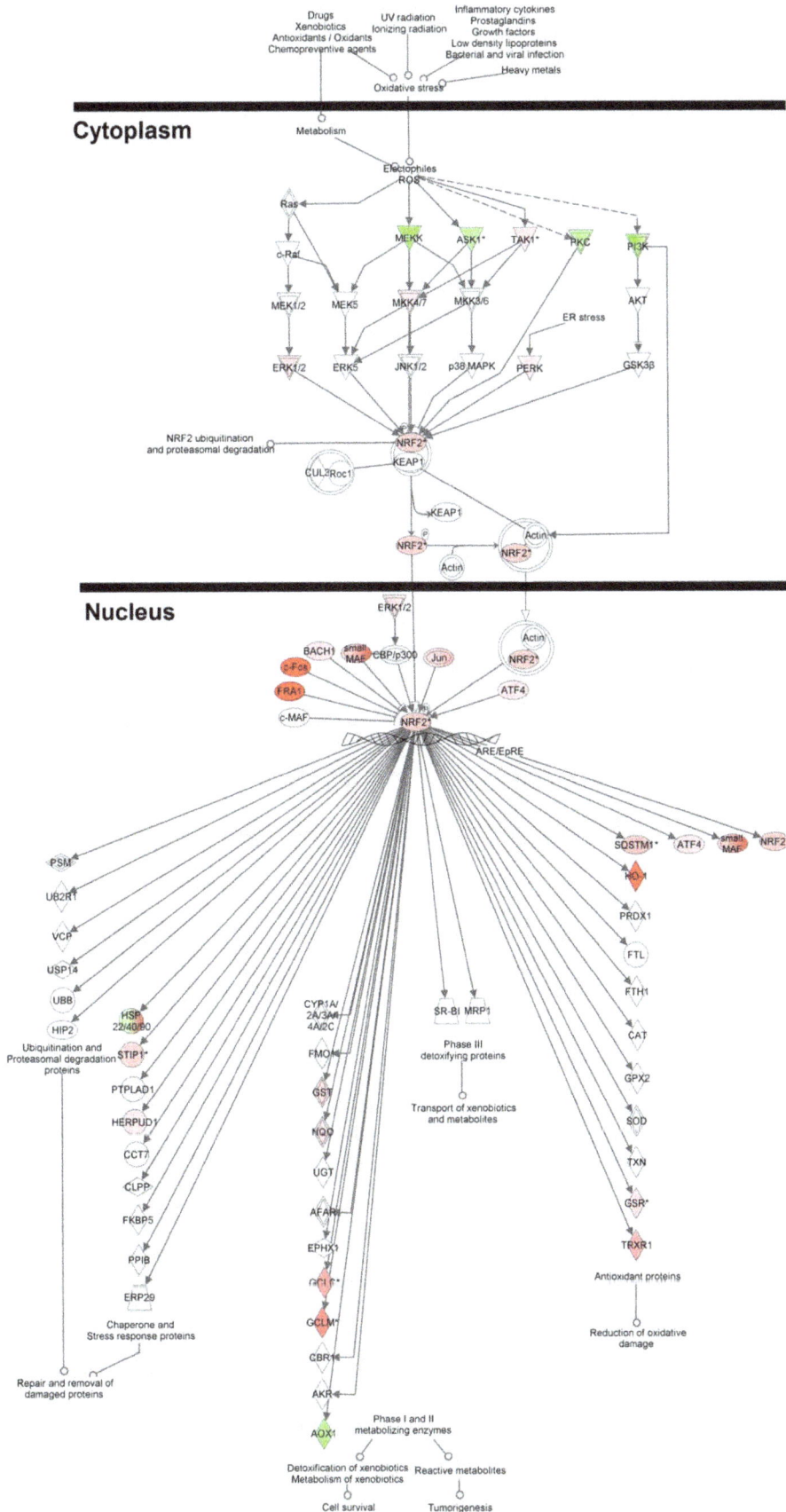

Figure 3. The Nrf2-mediated oxidative stress response pathway in IPA database. The red color and green color indicate the up- and down-regulated genes after treatment with high-concentration of SWT in this pathway, respectively.

Table 3. Top KEGG pathways enriched with differentially expressed genes and their corresponding Fisher's exact test *p* values.

Treatment	KEGG pathway name (Entry ID)	*p*-value
SWT at high concentration	MAPK signaling pathway (hsa04010)	4.81e-05
	TGF-beta signaling pathway (hsa04350)	7.76e-05
	Colorectal cancer (hsa05210)	9.76e-05
	Acute myeloid leukemia (hsa05221)	1.26e-04
	p53 signaling pathway (hsa04115)	8.88e-04
	Apoptosis (hsa04210)	9.54e-04
	Axon guidance (hsa04360)	1.28e-03
	Bladder cancer (hsa05219)	1.52e-03
	Glutamate metabolism (hsa00251)	2.60e-03
	Chronic myeloid leukemia (hsa05220)	2.73e-03
SWT at medium concentration	p53 signaling pathway (hsa04115)	4.36e-04
	Bladder cancer (hsa05219)	1.42e-03
	Prion disease (hsa05060)	2.49e-03
	Cell cycle (hsa04110)	3.12e-03
	Metabolism of xenobiotics by cytochrome P450 (hsa00980)	6.13e-03
	Small cell lung cancer (hsa05222)	1.12e-02
	Tetrachloroethene degradation (hsa00625)	3.76e-02
	Acute myeloid leukemia (hsa05221)	3.79e-02
SWT at low concentration	None of the pathways was significantly enriched with differentially expressed genes.	
Estradiol	Cell cycle (hsa04110)	1.00e-08
	Purine metabolism (hsa00230)	5.69e-04
	Porphyrin and chlorophyll metabolism (hsa00860)	3.18e-03
	Glycosphingolipid biosynthesis - globoseries (hsa00603)	3.70e-03
	p53 signaling pathway (hsa04115)	5.18e-03
	Pentose and glucuronate interconversions (hsa00040)	6.21e-03
	One carbon pool by folate (hsa00670)	6.24e-03
	Pyrimidine metabolism (hsa00240)	9.69e-03
	Thyroid cancer (hsa05216)	1.19e-02
	Bladder cancer (hsa05219)	1.49e-02

on the top 10 list (**Table 5**). In addition, the gene expression profiles resulting from treatments of three compounds, including butyl hydroxybenzoate, alpha-estradiol and genistein, were also on the top of the hit list. These compounds have been known to share the same molecular mechanisms of action with estradiol, mainly by regulating the hormonal signal transduction systems. Interestingly, the profile from treatment with fulvestrant, also known as ICI 182,780, turned out to be most contradictory to that from estradiol in our study, with a mean score of -0.806. This finding is consistent with the mechanistic role of fulvestrant, a pure estrogen receptor antagonist with no agonist effect for treating hormone receptor-positive metastatic breast cancer in postmenopausal women. These results from estradiol treatment indicated the value of the CMAP reference database and enhanced our confidence in the reliability of the microarray data from our study.

We also used the gene expression profiles of 100 up-regulated and 100 down-regulated genes from high-concentration SWT treatment and all the 53 differentially expressed genes from medium-concentration SWT treatment to query the CMAP database. For the low-concentration SWT treatment, CMAP search could not be performed because there were no down-regulated genes. The CMAP gene expression profile of MCF-7

treated with estradiol was the only one showing significant match (permutation *p*<0.00001) for both high- and medium-concentration SWT, indicating that SWT has an effect on MCF-7 cells similar to that of estradiol. This finding appeared to be consistent with SWT's widely claimed use as a TCM for women's diseases. The CMAP profiles of several other compounds (including phenoxybenzamine, withaferin A, 15-delta prostaglandin J2 and resveratrol) also showed high similarity to that of high-concentration SWT treatment. The pharmacological effects of these compounds are not similar to that of estradiol, suggesting that SWT has additional effects not seen with estradiol.

Validation of the microarray gene expression data by real-time RT-PCR

The differential expression of five genes in the Nrf2 pathway in response to SWT was validated by quantitative real-time RT-PCR on samples obtained from MCF-7 cells treated in a separate experiment. The selected genes are *HMOX1* (Heme oxygenase 1, HO-1), *GCLC* (glutamate-cysteine ligase, catalytic subunit), *GCLM* (glutamate-cysteine ligase, modifier subunit), *NQO1* (NAD(P)H:-quinine oxidoreductase 1) and *SLC7A11* [solute carrier family 7, (cationic amino acid transporter, y+ system) member 11]. The fold

Table 4. Top IPA pathways enriched with genes showing dose-responsive changes after SWT treatment and corresponding Fisher's exact test *p* values.

Ingenuity canonical pathways	p value	Total number of genes in IPA pathway	Ratio
Nrf2-mediated Oxidative Stress Response	4.9E-05	183	0.169
Chronic Myeloid Leukemia Signaling	0.0001	105	0.190
PPAR Signaling	0.0001	98	0.194
Glutamate Metabolism	0.0002	78	0.141
Cell Cycle: G1/S Checkpoint Regulation	0.0002	59	0.237
Small Cell Lung Cancer Signaling	0.0003	89	0.180
Protein Ubiquitination Pathway	0.0003	201	0.149
Molecular Mechanisms of Cancer	0.0004	372	0.126
mTOR Signaling	0.0005	156	0.154
PI3K/AKT Signaling	0.0007	137	0.153

*The ratio is calculated by dividing the number of differentially expressed genes found in the pathway by the total number of genes involved in the pathway.

changes of expression determined by RT-PCR for these genes were concordant with those obtained by microarrays (**Table 6**). The magnitude of the fold change from the RT-PCR assay was greater than that from the microarrays.

Effects of SWT on activation of Nrf2/ARE by dual luciferase reporter gene assay

In order to measure the activation of the Nrf2 pathway, a 39-bp ARE-containing sequence from the promoter region of the human *NQO1* gene was inserted into the cloning site of the luciferase plasmid pGL4.22 and then transiently transfected into MCF-7 cells. This assay was firstly established using HEK293 cells with sulforaphane as a positive control (**Figure 5A**). The transfected cells were then treated with SWT (SL, SM and SH) and the four individual herbal ingredients. A dual luciferase reporter gene assay was used in which a renilla luciferase gene was used as an internal control for normalization of the transfection efficiency and for toxicity induced during drug exposure. The high concentration of

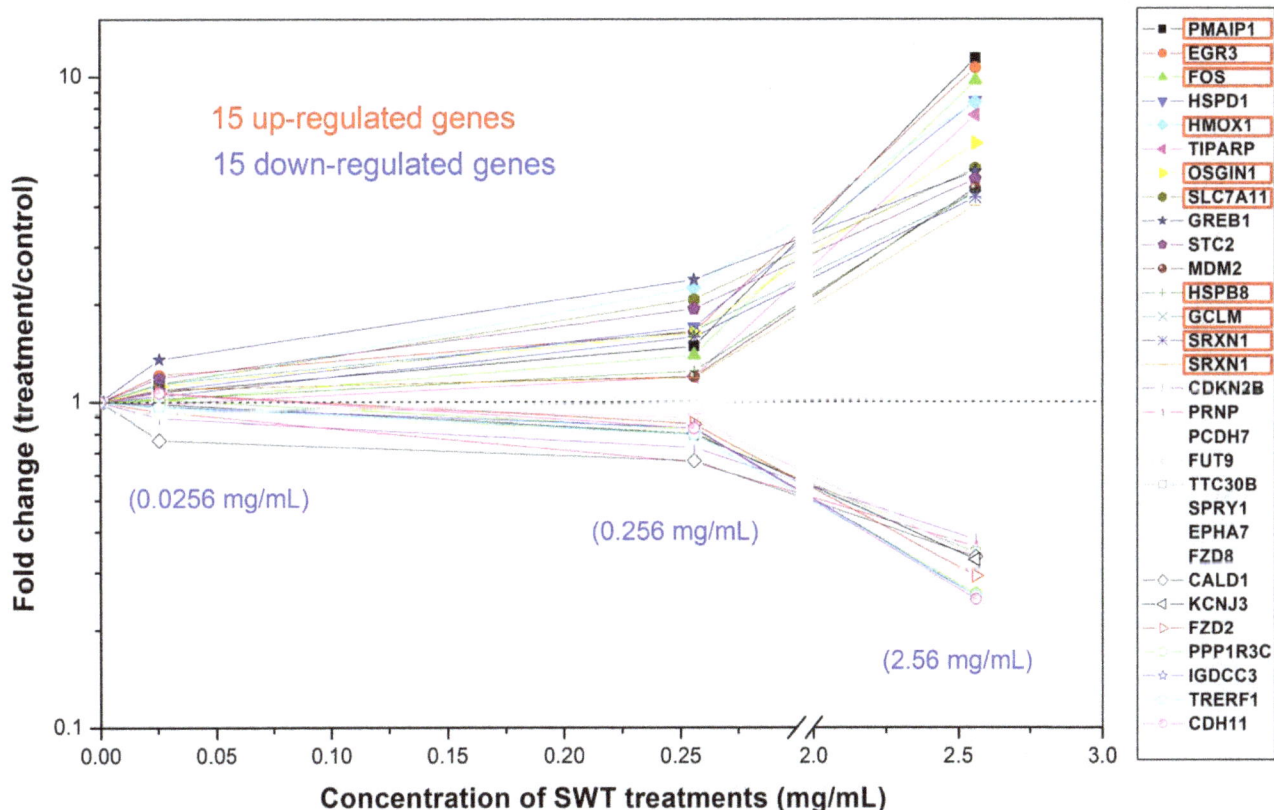

Figure 4. Dose-responsive genes with the largest fold changes. Among 15 dose-responsive up-regulated genes (probe sets) with the largest fold changes, ten are related to Nrf2 (highlighted in red box) according to PubMed literature search.

Table 5. Top CMAP hits correlated with SWT or estradiol treatment.

Treatment*	CMap chemical name and cell line	Mean score	p-value
SWT at high concentration	Phenoxybenzamine - MCF7	0.964	<0.00001
	Withaferin A - MCF7	0.885	<0.00001
	Securinine - MCF7	0.781	0.00002
	15-delta prostaglandin J2 - MCF7	0.697	<0.00001
	Thioridazine - MCF7	0.436	<0.00001
	Resveratrol - MCF7	0.432	<0.00001
	Estradiol - MCF7	0.345	<0.00001
	Tanespimycin - MCF7	0.188	<0.00001
	0317956-0000 - MCF7	−0.58	<0.00001
	Fulvestrant - MCF7	−0.698	<0.00001
SWT at medium concentration	Estradiol - MCF7	0.504	<0.00001
	Genistein - MCF7	0.452	<0.00001
	Valproic acid - MCF7	−0.367	0.00008
	Trichostatin A - HL60	−0.392	<0.00001
	LY-294002 − HL60	−0.428	<0.00001
	LY-294002 − MCF7	−0.445	0.00004
	Sirolimus - MCF7	−0.493	<0.00001
	Trichostatin A - MCF7	−0.658	<0.00001
	Vorinostat - MCF7	−0.608	0.00002
	Fulvestrant - MCF7	−0.765	<0.00001
SWT at low concentration	There were no down-regulated genes and CMap search could not be performed.		
Estradiol	Butyl hydroxybenzoate - MCF7	0.826	<0.00001
	Estradiol - MCF7	0.667	<0.00001
	Genistein - MCF7	0.632	<0.00001
	Alpha-estradiol - MCF7	0.544	<0.00001
	Trichostatin A - MCF7	−0.427	<0.00001
	0317956-0000 - MCF7	−0.434	<0.00001
	Vorinostat - MCF7	−0.457	<0.00001
	Phenoxybenzamine - MCF7	−0.496	<0.00001
	Pyrvinium - MCF7	−0.561	<0.00001
	Fulvestrant - MCF7	−0.806	<0.00001

*For high-concentration SWT and estradiol treatments, the query to CMAP search included 100 up-regulated and 100 down-regulated genes. For medium-concentration SWT treatment, all the 53 differentially expressed genes (3 down-regulated and 50 up-regulated) were used as the query for CMAP search.

Table 6. The gene expression fold changes of RT-PCR in comparison with the microarrays.

Gene	SL		SM		SH	
	Microarray	RT-PCR	Microarray	RT-PCR	Microarray	RT-PCR
SLC7A11	1.14±0.09	0.80±0.03	2.07±0.17**	1.33±0.16*	5.21±0.43**	8.38±0.13**
HMOX1	1.13±0.14	1.63±0.07	2.25±0.11**	5.73±0.55*	8.35±0.12**	45.99±0.53**
GCLC	1.01±0.08	3.58±0.12	1.42±0.02**	4.01±0.14*	3.12±0.06**	17.27±0.03**
GCLM	1.14±0.09*	1.06±0.12	1.65±0.07*	1.31±0.04*	4.38±0.33**	6.32±0.11**
NQO1	0.98±0.01	1.20	1.08±0.03	1.39	1.01±0.04	2.28

*$P<0.05$.
**$P<0.01$.
The standard deviation (SD) is not applicable for NQO1 gene, for which the PCR was performed for one time.

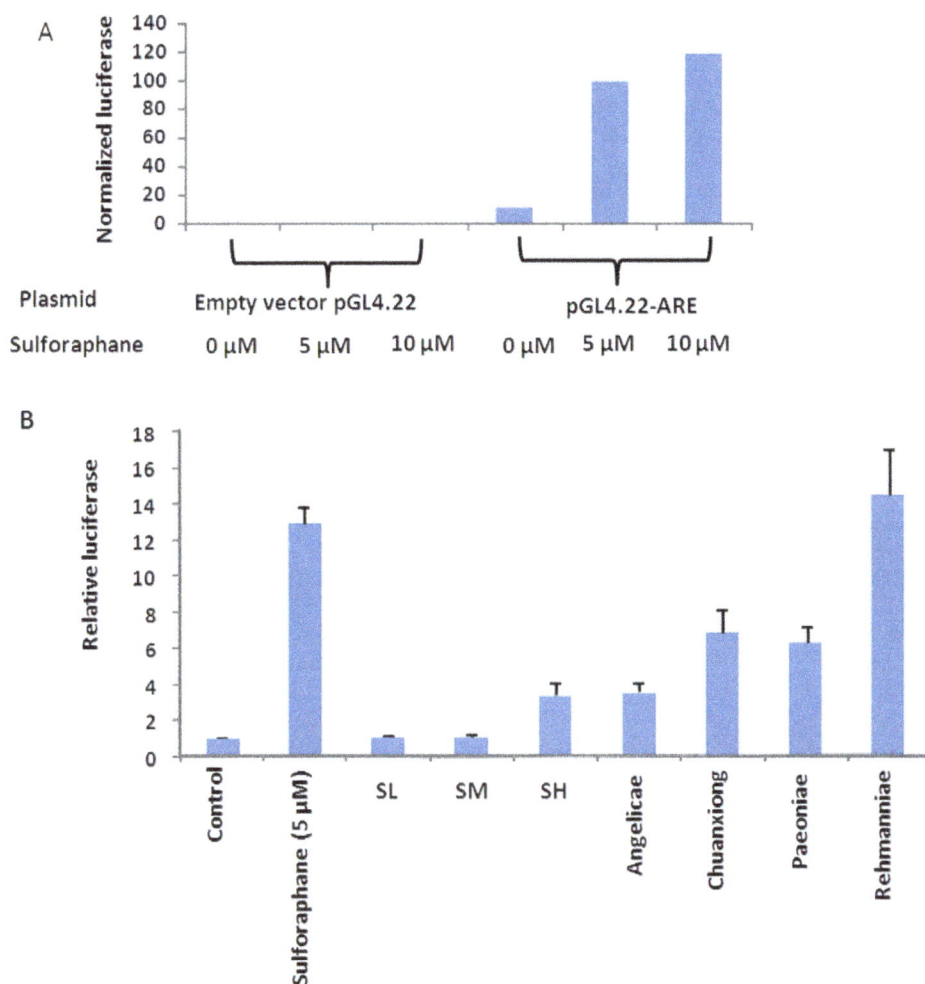

Figure 5. Luciferase assay results. (A) Luciferase assay established using HEK-293 cells co-transfected with a plasmid containing an ARE-luciferase reporter gene (pGL4.22-ARE) or empty vector (pGL4.22) and a plasmid encoding renillar luciferase (pGL4.74). The transfected cells were treated with sulforaphane for 24 hr prior to measurement of firefly and renillar luciferase activities using the dual luciferase reporter gene assay. (B) SWT (three doses SL, SM and SH in 0.0256, 0.256 and 2.56 mg/ml) and four herbal components of SWT (2.56 mg/ml) activated the Nrf2/ARE signaling pathway in MCF-7 cells.

SWT (SH) showed 3.4 ± 0.68-fold increase of the luciferase activity, while the individual herbs increased the luciferase activity to a higher degree (**Figure 5B**). Rehmanniae was found to be strongest activator for Nrf2/ARE transcription. Similar results have been obtained in another cell line HEK293 cells (data not shown). These results suggest that SWT and its ingredients may upregulate the expression of the Nrf2 target genes by activating the ARE on the promoters of these genes.

Discussion

The use of TCM is widespread in China and many Asian countries, and is also rapidly growing in Western countries [3]. Despite its long history of use, many questions remain to be answered due to lack of mechanistic understanding. In this study, we demonstrated, for the first time, a combined microarray gene expression and CMAP data mining approach to discover the mechanisms of action and to identify new therapeutic uses for TCM. We used a popular TCM formula SWT as a model to demonstrate the potential application of this approach.

The array data for 24 samples were firstly analyzed by hierarchical clustering analysis for a quality assessment of the array data and for a comparison of the treatment effects. The three

biological replicates in each treatment group showed a high reproducibility in the microarray experiments. The clustering results and the numbers of differentially expressed genes in each treatment group also revealed that the gene expression profile of MCF-7 cells was strongly changed by the treatment with estradiol and high-concentration of SWT, but not by FA and low-concentration SWT. The pathway analysis identified the Nrf2-mediated oxidative stress response as the pathway most significantly changed among differentially expressed genes showing dose-dependent response to SWT treatment. This new finding suggests that SWT could be cancer preventive. The real-time PCR data showed a similar but higher degree of gene upregulation of select genes in the Nrf2 pathway. When the gene expression profiles of MCF-7 cells resulting from SWT treatment were used to compare with those from 1,309 compounds in the CMAP database, the CMAP gene expression profile of estradiol-treated MCF-7 cells turned out to be the best match, consistent with SWT's widely claimed use for women's diseases and suggesting a potential phytoestrogenic effect. The CMAP profiles of several compounds with chemopreventive activity, i.e., withaferin A and resveratrol, also showed high similarity to the profiles of SWT.

One interesting finding is that the expression of genes involved in the Nrf2 signaling pathway was strongly impacted by SWT, but not by estradiol or ferulic acid treatment. The Nrf2 (nuclear factor erythroid 2 -related factor 2), a basic zip (bZIP) transcription factor, has been known as a key molecular target for chemopreventive agents, in particular, natural products and phytochemicals with activities in chemoprevention (for reviews, see [33] and [34]). Nrf2 plays a central role in the regulation of basal and/or inducible expression of phase II genes by binding to the antioxidant response elements (AREs) in their promoters [35]. Nrf2 is normally sequestered in the cytoplasm by Kelch-like ECH-associated protein 1 (Keap1). When activated upon exposure to inducers, it dissociates from Keap1, translocates to the nucleus, complexes with other nuclear factors, and binds to the ARE of genes. Chemopreventive Nrf2 inducers affect the interaction between Keap1 and Nrf2 through several mechanisms such as redox-sensitive modifications on cysteine residues of Keap1 or other cellular sensors and phosphorylation of Nrf2 [36]. Consistent with our results, the extract of *Angelicae Sinensis* (Dang Gui), one of the four herbal ingredients of SWT, has been shown to induce the expression of the detoxification enzyme NAD(P)H:quinine oxidoreductase 1 (NQO1), which is regulated by the Nrf2 pathway [37]. One of the active compounds, Z-ligustilide, was found with strong NQO1 inducing property by alkylating Keap1 [37]. We have also tested the effects of Z-liguistilide treatment on MCF-7 cells on Nrf2 gene expression and obtained the similar inducing effects (unpublished results).

The Nrf2-inducing activity of SWT represents an intriguing and interesting finding. SWT and its components, by affecting multiple Nrf2 target genes, could impact multiple components of the carcinogenic process. Many of the downstream target genes of Nrf2 are important in maintaining the cellular antioxidative response and amelioration of oxidative stress [38]. For example, the glutamate-cysteine ligase and SLC7A11 are essential in regulating the synthesis of glutathione, a very powerful endogenous antioxidant [39]. The NAD(P)H quinone oxidoreductase 1 (NQO1) catalyzes the reduction and detoxification of highly reactive quinones that can cause oxidative stress [40]. HO-1 (HMOX1) has been shown to protect from a variety of pathologies, including sepsis, hypertension, atherosclerosis, acute lung injury, kidney injury, and pain [41]. In addition, the effect of SWT on cytoprotective and detoxification pathways may explain other clinical effects of SWT. For example, its bone marrow protective effect on irradiated mice [27,28,42] may be attributed to the Nrf2-induding effects which may increase the radioresistance of bone marrow stem cells. It is also noted that many of Nrf2-regulated genes showed dose-dependent upregulation by SWT, but not by estrogen or ferulic acid. This suggests that the Nrf-2 activating effects of SWT may be separated from its phytoestrogenic effect. Further studies are needed to clarify the effect from different compounds compared to the whole SWT formula.

The identified differentially expressed genes in each treatment group were used in the comparison with the CMAP reference database [17]. We can directly compare the expression profiles of estradiol in our dataset and with those in the CMAP dataset due to the same cell line (MCF-7) and treatment time (6 hours). The gene expression profiles of SWT showed an excellent match to the CMAP gene expression profile of estradiol-treated MCF-7 cells (permutation $p<0.00001$). This finding is consistent with SWT's widely claimed use as an effective traditional Chinese medicine for women's diseases with a possible phytoestrogenic effect. The profile of SWT also shows similarity to the CMAP profiles of withaferin A, 15-delta prostaglandin J2 and resveratrol, which

have been reported to possess chemopreventive effects [43,44]. Results of KEGG pathway analysis found SWT and estradiol shared certain commonly regulated pathways of "cell cycle regulation", "p53 signaling" and "molecular mechanisms of cancer", further supporting SWT's phytoestrogenic effects. However, the gene expression profiles for SWT and estradiol also showed a significant difference. One of the most notable differences is that the ability to alter gene expression in the Nrf2 pathway only exists for SWT, but not for estradiol. The role of estrogens in the initiation and progression of breast cancer has been well known [45]. However, there is a large body of evidence that the consumption of phytoestrogens derived from plants and TCM can decrease the risk of cancer although they display estrogen-like activity [46]. These results support a notion that SWT may not have the cancer-causing effects of estradiol, but only have the beneficial cell protective activity.

Based on our previous work [25], the content of FA of the SWT extract was found to be 0.076%, corresponding to 0.0194, 0.194, and 1.94 µg/ml of FA, which were the concentrations tested in the present study. Such dosage selection allows a comparison of the activity of single compound (FA) with that of the TCM formulation (SWT). However, our data showed that FA in all the concentration tested only had subtle effects on global transcription in MCF-7 cells, although FA has been suggested as the chemical fingerprint for quality control of SWT products [29,30,31]. In view of lack of activity on gene expression, FA should not be used as a biological marker for activity of SWT.

The lack of expected gene expression change by FA may partially be explained by the statistical limitations of the approach: the sample size (n = 3 for each treatment group) and the fact that multiple tests of significance being done simultaneously may contribute to false positive/negative findings. Although the "multiple testing" corrections by False Discovery Rate (FDR) analysis were described in the text and Methods, such criteria may be too stringent to identify differentially expressed genes from treatment groups of FA and low concentration of SWT (Table 1). The biological limitations for this study, as is the case for almost all transcript profiling studies, is that there remains uncertainty about the relationship between mRNA and protein expression, and the relationship of both to function. Nevertheless, as indicated in Figure 5, a functional assay of Nrf2 pathway strongly supports the results obtained from microarray analysis.

In conclusion, gene expression profiles obtained by using microarrays combined with bioinformatic mining of the CMAP reference database can potentially shed light on the new molecular mechanism of SWT. If SWT can be shown to have cancer preventive potential, it has a great economic advantage because of its low cost and low toxicity, which will have a profound impact on human health. Further work is needed to determine the in vivo relevance of the in vitro findings obtained from the present study. This new approach proved to be powerful in an understanding of mechanisms of actions for TCM as exemplified by our study with SWT. In addition, the gene expression changes identified in this study could be used as biomarkers which can be used for assessing the intact quality of SWT. The genomic approach can be integrated with traditional chromatography-based fingerprinting method and metabolomics to obtain a more complete understanding of TCMs.

Materials and Methods

Compounds

Ferulic acid, 17 β-estradiol and DMSO were purchased from Sigma-Aldrich (St. Louis, MO, USA).

Preparation of SWT extracts

The SWT products were obtained from the School of Pharmacy, Chinese University of Hong Kong. These products were manufactured under GMP condition at the Hong Kong Institute of Biotechnology (Hong Kong, China) according to the protocol described in Chinese Pharmacopoeia 2005 [47] with modifications. Crude water extracts were prepared from powdered SWT. Fresh extracts were prepared right before the experiment. Three concentrations of SWT extract were prepared, 2.56 mg/ml, 0.256 mg/ml and 0.0256 mg/ml for high (SH), medium (SM), and low (SL) concentrations, respectively. The SH was prepared by dissolving 2.56 mg SWT powder into 1 ml of PBS buffer, followed by sonication for 30 min. The SM and SL were prepared by dilute the SH 10 and 100 times using PBS, respectively. As determined previously [25], the SL, SM and SH solutions contain 0.0194, 0.194, and 1.94 mg/ml of ferulic acid, respectively.

Cell lines and cell culture

The MCF-7 cells were purchased from American Type Culture Collection (ATCC, Manassas, VA, USA), cultured in Dulbecco's modified Eagle's medium (DMEM) supplemented with 10% fetal bovine serum (FBS), 1% non-essential amino acids, 100 unit/mL penicillin, 100 µg/mL streptomycin, 1 mM sodium pyruvate, and 2 mM L-glutamine in an atmosphere of 5% CO_2 at 37°C. The cells were seeded in 6-well plates at a density of 1×10^5 cells/ml. After incubating for 24 hours and at least 4 days before treatment, the medium was then replaced by hormone free medium which contains phenol-red free DMEM medium supplemented with 5% charcoal-dextrin stripped FBS (CD-FBS) to prevent the influence of hormones or estrogen-like compounds in the regular culture medium. The medium was changed every other day. The MCF-7 cells were then incubated with hormone free medium and treated by 0.001% DMSO (vehicle control group, C), 0.1 µM 17 β-estradiol (EM), 0.1, 1 or 10 µM of ferulic acid (equivalent to 0.0194, 0.194, and 1.94 mg/ml) (FL, FM and FH), 0.0256, 0.256, and 2.56 mg/ml SWT (SL, SM and SH) for 6 hours. Three replicates for each of the eight treatment groups were included, resulting in a total of 24 samples (wells). The detailed experimental information including names and concentrations of the treatments are shown in **Figure 1** and **Table 1**.

RNA extraction

Total RNA were extracted using RNeasy Mini Kit (QIAGEN, Valencia, California), following the manufacturer's protocol. The concentrations of RNA were measured by a NanoVue Plus (GE Healthcare, Piscataway, NJ, USA) and adjusted to 0.2 µg/µl. The RNA samples were stored at −80°C before further processing for microarray analysis.

Microarray processing

RNA quality was checked using the RNA 6000 LabChip and Agilent 2100 BioAnalyzer. Only high quality RNA with RNA Integrity Number (RIN) >9.0 were used for microarray experiments. The 24 RNA sample IDs were randomly ordered and were blinded to the microarray core facility, the Clinical Transcriptional Genomics Core at Cedars-Sinai Medical Center, in order to minimize the impact of potential confounding factors such as sample processing time and order. The gene expression data were generated using 24 Affymetrix Human Genome U133 Plus 2.0 arrays (Santa Clara, CA, USA). Each U133 Plus 2.0 array consists of 54,675 probe sets detecting over 47,000 transcripts.

The cRNA synthesis and labeling was carried out following Affymetrix one-cycle sample preparation protocol. Briefly, bioti-nylated cRNAs were prepared according to the standard Affymetrix GeneChip protocol. One µg of total RNA from each sample, along with poly A spikes (labeling control), were converted to double-stranded cDNA with GeneChip One-Cycle cDNA synthesis kit (Affymetrix). After second-strand synthesis, the cDNA was purified with the GeneChip sample cleanup module (Affymetrix). Biotinylated cRNAs were synthesized by in vitro transcription using the Affymetrix GeneChip 3'-Amplification kit. The A260/280 ratio and yield of each of the cRNAs were obtained. For each sample, 10 µg of biotinylated cRNA along spiked controls (bioB, bioC, bioD and cre) was hybridized to a Human Genome U133 Plus 2.0 array for 16 hours at 45°C. Following hybridization, arrays were washed, stained and then scanned with an Affymetrix GeneChip® 3000 7G scanner.

Real-time RT-PCR

To validate the microarray results, the MCF-7 cells were treated in a separate experiment using the identical experiment conditions and method as described above. One microgram of total RNA was incubated with DNase I, and reverse-transcribed with oligo dT using Superscript II RT-PCR (Invitrogen). One microliter of RT product was amplified by primer pairs specific for *HMOX1, NQO1, SLC7A11, GCLM* and *GCLC*. The *GAPDH* gene was used as a normalizing control. The primer sequences are available upon request. Relative gene expression was measured using the GeneAmp 7300 Sequence Detection system (Applied Biosystems, Foster City, CA, USA) using a SYBR Green protocol. For all amplifications, a standard amplification program was used (1 cycle of 50°C for 2 min, 1 cycle of 95°C for 10 min, 50 cycles of 95°C for 15 s and 60°C for 1 min). At the end of PCR cycling steps, data for each sample was displayed as a melting curve. The ABI SDS software was used to determine a ''Threshold Cycle' (Ct), which was the cycle number where the linear phase for each sample reached the threshold detection level.

Luciferase reporter gene assay

The luciferase reporter construct pGL4.22-ARE was a gift from Dr. Donna Zhang at the University of Arizona. It was generated by cloning a 39-bp antioxidant responsive element (ARE)-containing sequence from the promoter region of the NAD(P)H quinone oxidoreductase 1 (NQO1) into the pGL4.22 vector (Promega, Madison, WI, USA) [48]. The HEK293 or MCF-7 cells were transfected with the pGL4.22-ARE plasmid and a constitutively active renilla luciferase (pRL-TK-luc, from Promega; to correct for tranfection efficiency) (40:1 ratio) using FuGENE HD Transfection Reagent (Roche Applied Science, Indianapolis, IN, USA) according to the manufacturer's instructions. Twenty-four hours after transfection, the cells were exposed to the extracts of SWT or four herbal components for another 24 hours. Cell lysates were used for determining luciferase activities of both firefly and renilla by the dual luciferase reporter gene assay (Promega). Firefly luciferase activity was normalized to renilla luciferase activity. The experiment was carried out in triplicate and expressed as the mean ± SD.

Microarray data analysis

Microarray data specifically generated for this study are MIAME compliant. The raw data are available through the National Center for Biotechnology Information's Gene Expression Omnibus (GEO series accession number: GSE23610). The microarray gene expression data were imported to ArrayTrack [49], a software system developed by the U.S. Food and Drug Administration's National Center for Toxicological Research for the management, analysis, visualization and interpretation of microarray data (http://www.fda.gov/ArrayTrack/). The probe set-level expression data were summarized from probe-level data with Robust Multichip Average (RMA) [50] by taking all 24 microarrays together. Statistical testing and clustering analysis were conducted using ArrayTrack. Additional calculations were performed within JMP 7 (SAS Institute, Cary, NC, USA) and MATLAB 7.10 (MathWorks, Natick, MA, USA). For each probe set, log2-transformed intensity data were used in a two-sample t-test to obtain a p value and a fold change (FC).

Quality assessment of the microarray data

Hierarchical clustering analysis combined with heatmap was applied to evaluate the overall reproducibility and variation of 3 replicates within each group and the differences among the 8 groups. The $\log_2$-transformed expression intensities of 54,675 probe sets with RMA summarized data from 24 microarrays were used to calculate the correlation coefficients between two gene expression profiles and construct the heatmap. The quality of microarray data generated in this study is excellent for identifying differentially expressed genes.

Identification of differentially expressed genes

One important task in microarray data analysis is to identify a list of differentially expressed genes between two conditions (e.g. treatment versus control) [13,14]. Many methods have been used for selecting differentially expressed genes and the choice of the "best" gene selection methods has been under extensive debate [15,16]. In this study, genes differentially expressed between two sample groups were selected following the recommendations of the MAQC project [12,51]. Briefly, a t-test p value and a fold change comparing a treatment group and the control were calculated for each probe set. Probe sets with a p value greater than a pre-defined cutoff (e.g. $p>0.05$) were removed and the remaining probe sets were ranked according to the magnitude of fold changes. Genes measured by the probe sets with a fold change (FC) greater than a pre-defined threshold (e.g. FC>1.5) were considered as differentially expressed. This straightforward approach of combining a non-stringent p value filtering with a fold-change based ranking has been found to generate more reproducible and reliable differentially expressed genes [12,15,16,51,52]. The expression profiles of the differentially expressed genes have been used as an input to search reference gene expression data (i.e., CMAP database) for treatments with similar expression profiles or to identify pathways enriched with the differentially expressed genes. To reduce the number of false-positive differentially expressed genes among 54,675 probe sets, we controlled for the false-discovery rate (FDR) at the level of 0.05 as described previously [53]. However, the FDR criteria of 0.05 may be too stringent as more than half of the genes identified using the above criteria would be removed. Thus, although the criteria of $p<0.05$ and FC>1.5 were used with low stringency, this is expected to detect more genes truly associated with SWT at the expense of increasing the number of false-positives to be validated by other bioinformatic and experimental means.

Identification of pathways enriched with differentially expressed genes

The lists of differentially expressed genes were then imported to the Ingenuity Pathway Analysis (IPA) software (Ingenuity®

Systems, www.ingenuity.com) to identify pathways that are enriched with the genes. The probe sets were mapped to the HUGO gene symbols within IPA software. When multiple probe sets map to the same HUGO gene symbol, only the probe set with the maximal absolute log2 fold change value was kept for identifying enriched IPA canonical pathways. Probe sets that do not map to any HUGO genes were discarded. For each canonical pathway, the Fisher's exact test p value was calculated to measure the statistical significance of enrichment of the pathway of the differentially expressed genes in relation with what would be expected by chance from the total number of unique genes in the input list. In addition, the ratio of the number of input genes that are in the pathway to the total number of genes in the pathway was calculated. The p value and the ratio indicate the levels of impact the treatment has on the pathway. The pathways were ranked according to p values, with the most significantly impacted pathways are shown on the top.

The lists of differentially expressed genes were also imported to the Kyoto Encyclopedia of Genes and Genomes (KEGG) database [54,55,56]. The probe sets in each treatment group were mapped to the HUGO gene symbols within the KEGG database, and the pathways enriched with the differentially expressed genes according to the Fisher's exact test p values are considered to be impacted by the treatments.

Comparison of gene expression profiles with the CMAP reference database

To help better understand the underlying mechanisms of the therapeutic effects of SWT, we used the gene expression profiles of SWT treatments as queries to search the "Connectivity Map" (CMAP, http://www.broadinstitute.org/cMAP/) reference database (Build 02), which contains more than 7,000 expression profiles (instances) mainly from three cell lines (MCF-7, HL60 and PC3) treated with 1,309 compounds [17]. The query to CMAP is two lists of differentially expressed genes (listed as Affymetrix probe sets), one for up-regulation and the other for down-regulation, in which genes are ranked by the absolute log2 fold change values with descending order. The similarity between the gene expression profile of the query signature and that of a CMAP instance is measured by the connectivity score, ranging from -1 to 1. A high positive connectivity score indicates that the corresponding perturbagen in the CMAP database may similarly induce the expression change as the query agent. A high negative connectivity score indicates that the corresponding perturbagen in the CMAP database may reverse the expression effects of the query agent. Multiple profiles may exist for the same CMAP chemical name (due to different treatment concentrations, cell lines, or batches). CMAP allows individually matched instances consolidated by CMAP chemical name and cell line. Each combination of chemical names and cell lines combination comes with a mean connectivity score and a permutation p value, which indicates the probability of enrichment of a set of instances in a list of all instances by chance.

Author Contributions

Conceived and designed the experiments: MSSC LS YH Z. Wang CW ZZ. Performed the experiments: Z. Wang SW RR XJ. Analyzed the data: Z. Wen LS YH Z. Wang LY CW. Contributed reagents/materials/ analysis tools: ZZ MC CW. Wrote the paper: YH MSSC LS Z. Wen.

References

1. Efferth T, Li PC, Konkimalla VS, Kaina B (2007) From traditional Chinese medicine to rational cancer therapy. Trends Mol Med 13: 353–361.

2. Wang L, Zhou GB, Liu P, Song JH, Liang Y, et al. (2008) Dissection of mechanisms of Chinese medicinal formula Realgar-Indigo naturalis as an

effective treatment for promyelocytic leukemia. Proc Natl Acad Sci U S A 105: 4826–4831.

3. Chow MS, Huang Y (2010) Utilizing chinese medicine to improve cancer therapy - fiction or reality? Curr Drug Discov Technol 7: 1.

4. Chavan P, Joshi K, Patwardhan B (2006) DNA microarrays in herbal drug research. Evid Based Complement Alternat Med 3: 447–457.

5. Kang JX, Liu J, Wang J, He C, Li FP (2005) The extract of huanglian, a medicinal herb, induces cell growth arrest and apoptosis by upregulation of interferon-beta and TNF-alpha in human breast cancer cells. Carcinogenesis 26: 1934–1939.

6. Chan E, Tan M, Xin J, Sudarsanam S, Johnson DE (2010) Interactions between traditional Chinese medicines and Western therapeutics. Curr Opin Drug Discov Devel 13: 50–65.

7. Zhang J, Zuo G, Bai Q, Wang Y, Yang R, et al. (2009) Microarray expression profiling of Yersinia pestis in response to berberine. Planta Med 75: 396–398.

8. Wang CY, Staniforth V, Chiao MT, Hou CC, Wu HM, et al. (2008) Genomics and proteomics of immune modulatory effects of a butanol fraction of echinacea purpurea in human dendritic cells. BMC Genomics 9: 479.

9. Cheng WY, Wu SL, Hsiang CY, Li CC, Lai TY, et al. (2008) Relationship Between San-Huang-Xie-Xin-Tang and its herbal components on the gene expression profiles in HepG2 cells. Am J Chin Med 36: 783–797.

10. Yang NS, Shyur LF, Chen CH, Wang SY, Tzeng CM (2004) Medicinal herb extract and a single-compound drug confer similar complex pharmacogenomic activities in mcf-7 cells. J Biomed Sci 11: 418–422.

11. Pon D, Wang Z, K. L, Chow MS (2010) Harnessing traditional Chinese medicine to improve cancer therapy: issues for future development. Therapeutic Delivery 1: 335–344.

12. Shi L, Reid LH, Jones WD, Shippy R, Warrington JA, et al. (2006) The MicroArray Quality Control (MAQC) project shows inter- and intraplatform reproducibility of gene expression measurements. Nat Biotechnol 24: 1151–1161.

13. Allison DB, Cui X, Page GP, Sabripour M (2006) Microarray data analysis: from disarray to consolidation and consensus. Nat Rev Genet 7: 55–65.

14. Simon R (2009) Analysis of DNA microarray expression data. Best Pract Res Clin Haematol 22: 271–282.

15. Shi L, Jones WD, Jensen RV, Harris SC, Perkins RG, et al. (2008) The balance of reproducibility, sensitivity, and specificity of lists of differentially expressed genes in microarray studies. BMC Bioinformatics 9(Suppl 9): S10.

16. Shi L, Perkins RG, Tong W (2008) The Current Status of DNA Microarrays. In: Dill K, Liu R, Grodzinski P, eds. Microarrays: Preparation, Microfluidics, Detection methods, and Biological Applications. New York: Springer. pp 3–24.

17. Lamb J, Crawford ED, Peck D, Modell JW, Blat IC, et al. (2006) The Connectivity Map: using gene-expression signatures to connect small molecules, genes, and disease. Science 313: 1929–1935.

18. Hieronymus H, Lamb J, Ross KN, Peng XP, Clement C, et al. (2006) Gene expression signature-based chemical genomic prediction identifies a novel class of HSP90 pathway modulators. Cancer Cell 10: 321–330.

19. Bhattacharyya RP, Remenyi A, Good MC, Bashor CJ, Falick AM, et al. (2006) The Ste5 scaffold allosterically modulates signaling output of the yeast mating pathway. Science 311: 822–826.

20. De Preter K, De Brouwer S, Van Maerken T, Pattyn F, Schramm A, et al. (2009) Meta-mining of neuroblastoma and neuroblast gene expression profiles reveals candidate therapeutic compounds. Clin Cancer Res 15: 3690–3696.

21. Gheeya J, Johansson P, Chen QR, Dexheimer T, Metaferia B, et al. (2010) Expression profiling identifies epoxy anthraquinone derivative as a DNA topoisomerase inhibitor. Cancer Lett 293: 124–131.

22. Yeh LL, Liu JY, Lin KS, Liu YS, Chiou JM, et al. (2007) A randomised placebo-controlled trial of a traditional Chinese herbal formula in the treatment of primary dysmenorrhoea. PLoS One 2: e719.

23. Ohta H, Ni JW, Matsumoto K, Watanabe H, Shimizu M (1993) Peony and its major constituent, paeoniflorin, improve radial maze performance impaired by scopolamine in rats. Pharmacol Biochem Behav 45: 719–723.

24. Watanabe H (1998) Protective effect of a traditional medicine, shimotsu-to, on brain lesion in rats. J Toxicol Sci 23(Suppl 2): 234–236.

25. Wang ZJ, Wo SK, Wang L, Lau CB, Lee VH, et al. (2009) Simultaneous quantification of active components in the herbs and products of Si-Wu-Tang by high performance liquid chromatography-mass spectrometry. J Pharm Biomed Anal 50: 232–244.

26. Zhang H, Shen P, Cheng Y (2004) Identification and determination of the major constituents in traditional Chinese medicine Si-Wu-Tang by HPLC coupled with DAD and ESI-MS. J Pharm Biomed Anal 34: 705–713.

27. Liang QD, Gao Y, Tan HL, Guo P, Li YF, et al. (2006) Effects of four Si-Wu-Tang's constituents and their combination on irradiated mice. Biol Pharm Bull 29: 1378–1382.

28. Hsu HY, Ho YH, Lin CC (1996) Protection of mouse bone marrow by Si-WU-Tang against whole body irradiation. J Ethnopharmacol 52: 113–117.

29. Lv G, Cheng S, Chan K, Leung KS, Zhao Z (2010) [Determination of free ferulic acid and total ferulic acid in Chuanxiong by high-performance liquid chromatography for quality assessment]. Zhongguo Zhong Yao Za Zhi 35: 194–198.

30. Chang CJ, Chiu JH, Tseng LM, Chang CH, Chien TM, et al. (2006) Modulation of HER2 expression by ferulic acid on human breast cancer MCF7 cells. Eur J Clin Invest 36: 588–596.

31. Chang CJ, Chiu JH, Tseng LM, Chang CH, Chien TM, et al. (2006) Si-Wu-Tang and its constituents promote mammary duct cell proliferation by up-regulation of HER-2 signaling. Menopause 13: 967–976.

32. Wang L, Wang Z, Wo S, Lau CB, Chen X, et al. (2011) A bio-activity guided in vitro pharmacokinetic method to improve the quality control of Chinese medicines, application to Si Wu Tang. Int J Pharm 406: 99–105.

33. Kwak MK, Kensler TW (2009) Targeting NRF2 signaling for cancer chemoprevention. Toxicol Appl Pharmacol 244: 66–76.

34. Wang S, Penchala S, Prabhu S, Wang J, Huang Y (2010) Molecular basis of traditional Chinese medicine in cancer chemoprevention. Curr Drug Discov Technol 7: 67–75.

35. McMahon M, Itoh K, Yamamoto M, Chanas SA, Henderson CJ, et al. (2001) The Cap'n'Collar basic leucine zipper transcription factor Nrf2 (NF-E2 p45-related factor 2) controls both constitutive and inducible expression of intestinal detoxification and glutathione biosynthetic enzymes. Cancer Res 61: 3299–3307.

36. Sun Z, Huang Z, Zhang DD (2009) Phosphorylation of Nrf2 at multiple sites by MAP kinases has a limited contribution in modulating the Nrf2-dependent antioxidant response. PLoS One 4: e6588.

37. Dietz BM, Liu D, Hagey GK, Yao P, Schinkovitz A, et al. (2008) Angelica sinensis and its alkylphthalides induce the detoxification enzyme NAD(P)H: quinone oxidoreductase 1 by alkylating Keap1. Chem Res Toxicol 21: 1939–1948.

38. Li W, Kong AN (2009) Molecular mechanisms of Nrf2-mediated antioxidant response. Mol Carcinog 48: 91–104.

39. Huang Y, Dai Z, Barbacioru C, Sadee W (2005) Cystine-glutamate transporter SLC7A11 in cancer chemosensitivity and chemoresistance. Cancer Res 65: 7446–7454.

40. Venugopal R, Jaiswal AK (1996) Nrf1 and Nrf2 positively and c-Fos and Fra1 negatively regulate the human antioxidant response element-mediated expression of NAD(P)H:quinone oxidoreductase1 gene. Proc Natl Acad Sci U S A 93: 14960–14965.

41. Jarmi T, Agarwal A (2009) Heme oxygenase and renal disease. Curr Hypertens Rep 11: 56–62.

42. Lee SE, Oh H, Yang JA, Jo SK, Byun MW, et al. (1999) Radioprotective effects of two traditional Chinese medicine prescriptions: si-wu-tang and si-jun-zi-tang. Am J Chin Med 27: 387–396.

43. Vanaja DK, Grossmann ME, Celis E, Young CY (2000) Tumor prevention and antitumor immunity with heat shock protein 70 induced by 15-deoxy-delta12,14-prostaglandin J2 in transgenic adenocarcinoma of mouse prostate cells. Cancer Res 60: 4714–4718.

44. Bancos S, Baglole CJ, Rahman I, Phipps RP (2010) Induction of heme oxygenase-1 in normal and malignant B lymphocytes by 15-deoxy-Delta(12,14)-prostaglandin J(2) requires Nrf2. Cell Immunol 262: 18–27.

45. Riggs BL, Hartmann LC (2003) Selective estrogen-receptor modulators – mechanisms of action and application to clinical practice. N Engl J Med 348: 618–629.

46. Moiseeva EP, Manson MM (2009) Dietary chemopreventive phytochemicals: too little or too much? Cancer Prev Res (Phila) 2: 611–616.

47. (2005) The state pharmacopoeia commission of P.R.China. Pharmacopoeia of the People's REpublic of China. Beijing: Chemical Industry Press.

48. Kronke G, Bochkov VN, Huber J, Gruber F, Bluml S, et al. (2003) Oxidized phospholipids induce expression of human heme oxygenase-1 involving activation of cAMP-responsive element-binding protein. J Biol Chem 278: 51006–51014.

49. Tong W, Cao X, Harris S, Sun H, Fang H, et al. (2003) ArrayTrack–supporting toxicogenomic research at the U.S. Food and Drug Administration National Center for Toxicological Research. Environ Health Perspect 111: 1819–1826.

50. Irizarry RA, Wu Z, Jaffee HA (2006) Comparison of Affymetrix GeneChip expression measures. Bioinformatics 22: 789–794.

51. Guo L, Lobenhofer EK, Wang C, Shippy R, Harris SC, et al. (2006) Rat toxicogenomic study reveals analytical consistency across microarray platforms. Nat Biotechnol 24: 1162–1169.

52. Shi L, Tong W, Fang H, Scherf U, Han J, et al. (2005) Cross-platform comparability of microarray technology: intra-platform consistency and appropriate data analysis procedures are essential. BMC Bioinformatics 6 (Suppl 2): S12.

53. Benjamini Y, Hochberg Y (1995) Controlling the False Discovery Rate: a practical and powerful approach to multiple testing. J Royal Stat Soc, B 57: 289–300.

54. Wixon J, Kell D (2000) The Kyoto encyclopedia of genes and genomes–KEGG. Yeast 17: 48–55.

55. Masoudi-Nejad A, Goto S, Endo TR, Kanehisa M (2007) KEGG bioinformatics resource for plant genomics research. Methods Mol Biol 406: 437–458.

56. Kanehisa M, Goto S, Furumichi M, Tanabe M, Hirakawa M (2009) KEGG for representation and analysis of molecular networks involving diseases and drugs. Nucleic Acids Res 38: D355–360.

3

Validation of Orthopedic Postoperative Pain Assessment Methods for Dogs: A Prospective, Blinded, Randomized, Placebo-Controlled Study

Pascale Rialland[1], Simon Authier[1,2], Martin Guillot[1], Jérôme R. E. del Castillo[1], Daphnée Veilleux-Lemieux[1], Diane Frank[3], Dominique Gauvin[1], Eric Troncy[1]*

1 Groupe de Recherche en Pharmacologie Animale du Québec (GREPAQ), Department of Biomedical Sciences, Faculty of veterinary medicine, Université de Montréal, Saint-Hyacinthe, Quebec, Canada, 2 CiToxLAB North America, Laval, Quebec, Canada, 3 Department of Clinical Sciences; Faculty of veterinary medicine, Université de Montréal, Saint-Hyacinthe, Quebec, Canada

Abstract

In the context of translational research, there is growing interest in studying surgical orthopedic pain management approaches that are common to humans and dogs. The validity of postoperative pain assessment methods is uncertain with regards to responsiveness and the potential interference of analgesia. The hypothesis was that video analysis (as a reference), electrodermal activity, and two subjective pain scales (VAS and 4A-VET) would detect different levels of pain intensity in dogs after a standardized trochleoplasty procedure. In this prospective, blinded, randomized study, postoperative pain was assessed in 25 healthy dogs during a 48-hour time frame (T). Pain was managed with placebo (Group 1, n = 10), preemptive and multimodal analgesia (Group 2, n = 5), or preemptive analgesia consisting in oral tramadol (Group 3, n = 10). Changes over time among groups were analyzed using generalized estimating equations. Multivariate regression tested the significance of relationships between pain scales and video analysis. Video analysis identified that one orthopedic behavior, namely 'Walking with full weight bearing' of the operated leg, decreased more in Group 1 at T24 (indicative of pain), whereas three behaviors indicative of sedation decreased in Group 2 at T24 (all $p<0.004$). Electrodermal activity was higher in Group 1 than in Groups 2 and 3 until T1 ($p<0.0003$). The VAS was not responsive. 4A-VET showed divergent results as its orthopedic component (4A-VETleg) detected lower pain in Group 2 until T12 ($p<0.0009$), but its interactive component (4A-VETbeh) was increased in Group 2 from T12 to T48 ($p<0.001$). Concurrent validity established that 4A-VETleg scores the painful orthopedic condition accurately and that pain assessment through 4A-VETbeh and VAS was severely biased by the sedative side-effect of the analgesics. Finally, the video analysis offered a concise template for assessment in dogs with acute orthopedic pain. However, subjective pain quantification methods and electrodermal activity need further investigation.

Editor: Giorgio F. Gilestro, Imperial College London, United Kingdom

Funding: This study was supported in part by a grant from Vétoquinol Laboratories, Lure, France (http://www.vetoquinol.fr/); an ongoing New Opportunities Fund grant from the Canada Foundation for Innovation (#9483) for the pain/function equipment (http://www.innovation.ca); a Discovery grant from the Natural Sciences and Engineering Research Council of Canada (#327158-2008) as operating fund for pain biomarkers (http://www.nserc-crsng.gc.ca). The funders had no role in study design, data collection and analysis, decision to publish, or preparation of the manuscript.

Competing Interests: The authors received funding for this work from a commercial source (Vétoquinol Laboratories) and with regards to their agreement with this company. Moreover, the authors contracted the realization of the experiments in a Contract Research Organization, named CiToxLAB North America, and one author, Simon Authier at the time a Ph.D. student under supervision and actually Head of Veterinary Services at this company, participated actively in the study's realization as well as edition of the manuscript.

* E-mail: eric.troncy@umontreal.ca

Introduction

Postoperative pain remains the main cause of morbidity related to surgery. Spontaneous nociceptive pain has been associated with both skin incisions [1] and deep surgery [2]. Using a rodent knee surgery model, Buvanendran *et al.* [3] also characterized some functional (behavioral) outcomes. In addition, nociceptive stimulation and neuronal changes might differ between those observed in models of acute postsurgical pain [2] and chemical models of acute inflammation like sodium urate-induced synovitis in dogs [4,5,6]. In this context, a standardized and technically well-recognized canine orthopedic surgery might be a stronger surrogate of surgical pain than a chemically inflammatory pain

model in dogs. Altogether, rodent models and chemical models would present a limited approach to the complex process of pain associated with orthopedic surgery. Veterinary surgeons, on the other hand, manage many natural painful disease processes that are common to both dogs and human beings [7], and they perform preclinical and clinical orthopedic procedures in dogs, some of which are directly derived from procedures used in human beings [8]. Consequently, we argue that common orthopedic dog surgeries, as trochleoplasty, are valid surrogates for the investigation of human surgical pain [9,10]. However, methods of pain assessment in dogs are not extensively documented or standardized [11,12,13]. Inadequate pain assessment for dogs decreases the validity of canine pain models and hampers the comparison of pain studies.

Both owners [14] and veterinarians [15,16] associate orthopedic surgery with a high degree of pain. Behavioral (guarding, interaction with owner, reaction to palpation, etc.) and physiological (cardiovascular indices and stress response) indicators are commonly used to assess pain in non-verbal patients [17]. Composite pain scales and multidimensional questionnaires have been developed for use in a wide range of canine postoperative pain conditions [11,12,13]. According to the Cohen's classification [18], both postoperative pain scales Glasgow Composite Pain Scale and University of Melbourne Pain Scale were developed in compliance with the psychometrics rules. However, these instruments did not differentiate the analgesic effect of the standard non-steroidal anti-inflammatory drugs (NSAID) from this of the Coxib [19] or fentanyl [20] in pain studies with canine orthopedic surgery. In contrast, kinetic gait analysis using a force plate or a pressure-sensing weight mattress decreased following sodium urate-induced acute synovitis in dogs [21,22] and improved following NSAID drug administration [21,23,24]. Kinetic gait analysis did no correlate well with the subjective lameness scoring in dogs [25,26,27,28], which supported the kinetic analysis to be a more sensitive indicator of joint pain than subjective lameness scoring. Even if kinetic gait analysis is a great asset in lameness study, it might not capture the broader aspects of pain [29] and is not available in every clinical center. Recently, the behavioral assessment of rodent pain has evolved with the use of semi-automated behavioral video analysis [30] and standardized behavioral facial expression coding systems [31]. Previously, video analysis of spontaneous behaviors in dogs after ovariohysterectomy allowed unique discrimination between pain-related behaviors and drug side effects, such as sedation [32,33], but this pain monitoring method has not yet been used following canine orthopedic surgery.

The purpose of the present study was to evaluate methods of pain assessment following canine orthopedic surgery. The hypothesis was that the effects of three different levels of analgesia would be reflected and therefore recognizable by the behavioral and physiological changes they elicit on a standardized canine postoperative pain model. Several methods (video analysis of spontaneous behaviors, electrodermal activity [EDA], visual analogue scale [VAS], and composite pain scale [4A-VET pain scale]) were used for the assessment of postoperative pain to evaluate their reliability and responsiveness. The concurrent validity of the behavioral pain assessment tools was tested using video analysis as the reference method.

Results

Rescue Analgesia

Rescue analgesia was provided for 25% of all dogs. Rescue analgesia requirements were distributed as follows: three dogs from Group 1 at Time (T)0.41, T6.01 and T6.31, one dog from Group 2 at T24.01, and two dogs from Group 3 at T1.19 and T6.19 hours postoperatively, with T0 being the extubation time.

Video Analysis of Spontaneous Behaviors

Of all the spontaneous behaviors identified in our ethogram (Appendix S1), fourteen that occurred frequently were statistically analyzed and their reliability tested (Table 1). Eleven behaviors presented a moderate to high inter-observer reliability, as their intraclass correlation coefficient ranged from 0.50 to 0.99.

For 'Walking with full weight bearing', 'Howling', 'Sniffing', and 'Licking lips', generalized estimating equation (GEE) analysis indicated significant main effects for time and group, as well as a

significant interaction between group and time (Table 2). For the occurrence rates of 'Standing with full weight bearing', and 'Dog in front of the kennel,' there was no group effect, but there were significant effects of time and a significant interaction between group and time (Table 2). There were no significant interactions between group and time for the remaining behaviors, thus explaining why they were discarded from further analyses.

The planned comparison analysis over time indicated that the occurrence rates of the remaining behaviors (as listed in Table 3) were not different across groups at baseline: T-96 (all $p>0.08$). From T-96 to T24, the occurrence rate decreased for 'Walking with full weight bearing', 'Standing with full weight bearing', 'Howling', and 'Sniffing' in all treatment groups (all $p<0.0001$, Table 3). Furthermore, for 'Licking lips' and 'Dog in front of the kennel', the occurrence rates declined in Group 2 ($p<0.0001$, and $p<0.0001$, respectively) and Group 3 ($p=0.001$, and $p=0.0002$, respectively) from T-96 to T24 (Table 3) but did not change in Group 1 ($p=0.69$, and $p=0.09$, respectively).

At T24, the estimated occurrence of 'Walking with full weight bearing' was 43.3 (95% confidence interval [95%CI]: 11.1, 170.7; $p<0.0001$), and 36.2 (95%CI: 4.5, 285.7; $p=0.0007$) times higher in Group 3 than in Groups 1 and 2, respectively (Table 3). Also at T24, the estimated occurrences of 'Howling', 'Licking lips', and 'Dog in front of the kennel' were 29.0 (95%CI: 3.5, 235.4; $p=0.001$), 23.6 (95%CI: 8.6, 65.0; $p<0.0001$), and 7.7 (95%CI: 3.1, 18.9; $p=0.003$) times higher, respectively, in Group 1 than in Group 2. Moreover, the observed difference between Groups 1 and 2 for 'Licking lips' persisted at T48 with an estimated risk ratio of 10.4 (95%CI: 3.9, 27.8; $p<0.0001$) (Table 3). The occurrence of 'Licking lips' was also higher in Group 3 than in Group 2 both at T24 and T48, with estimated risk ratios of 13.9 (95%CI: 5.1, 38.3; $p<0.0001$) and 10.9 (95%CI: 4.1, 28.8; $p<0.0001$), respectively (Table 3).

Electrodermal Activity

The EDA measurements at T-96 were not correlated with those at T-5 (Spearman's rank correlation (rho_s) = 0.001, $p=0.87$), and Cohen's kappa coefficient (κ) could not be computed. The EDA measurement analysis indicated an overall time effect ($p<0.0001$), and a significant interaction between group and time ($p<0.0001$), but there was no significant group effect ($p=0.40$). The planned comparisons showed that the EDA measurements of Group 1 were higher than those of Groups 2 and 3 at T0.5 ($p<0.0001$, and $p<0.0001$, respectively) and T1 ($p<0.0001$, and $p=0.0003$, respectively) (Figure 1).

Pain Scales

The VAS reliability was not estimated, because all of the scores were 0 at T-96 and T-5. For the composite pain scale, namely 4A-VET pain scale, scores at T-96 and T-5 were correlated ($rho_s - 0.52$; $p=0.008$) and demonstrated fair agreement ($\kappa = 0.33$, 95%CI: 0.08, 0.57) [34]. Cronbach's alpha coefficient was 0.7, indicating that the items of the 4A-VET pain scale were homogeneous.

An analysis of the VAS scores indicated overall effects of time ($p<0.0001$) and group ($p=0.003$), as well as a significant interaction between group and time ($p<0.0001$). At T24, Group 2 presented higher pain scores than Groups 1 and 3 ($p<0.0001$, and $p<0.0001$, respectively) (Figure 2A).

An analysis of the 4A-VET scores indicated overall effects of time ($p<0.0001$) and group ($p<0.0001$), as well as a significant interaction between group and time ($p<0.0001$). Group 2 presented lower scores than Groups 1 and 3, at T0.5 (both

Table 1. Interobserver reliability of the video-analysis.

Spontaneous behaviour Observer	Number #1	Number #2	Mean (SD) #1	Mean (SD) #2	ICC
Standing with no weight bearing	6	4	4.3 (3.6)	6.7 (3.6)	**0.74**
Walking with full weight bearing	4	3	136.2 (141.9)	54.6 (30.1)	**0.99**
Standing with full weight bearing	4	3	83.0 (105.8)	67.0 (93.5)	**0.97**
Sitting normal with equal weight on limbs	4	3	11.7 (15.0)	7.3 (3.5)	**0.84**
Immobile with head down	4	3	49.5 (24.7)	17.0 (10.0)	**0.52**
Silent	5	5	63.2 (49.0)	46.8 (48.7)	0.01
Howling	5	5	63.4 (51.8)	24.0 (41.5)	**0.50**
Sniffing	8	8	182.1 (138.8)	87.0 (47.7)	**0.98**
Immobile with head up	8	8	167.1 (123.2)	31.3 (17.3)	**0.91**
Immobile while looking around	8	8	32.2 (23.7)	34.0 (21.07)	0.39
Licking lips	6	6	50.8 (51.9)	19.8 (20.1)	**0.92**
Ears twitching	6	5	6.1 (3.6)	4.6 (2.6)	0.01
Ears normal	8	8	69.1 (47.8)	25.5 (15.5)	**0.87**
Dog in front of the kennel	8	8	34.7 (28.2)	36.3 (30.5)	**0.99**

Data presents the number of videotapes (Number) for which the behaviour was recorded by both independent observers (#1 and #2) blinded to treatment groups for 10% of all videos (n = 8). Mean (SD) of the occurrence rate is presented for each observer (#1 and #2). Intraclass correlation coefficients (ICC) were calculated from a set of 10% randomized videotapes.

$p < 0.0001$), T1 (both $p < 0.0001$) and T2 ($p = 0.0009$, and $p = 0.0012$, respectively) (Figure 2B).

An analysis of the behavioral component of 4A-VET (4A-VETbeh) scores showed overall effects of time ($p < 0.0001$) and group ($p < 0.0003$), as well as a significant interaction between group and time ($p < 0.0001$). Group 2 had higher 4A-VETbeh scores than Groups 1 and 3, at T12 ($p = 0.0001$, and $p = 0.0003$, respectively), T36 ($p = 0.0002$, and $p = 0.0003$, respectively), and T48 ($p = 0.0011$, and $p < 0.0001$, respectively) (Figure 2C). In addition, the 4A-VETbeh scores of Group 2 were higher than those of Group 3 at T9 ($p = 0.0015$) and those of Group 1 at T24 ($p = 0.0002$) (Figure 2C).

An analysis of the orthopedic component of 4A-VET (4A-VETleg) scores indicated main effects of time ($p < 0.0001$) and group ($p < 0.0001$), as well as a significant interaction between group and time ($p < 0.0001$). Group 2 presented significantly lower 4A-VETleg scores than Groups 1 and 3, at T0.5 (both $p < 0.0001$), T1 (both $p < 0.0001$), T2 ($p = 0.0002$, and $p = 0.0009$, respectively), T6 ($p < 0.0001$, and $p = 0.0002$, respectively), and T12 (both $p < 0.0001$) (Figure 2D). Additionally, the 4A-VETleg scores of Group 2 were lower than those of Group 3 at T3 ($p = 0.0008$) (Figure 2D).

Concurrent Validity

A multivariate GEE regression analysis indicated that all of the pain scores were negatively associated with the administration of rescue analgesia (β estimate$\pm$SE: -0.92 ± 0.30; $p = 0.002$ for VAS, -2.19 ± 0.58; $p = 0.0002$ for 4A-VET, -2.20 ± 1.04; $p = 0.04$ for 4A-VETbeh, and -0.92 ± 0.30; $p = 0.002$ for 4A-VETleg). Except for 4A-VETbeh, all pain scores were positively associated with

Table 2. Wald statistics for Type 3 GEE[1] analyses of video-analysis.

Spontaneous behaviour	Time ChiSq (p)	Group ChiSq (p)	Group × Time ChiSq (p)
Standing with no weight bearing	198.91 (<.0001)	35.8 (<.0001)	5.77 (0.21)
Walking with full weight bearing	**920.21 (<.0001)**	**16.15 (0.0003)**	**33.57 (<.0001)**
Standing with full weight bearing	*1692.66 (<.0001)*	*4.27 (0.12)*	*11.47 (0.022)*
Sitting normal with equal weight on limbs	996.06 (<.0001)	2.23 (0.33)	5.36 (0.25)
Immobile with head down	3214.42 (<.0001)	4.72 (0.09)	3.61 (0.46)
Howling	**1800.35 (<.0001)**	**7.1 (0.03)**	**170.58 (<.0001)**
Sniffing	**4141.17 (<.0001)**	**19.74 (<.0001)**	**9.49 (0.05)**
Immobile with head up	4564.48 (<.0001)	10.34 (0.006)	6.4 (0.17)
Licking lips	**834.88 (<.0001)**	**17.76 (0.0001)**	**29.71 (<.0001)**
Ears normal	1485.69 (<.0001)	3.05 (0.22)	2.49 (0.65)
Dog in front of the kennel	*2745.23 (<.0001)*	*0.75 (0.69)*	*36.02 (<.0001)*

[1]Generalized estimating equation. For each behaviour, the results of GEE analysis are presented as the Chi-square result (ChiSq) and the p-value (p) of the main effect for Time, Group and the Group × Time interaction. Significant main effect for Group × Time interaction is presented in bold. Italics for the behaviours indicated in bold is indicative of no significant Group effect.

Table 3. Descriptive statistics of spontaneous behaviour during video-analysis.

Spontaneous behaviour	Group	T-96 Med (min-max)	Freq (%)	T24 Med (min-max)	Freq (%)	T48 Med (min-max)	Freq (%)
Walking with full weight bearing							
	1	186 (40–308)	*16.9^x*	0 (0–2)	*0.05^a*	64 (0–228)	10.78
	2	139 (9–321)	*27.64^x*	0 (0–3)	*0.12^a*	1 (0–109)	6.94
	3	250 (81–332)	*24.25^x*	3 (0–117)	*2.4^b*	6 (0–145)	4.81
Standing with full weight bearing							
	1	52(7–128)	*6.02^x*	4 (0–25)	0.57	22 (0–103)	3.69
	2	45 (5–179)	*11.84^x*	4 (0–4)	0.48	3 (0–21)	1.63
	3	57 (25–304)	*11.22^x*	4 (0–10)	0.42	6 (0–24)	0.74
Howling							
	1	1 (0–192)	*2.25^x*	0 (0–33)	*0.58^a*	3 (0–73)	1.38
	2	13 (0–111)	*8.48^x*	0 (0–1)	*0.04^b*	0 (0–4)	0.25
	3	21 (0–115)	*4.02^x*	1 (0–13)	*0.40^{ab}*	2 (0–43)	0.72
Sniffing							
	1	208 (78–373)	*23.86^x*	89 (17–213)	9.49	178 (8–395)	21.47
	2	147 (98–295)	*37.92^x*	10 (0–93)	4.76	77 (9–130)	18.25
	3	301 (112–483)	*31.06^x*	124 (1–269)	13.38	98 (1–374)	12.27
Licking lips							
	1	7 (0–23)	*1.12*	7 (0–52)	*1.42^a*	17 (0–72)	*2.88^a*
	2	10 (2–116)	*5.80^x*	1 (0–1)	*0.12^b*	3 (0–5)	*0.63^b*
	3	10 (7–11)	*2.80^x*	7 (0–30)	*0.96^a*	18 (0–68)	*2.54^a*
Dog in front of the kennel							
	1	28 (6–130)	3.98	9 (2–72)	*2.12^a*	23 (4–57)	3.47
	2	27 (2–181)	*10.68^x*	2 (1–12)	*0.84^b*	18 (1–85)	7.63
	3	78 (12–219)	*9.32^x*	7 (1–55)	*1.79^{ab}*	21 (1–75)	2.20

Data are presented as the median (Med), minimum (min), maximum (max) and relative frequency (Freq) in percentage (%) of spontaneous behaviour by group and time (T) −96, 24 and 48 hours. Superscript case (x): significant difference when −96 h is compared to 24 h; At each time point, different letters (higher case (a) or (b)) indicate significantly different values among treatment groups. Significant differences are presented in bold. Bonferroni-corrected alpha level was of 0.0041.

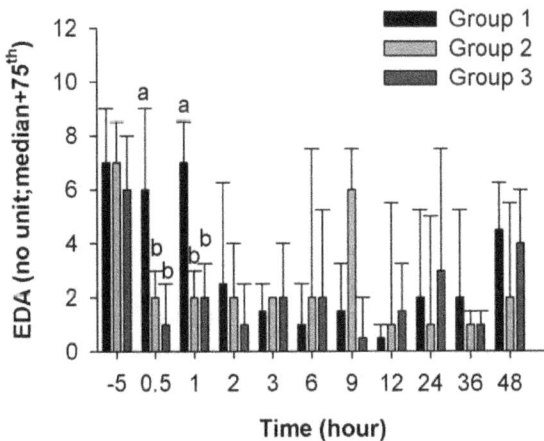

Figure 1. Electrodermal activity. EDA (no unit) by group over time. Data are presented as the median and 75th percentile for groups of n = 5 to 10 dogs over time. At each time point, different letters (higher case (a) or (b)) indicate significantly different values among treatment groups. Bonferroni-corrected alpha level was of 0.0015.

time (0.79±0.14; p<0.0001 for VAS, 0.89±0.29; p = 0.002 for 4A-VET, and 0.79±0.14; p<0.0001 for 4A-VETleg). In addition, VAS scores were negatively associated with the occurrence of two behaviors: 'Walking with full weight bearing on the operated limb' (−0.13±0.04; p = 0.0003) and 'Dog in front of the kennel' (−0.14±0.06; p = 0.03), while 4A-VET scores were negatively associated with 'Walking with full weight bearing' (−0.22±0.03; p<0.0001). 4A-VETbeh scores were positively associated with 'Immobile with head down' (0.42±1.04; p = 0.02) and negatively associated with 'Sniffing' (−0.43±0.10; p<0.001). Finally, 4A-VETleg scores were positively associated with 'Standing with no weight bearing on the operated limb' (0.73±0.25; p = 0.004) and negatively associated with both 'Walking with full weight bearing' (−0.20±0.06; p = 0.002) and 'Sitting normally with equal weight on limbs' (−0.57±0.26; p = 0.04).

Discussion

In this model, the hypothesis was that Group 1 would present the most pain, Group 2 the least, and Group 3 intermediate pain. The results partially support this hypothesis although no behavioral or physiological assessment demonstrated the expected gradient of pain response (Group 1>Group 3>Group 2). Group 1 did present more pain than the other two groups, as demonstrated clearly by one video analysis criterion, namely 'Walking with full weight bearing' (Group 1 ≠ Group 3, at T24),

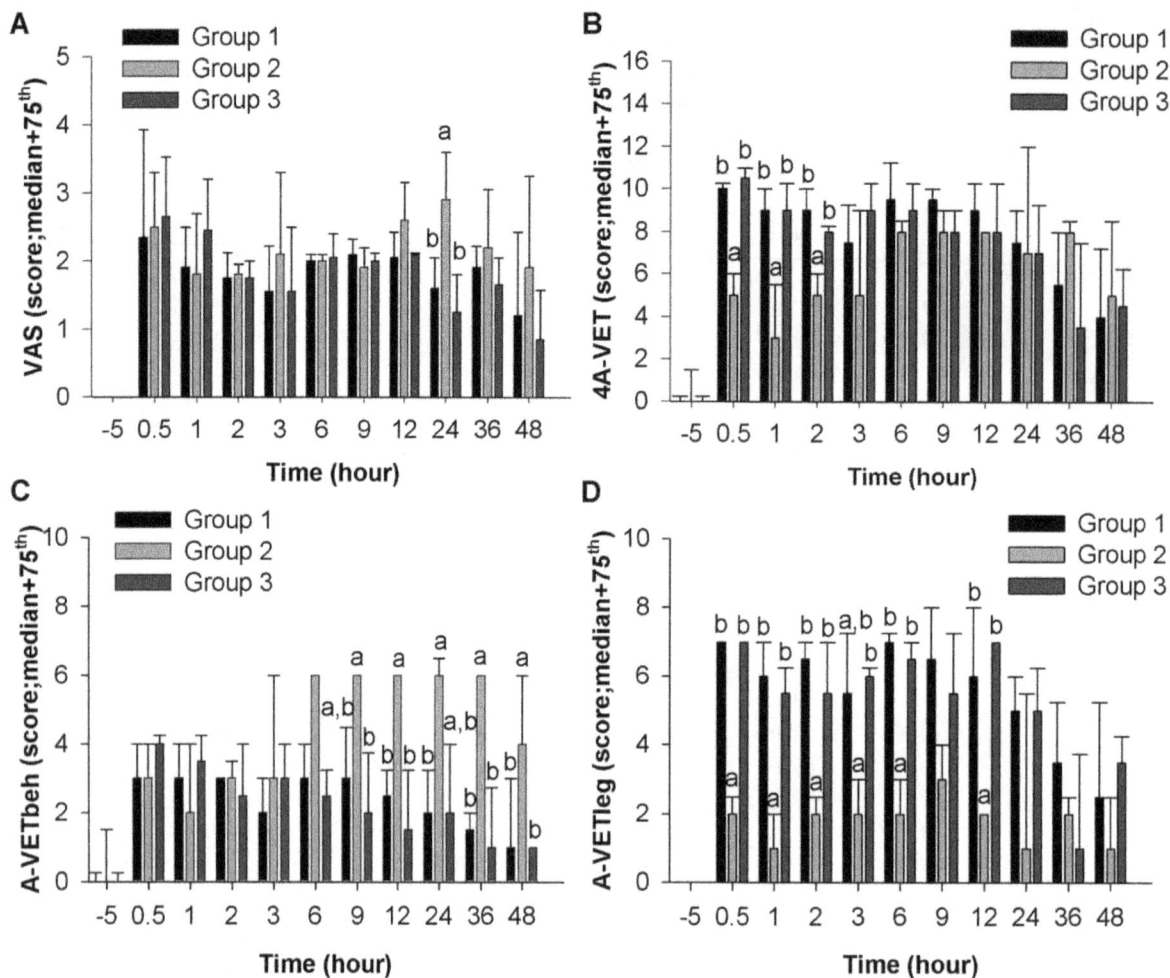

Figure 2. Pain scales. A) Visual analogue scale, **B)** the 4A-VET pain scale, **C)** 4A-VETbeh subscale, and **D)** 4A-VETleg subscale by group over time. Data are presented as the median and 75th percentile for groups of n = 5 to 10 dogs at each time points. At each time point, different letters (higher case (a) or (b)) indicate significantly different values among treatment groups. Bonferroni-corrected alpha level was of 0.0015.

as well as by 4A-VETleg (Group 2 ≠ Groups 1 and 3, at T0.5, 1, 2, 3, 6, and 12) and EDA (Group 1 ≠ Groups 2 and 3, at T0.5, and 1). Heavy sedation appears to explain the lack of specificity in pain detection by the other methods (namely VAS and 4A-VETbeh). Most interestingly, the multimodal analgesia group (#2) was higher than would be expected for VAS at T24 and for 4A-VETbeh at T9, 12, 24, 36, and 48. This was definitively a concurring and surprising discovery. Inclusion of anesthesia/drug controls would have assisted in determining the effects of sedation. In fact, video analysis confirmed that analgesic drug-induced sedation decreased some behaviors because dogs in Group 2 spent less time acting interested to their environment ('Dog in front of the kennel'), or trying to attract attention ('Howling'), and making facial expressions ('Licking lips'). With regards to our specific objectives, we observed good reliability for eleven behaviors in the video analysis (see Table 1) and for the 4A-VET pain scale. We could not evaluate VAS reliability, and EDA reliability was poor. Establishing measurement reliability was an obligatory step before we could assess responsiveness and concurrent validity.

In animal video analysis, there are numerous methods for recording behavioral changes. In this study, we performed a microanalysis approach of events based on a quantitative

description of an animal's normal behavior. The method generated a wide range of behaviors and occurrences. Only behaviors that demonstrated significant occurrence rates and high inter-observer reliability were selected as final endpoints. This selection method could be considered quite limiting, particularly as the duration of video was a one hour-period, and the inter-observer reliability was tested on 10% of randomized videotapes. We deemed that these strict behavioral criteria would be strongly representative of postsurgical orthopedic pain.

A decreased occurrence rate of 'Walking with full weight bearing' was demonstrated in all treatment groups following trochleoplasty compared to normal behavior. At T24, this decrease was higher in Group 1 than in Group 3, suggesting that tramadol in the latter group provided some analgesia-related use of the operated limb. Intuitively, it makes sense to measure the occurrence rate of 'Walking with full weight bearing on the operated limb' as a measure of orthopedic pain (or, at least as a measure of an absence of lameness) but no previous study has investigated this measurement as an indicator of pain.

So far, it was postulated that the degree of pain would correlate to the degree of weight bearing using force plate systems. Unexpectedly, the occurrence rate of the spontaneous behavior

'Standing/walking/trotting with no or partial weight bearing' (as indicator of lameness) did not discriminate different levels of pain and indicated the lack of specificity of this measurement using video-analysis. It is also possible that the observer-reported behavior was less accurate in quantifying lameness than evaluating absence of lameness in dogs. This hypothesis would be in accordance with previous publications reporting a lack of correlation between subjective lameness scores and weight bearing measurements recorded through kinetic gait analysis in canine studies [25,26,27,35]. Nevertheless, postoperative pain was correlated to a decrease in the occurrence rate of a normal behavior 'Walking with full weight bearing of the operated leg', suggesting that this latter behavior was a specific pain-free behavior. Our result supported that first, painful dogs were less active (walk, trot); second, the dogs were either lame or not lame when they were active; and third, the naturally occurring behavior of severity of lameness was not correlated to pain severity using video-analysis. Altogether, recording of a spontaneous behavior should not be interpreted in the same way as kinetic gait analysis. Kinetic gait analysis was currently performed when dogs were compelled to walk or trot, suggesting a sustained nociceptive firing during limb use. Indeed, video-analysis would summarize the way the dogs behaved and responded to postoperative pain, suggesting a cognitive adaptation to pain. Therefore the sensitivity of the behavioral quantification of 'Walking with full weight bearing of the operated leg' supports its use for further study as a new surrogate for assessing pain in clinical conditions.

'Howling' frequency differentiated Group 2 from Group 1 at T24, and the difference between Groups 2 and 3 approached significance ($p = 0.006$– Table 3). It is generally acknowledged that increased vocalization is associated with postoperative pain expression in the dog as reflected by the inclusion of this behavior in many canine postoperative pain scales [13,36,37]. However, a decrease in 'Howling' in all three groups could indicate that postoperative pain decreased the occurrence rate of 'Howling', particularly for Group 1. That the decrease was more pronounced in Group 2 suggests that the use of a multimodal analgesic protocol may have contributed more to the decrease than did pain. Indeed, the occurrence rate did not return to its baseline value in any group. This finding supports vocalization's lack of sensitivity to postoperative pain intensity, as was observed in a previous study [38].

The occurrence rates of both 'Dog in front of the kennel' and 'Licking lips' behaviors decreased in Group 2 when compared to Group 1 and decreased in both analgesic groups over time, while remaining stable over the same period in Group 1. Moreover, Group 2 spent less time 'Licking lips' during the overall postoperative period. Altogether, the decreased occurrence rate observed in both pharmacologically treated groups, and mostly in Group 2, may simply not be related to a pain-controlling effect but rather may be related to a sedative effect of the different opioids (fentanyl patch, epidural morphine, and oral tramadol). Similar results were previously observed following administration of butorphanol in a canine pain study [32]. These results highlight the major interference of the neuropharmacological effects of commonly used analgesic (opioid) drugs in the apparent expression of postoperative pain. The frequency of these two behaviors did not change over time in Group 1, suggesting that they were not affected by postoperative pain. Thus, the observations regarding restlessness/interest in the environment indicated by 'Dog in front of the kennel' and 'Licking lips' behaviors should be analyzed with caution and may not demonstrate assay sensitivity for comparing analgesic protocols.

Altogether, video analysis was a powerful method that provided evidence of pain related behaviors and identified behaviors related to drug side-effects. The low number of selected and validated spontaneous behaviors is related to inter-subject variability in pain expression and to the difficulty associated with standardizing a behavioral observation for assessing pain. These results support the use of video analysis as a valid pain assessment tool because of its ability to test concurrent validity with subjective behavioral pain assessments. The concurrent validity analysis completed in this study confirmed sedation's major influence not only on video analysis but also on VAS and 4A-VETbeh scores.

In this study, EDA and 4A-VET were responsive to multimodal analgesia in the immediate postoperative period by reporting decreased skin conductance, a known method for indirectly quantifying sympathetic activity and decreased (4A-VET) pain scores, respectively, in Group 2. There were slight discordant responses between EDA measurements and 4A-VET scoring. With EDA, Group 1 demonstrated higher pain intensity compared to Groups 2 and 3, whereas with 4A-VET, the intensity of pain was lower in Group 2 than in both Groups 1 and 3 at similar time points.

The most plausible explanation for the decreased EDA intensity in Groups 2 and 3 was the analgesia/anxiolysis induced by either treatment. This analgesic detection is supported by a study where the EDA intensity correlated significantly with kinetic gait analysis, telemetered motor activity and subjective scoring to demonstrate analgesic effect of a bisphosphonate in an experimental dog osteoarthritis model [39]. Hypothetically, the EDA decrease could also be related to other pharmacological interactions with sympathetic activity [40,41,42]. Moreover, the sensitivity of EDA was not important, as highlighted by the absence of a difference between Groups 2 and 3 and the short duration of its effectiveness to differentiate Group 1 from both Groups 2 and 3. This low psychometric quality added to the previously reported lack of specificity in a rodent model of surgical pain [43]. Further investigation is needed before considering increasing the clinical use of EDA.

Although other canine pain studies have validated the pain VAS [44,45], different treatment effects on mean VAS scores following trochleoplasty were not demonstrated in this study. The VAS might have provided systematic error, particularly when measuring pain at baseline (floor effect) and during the postoperative period (ceiling effect). The VAS observer could not be blinded to the presence or the absence of surgery because sham dogs were not included, and therefore this was an evident first source of bias (explaining the floor effect). Furthermore, increased VAS scores in Group 2 at T24 suggested that sedative side-effects of analgesics might interfere with VAS scoring. Confounding effect of analgesic side effect on VAS score (increasing it) was previously observed [46,47]. This could explain the lack of sensitivity in postoperative pain quantification using the VAS and the absence of a treatment effect using this method. Altogether, these findings urge for caution in the use and interpretation of observer-reported VAS pain scoring as a standardized pain assessment method with experimental animals as it could be biased and not specific for pain.

The 4A-VET pain scale showed acceptable reliability and, as reported earlier, was partially responsive to treatments. Nevertheless, like EDA, 4A-VET demonstrated weak performance because of its apparent low sensitivity (no difference between Groups 1 and 3) and short duration (initial 2 hours post-surgery) of effective responsiveness in favor of Group 2. Interestingly, the weak performance of the 4A-VET pain scale could be explained by the response divergence between its two main components, namely

4A-VETbeh and 4A-EVTleg. The 4A-VETleg scores indicated significantly lower pain in Group 2 compared to Groups 1 and 3 at T0.5, 1, 2, 3, 6, and 12. Conversely, 4A-VETbeh scores indicated increased pain for Group 2 compared to Groups 1 and 3 at T9, 12, 24, 36, and 48. Considered together, these results suggest that non-analgesic effects of the multimodal analgesia protocol used in Group 2 may have been a potential confounder in pain assessment, as has been observed in previous canine postoperative pain studies [38,44]. The differences between the mean scores of 4A-VETbeh and 4A-VETleg might also illustrate differences in scale construction. This is a strong argument for choosing 4A-VETleg as a standard measure of orthopedic postoperative pain. Nevertheless, 4A-VETleg had some limitations because it was not as responsive at T24 as was the video analysis, suggesting that 4A-VETleg was valid during at least the first twelve hours following surgery. At this point, the validity of behavioral pain assessment based on pain scoring systems is uncertain because many questions remain in relation to measurement errors and the difficulty of weighing the consequence of sedation against those of unrelieved pain, as has already been observed [48].

Using video analysis, 'Walking with full weight bearing' of the operated limb was the only validated behavior to support the analgesic efficacy of tramadol as well as to indicate the presence of pain in Group 1. Analgesic side-effects strongly associated with behavioral changes. Regression methods were used to test the concurrent validity of the pain scales scores with video analysis as the standard of the behavioral pain assessment. Of all displayed behaviors, 'Walking with full weight bearing on the operated limb' was the behavior that was most correlated with the VAS, 4A-VET and 4A-VETleg pain scores. It is possible that the relationship between the pain scales and 'Walking with full weight bearing' occurred for several reasons: 1) this behavior was more frequent; 2) this higher frequency could be attributed to a more conservative and well-understood definition, allowing it to be observed with more accuracy; and 3) recording during daytime might have improved the robustness of the occurrence rate of 'Walking with full weight bearing' in relation to the dog's level of daylight activity.

Additionally, it appears this behavior ('Walking with full weight bearing') is unconsciously linked to pain-free behavior for VAS and 4A-VETleg. Moreover, for the latter, pain intensity was clearly linked to lameness (reflected by 'Standing with no weight bearing'), thus reinforcing the conceptual validity of 4A-VETleg scores. Interestingly, the regression analysis in this study confirmed the previously suspected limitations in the pain scoring systems. First, sedative side-effect of the drug(s) was a confounding factor for assessing pain with VAS because VAS was linked to the spontaneous behavior 'Dog in front of the kennel' that changed in response to the side-effect of the analgesic. Second, the regression models revealed that 4A-VETbeh scores were related to two spontaneous behaviors, 'Immobile with head down' and 'Sniffing', which were not validated by the video analysis and were assumed to be included in the communicative category. The video analysis confirmed that the present 4A-VETbeh was not an accurate method for pain evaluation in this study. The results also showed strong evidence that the large number of items in the composite 4A-VET pain scale introduces noise into this pain scoring system.

Pain expression may hypothetically differ when an animal is observed directly as opposed to being filmed without a person in the environment. This could, evidently, lead to differences in pain observation using various methods. The advantage of video analysis for pain expression is that it can be used as a reference method to introduce further development of pain scales [49], as has been previously performed in dogs [48]. It is important to consider that many factors can influence the measurement of pain. It has been proposed that not only the pain stimulus itself, but observer characteristics, environmental and social interaction effects, and intra-subject factors can all influence the measurement of pain. This can occur *via* effects on the pain experience, as well as on its expression [49]. In this study, the standardization of procedures allowed us to control all of these aspects, except the intra-subject experience.

An important limitation of the study was the apparent moderate intensity of postoperative pain generated by the trochleoplasty procedure, as reflected by the low levels of pain scale scoring, as well as the low use of rescue analgesia in Groups 1 and 3. This could be related to an inadequate sensitivity of pain scales. A higher intensity of pain would surely have contributed to better discrimination in pain assessment method responsiveness.

In conclusion, the video analysis provided strong evidence of responsiveness and validity of the 4A-VETleg pain scale for assessing acute orthopedic pain. The alteration of normal gait behavior, as observed by changes in 'Walking with full weight bearing,' is likely to be the best behavioral orthopedic pain assessment method. The current results will hopefully contribute to the generation of a refined and validated method of orthopedic pain assessment. This study also clearly establishes the major interference of analgesic side effects on dog behaviors. This is a major finding with regards to the use of opioid drugs as a staple in the surgical analgesic arsenal in veterinary and human medicine. Such interference could potentially contribute to the overdosing of opioids.

Methods

Ethics Statement, Animals and Experimental Design

The Institutional Animal Care and Use Committee approved the study protocol (# Rech-1220), and the Canadian Council on Animal Care guidelines were followed regarding care and handling of the dogs. This study also adhered to the guidelines of the Committee for Research, Ethical Issues of the IASP [17] and the ARRIVE checklist [50]. Twenty-five healthy male beagle dogs (15.2 (3.3) [mean (SD)] months old and weighing 9.9 (1.4) kg) belonging to the colony of a contract research organization (CiToxLAB North-America, Inc.) accredited by the Association for Assessment and Accreditation of Laboratory Animal Care International were included. Dogs were acclimated for 1 week and housed in individual kennels under standard laboratory conditions in a 12 h light/dark cycle with food and water provided *ad libitum*. Dogs were maintained in standard environmental conditions (humidity, temperature, and ventilation).

Baseline evaluations were carried out before surgery at –96 h (video analysis occurrence rate of spontaneous behaviors, EDA measurements and pain scales scores) and –5 h (EDA measurements and pain scales scores). Then, the dogs were subjected to a standardized trochleoplasty and general anesthesia. The time of tracheal extubation was defined as the time "zero" (T0) hour post-surgery. Video recording of the spontaneous behaviors was also performed at T24 and T48 post-surgery. Measurements of EDA and pain scales scores were recorded at T0.5, 1, 2, 3, 6, 9, 12, 24, 36, and 48 post-surgery. One observer (SAU), blinded to dog group attribution, performed live assessments in the following sequential order: VAS, 4A-VET, and EDA. Another observer (DVL) performed the video analysis of the spontaneous behaviors.

The dogs were randomized into three groups. Group 1 dogs (n = 10), received an oral placebo (Dextrose, Sigma-Aldrich Canada Ltd., Oakville, ON, Canada) between 3 to 2.5 h before T0 (*i.e.*, approximately 1.5 h before starting surgery), and the administration was repeated every 6 h until study completion. Group 2 dogs ($n = 5$) received a multimodal pre-emptive analgesia consisting of the following: 1) a transdermal fentanyl patch (2–3 µg/kg, Duragesic™ 50, Janssen-Ortho Inc., Toronto, ON, Canada) applied to the skin 24 h prior to the surgery and maintained in place until study completion; 2) an epidural mixture injection of morphine sulfate (0.1 mg/kg, Morphine HP®25, Sandoz, QC, Canada) and ropivacaine (1 mg/kg Naropin™ 0.2%, AstraZeneca Canada Inc., Mississauga, ON, Canada), administered 20 min prior to the surgery, followed by an 0.1 mg/kg epidural morphine sulfate injection given at 12, 24, and 36 h after extubation; 3) a subcutaneous (SC) tolfenamic acid injection (4 mg/kg Tolfedine™ 4%, Vetoquinol Inc., Lure, France) administered 1 h prior to the surgery and repeated after 24 and 48 h; and 4) an oral administration of tramadol (10 mg/kg, V1002, Vetoquinol Inc., Lure, France) started 3 to 2.5 h prior to T0 and repeated every 6 h until study completion. Group 3 dogs ($n = 10$) received 10 mg/kg of tramadol orally between 3 to 2.5 h prior to T0 and every 6 h until study completion. The dogs in Groups 1 and 3 also received a sham or placebo for the transdermal, epidural, and subcutaneous administrations. Rescue analgesia (0.1 mg/kg hydromorphone intravenously [IV], 25–50 µg/h fentanyl patch, and 4 mg/kg SC tolfenamic acid) was provided if the VAS score exceeded 6.5 (out of 10), and/or the 4A-VET score exceeded 11 (out of a total score of 18).

At the end of the experiment at T54, all dogs were euthanized using an IV overdose of sodium pentobarbital (Euthanyl™, Bimeda-MTC Animal Health Inc., Cambridge, ON, Canada).

Anesthesia and Surgery Procedures

Anesthesia was induced with IV propofol to effect (up to 8 mg/kg, Propoflo™ 1%, Abbott Animal Health, North Chicago, IL, USA). Lidocaine spray (10% w/w, Lidodan™, Odan Laboratories Ltd., Pointe-Claire, QC, Canada) was administered onto the glottis prior to tracheal intubation. Volatile anesthesia was initiated with isoflurane (AErrane™, Baxter Corporation, Mississauga, ON, Canada) in oxygen (oxygen flow originally set at 200 ml/kg/min and isoflurane vaporizer set at 3%) using a Bain coaxial system. Then, volatile anesthesia was maintained using mechanical ventilation set at a respiratory rate between 8–12 breaths/min and using a peak inspiratory pressure of less than 20 cm H_2O to achieve a constant end-tidal carbon dioxide of approximately 40 mmHg. End-tidal isoflurane was maintained at 1.7%. Lactated Ringer's solution (Baxter Corporation, Toronto, ON, Canada) was IV-administered at a rate of 10 ml/kg/h throughout the anesthesia procedure. Cefazolin (25 mg/kg, Novopharm™ Toronto, ON, Canada) was IV-administered 1 hour prior to surgery and repeated 6 to 8 hours up to the end of the study.

The standardized trochleoplasty was performed in the right femorotibial joint. A skin incision of 8 cm was made at the anterolateral aspect of the femorotibial joint. After incision of the articular capsule and medial stabilization of the patella, a rectangular abrasion (2 × 1 cm dimensions) trochleoplasty was performed in the right femoral trochlea. Next, the arthrotomy was sutured using 3–0 polydioxane absorbable sutures for the articular capsule, 3–0 polyglecaprone 25 polydioxanone absorbable sutures for the subcutaneous tissue, and 3–0 nylon sutures for the skin.

Video Analysis of the Spontaneous Behaviors

We constructed a useful ethogram (Appendix S1) based on previous observations from pain research in the canine population [32,33], personal observations and selection by a veterinary behaviorist (DFR). Behaviors were categorized using operational definitions. Categories were mutually exclusive and consisted of "Location in the kennel", "Body position", "Facial expression", "Motor activity", "Tail position", and "Self-care". The dogs were video-recorded during the same one-hour daylight period per session using a camera placed in front of the kennel. An automated video behavioral analysis system (The Observer® XT, Noldus Information Technology, Tracksys Ltd., Nottingham, United Kingdom) was used to collect expression of spontaneous dog behaviors. Ten percent of the videos were selected randomly and reviewed by two independent observers (DVL, DFR). The occurrence rate of spontaneous behaviors was quantified for each video-recording session.

Electrodermal Activity

EDA measures sympathetic response and is associated with pain and stress behavior [51,52]. The portable device (Pain Gauge®, PHIS Inc., Dublin, OH, USA) converts electrical signals measured on the dry principal pad of the right thoracic limb to numerical values ranging from 0.1 (lowest value of stress and pain) to 9.9. Measurements of EDA were recorded in triplicate and averaged.

Pain Scales

A VAS was used as a linear intensity pain scale with words that convey "no pain" (0-value) up to "worst pain" (100-value). The observer placed a mark along the line indicating the dog's estimated pain intensity.

The composite 4A-VET pain scale recently tested by our group [48] was used again. It is composed of two sections. The first focuses on behavioral expressions of pain (4A-VETbeh) consisting of the "Global subjective appreciation", "General attitude" and "Interactive behavior" subscales (Appendix S2). The second (4A-VETleg) includes orthopedic components of pain with "Gait evaluation", "Reaction to handling of the surgical wound" and "Intensity of this reaction" subscales (Appendix S2). Each subscale scored pain intensity from 0 (no pain) to 3 (worst pain) and therefore, the total 4A-VET pain scale intensity ranged from 0 (no pain) to 18 (worst pain). Pain evaluation using the 4A-VET pain scale was performed in three successive and standardized phases: an initial, undisturbed observation of the dog, an interactive period of handling and encouragement and finally, a phase of systematic palpation of the incision and surrounding area of the operated leg.

Statistical Analyses

The numbers and times of required rescue analgesia were described for each group. The data are reported as the median plus the 75th percentile, unless otherwise specified.

The intra-observer reliabilities of the pain scales and repeatability of EDA were calculated based on the –96 h and –5 h evaluations using a weighted Cohen's kappa coefficient and Spearman's rank correlations [53]. The inter-observer reliabilities of the video-recording spontaneous behavior assessment were calculated based on the 10% random set of spontaneous behavior changes using an intraclass correlation coefficient tested on log-transformed (to fulfill homoscedasticity and Wilk-Shapiro test normality requirements) data [54]. The internal consistency of the 4A-VET pain scale was assessed using a Cronbach's alpha coefficient [55].

Pain assessment scores were modeled over time using GEE for repeated measures [56,57]. Data distribution was assessed and followed a negative binomial distribution (video analysis of spontaneous behavior), a Poisson distribution (VAS and 4A-VET pain scores and EDA measures) and a multinomial distribution (4A-VETbeh and 4A-VETleg scores). Model adequacy was verified using a thorough residual analysis [58]. For the negative binomial model, pairwise differences of mean estimates were expressed using estimated risk ratios along with a 95% confidence interval. To adjust for the multiple comparison tests performed, an adjusted-alpha level was set using the Bonferroni correction (original alpha-value divided by the number of comparisons of interest): 0.0041 for the video analysis of spontaneous behaviors (0.05/12), and 0.0015 for the EDA measurements and the pain scores (0.05/33).

To test the concurrent validity, multivariate GEE logistic regression models were used to assess the ability of each filmed spontaneous behavior to predict the pain scales scores. In addition, the regression models tested the following covariates: time, age, body weight and the use of rescue analgesia. The statistical significance of the above predictor variables and all of their possible dual interactions was tested with a stepwise-forward algorithm, using a threshold of $p = 0.15$ for including these factors in the multivariate model and a threshold of $p = 0.20$ for their removal [59]. A thorough residual analysis was performed for each model. The predictor variables showing clear non-linear relationships with the response variables were mathematically transformed to improve regression fit. Each final model was selected based on the best scatter of residuals over the regression line, coefficient of determination (R^2) and quasi-likelihood information criterion [60]. The robust standard errors were calculated for all GEE estimates [61]. All analyses were conducted using a statistical software program (SAS system, version 9.2, SAS Institute Inc.); all tests were two-sided with an α threshold of 0.05.

Supporting Information

Appendix S1 Ethogram of dog behaviors used for pain assessment. **Spontaneous behaviors** were defined collegially by Pascale Rialland, Daphnée Veilleux-Lemieux, Diane Frank, Dominique Gauvin, and Eric Troncy. Behaviors were categorized using operational definitions. Categories were mutually exclusive and consisted of "Location in the kennel", "Body position",

"Facial expression", "Motor activity", "Tail position", and "Self-care". The corresponding definitions are presented in the Appendix, as well as the Modifiers applicable to the different categories.

Appendix S2 The 4A-VET pain scale. The VETerinary Association for Animal Anesthesia and Analgesia (4A-VET) launched a composite multifactorial post-operative pain scale for dogs the 01/01/01. Originally created by Drs Patrick Verwaerde, Eric Troncy, Marc Gogny and Christophe Desbois, the 4A-VET pain scale had content validation by a panel of experts (Moens, Y.; Deschamps, J.-Y.; Cuvelliez, S.G., and Coppens, P.). The canine 4A-VET post-operative pain scale is composed of two sections. The first focuses on behavioral expressions of pain (4A-VETbeh) consisting of the "Global subjective appreciation", "General attitude" and "Interactive behavior" subscales. The second (4A-VETleg) includes orthopedic components of pain with "Gait evaluation", "Reaction to handling of the surgical wound" and "Intensity of this reaction" subscales. Each subscale scores pain intensity from 0 (no pain) to 3 (worst pain) and therefore, the total 4A-VET pain scale intensity ranged from 0 (no pain) to 18 (worst pain).

Acknowledgments

The authors thank Dr. Guy Beauchamp for his assistance in statistical analysis.

Author Contributions

Conceived and designed the experiments: PR SA DF ET. Performed the experiments: SA DVL ET. Analyzed the data: PR MG JdC DF ET. Contributed reagents/materials/analysis tools: PR SA DG ET. Wrote the paper: PR SA DVL DF ET. Contributed to statistical analysis: MG JdC DG. Critical review of the manuscript: MG JdC DG.

References

1. Brennan TJ, Zahn PK, Pogatzki-Zahn EM (2005) Mechanisms of Incisional Pain. Anesthesiol Clin 23: 1–20.
2. Xu J, Brennan TJ (2009) Comparison of skin incision vs. skin plus deep tissue incision on ongoing pain and spontaneous activity in dorsal horn neurons. Pain 144: 329–339.
3. Buvanendran A, Kroin JS, Kari MR, Tuman KJ (2008) A new knee surgery model in rats to evaluate functional measures of postoperative pain. Anesth Analg 107: 300–308.
4. Budsberg SC, Torres BT, Zwijnenberg RJ, Eppler CM, Clark JD, et al. (2011) Effect of perzinfotel and a proprietary phospholipase A2 inhibitor on kinetic gait and subjective lameness scores in dogs with sodium urate-induced synovitis. Am J Vet Res 72: 757–763.
5. Punke JP, Speas AL, Reynolds LR, Claxton RF, Budsberg SC (2007) Kinetic gait and subjective analysis of the effects of a tachykinin receptor antagonist in dogs with sodium urate-induced synovitis. Am J Vet Res 68: 704–708.
6. Schumacher H, Phelps P, Agudelo C (1974) Urate crystal induced inflammation in dog joints: sequence of synovial changes. J Rheumatol 1: 102–113.
7. Quessy SN (2010) The Challenges of Translational Research for Analgesics: The State of Knowledge Needs Upgrading and Some Uncomfortable Deficiencies Remain to be Urgently Addressed. J Pain 11: 698–700.
8. Liska WD, Doyle ND (2009) Canine Total Knee Replacement: Surgical Technique and One-Year Outcome. Vet Surg 38: 568–582.
9. Mann KA, Miller MA, Khorasani M, Townsend KL, Allen MJ (2012) The dog as a preclinical model to evaluate interface morphology and micro-motion in cemented total knee replacement. Vet Comp Orthop Traumatol 25: 1–10.
10. Ji Z, Ma Y, Li W, Li X, Zhao G, et al. (2012) The Healing Process of Intracorporeally and In Situ Devitalized Distal Femur by Microwave in a Dog Model and Its Mechanical Properties in vitro. PLoS One 7: e30505.
11. Holton L, Pawson P, Nolan A, Reid J, Scott EM (2001) Development of a behaviour-based scale to measure acute pain in dogs. Vet Rec 148: 525–531.
12. Laboissière B (2006) Statistical validation of 4A-VET'S postoperative pain scale in dogs and cats [Thesis]. Nantes: École Nationale Vétérinaire de Nantes. 229 p.

13. Reid J, Nolan AM, Hughes JML, Lascelles D, Pawson P, et al. (2007) Development of the short-form Glasgow composite measure pain scale (CMPS-SF) and derivation of an analgesic intervention score. Animal Welfare 16: 97–104.
14. Väisänen MAM, Tuomikoski-Alin SK, Brodbelt DC, Vainio OM (2008) Opinions of Finnish small animal owners about surgery and pain management in small animals. J Small Anim Pract 49: 626–632.
15. Hugonnard M, Leblond A, Keroack S, Cadore JL, Troncy E (2004) Attitudes and concerns of French veterinarians towards pain and analgesia in dogs and cats. Vet Anaesth Analg 31: 154–163.
16. Williams VM, Lascelles BD, Robson MC (2005) Current attitudes to, and use of, peri-operative analgesia in dogs and cats by veterinarians in New Zealand. N Z Vet J 53: 193–202.
17. Zimmermann M (1983) Ethical guidelines for investigations of experimental pain in conscious animals. Pain 16: 109–110.
18. Cohen LL, La Greca AM, Blount RL, Kazak AE, Holmbeck GN, et al. (2008) Introduction to Special Issue: Evidence-based Assessment in Pediatric Psychology. J Pediatr Psychol 33: 911–915.
19. Gruet P, Seewald W, King JN (2011) Evaluation of subcutaneous and oral administration of robenacoxib and meloxicam for the treatment of acute pain and inflammation associated with orthopedic surgery in dogs. Am J Vet Res 72: 184–193.
20. Lafuente MP, Franch J, Durall I, Diaz-Bertrana MC, Marquez RM (2005) Comparison between meloxicam and transdermally administered fentanyl for treatment of postoperative pain in dogs undergoing osteotomy of the tibia and fibula and placement of a uniplanar external distraction device. J Am vet Med Assoc 227: 1768–1774.
21. Hazewinkel HA, van den Brom WE, Theijse LF, Pollmeier M, Hanson PD (2003) Reduced dosage of ketoprofen for the short-term and long-term treatment of joint pain in dogs. Vet Rec 152: 11–14.

22. Borer LR, Peel JE, Seewald W, Schawalder P, Spreng DE (2003) Effect of carprofen, etodolac, meloxicam, or butorphanol in dogs with induced acute synovitis. Am J Vet Res 64: 1429–1437.

23. Lipscomb VJ, Pead MJ, Muir P, AliAbadi FS, Lees P (2002) Clinical efficacy and pharmacokinetics of carprofen in the treatment of dogs with osteoarthritis. Vet Rec 150: 684–689.

24. Hazewinkel HAW, van den Brom WE, Theyse LFH, Pollmeier M, Hanson PD (2008) Comparison of the effects of firocoxib, carprofen and vedaprofen in a sodium urate crystal induced synovitis model of arthritis in dogs. Res Vet Sci 84: 74–79.

25. Horstman CL, Conzemius MG, Evans R, Gordon WJ (2004) Assessing the Efficacy of Perioperative Oral Carprofen after Cranial Cruciate Surgery Using Noninvasive, Objective Pressure Platform Gait Analysis. Vet Surg 33: 286–292.

26. Waxman AS, Robinson DA, Evans RB, Hulse DA, Innes JF, et al. (2008) Relationship Between Objective and Subjective Assessment of Limb Function in Normal Dogs with an Experimentally Induced Lameness. Vet Surg 37: 241–246.

27. Quinn MM, Keuler NS, Maria YL, Faria LE, Muir P, et al. (2007) Evaluation of Agreement Between Numerical Rating Scales, Visual Analogue Scoring Scales, and Force Plate Gait Analysis in Dogs. Vet Surg 36: 360–367.

28. Oosterlinck M, Bosmans T, Gasthuys F, Polis I, Van Ryssen B, et al. (2011) Accuracy of pressure plate kinetic asymmetry indices and their correlation with visual gait assessment scores in lame and nonlame dogs. Am J Vet Res 72: 820–825.

29. Melzack R, Wall P (1965) Pain mechanisms: a new theory. Science 150: 971–979.

30. Roughan JV, Flecknell PA (2006) Training in behaviour-based post-operative pain scoring in rats - an evaluation based on improved recognition of analgesic requirements. Appl Anim Behav Sci 96: 327–342.

31. Langford DJ, Bailey AL, Chanda ML, Clarke SE, Drummond TE, et al. (2010) Coding of facial expressions of pain in the laboratory mouse. Nat Methods 7: 447–449.

32. Fox SM, Mellor DJ, Stafford KJ, Lowoko CRO, Hodge H (2000) The effects of ovariohysterectomy plus different combinations of halothane anaesthesia and butorphanol analgesia on behaviour in the bitch. Res Vet Sci 68: 265–274.

33. Kyles AE, Hardie EM, Hansen BD, Papich MG (1998) Comparison of transdermal fentanyl and intramuscular oxymorphone on post-operative behaviour after ovariohysterectomy in dogs. Res Vet Sci 65: 245–251.

34. Landis JR, Koch GG (1977) The Measurement of Observer Agreement for Categorical Data. Biometrics 33: 159–174.

35. Hoelzler MG, Millis DL, Francis DA, Weigel JP (2004) Results of arthroscopic versus open arthrotomy for surgical management of cranial cruciate ligament deficiency in dogs. Vet Surg 33: 146–153.

36. Firth AM, Haldane SL (1999) Development of a scale to evaluate postoperative pain in dogs. J Am Vet Med Assoc 214: 651–659.

37. Hansen BD (2003) Assessment of pain in dogs: veterinary clinical studies. ILAR J 44: 197–205.

38. Dzikiti TB, Joubert KE, Venter LJ, Dzikiti LN (2006) Comparison of morphine and carprofen administered alone or in combination for analgesia in dogs undergoing ovariohysterectomy. J S Afr Vet Assoc 77: 120–126.

39. Moreau M, Rialland P, Pelletier JP, Martel-Pelletier J, Lajeunesse D, et al. (2011) Tiludronate treatment improves structural changes and symptoms of osteoarthritis in the canine anterior cruciate ligament model. Arthritis Research & Therapy. 13: R98.

40. Guedes AG, Papich MG, Rude EP, Rider MA (2007) Pharmacokinetics and physiological effects of two intravenous infusion rates of morphine in conscious dogs. J Vet Pharmacol Ther 30: 224–233.

41. Valtolina C, Robben JH, Uilenreef J, Murrell JC, CJohn B, et al. (2009) Clinical evaluation of the efficacy and safety of a constant rate infusion of dexmedetomidine for postoperative pain management in dogs. Vet Anaesth Analg 36: 369–383.

42. Vettorato E, Zonca A, Isola M, Villa R, Gallo M, et al. (2010) Pharmacokinetics and efficacy of intravenous and extradural tramadol in dogs. Vet J 183: 310–315.

43. Richardson CA, Niel L, Leach MC, Flecknell PA (2007) Evaluation of the efficacy of a novel electronic pain assessment device, the Pain Gauge, for measuring postoperative pain in rats. Lab Anim 41: 46–54.

44. Shih AC, Robertson S, Isaza N, Pablo L, Davies W (2008) Comparison between analgesic effects of buprenorphine, carprofen, and buprenorphine with carprofen for canine ovariohysterectomy. Vet Anaesth Analg 35: 69–79.

45. Marucio RL, Luna SPL, Neto FJT, Minto BW, Hatschbach E (2008) Postoperative analgesic effects of epidural administration of neostigmine alone or in combination with morphine in ovariohysterectomized dogs. Am J Vet Res 69: 854–860.

46. Kona-Boun JJ, Cuvelliez S, Troncy E (2006) Evaluation of epidural administration of morphine or morphine and bupivacaine for postoperative analgesia after premedication with an opioid analgesic and orthopedic surgery in dogs. J Am Vet Med Assoc 229: 1103–1112.

47. Pacharinsak C, Greene SA, Keegan RD, Kalivas PW (2003) Postoperative analgesia in dogs receiving extradural morphine plus medetomidine. J Vet Pharmacol Ther 26: 71–77.

48. Guillot M, Rialland P, Nadeau MÈ, del Castillo JRE, Gauvin D, et al. (2011) Pain induced by a minor medical procedure (bone marrow aspiration) in dogs: comparison of pain scales in a pilot study. J Vet Intern Med 25: 1050–1056.

49. Hadjistavropoulos T, Craig KD (2002) A theoretical framework for understanding self-report and observational measures of pain: a communications model. Behav Res Ther 40: 551–570.

50. Kilkenny C, Browne W, Cuthill IC, Emerson M, Altman DG (2010) Animal research: Reporting in vivo experiments: The ARRIVE guidelines. B J Pharmacol 160: 1577–1579.

51. Critchley HD (2002) Electrodermal Responses: What Happens in the Brain. Neuroscientist 8: 132–142.

52. Storm H (2008) Changes in skin conductance as a tool to monitor nociceptive stimulation and pain. Curr Opin Anaesthesiol 21: 796–804.

53. Brennan P, Silman A (1992) Statistical methods for assessing observer variability in clinical measures. BMJ 304: 1491–1494.

54. Berk RA (1979) Generalizability of behavioral observations: a clarification of interobserver agreement and interobserver reliability. Am J Ment Defic 83: 460–472.

55. Streiner DL, Norman GR (2003) Health measurement scales: a practical guide to their development and use; Streiner DL, Norman GR, editors. New York: Oxford University Press. 283 p.

56. Liang KY, Zeger SL (1986) Longitudinal data analysis using generalized linear models. Biometrika 73: 13–22.

57. Ziegler A, Kastner C, Blettner M (1998) The Generalised Estimating Equations: An Annotated Bibliography. Biom J 40: 115–139.

58. Stokes ME, Davis CS, Koch GG (2000) Categorical data analysis using the SAS system; Wiley, editor. Cary, N.C: SAS Publishing Inc. 634 p.

59. Hosmer D, Lemeshow S (1989) Applied Logistic Regression. New York: Wiley. 307 p.

60. Pan W (2001) Akaike's information criterion in generalized estimating equations. Biometrics 57: 120–115.

61. Hanley JA, Negassa A, Edwardes MDd, Forrester JE (2003) Statistical Analysis of Correlated Data Using Generalized Estimating Equations: An Orientation. Am J Epidemiol 157: 364–375.

4

Effectiveness of Biosecurity Measures in Preventing Badger Visits to Farm Buildings

Johanna Judge[1]*, **Robbie A. McDonald**[1,2], **Neil Walker**[1], **Richard J. Delahay**[1]

1 The Food & Environment Research Agency, Sand Hutton, York, Yorkshire, United Kingdom, **2** Environment and Sustainability Institute, University of Exeter, Cornwall Campus, Penryn, Cornwall, United Kingdom

Abstract

Background: Bovine tuberculosis caused by *Mycobacterium bovis* is a serious and economically important disease of cattle. Badgers have been implicated in the transmission and maintenance of the disease in the UK since the 1970s. Recent studies have provided substantial evidence of widespread and frequent visits by badgers to farm buildings during which there is the potential for close direct contact with cattle and contamination of cattle feed.

Methodology: Here we evaluated the effectiveness of simple exclusion measures in improving farm biosecurity and preventing badger visits to farm buildings. In the first phase of the study, 32 farms were surveyed using motion-triggered infrared cameras on potential entrances to farm buildings to determine the background level of badger visits experienced by each farm. In the second phase, they were divided into four treatment groups; "Control", "Feed Storage", "Cattle Housing" and "Both", whereby no exclusion measures were installed, exclusion measures were installed on feed storage areas only, cattle housing only or both feed storage and cattle housing, respectively. Badger exclusion measures included sheet metal gates, adjustable metal panels for gates, sheet metal fencing, feed bins and electric fencing. Cameras were deployed for at least 365 nights in each phase on each farm.

Results: Badger visits to farm buildings occurred on 19 of the 32 farms in phase one. In phase two, the simple exclusion measures were 100% effective in preventing badger entry into farm buildings, as long as they were appropriately deployed. Furthermore, the installation of exclusion measures also reduced the level of badger visits to the rest of the farmyard. The findings of the present study clearly demonstrate how relatively simple practical measures can substantially reduce the likelihood of badger visits to buildings and reduce some of the potential for contact and disease transmission between badgers and cattle.

Editor: Justin David Brown, University of Georgia, United States of America

Funding: This work was funded by Defra project number SE3119, http://www.defra.gov.uk/. The funders had no role in study design, data collection and analysis, decision to publish, or preparation of the manuscript.

Competing Interests: The authors have declared that no competing interests exist.

* E-mail: johanna.judge@fera.gsi.gov.uk

Introduction

Agricultural buildings may be attractive to wildlife for a variety of reasons. They can provide shelter, particularly during the winter to escape harsh temperatures [1]. Foraging opportunities arise from the availability of stored livestock feed and harvested crops, particularly for rodents which in turn may attract predators [2,3]. In addition to the potential for costly losses of stored feed and crops, wildlife activity may also increase the risk of spreading pathogens of agricultural and zoonotic importance such as *Brucella*, *Trichinella* [4], *Mycobacterium avium paratuberculosis* [5] and *Cryptosporidium* [6]. Disease risks may arise as a result of direct contact between wildlife and livestock or contamination by wildlife of buildings, equipment and feed. For example, it has been estimated that individual cattle or sheep could come into contact with 1626 and 814 rodent or bird droppings respectively in stored feed over one winter [7]. Developing simple methods of excluding wildlife from farm buildings may therefore be a useful tool in the mitigation of disease transmission risk between livestock and wild hosts.

The Eurasian badger (*Meles meles*) is the principal wildlife reservoir of *Mycobacterium bovis* (the causative agent of bovine tuberculosis infection) in the UK and Ireland [8,9]. The failure to eradicate bovine tuberculosis (TB) from cattle in these countries is hampered by the transmission of infection between badgers and cattle. Infectious badgers can excrete *M. bovis* bacilli in faeces, urine, sputum and exudate from wounds and abscesses [10]. Contact with badgers or their excretions may therefore present opportunities for the infection of cattle [11,12].

The principal route by which infection is transmitted from badgers to cattle is not clear. From the few studies that have been conducted, direct contact between badgers and grazing cattle appears relatively infrequent [13,14]. In contrast, several studies have demonstrated contamination of pasture with badger faeces and urine [12,13,15–17], and subsequent calculations suggest potentially significant risks of exposure to cattle [18]. More recent research suggests that the potential for disease transmission to cattle as a result of badger activity in farm buildings may also be substantial. Several studies have now demonstrated that badger visits to farm buildings are frequent and widespread in the southwest of England [19-23]. During these visits badgers have been observed foraging on stored feed, invertebrates and vertebrate prey, collecting bedding, and coming to within 2m of housed cattle [19,21,24]. Observations of badgers defecating, urinating and grooming in buildings, sometimes in direct contact with cattle feed, provide evidence of the potential for indirect transmission of *M. bovis* via contamination of this environment [19,21,24].

Numerous studies have been conducted to investigate methods of reducing contact between wildlife and livestock on pasture, with varying degrees of success. For example fitting electric shock collars to wolves, which were activated when the wolves came within a certain distance of the protected area [25] and using acoustic frightening devices to deter coyotes [26] in order to reduce predation on sheep, ultrasonic devices and water jets to deter badgers [27], lasers to disperse deer [28,29] and electric fencing to keep deer [30] and badgers [31] out of crop fields. However, to date, little research has been aimed specifically at keeping wildlife out of farm buildings, although a notable exception was the localised evaluation of the use of electric fencing to reduce badger visits [32].

Here we describe the results of an experimental study to investigate the effectiveness of a range of simple exclusion measures on the level and frequency of badger visits to farm yards and buildings. The aims were to determine (i) if simple exclusion measures deter badger visits to farmyards and buildings and (ii) if exclusion measures cause displacement of badger activity to unprotected buildings.

Methods

Study farm selection

The study was undertaken in Gloucestershire, a county of southwest England with a high incidence of bovine TB in cattle. Potential study farms that had not been the subject of badger culling during the Randomised Badger Culling Trial (RBCT) from 1998 to 2005 inclusive (Bourne et al. 2007), and which were under annual TB testing of their cattle herds, were randomly selected from VETNET (The UK Department for the Environment, Food and Rural Affairs (Defra) bovine TB control and surveillance database). From this sample, we selected 32 farms with a herd size of at least 30 animals, which were kept indoors for at least part of the year, and where concentrates or cereal feed (e.g. cake, grain, barley, sugar beet) were stored on site but separately from housed cattle.

Experimental design

The experiment consisted of two phases, both lasting at least 365 days on each farm. During an initial surveillance phase (between 1st February 2007 and 31st August 2008) we established the background frequency of badger visits to all farms. During the second phase (between 1st February 2008 and 31st August 2009) we investigated the effect on badger visits of installing exclusion measures on farm buildings. For logistical reasons surveillance was initiated on different dates on individual farms, and consequently the periods of surveillance on each farm were not simultaneous.

Clearly we could only measure the effects of exclusion measures on farms where badgers were found to visit. Hence, while all 32 farms were monitored in both the first and second phases of the experiment, only those which experienced badger visits during the first background surveillance phase are included in the statistical analyses described below.

Surveillance

Infra-red, motion-triggered, digital still cameras (Leaf River IR3-BU, Vibrashine Inc., Taylorsville MS, USA; Stealth Cam

1430IR, Stealth Cam LLC, Grand Prairie TX, USA and Game Spy I40, Moultrie Feeders, Alabaster AL, USA) were deployed at potential badger access points to cattle sheds, feed stores, and silage clamps on all study farms. The positioning of cameras was constrained by the need to avoid them being damaged by livestock or machinery during normal farm working practices. Between four and thirteen cameras were deployed on each farm, depending on the size and the number of buildings and potential entrance points for badgers. The cameras were operational nightly throughout both phases of the experiment.

Memory cards, with at least 1Gb of storage capacity and batteries were replaced every two weeks. Images were downloaded from retrieved memory cards and all observations of badgers and other wildlife were catalogued using Extensis Portfolio 8 software (Extensis, Portland OR, USA). The date, time, farm ID, individual camera identity, type of building (feed store, silage clamp or cattle housing), and species observed was recorded for each observation. During phase 2, if an image clearly showed the exclusion measure was not in use, or otherwise allowed badger access (e.g. was damaged), on particular nights, this was also recorded. Images documenting badger visits were also allocated to one of two categories. Where a badger was clearly evident either entering or already inside a building, the observation was classified as a 'building visit', but where it was neither inside nor entering a building this was deemed a 'farmyard visit'.

Badger exclusion measures

In order to investigate the effects of installing badger exclusion measures on farm buildings, the study employed a factorial design (Table 1). Each farm was allocated to one of four experimental treatments where farms had: no exclusion measures, measures to reduce visits to cattle housing and associated feed troughs only, measures to reduce visits to feed stores (including silage clamps) only or measures to reduce visits to cattle housing (including feed troughs), and feed stores (including silage clamps). These treatments were each replicated eight times (n = 32 farms). Treatment was allocated to each farm towards the end of the initial surveillance phase, using a randomised complete block design to ensure an even distribution of farms with respect to the frequency of badger visits in phase 1 across the four treatment groups.

The badger exclusion measures were individually tailored to fit the requirements of each farm and sought to secure every potential entrance point on each selected facility. The five main exclusion measures used were galvanised aluminium sheeted metal gates, adjustable galvanised aluminium sheeted panels (which could be moved up or down) on gates, galvanised aluminium sheeted fencing, aluminium feed bins and electric fencing (Figure 1). A full list of measures employed on each farm is given in Table S1. Other measures installed on some farms included sheeted gates

Table 1. The factorial design of the study, showing the exclusion measure combinations by treatment.

	Treatment			
	Control	Cattle Housing	Feed Stores	Both
Measures on:				
Cattle Housing	No	Yes	No	Yes
Feed Stores	No	No	Yes	Yes

with hinged flaps, roller doors, metal sheets attached to angled feed troughs and sheeted wheeled barriers. Gates and fences were constructed and fitted so that the gap between the bottom and the ground was less than approximately 7.5cm as this was considered to be sufficiently low to prevent badger access. Gates with two or three adjustable solid panels that could be raised or lowered were employed on uneven ground and deep litter.

Electric fencing (either fixed or retractable) was installed on farms where permanent gates or panels were not suitable, such as on very uneven ground or in areas where farm machinery access would have been compromised. The area beneath fixed-position electric fences over rough ground was sprayed with herbicide to retard vegetation growth which could otherwise cause the fence to short-circuit. Retractable electric fences were installed on silage clamps and across farmyards that were too wide for conventional gates and required frequent farm machinery access. The electric fence strands were held on self-tensioning reel systems, fixed to an insulated rod, which could be pulled across gaps of up to 20 metres. The height of the bottom three strands of fencing were 10, 15 and 20 cm above the ground as specified in designs that have been demonstrated to effectively exclude badgers [31,32]. A fourth non-electrified strand was placed at a height of approximately 122cm to increase the visibility of the fence as a safety measure to prevent farm workers accidentally driving through, or tripping over, the lower strands.

During the fortnightly building surveys, any observed damage to badger exclusion measures was recorded. In addition, details of whether the measures were maintained *in situ* by farmers were also recorded from the images taken during camera trapping where possible. Although this study was not designed to quantify the extent to which exclusion measures were employed and maintained by farmers, we attempted to gain some insights by calculating the number of nights that any measure was observed (from digital images) to be in use as a percentage of the total number of nights when the camera was activated. A conservative approach was employed, whereby all digital images from nights when multiple images suggested that measures were only adequately employed for part of the night were excluded. In addition, as we would expect more wildlife visits to take place (and therefore to be recorded in digital images) when exclusion

measures were not adequately employed, we also excluded all images which contained wildlife. Hence, all remaining images were likely to have been triggered by non-wildlife events (e.g. wind-blown leaves) which are likely to have taken place independently of whether exclusion measures were correctly employed. This approach yielded a minimum estimate of the number of nights when exclusion measures were not adequately employed because we were unable to determine if the measures had been in use on those nights when cameras were not triggered.

Statistical Analyses

Camera level analyses. In order to assess the effect of fitting exclusion measures on buildings, images from each camera were examined for evidence of badger visits. Each observation in this analysis represented whether or not a badger visit was observed by a given camera on a given night (a camera-night). If a camera was known not to have been working on specific nights, those nights for that camera were omitted from the analyses.

Variations in the binary variable "building visit" (1 = 1 or more visits observed on a given camera night and 0 = no visits observed on a given camera night) were related to potential explanatory variables using a Generalised Linear Mixed Model (GLMM; GenStat for Windows, Version 13, VSN International, Hemel Hempstead, UK). Factors affecting the probability of a building visit were modelled with a binomial distribution using a logit-link transformation [33]. Fixed effect explanatory variables were season (spring = March to May, summer = June to August, autumn = September to November and winter = December to February inclusive), experimental phase (1 = pre-treatment phase, 2 = treatment phase) and building type (cattle housing or feed store). The model included all observations from phase 1 and phase 2 in order to allow for within-farm and year-to-year variation to be accounted for. A further explanatory variable was treatment status, which described whether any exclusion measures were in place on the entire farm (i.e. either no exclusion measures were present, measures were in place on the building covered by that camera, or they were in place somewhere else on the farm). For the purposes of these analyses, all exclusion measures were considered to be in place on the relevant buildings on all nights in phase 2 of the experiment. However, in reality there were nights

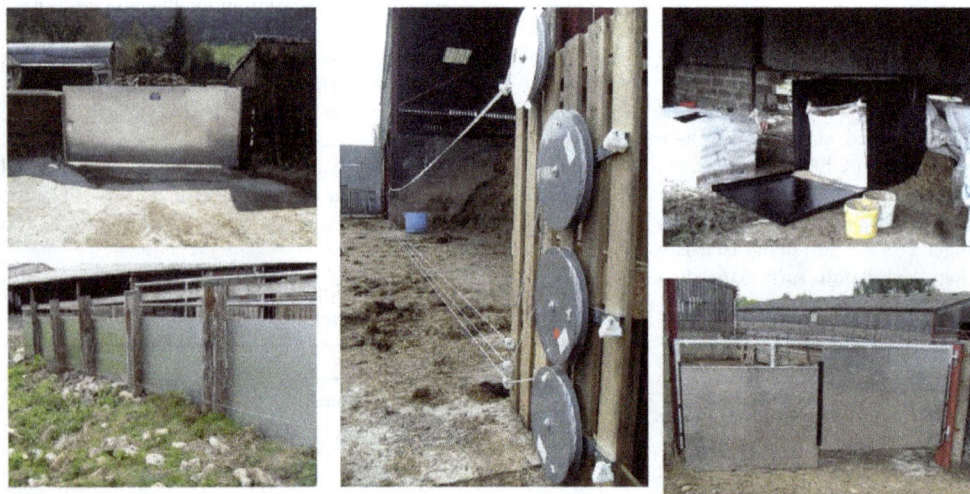

Figure 1. Examples of badger exclusion measures: solid aluminium sheeted gate (top left), aluminium sheeting installed on rail fence (bottom left), retractable electric fencing (middle), front and top opening aluminium feed bin (top right) and rail gate with adjustable galvanised aluminium panels (bottom right).

where the installed measures had not been used or were not properly maintained which may, therefore, have allowed badger access. Categorical variables representing individual farms and cameras were incorporated as random effects in the model to account for potential correlation between observations recorded from the same source. Wald tests (using chi-squared statistics) were used to make inference on the main variables and Z-tests were used to make inference on comparisons between different levels of a given variable. Statistical significance was inferred when the associated p-value was less than 5%.

Farm level analyses. In order to investigate sources of variation in the likelihood of treatments affecting badger visits to any part of a single farmyard (whether to a specific building or elsewhere), data were aggregated across all cameras for each farm-night. Hence each binary observation in this analysis comprised of a record indicating whether there was photographic evidence of any badgers visiting a given farm on a given night (1) or not (0).

A similar GLMM approach was used to relate variation in the likelihood of a badger visit on any given farm-night to the series of explanatory variables as described above. In order to examine whether there was any displacement of badger activity from protected to unprotected buildings in the farmyard, the effect of treatment status on badger visits was examined at two levels, which were tested independently. First, we tested the effect on badger visits of whether the farm had any exclusion measures in place (regardless of location), compared to where no exclusion measures were in place. Second, the difference in badger visits between the three levels of exclusion treatment (i.e. on feed stores, cattle sheds or both) was investigated. The $\log_e$ of the number of active cameras was included as a fixed effect covariate as this was analogous to sampling effort and might influence the chance of a positive observation. A term for the individual farm was included as a random effect. All significance-testing was carried out as described above except for post-hoc tests between the different treatments, which were based on chi-squared statistics.

Results

In phase one (i.e. with no exclusion measures in place on any farms) badger visits occurred on 19 of the 32 farms and on between 0.3% and 71% of the total number of surveillance nights on each farm (Figure 2). Overall, feed storage areas received more than double the number of visits to cattle housing (Table S2). Badger visits to farms occurred throughout the year, but frequency varied significantly with month (GLMM, d.f. = 11, $\chi^2 = 142.8$, p<0.001). The highest numbers of nights with recorded badger visits were in April, May and June and the lowest in December and January.

The installation of simple exclusion measures on farm buildings significantly reduced levels of badger visits compared to buildings with no protection installed (GLMM, Z = -8.3, p<0.001). Over the two phases, the percentage of nights with incursions into feed stores reduced from 11.2% when no exclusion measures were installed to 0.5% when exclusion measures were installed; for cattle housing the percentage of incursions reduced from 3.5% to 1.2% (Figure S1). With exclusion measures installed there was a highly significant reduction in the frequency of visits to all types of facility, though the reduction in entry to feed stores was greater than in cattle housing (Table 2).

During phase two of the experiment there were only 58 recorded entries into buildings which had exclusion measures installed. All of these incursions could be attributed either to the measure not being adequately employed (7 occasions) or maintained (51 occasions). This latter category also included

occasions when badger access was possible through damage to other areas of the buildings which had not been repaired. Badger incursions into farm buildings were completely eliminated when exclusion measures were in place and were adequately maintained.

The frequency of badger visits to farms as a whole (both incursions into buildings and observations anywhere in the farmyard) declined significantly when exclusion measures were installed anywhere on a farm (Table 3). Furthermore, the presence of exclusion measures on both feed stores and cattle housing resulted in a significantly greater protective effect, compared to where they were present on only one type of building (Table 3).

The installation of exclusion measures on some buildings also resulted in a significant reduction in recorded incursions into unprotected buildings on the same farm (GLMM, Z = −6.1, p<0.001). Incursions into buildings on farms with no measures installed occurred on 2.6% of all nights surveyed whereas incursions into unprotected buildings on farms with measures installed elsewhere on the farm occurred on 2.1% of nights. (Figure S1). While the number of visits to unprotected buildings was significantly reduced by installing measures on either feed stores or cattle housing, the reduction in visits to cattle housing when measures were only installed on feed stores was greater than *vice versa*.

The percentage of nights when exclusion measures were adequately employed and maintained varied considerably among farms (from 12% to 98%). However, over half the farms with measures installed (13/24) employed them on over 60% of nights (Figure 3). The results of a simple linear regression indicated that there was no relationship between the frequency of badger visits to a farm in the first phase of the study and the level of farmer compliance during the second ($F_{1,22} = 2.2$, p = 0.2).

Discussion

This study provides the clearest evidence to date that, in this region, badger visits to farm buildings are a common occurrence. Intensive surveillance over a full year demonstrated that badgers visited buildings at least occasionally on 19 of 32 (59%) farms in our sample. On 3 of the 32 farms (approximately 1 in 10), visits were very frequent, occurring on more than 60% of nights. Badgers visited feed stores and cattle housing, with visits to feed stores being more frequent. While badger visits to farmyards occurred all year round, they peaked in late spring/early summer.

Badgers were successfully excluded from farm buildings with the use of relatively simple, practical exclusion measures. These measures were 100% effective in preventing badger entry into farm buildings when properly used and maintained, such that the only recorded incursions occurred when measures were not employed adequately. Furthermore, the installation of exclusion measures not only stopped entry into buildings but also reduced the level of badger visits to the farmyard as a whole.

The reduction in visits to the farmyard which accompanied protection of one building type (i.e. just feed stores or just cattle housing) was most evident when feed stores were protected. This apparent 'deterrent effect', was also observed by Tolhurst et al.[32], who found that the use of electric fencing around feed stores resulted in a reduction in visits to unfenced facilities on the same farms. Tolhurst et al. also radio-tracked the badgers using these farms and demonstrated that excluded badgers simply exploited other food sources within their pre-existing territories, suggesting that farm-derived food may not be vital for the local badger population, at least not in the short term. This hypothesis may be further supported by our finding that installation of

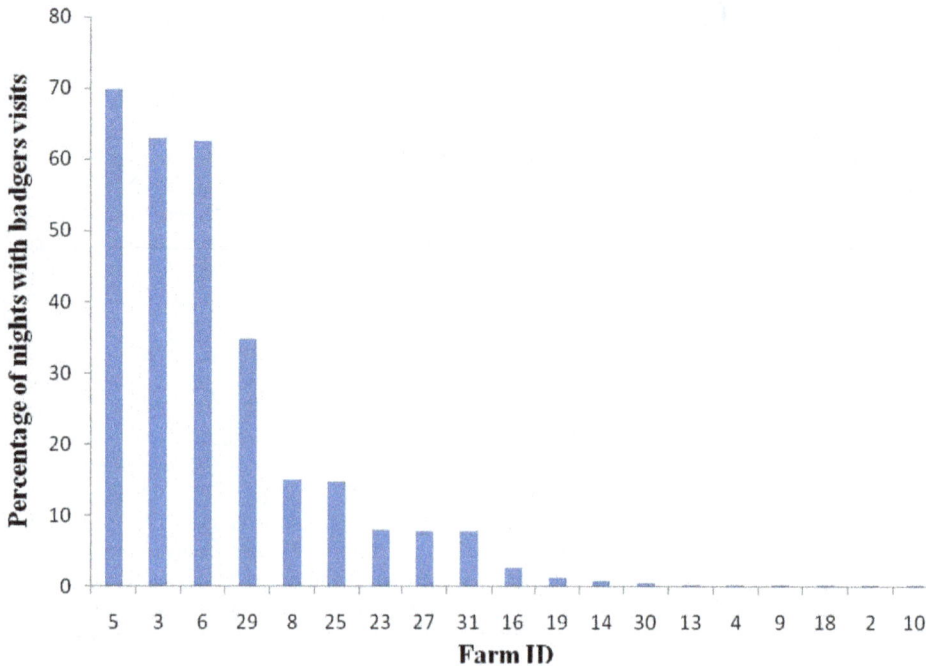

Figure 2. Percentage of nights on which badger visits to farmyards and farm buildings were observed during surveillance phase 1. Observations were made prior to any exclusion measures being installed on study farms.

Table 2. Results of a GLMM to identify factors associated with variations in the number of nights with badger entry into buildings.

Variable	Level	Number of nights with badger visits/Number of nights surveyed (%)	factors		levels	
			beta	Chi-square (df)	Z-statistic (1 df)	p-value
Season				156.4 (3)		<0.001
	spring	546/4048 (13.5%)	0			
	summer	346/4075 (8.5%)	−0.74		−8.6	<0.001
	autumn	240/3458 (6.9%)	−0.96		−10.1	<0.001
	winter	213/3425 (6.2%)	−0.95		−9.8	<0.001
Phase	1	738/7111 (10.4%)	0			
	2	607/7895 (7.7%)	+0.51		4.5	<0.001
Treatment status on night of observation						
	Treatment vs. No Treatment		−2.02		−8.3	<0.001
	Difference between three treatments			39.8 (2)		<0.001
	Individual treatment effects					
	No treatment	1066/9238 (11.54%)	0			
	CH	175/1699 (10.30%)	−1.34		−7.7	<0.001
	FS	70/2421 (2.89%)	−2.62		−13.3	<0.001
	B	34/1648 (2.06%)	−2.02		−8.3	<0.001
	post-hoc comparisons					
	FS vs. CH		−1.28	32.4 (1)		<0.001
	FS vs. B		−0.60	7.6 (1)		0.01
	CH vs. B		+0.68	10.5 (1)		0.001

CH = Cattle Housing, FS = Feed Store, B = Both building types, C = Control.

Table 3. Results of a GLMM to identify factors associated with variations in the number of nights with any badger visits, including both incursions into buildings and observations of badgers within the farmyard (but not entering buildings).

variable	level	Number of nights with badger visits/ Number of nights surveyed (%)	factors		levels	
			beta	Chi-square (df)	Z-statistic (1 df)	p-value
Season				184.7 (3)		<0.001
	Spring	759/4048 (18.75%)	0			
	Summer	583/4075 (14.31%)	−0.51		−7.0	<0.001
	Autumn	414/3458 (11.97%)	−0.73		−9.1	<0.001
	Winter	299/3425 (8.73%)	−1.09		−12.8	<0.001
Phase						
	1	1095/7111 (15.4%)	0			
	2	960/7895 (12.2%)	+0.54		4.9	<0.001
Treatment status on night of observation						
	Treatment vs. No Treatment		−2.28		−12.4	<0.001
	Difference between three treatments			31.6 (2)		<0.001
	Individual treatment effects					
	No treatment	1465/9238 (15.9%)	0			
	CH	239/1699 (14.17%)	−1.60		−10.0	<0.001
	FS	240/2421 (9.9%)	−1.25		−8.0	<0.001
	B	111/1648 (6.7%)	−2.28		−12.4	<0.001
	post-hoc comparisons					
	FS vs. CH		+0.35	3.1 (1)		0.1
	FS vs. B		+1.02	27.6 (1)		<0.001
	CH vs. B		+0.68	12.2 (1)		<0.001

CH = Cattle Housing, FS = Feed Store, B = Both building types, C = Control.

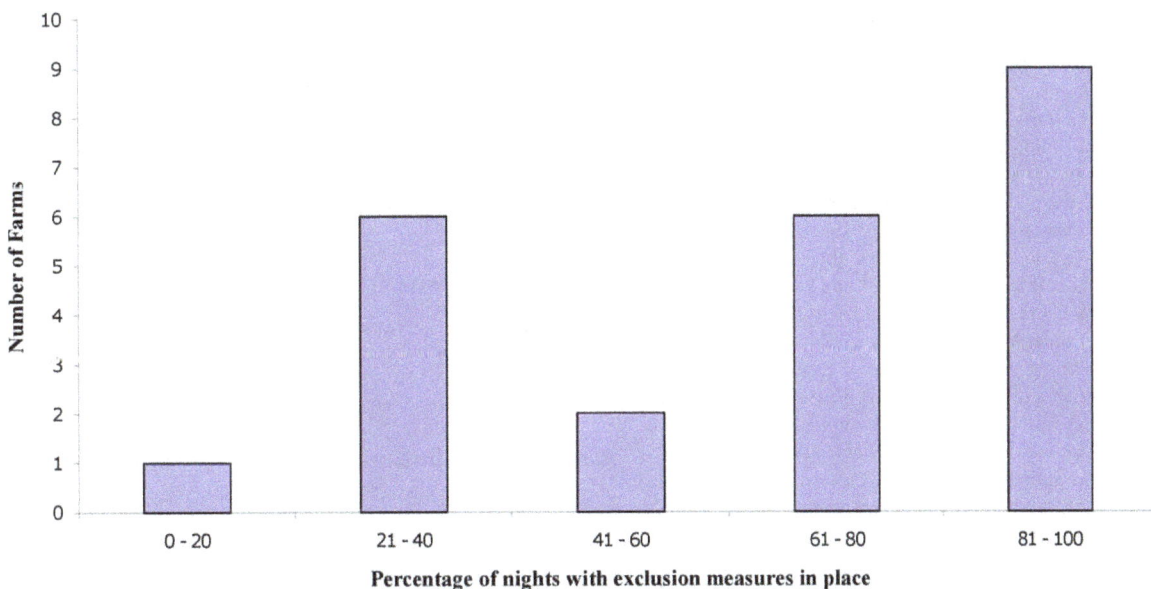

Figure 3. Frequency distribution showing the percentage of surveillance nights on which exclusion measures were observed to be adequately employed. This includes permanent, non-moveable measures, which will always be observed to be in use unless damaged.

exclusion measures reduced the overall level of visits to the farmyard, indicating that when cattle feed is not readily accessible badgers may spend more time in other areas of their territories rather than persistently attempting to gain access to farm-derived feed. If farms were an essential source of food it would be expected that badgers would increase their attempts to gain access to stored feed or, alternatively, that their attentions would turn from protected to unprotected buildings, but neither phenomenon was observed here.

From the camera trap images it was possible to determine that badgers were only able to enter buildings that had exclusion measures installed when the measures were not adequately employed. For example, when gates were left open, when adjustable panels/flaps were not lowered sufficiently or when a new potential entrance point appeared in the building and was not repaired. On average, farmers only used badger exclusion measures that were installed on their farms on approximately 59% of nights, while electric fencing was only used on 48% of nights. On one farm, the retractable electric fencing was only used on 7% of nights. One farmer completely removed some gates that had been installed and on two other farms, walls were almost completely destroyed by cattle or machinery but were not rebuilt, thus negating the exclusion measures that had been installed.

Previous studies have found that farmers rarely employ measures to reduce direct and indirect contact opportunities between badgers and livestock [23,34]. In the present study exclusion measures were purchased and installed at no cost to the farmer, and yet the extent to which they were adequately employed varied widely, with some farmers diligently using measures almost every night, and others deploying them only rarely. This variation was not related to the background level of badger activity observed during the first phase of our study, even though farmers had been made aware that badgers were visiting their buildings. Measures that required adjustments to existing working practices (e.g. pulling retractable electric fences across, closing feed bin lids, dropping flaps on gates or shutting a gate that was previously not operational) were less likely to be used consistently, as were those that required maintenance (e.g. retractable or fixed electric fencing). Solid metal gates that were installed where gates had previously been situated were used most consistently.

The size and design of farmyards and buildings varies widely, so whilst a suite of badger exclusion measures are available, the number, distribution and nature of their deployment will differ among farms. The uniqueness of each farm also makes it impossible to quote a standard cost for the implementation of badger exclusion measures. For the farms in our study in 2008 the costs of installing exclusion measures ranged from approximately £600 to £12500, with an average cost for their purchase and installation on both cattle housing and feed stores of £3840 per farm. However, this figure should be used with caution as it is derived from a small sample size (n = 8) and costs will vary widely amongst farms depending on their individual characteristics. By comparison, the average cost of a cattle herd breakdown (CHB) in 2010/11 was estimated at £30,000 [35]. Unfortunately, it is not currently possible to conduct a cost-benefit analysis for the installation of badger biosecurity measures as we have no data on the contribution of such measures towards reducing risk of TB in cattle. Due to the relatively small sample size and short duration of the study described here, even if all breakdowns were prevented solely by the use of exclusion measures, there would be insufficient statistical power to detect any significant effect on cattle disease incidence. Nevertheless, intuitively, reducing the potential for direct or indirect contact between badgers and cattle should reduce the risk of disease transmission between the two species.

Conclusions

Wildlife populations can be a source of infectious diseases of importance to livestock. Where opportunities for transmission arise because of direct or indirect contact in well-defined areas then management of disease risks by using physical barriers may be a practical option. This study clearly demonstrates how relatively simple practical measures can substantially reduce the likelihood of badger visits to buildings. Given the opportunities that visits to farm facilities may present for the transmission of *M. bovis* between badgers and cattle, these measures could potentially have an important role to play in reducing the incidence of TB in cattle. However, we observed wide variation in the extent to which exclusion measures were employed by farmers. In addition, the frequency of badger visits amongst farms varied independently of the presence of exclusion measures, suggesting that badgers are more attracted to some farms than to others and hence that the potential benefits of exclusion measures will also vary. Consequently, the identification of factors that might determine the likelihood of badger visits to farm premises would be a useful aid to individual farmers in making decisions about whether to spend their time and money on installing and maintaining badger exclusion measures.

Supporting Information

Figure S1 The percentage of total surveillance nights over both phases when badger incursions into buildings were recorded with (■) and without (■) exclusion measures in place.

Table S1 Description of exclusion measures installed on each farm.

Table S2 The number of nights when badgers visited the farm (but not necessarily entering farm buildings), entered cattle housing or entered feed stores in both phases. Values in brackets are percentage of nights surveyed with badger visits.

Acknowledgments

We wish to thank the farmers involved in the study for their kind cooperation. We also thank the members of the Woodchester Park field team who carried out survey and monitoring work, in particular Ian Vernon, Carol Christie, Clare Wigmore, Tim Glover and Phil Court.

Author Contributions

Conceived and designed the experiments: JJ RJD NW. Performed the experiments: JJ. Analyzed the data: NW. Wrote the paper: JJ RJD RM.

References

1. Glueck TF, Clark WR, Andrews RD (1988) Racoon movement and habitat use during the fur harvest season. Wildlife Society Bulletin 16(1): 6–11.

2. Birks JDS (1998) Secondary rodenticide poisoning risk arising from winter farmyard use by the European polecat *Mustela putorius*. Biological conservation 85: 233–240.

3. Tolhurst BA, Ward AI, Delahay RJ. A study of fox (*Vulpes vulpes*) visits to farm buildings and the implications for disease management. European Journal of Wildlife Research, (in press).

4. Gortázar C, Ferroglio E, Höfle U, Frölich K, Vicente J (2007) Diseases shared between wildlife and livestock: a European perspective. European Journal of Wildlife Research 5: 241–256.

5. Greig A, Stevenson K, Perez V, Pirie AA, Grant JM, et al. (1997) Paratuberculosis in wild rabbits (*Oryctolagus cuniculus*). Veterinary Record 140: 141–143.

6. Webster JP, Macdonald DW (1995) Parasites of wild brown rats (*Rattus norvegicus*) on UK farms. Parasitology 111: 247–255.

7. Daniels MJ, Hutchings MR, Grieg A (2003) the risk of disease transmission to livestock posed by contamination of farm stored feed by wildlife excreta. Epidemiology and Infection 130: 561–568.

8. Bourne FJ, Donnelly C, Cox D, Gettinby G, McInerney J, et al. (2007) Bovine TB: The Scientific Evidence, A Science Base for a Sustainable Policy to Control TB in Cattle, An Epidemiological Investigation into Bovine Tuberculosis. Final Report of the Independent Scientific Group on Cattle TB. London: Department for Environment, Food and Rural Affairs.

9. Griffin JM, Williams DH, Kelly GE, Clegg TA, O'Boyle IO, et al. (2005) The impact of badger removal on the control of tuberculosis in cattle herds in Ireland. Preventive Veterinary Medicine 67: 237–266.

10. Clifton-Hadley RS, Wilesmith JW, Stuart FA (1993) *Mycobacterium bovis* in the European badger (*Meles meles*): epidemiological findings in tuberculous badgers from a naturally infected population. Epidemiology and Infection 111: 9–19.

11. Muirhead RH, Gallagher J, Burn KJ (1974) Tuberculosis in wild badgers in Gloucestershire: Epidemiology. Veterinary Record 95: 552–555.

12. MAFF (1979) Bovine tuberculosis in badgers. Third report by the Ministry of Agriculture, Fisheries and Food. London: MAFF.

13. Benham PFJ, Broom DM (1989) Interactions between cattle and badgers at pasture with reference to bovine tuberculosis transmission. British Veterinary Journal 145: 226–241.

14. Böhm M, Hutchings MR, White PCL (2009) Contact networks in a wildlife-livestock host community: identifying high-risk individuals in the transmission of bovine TB among badgers and cattle. PLoS ONE 4(4): e5016. doi:10.1371/journal.pone.0005016.

15. Benham PFJ (1985) a study of cattle and badger behaviour and farm husbandry practices relevant to the transmission of bovine tuberculosis (Mycobacterium bovis). Report to MAFF Chief Scientist's Group (1982-1985).

16. Cheeseman CL, Mallinson PJ (1981) Behaviour of badgers (*Meles meles*) infected with bovine tuberculosis. Journal of Zoology 194: 284–289.

17. Hutchings MR, Harris S (1997) Effects of farm management practices on cattle behaviour and the potential for transmission of bovine tuberculosis from badgers to cattle. The Veterinary Journal 153: 149–162.

18. Hutchings MR, Harris S (1999) Quantifying the risks of TB infection to cattle posed by badger excreta. Epidemiology and Infection 122: 167–174.

19. Garnett BT, Delahay RJ, Roper TJ (2002) Use of cattle farm resources by badgers (*Meles meles*) and risk of bovine tuberculosis (*Mycobacterium bovis*) transmission to cattle. Proceedings of the Royal Society 269B: 1487–1491.

20. Garnett BT, Roper TJ, Delahay RJ (2003) Use of cattle troughs by badgers (*Meles meles*) a potential route for the transmission of bovine tuberculosis (*Mycobacterium bovis*) to cattle. Applied Animal Behaviour Science 80: 1–8.

21. Tolhurst BA (2006) Behaviour of badgers (*Meles meles*) in farm buildings, in relation to the transmission of bovine tuberculosis (*Mycobacterium bovis*) between badgers and cattle. Unpublished PhD Thesis. University of Sussex.

22. Tolhurst BA, Delahay RJ, Walker NJ, Ward AI, Roper TJ (2009) Behaviour of badgers (*Meles meles*) in farm buildings: Opportunities for transmission of *Mycobacterium bovis* to cattle. Applied Animals Behavioural Science 117: 103–113.

23. Ward AI, Tolhurst BA, Walker NJ, Roper TJ, Delahay RJ (2008) Survey of badger access to farm buildings and facilities in relation to contact with cattle. Veterinary Record 163: 107–111.

24. Roper TJ, Garnett BT, Delahay RJ (2003) Visits to farm buildings and cattle troughs by badgers (*Meles meles*): a potential route for transmission of bovine tuberculosis (*Mycobacterium bovis*) between badgers and cattle. Cattle Practice 11: 9–12.

25. Gehring TM, Hawley JE, Davidson SJ, Rossler ST, Cellar AC, et al. (2006) Are viable non-lethal management tools available for reducing wolf–human conflict? Preliminary results from field experiments. In: Timm RM, O'Brien JM, eds. Proceedings of the 22nd Vertebrate Pest Conference. California: University of California: Davis. pp 2–6.

26. VerCauteren KC, Lavelle MJ, Moyles S (2003) Coyote-activated frightening devices for reducing sheep predation on open range. Proceedings of Wildlife Damage Management 10: 146–151.

27. Ward AI, Pietravalle S, Cowan DP, Delahay RJ (2008) Deterrent or dinner bell? Alteration of badger activity and feeding at baited plots using ultrasonic and water jet devices. Applied Animal Behaviour Science 115: 221–232.

28. VerCauteren KC, Gilsdorf JM, Hygnstrom SE, Fioranelli PB, Wilson JA, et al. (2003) Green and Blue Lasers are Ineffective for Dispersing Deer at Night. Wildlife Society Bulletin 34(2): 371–374.

29. VerCauteren KC, Hygnstrom SE, Pipas MJ, Fioranelli PB, Werner SJ, et al. (2006) Red Lasers Are Ineffective for Dispersing Deer at Night. Wildlife Society Bulletin 34(2): 371–374.

30. Seamans TW, VerCauteren KC (2006) Evaluation of ElectroBraid™ Fencing as a White-Tailed Deer Barrier. Wildlife Society Bulletin 34(1): 8–15.

31. Poole DW, McKillop IG, Western G, Hancocks PJ, Packer JJ (2002) Effectiveness of an electric fence to reduce badger (*Meles meles*) damage to field crops. Crop Protection 21: 409–417.

32. Tolhurst BA, Ward AI, Delahay RJ, MacMaster AM, Roper TJ (2008) The behavioural responses of badgers (*Meles meles*) to exclusion from farm buildings using an electric fence. Applied Animal Behavioural Science 113(1-3): 224–235.

33. Collett D (2002) Modelling Binary Data (2nd Edition). London: Chapman & Hall.

34. Bennett R, Cooke R (2005) Control of bovine TB: preferences of farmers who have suffered a TB breakdown. Veterinary Record 156: 143–145.

35. Defra (2011) Bovine TB eradication programme for England. Available: http://www.defra.gov.uk/publications/files/pb13601-bovinetb-eradication-programme-110719.pdf..

5

Development and Validation of Real-Time PCR for Rapid Detection of *Mecistocirrus digitatus*

Subhra Subhadra, Mohanraj Karthik, Muthusamy Raman*

Department of Veterinary Parasitology, Madras Veterinary College, Tamil Nadu Veterinary and Animal Sciences University, Chennai, Tamil Nadu, India

Abstract

Hematophagous activity of *Mecistocirrus digitatus*, which causes substantial blood and weight loss in large ruminants, is an emerging challenge due to the economic loss it brings to the livestock industry. Infected animals are treated with anthelmintic drugs, based on the identification of helminth species and the severity of infection; however, traditional methods such as microscopic identification and the counting of eggs for diagnosis and determination of level of infection are laborious, cumbersome and unreliable. To facilitate the detection of this parasite, a SYBR green-based real-time PCR was standardized and validated for the detection of *M. digitatus* infection in cattle and buffaloes. Oligonucleotides were designed to amplify partial Internal Transcribed Spacer (ITS)-1 sequence of *M. digitatus*. The specificity of the primers was confirmed by non-amplification of DNA extracted from other commonly occurring gastrointestinal nematodes in ruminants. Plasmids were ligated with partial ITS-1 sequence of *M. digitatus*, serially diluted (hundred fold) and used as standards in the real-time PCR assay. The quantification cycle (Cq) values were plotted against the standard DNA concentration to produce a standard curve. The assay was sensitive enough to detect one plasmid containing the *M. digitatus* DNA. Clinical application of this assay was validated by testing the DNA extracted from the faeces of naturally infected cattle (n = 40) and buffaloes (n = 25). The results were compared with our standard curve to calculate the quantity of *M. digitatus* in each faecal sample. The Cq value of the assay depicted a strong linear relationship with faecal DNA content, with a regression coefficient of 0.984 and efficiency of 99%. This assay has noteworthy advantages over the conventional methods of diagnosis because it is more specific, sensitive and reliable.

Editor: Justin David Brown, University of Georgia, United States of America

Funding: The work was supported by TANUVAS funding (http://www.tanuvas.tn.nic.in/). The funders had no role in study design, data collection and analysis, decision to publish, or preparation of the manuscript.

Competing Interests: The authors have declared that no competing interests exist.

* E-mail: raman@tanuvas.org.in

Introduction

Sub-clinical parasitism due to gastrointestinal nematodes (GINs) is a major problem in ruminant livestock because it leads to huge financial losses. Among the GINs affecting large ruminants, *Mecistocirrus digitatus*, commonly known as a large stomach worm, is a bloodsucking helminth found in the abomasum of Asian zebu cattle (*Bos indicus*) and buffalo (*Bubalis bubalis*) [1]. In the abomasum of infected animals, this nematode is reported to cause severe micro- and macroscopic lesions such as mucosal inflammation, haemorrhage, ulcers and necrosis [2]. Occurrence of *M. digitatus* was recorded as early as the 1920s, from the abomasum of cattle in India [3,4]. Various studies have confirmed the presence of *M. digitatus* infection in cattle and buffaloes in different parts of India [5,6,7,8]. *M. digitatus* may be found in mixed infection in ruminants along with other GINs such as *Ostertagia ostertagi*, *Trichostrongylus spp.*, *Haemonchus placei*, *Cooperia spp.*, etc., which makes the eradication of GINs a difficult task using chemotherapeutic agents [9]. In spite of the studies on the biology [10] and geographical distribution of this parasite [11,12,13], there is a dearth of information on detection and control strategies. Furthermore, the longer pre-patent period (up to 60 days) of this bloodsucking GIN [14] affects early detection.

The diagnosis of this bloodsucking nematode is done by identification of eggs in the faeces of infected animals and infective L3 larvae after coproculture. Given the fact that the average length of *M. digitatus* egg (95–122 µm) [10,11] is either the same as or slightly larger than other trichostrongylid nematode eggs, the conventional morphometric and microscopic examination fails to differentiate between trichostrongyle eggs. This problem calls for a more sensitive and reliable assay to provide information on the preponderance and relative abundance of this nematode. Molecular techniques are extensively used for sensitive and specific detection of common GINs, including *M. digitatus* [15,16,17,18]. In 2002, Samson-Himmestjerna *et al.* [19] developed the TaqMan based qPCR assay to detect and quantify common GINs such as *Haemonchus contortus*, *Ostertagia leptospicularis*, *Trichostrongylus colubriformis* and *Cooperia curticei* based on ITS-2 sequence of ribosomal DNA (rDNA). Later, Bott *et al.* [20] developed a SYBR green-based real-time assay for the detection of strongylids such as *H. contortus*, *Teladorsagia circumcincta*, *Trichostrongylus spp.*, *Cooperia oncophora*, *Oesophagostomum columbianum* and *Oesophagostomum venulosum*. More recently, during 2009, the TaqMan based real-time assay was developed and validated for the detection of *H. contortus* and *T. circumcincta* [21]. The aim of the present study was to standardize a SYBR green-based real-time PCR for the detection and quantification of *M. digitatus* infection and validate the assay in naturally infected large ruminants such as non-descript cattle (NDC), cross-bred jersey cattle (CBJC), cross-bred Holstein

Friesian cattle (CBHFC), non-descript buffaloes (NDB) and graded Murrah buffaloes (GMB).

Materials and Methods

Ethics Statement

Permission was obtained from the chief health officer of Chennai Corporation to collect adult worms from the abomasum of cattle (NDC, CBJC and CBHFC) and buffaloes (NDB and GMB) for research purpose at the corporation's slaughter house in Perambur. The collection of faecal samples for this work was conducted in accordance with the guidelines and approval of the Institutional Animal Ethical Committee of the Tamil Nadu Veterinary and Animal Sciences University in Chennai, India (approval#318/DFBS/IAEC/2010).

Extraction of gDNA from Adult *M. digitatus* Worms

Adult *M. digitatus* worms (n = 25) were collected from the abomasum of cattle (n = 15) and buffaloes (n = 10) at the Chennai Corporation slaughter house in Perambur. The worms were individually identified, on the basis of copulatory bursa and spicules, by light microscopy [5] and the keys provided by Whitlock (1960) [22]. The DNA was extracted, as described by Sambrook and Russell (2001) [23], with minor modifications. The purified DNA was eluted with TE buffer and stored at $-20°C$ until being used as a positive control.

Extraction of gDNA from Faecal Samples

Faecal samples (n = 65) were collected, i.e., 40 samples from cattle (NDC-23 samples, CBJC-7 samples and CBHFC-10 samples) and 25 samples from buffaloes (NDB-18 samples and GMB-7 samples) showing symptoms of diarrhoea from villages across the districts of Chennai, Tanjore, Tiruchirappalli, Thiruvarur, Ernakulam, Vijayawada, Nellore, Nagapattinam and Kodaikanal in Southern India. The faecal samples were transported under cold condition to the laboratory. The DNA was extracted by using QIAmp stool DNA kit (Qiagen, Germany) as per the manufacturer's protocol. The PCR inhibitors present in the faecal samples were removed by the use of InhibitEX tablet provided in the kit in order to increase the sensitivity of the subsequent PCR assays. The purified DNA was stored in TE buffer at –20°C till use.

Primer Design

A pair of oligonucleotides was designed to amplify part of the ITS-1 region of *M. digitatus* rDNA. The forward and reverse primers were chosen manually from sequences available in NCBI, GenBank (GenBank AB222059.1). The primers are MD ITSF (5′-TCACTTTGATTACGAGAATCCAACAG) and MD ITSR (5′-GTCTAAATCTCAACTATCATTAAACGTGA).

Standardization of Conventional PCR

The purified *M. digitatus* gDNA was subjected to gradient PCR (55–65°C), using Taq DNA polymerase 2X Master Mix Red (containing 0.2 units/µl Ampliqon Taq DNA polymerase, 0.4 mM dNTPs and 3.0 mM MgCl$_2$) (Ampliqon, Bie & Berntsen, Herlev, Denmark) and 10 picomole of each forward and reverse primer (Eurofins MWG Operon, Germany). PCR cycling conditions were as follows: one cycle of initial denaturation at 94°C for 5 minutes; followed by 40 cycles of (94°C, 55–65°C and 72°C for 30 seconds each) followed by final extension step of 72°C for 10 minutes. No-template control (NTC) and negative amplification control (NAC) were also included with each run. The specificity of the primers was checked with DNA extracted

from eight other nematodes viz., *H. contortus*, *Trichostrongylus spp.*, *O. ostertagi*, *Oesophagostomum radiatum*, *Cooperia spp.*, *Nematodirus spp.*, *Bunostomum spp.* and *Trichuris spp.*, which are prevalent in this geographical location. The PCR product was electrophoresed through 2% agarose gel to check for positive PCR amplification.

Purification, Cloning and Sequencing of PCR Product

The desired PCR product was purified using QIAQuick PCR purification kit (Qiagen, Hilden, Germany). The purified product was ligated into plasmid (pTZ57R/T) and transferred into *E. coli* DH5α cells using InsTAclone PCR cloning kit (Fermentas, European Union). Plasmid DNA was purified using Fast Plasmid mini-kit (Eppendorf, Germany) and was sequenced on both strands using the Big Dye Terminator v. 1.1 Cycle sequencing kit (Applied Biosystems, Foster City, CA) on a PRISM 3100 Genetic Analyzer.

Standard DNA for Real-time PCR

Recombinant plasmids containing partial ITS-1 sequence of *M. digitatus* were quantified using Biophotometer plus (Eppendorf, Germany) and were used as standards for real-time PCR assay. Serial hundred fold dilutions of the plasmid representing 1.5×10^8 to 1.5×10^{-6} plasmid molecules/µl were made and aliquots of each dilution were stored at $-20°C$.

Standardization of Real-time PCR for Detection of *M. digitatus*

Real-time PCR assay was performed in Bio-Rad CFX-96 real-time PCR machine (Bio-Rad Laboratories, Hercules, CA) and the data generated were analyzed with the CFX Manager^{TM} Software (version 2.0). The assay was carried out in a total reaction volume of 10 µl that consisted of 5.0 µl of 2X SsoAdvanced SYBR green super mix (containing dNTPs, Sso7d fusion polymerase, MgCl$_2$, SYBR green I)(Bio-Rad Laboratories, Hercules, CA), 5.0 pico-moles of each primer (Eurofins MWG Operon, Germany) and 1.0 µl of DNA template. All the samples, including the standards, NTC and NAC, were run in triplicates and all experiments were repeated at least twice. The protocol was as follows: 5 minutes at 95°C, 40 cycles at 95°C for 5 seconds, 58°C for 20 seconds and 72°C for 10 seconds. Amplicons were subjected to melt curve analysis by increasing the temperature from 58°C to 95°C at an increment of 0.5°C per second.

Testing of Faecal Samples Collected from Naturally Infected Cattle and Buffaloes

Triplicates of DNA extracted from faecal samples collected from naturally infected cattle (n = 40) and buffaloes (n = 25) were used to detect and quantify *M. digitatus* infection by standardized real-time PCR assay as described above. The mean Cq values were compared with the standard curve data to calculate the quantity of DNA in each sample.

Results

Standardization of Conventional PCR

Specific amplification of 182 bp was observed with the positive control at 58°C and 1.5 mM MgCl$_2$, while the NTC did not show any amplification. No amplification was observed with DNA extracted from eight other nematode species (Fig. 1). The PCR detected as low as 1.5×10^2 plasmid molecules/µl of DNA (Fig. 2). The newly designed primers were found to be both species specific and sensitive. A BLAST search of the sequence result was carried out to confirm the identity of the sequence, which revealed a 98%

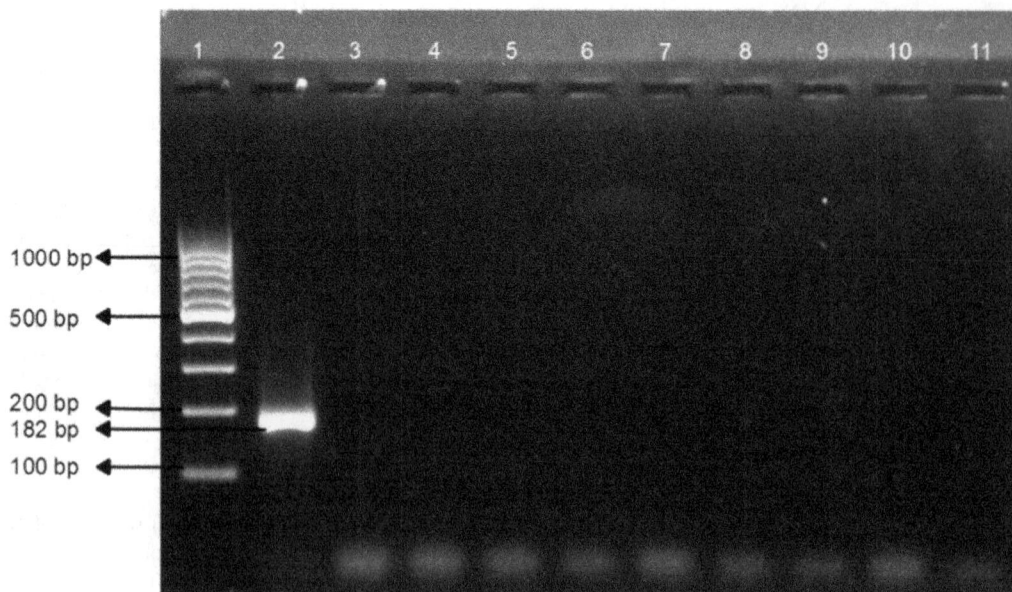

Figure 1. Species-specific PCR for detection of *M. digitatus*. Lane 1:100–1000 bp DNA ladder, Fermentas Lane 2: *Mecistocirrus digitatus* DNA (182 bp) Lane 3: *Haemonchus contortus* DNA Lane 4: *Trichostrongylus spp.* DNA Lane 5: *Ostertagia ostertagi* DNA Lane 6: *Oesophagostomum radiatum* DNA Lane 7: *Cooperia spp.* DNA Lane 8: *Nematodirus spp.* DNA Lane 9: *Trichuris spp.* DNA Lane 10: *Bunostomum spp.* DNA Lane 11: No Template Control.

identity with the existing *M. digitatus* sequences in GenBank, NCBI, thus confirming the identity of the species. The sequence was submitted in the EMBL-EBI database under the accession number HE974385.

Standardization of Real-time PCR for Detection of *M. digitatus*

Standard curves generated by the software were analyzed. A rise in Cq value was associated with a decrease in DNA content, pointing to a strong linear relationship between fluorescence and target copy number. The reaction was highly reproducible over a range of 10^8 to a single copy number of the plasmid DNA, with a correlation coefficient (r^2) of 0.984 and 99.0% efficiency (Fig. 3). No Cq value was observed for NAC and NTC. The assay detected as low as one plasmid molecule/μl of DNA. Amplified products were also subjected to melt curve analysis to confirm the presence of a single PCR product. Neither primer-dimer nor non-specific amplification products were observed on melt curve analysis (Fig. 4) or by gel electrophoresis (results not shown).

Testing of Faecal Samples Collected from Naturally Infected Cattle and Buffaloes

Out of the total 65 samples screened, 41 were found positive for *M. digitatus* by the assay. The positive samples were quantified by the system based on the standard curve generated. The amplification plot for standard and unknown samples is shown in Fig. 5. The quantity of DNA in those samples ranged from 2.387 to 7.70×10^4 molecules/μl (Table S1).

Discussion

To date, there is no study reporting the use of real-time PCR for the detection of *M. digitatus*. Advances in nucleic acid testing offer more efficient and reliable methods like PCR-based assays, which have been used for detecting various parasites that affect livestock

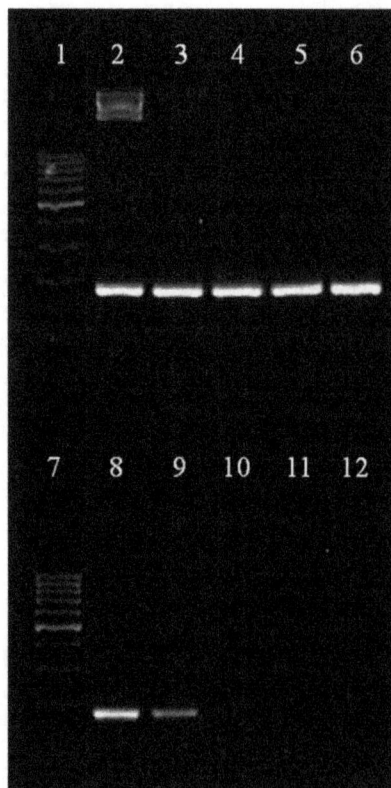

Figure 2. Sensitivity PCR to detect quantity of *M. digitatus* DNA. Lane 1&7:100–1000 bp DNA ladder, Fermentas Lane 2–11: Serial 10 fold dilution of plasmid DNA (1.5×10^8 to 1.5×10^0 molecules/μl) Lane 12: No Template Control.

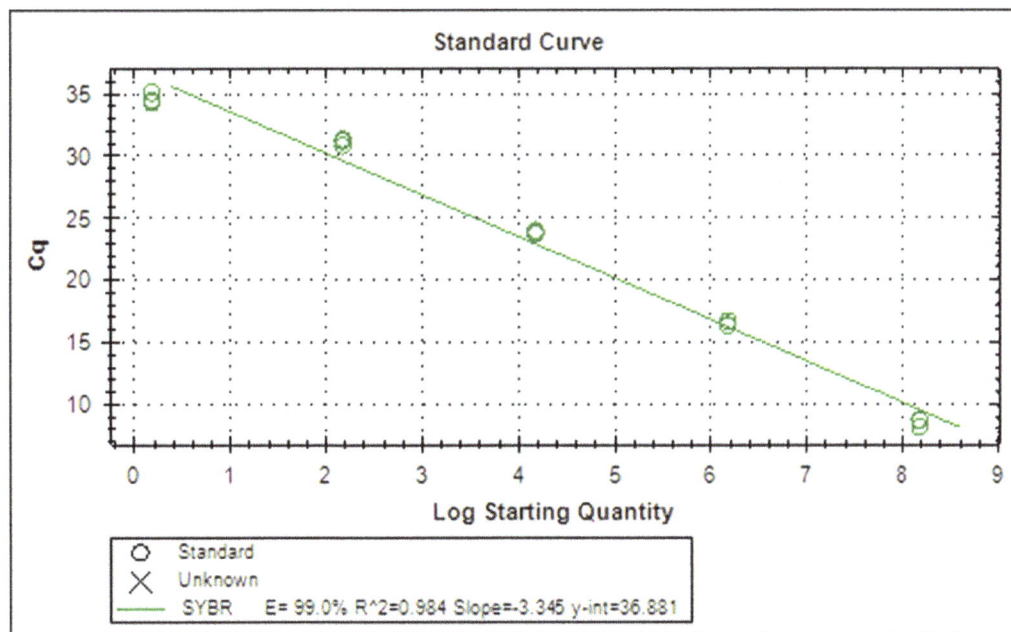

Figure 3. Standard curve of serial 100 fold dilutions of the plasmid representing 1.5×10^8 to 1.5×10^{-6} molecules/µl.

[18,24]. The sequences of ITS-1 and ITS-2 of rDNA have been used extensively as a genetic marker for diagnostic purposes across a diverse range of organisms [19,25,26,27,28]. This study was undertaken to amplify the partial ITS-1 sequence in rDNA of *M. digitatus* using SYBR green as the fluorophore. The 182 bp PCR product was sequenced to confirm *M. digitatus*, and no amplification was observed with DNA from eight closely related species, i.e., *H. contortus*, *Trichostrongylus spp.*, *O. ostertagi*, *Oesophagostomum radiatum*, *Cooperia spp.*, *Nematodirus spp.*, *Bunostomum spp.* and *Trichuris spp.* The conventional PCR detects 150 plasmids, whereas real-time PCR

detects as low as one plasmid. In comparison to conventional PCR, the real-time assay was found to be sensitive and specific. Moreover, an evaluation of our real-time PCR assay using faecal DNA from cattle (n = 40) and buffaloes (n = 25) with naturally acquired trichostrongylid infections showed a significant correlation between Cq values and DNA amounts. In 2009, Learmount *et al.* [21] validated a qPCR assay for diagnosis of sheep nematodes *T. circumcincta* and *H. contortus* by harvesting eggs from the faecal samples. Whereas, in our study, we validated our qPCR assay by using the DNA extracted directly from faeces. The assay was good

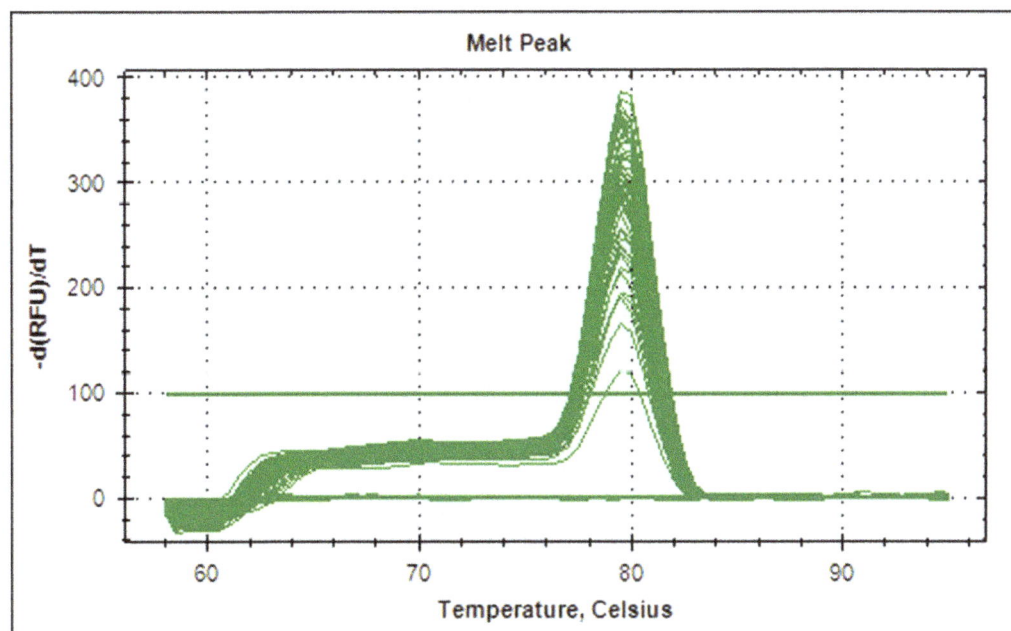

Figure 4. Melt curve analysis of PCR products.

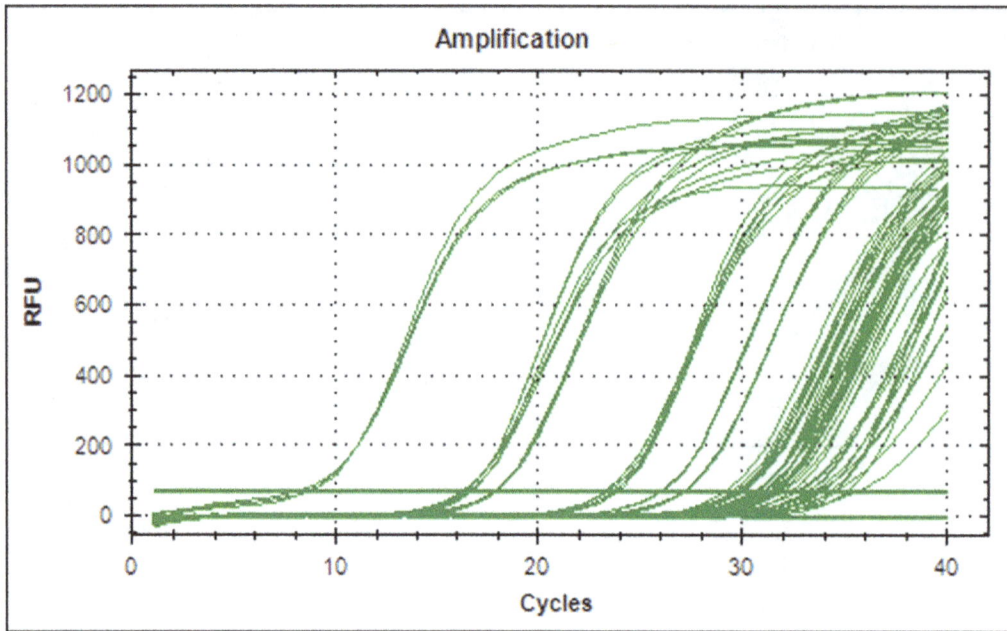

Figure 5. Fluorescence profile for standards and clinical samples used in real-time PCR assay.

enough to produce reproducible results to detect the infection directly from faeces, thus reducing the time (3–5 days) needed for harvesting eggs by coproculture.

Currently, there is limited information available on the status of *M. digitatus* infection and its effect on the growth and reproductive parameters of cattle and buffaloes. This underpins the need for early and specific diagnostic assays. The present quantitative PCR-based assay was found to be specific and sensitive for the detection of *M. digitatus* from faecal samples. However, more such studies are needed in other countries to confirm the present finding. In addition to this, the real-time PCR assay can be used for large-scale epidemiological and population biology based studies [19,29]. In conclusion, the developed qPCR assay will be useful to enhance our understanding on the severity of *M. digitatus* infection in large ruminants which in turn will be helpful in its treatment and control programs.

Supporting Information

Table S1   Validation of qPCR by testing faecal samples collected from cattle and buffaloes. The Cq value and

copies per µl of standard and unknown samples are mean values of the triplicates N/A- Not Applicable; *Tm*- Melting temperature.

Acknowledgments

The authors are grateful to the authorities of the Tamil Nadu Veterinary and Animal Sciences University and the Dean of Madras Veterinary College for the facilities provided. The authors also thank Dr. Arvind Prasad from the Indian Veterinary Research Institute (IVRI) in Bareilly, India, for providing known positive DNA of GINs. The authors are grateful to Dr. Subrat Kumar, Dr. A. Nambi and Siddhartha Tripathy, for their contribution and helpful comments in the preparation of the manuscript.

Author Contributions

Conceived and designed the experiments: SS MK. Performed the experiments: SS MK. Analyzed the data: SS MK. Contributed reagents/materials/analysis tools: MR MK SS. Wrote the paper: SS MK MR.

References

1. Van Aken D, Vercruysse J, Dargantes AP, Lagapa JT, Shaw DJ (1998) Epidemiology of *Mecistocirrus digitatus* and other gastrointestinal nematode infections in cattle in Mindanao, Philippines. Vet Parasitol 74(1): 29–41.
2. Gaur SNS, Dutt SC (1973) Tissue responses to *Mecistocirrus digitatus* infection in cattle. Philipp. J Vet Med 12: 64–68.
3. Baylis HA, Daubney R (1923) A further report on the parasitic nematodes in the collection of the zoological survey of India. Rec Indian Mus 25: 575.
4. Bhalerao GD (1933) The most practical methods of combating parasitic gastritis and fluke infestation of ruminants under faecal conditions in India. Agric Live-stock India 3: 354–360.
5. Bandyopadhyay S (2010) Economic analysis of risk of gastrointestinal parasitic infection in cattle in north eastern states of India. Trop Anim Health Prod 42: 1481–1486.
6. Laha R (2013) Gastrointestinal parasitic infections in organized cattle farms of Meghalaya. Vet world 6(2): 109–112.
7. Sreedhar S, Madan EM, Suresh Babu D (2009) Prevalence of parasitic infections in cattle and buffaloes of Anantapur district of Andhra Pradesh. Indian J Anim Res 43(3): 230–231.
8. Wadhwal A, Tanwar RK, Singla LD, Eda S, Kumar N, et al. (2011) Prevalence of gastrointestinal helminthes in cattle and buffaloes. Vet World 4(9): 417–419.
9. Raman M, Anandan R, Joseph SA (1996) Prevalence of different strongyle larvae in dairy cattle around Madras. Indian J Anim Sci 66(10): 1010–1011.
10. Fernando ST (1965) Morphology, systematics and geographic distribution of *Mecistocirrus digitatus*, a trichostrongylid parasite of ruminants. J Parasitol 51: 149–155.
11. Soulsby EJL (1982) Helminths, Arthropods and Protozoa of Domesticated Animals. Balliere, Tindall and Cassell, London.
12. Abdel-Rahman MS, Hassanian MA, Fahmy MM, Tawfik OM (1991) Nematode worm-burden of cattle in Egypt. Vet Med J Giza 39: 119–128.
13. Ivashkin VM (1947) Characteristics of the biological cycle of the nematode *Mecistocirrus digitatus* (Linstow 1901) a parasite of the abomasum of ruminants. Dokladi Akad. NaukSSR 56 (Translation): 1251–1252.
14. Van Aken D, Vercruysse J, Dargantes AP, Lagapa JT, Raes S, et al. (1997) Pathophysiological aspects of *Mecistocirrus digitatus* (Nematoda: Trichostrongyli-dae) infection in calves. Vet Parasitol 69: 255–26.

15. Hoste H, Gasser RB, Chilton NB, Mallet S, Beveridge I (1993) Lack of intra-specific variation in second internal transcribed spacer (ITS-2) of *Trichostrongylus colubriformis* ribosomal DNA. Int J Parasitol 23: 1069–1071.

16. Stevenson LA, Chilton NB, Gasser RB (1995) Differentiation of *Haemonchus placei* from *H. contortus* (Nematoda: Trichostrongylidae) by the ribosomal DNA second internal transcribed spacer. Int J Parasitol 25: 483–488.

17. Zarlenga DS, Chute MB, Gasbarre LC, Boyd PC (2001) A multiplex PCR assay for differentiating economically important gastrointestinal nematodes of cattle. Vet Parasitol 97: 199–209.

18. Mochizuki R, Endoh D, Onuma M, Fukumoto S, (2005) PCR-based species-specific amplification of ITS of *Mecistocirrus digitatus* and its application in identification of GI nematode eggs in bovine faeces. J Vet Med Sci 68(4): 345–351.

19. Samson-Himmestjerna G, Harder A, Schnieder T (2002) Quantitative analysis of ITS2 sequences in trichostrongyle parasites. Int J Parasitol 32: 1529–1535.

20. Bott NJ, Campbell BE, Beveridge I, Chilton NB, Rees D, et al. (2009) A combined microscopic-molecular method for the diagnosis of strongylid infections in sheep. Int J Parasitol 39: 1277–1287.

21. Learmount J, Conyers C, Hird H, Morgan C, Craig BH, et al. (2009) Development and validation of real-time PCR methods for diagnosis of *Teladorsagia circumcincta* and *Haemonchus contortus* in sheep. Vet Parasitol 166: 268–274.

22. Whitlock JH (1960) Diagnosis of Veterinary Parasitisms. Lea & Febiger Publisher, Philadelphia.

23. Sambrook J, Russell DW (2001) Molecular cloning: a laboratory manual. Third Edition. Cold Spring Harbor Laboratory Press, Cold Spring Harbour, New York.

24. Roeber F, Larsen JW, Anderson N, Campbell AJ, Anderson GA, et al.(2012) A molecular diagnostic tool to replace larval culture in conventional faecal egg count reduction testing in sheep. PLoS One 7(5): e37327.

25. Zarlenga DS, Chute MB, Martin A, Kapel CMO (1999) A multiplex PCR for unequivocal differentiation of all encapsulated and non-encapsulated genotypes of Trichinella. Int J Parasitol 29: 1859–1867.

26. Caldeira RL, Carvalho OS, Mendonca CLFG, Graeff-Teixeira C, Silva MCF, et al. (2003) Molecular differentiation of *Angiostrongylus costaricensis*, *A. cantonensis* and *A. vasorum* by polymerase chain reaction-restriction fragment length polymorphism. Mem Inst Oswaldo Cruz 98: 1039–1043.

27. Marek M, Zouhar M, Rysanek P, Havranek P (2005) Analysis of ITS sequences of nuclear rDNA and development of a PCR-based assay for the rapid identification of the stem nematode *Ditylenchus dipsaci* (Nematoda: Anguinidae) in plant tissues. Helminthologia 42: 49–56.

28. Jefferies R, Morgan ER, Shaw SE (2009) A SYBR green real-time PCR assay for the detection of nematode *Angiostrongylus vasorum* in definitive and intermediate hosts. Vet Parasitol 166: 112–118.

29. Gasser RB, Newton SE (2000) Genomic and genetic research on bursate nematodes: significance, implications and prospects. Int J Parasitol 30: 509–534.

6

Using Informatics and the Electronic Medical Record to Describe Antimicrobial Use in the Clinical Management of Diarrhea Cases at 12 Companion Animal Practices

R. Michele Anholt[1]*, John Berezowski[2], Carl S. Ribble[1,3], Margaret L. Russell[4], Craig Stephen[1,3]

1 Faculty of Veterinary Medicine, University of Calgary, Calgary, Alberta, Canada, 2 Veterinary Public Health Institute, University of Bern, Bern, Switzerland, 3 Centre for Coastal Health, Nanaimo, British Columbia, Canada, 4 Community Health Sciences, University of Calgary, Calgary, Alberta, Canada

Abstract

Antimicrobial drugs may be used to treat diarrheal illness in companion animals. It is important to monitor antimicrobial use to better understand trends and patterns in antimicrobial resistance. There is no monitoring of antimicrobial use in companion animals in Canada. To explore how the use of electronic medical records could contribute to the ongoing, systematic collection of antimicrobial use data in companion animals, anonymized electronic medical records were extracted from 12 participating companion animal practices and warehoused at the University of Calgary. We used the pre-diagnostic, clinical features of diarrhea as the case definition in this study. Using text-mining technologies, cases of diarrhea were described by each of the following variables: diagnostic laboratory tests performed, the etiological diagnosis and antimicrobial therapies. The ability of the text miner to accurately describe the cases for each of the variables was evaluated. It could not reliably classify cases in terms of diagnostic tests or etiological diagnosis; a manual review of a random sample of 500 diarrhea cases determined that 88/500 (17.6%) of the target cases underwent diagnostic testing of which 36/88 (40.9%) had an etiological diagnosis. Text mining, compared to a human reviewer, could accurately identify cases that had been treated with antimicrobials with high sensitivity (92%, 95% confidence interval, 88.1%–95.4%) and specificity (85%, 95% confidence interval, 80.2%–89.1%). Overall, 7400/15,928 (46.5%) of pets presenting with diarrhea were treated with antimicrobials. Some temporal trends and patterns of the antimicrobial use are described. The results from this study suggest that informatics and the electronic medical records could be useful for monitoring trends in antimicrobial use.

Editor: Herman Tse, The University of Hong Kong, Hong Kong

Funding: This research was partially funded by the University of Calgary (www.ucalgary.ca) and The Centre for Coastal Health (www.centreforcoastalhealth.ca). The funders had no role in study design, data collection and analysis, decision to publish, or preparation of the manuscript.

Competing Interests: The authors have declared that no competing interests exist.

* Email: rmanholt@ucalgary.ca

Introduction

Diarrhea is a common clinical presentation in companion animals [1]. The pathophysiology of diarrhea is complex, poorly understood and can involve a wide array of infectious and non-infectious etiologies [2,3]. Clinical evaluation of ill animals directs the selection of diagnostic procedures such as parasite studies, microbiological examinations and/or toxin testing. Clinicians must weigh the cost of diagnostic procedures, the owner's willingness to pay for them and the time spent waiting for a result against the likelihood that the results of a diagnostic test will affect their therapeutic recommendations. This cost-benefit analysis often results in diarrhea in pets being managed by empirical therapy with antihelmintics and antimicrobials [4].

Infectious disease specialists advocate restricting antimicrobial use (AMU) to cases where there is evidence that AMU will result in improved clinical outcomes [3,5,6]. Warnings against indiscriminate AMU in animals are increasing because the consequences of AMU include antimicrobial resistance (AMR) with decreased efficacy of important antimicrobials against significant animal and human pathogens [7,8]. In their closely shared environment, pets may be a source of antimicrobial resistant enteric bacteria or resistance genes for their owners [9–11].

Understanding the clinical management of common veterinary problems and patterns of AMU may provide the necessary exposure information to help interpret AMR trends, identify potential problem areas in prescribing practices and provide evidence-based practice guidelines for practitioners [12–16]. Collecting clinical management and AMU data at the veterinary patient level has not been legislated in Canada and remains a challenge in veterinary medicine in Canada [11,17,18].

The uptake of the electronic medical record (EMR) by companion animal practitioners provides an opportunity for accessing case management and AMU data. Informatics is "the application of information and computer science technology to public health practice, research and learning" [19]. Informatics has been applied elsewhere to text-based clinical records to describe disease-drug associations by physicians [20]. In this paper we used the EMR's from a participating practice network and explored text mining for accessing and analyzing the textual orders for diagnostic testing and AMU in the medical records.

The objectives of this study were to:

1. Apply and evaluate text-mining technology of EMR's to characterize the clinical management of diarrhea cases by companion animal veterinarians in a network of participating veterinary practices.

2. Describe the diagnostic management of diarrhea in companion animals and the proportion of cases for which there was documented evidence of an infectious process.

3. Describe the use of antimicrobials in the management of diarrhea cases.

4. Describe the temporal patterns of the use for each antimicrobial class used in the treatment of diarrhea cases for a 4 year period (January 1, 2007 to December 31, 2010).

Materials and Methods

Study area and data

The study area included 6 communities in the province of Alberta, Canada including: Calgary, Cochrane, Airdrie, Chestermere, Strathmore and Okotoks. A survey of all of the companion animal practices in the study area identified the practices that had completely computerized medical records and the same veterinary practice management software. Twelve of the 20 eligible practices agreed to participate in this project; a sample of convenience. A data sharing agreement was signed by each of the practice's managing partners and the author (Anholt). Approval from the University of Calgary Conjoint Faculties Research Ethics Board did not require permission from the pet owners.

A custom-built data extraction program was used to extract the anonymized electronic medical records (n = 428,783) from the veterinary practice management programs from January 1, 2007 to December 31, 2010. All records were stored in a secure data warehouse at the University of Calgary. The appointment schedule, medical notes (history, clinical exam, interpretations of diagnostic tests, assessment, differential diagnoses, and treatment) and prescription data for each case were combined into one free-text variable named 'Note', in the data file. Data was stored and managed using Microsoft Office Excel 2007 (Microsoft Corporation, Redmond, Washington) and Konstanz Information Miner 2.2.2 (Knime, http://www.knime.org). The features of the participating practices, data extraction and management of the warehoused data have been described elsewhere [21].

Linguistics-based text-mining software (QDAMiner3.1/WordStat6, Provalis Research, Montreal, QC), was used in this study. Text, in the form of individual words or phrases was organized into categorization dictionaries which were used to identify and retrieve cases. A categorization dictionary was applied to the 'Note' variable in the warehoused records to identify and retrieve records that met the case definition of any companion animal species (dog, cat, small mammal, bird, reptile) with clinical diarrhea or a description of feces consistent with diarrhea (n = 18,827 records). The case definition and the development, optimization and validation of the text miner to identify and retrieve records of diarrhea is further described in Anholt et al.[22].

Each of the 18,827 records represented a uniquely identified patient classified as having diarrhea, seen at a participating practice on a recorded date. After the initial visit, animals may have been hospitalized, returned for re-examination or there may have been a telephone consultation with the owners for the same complaint. To minimize repeated counts of the same case of diarrhea, all records of veterinary utilization (consultations, hospitalizations, laboratory results) for the same animal within 14 days of the initial visit were combined to represent one diarrhea case. There were 15,928 diarrhea cases in this study.

Development of the categorization dictionary in the text miner

Text mining was used to identify and retrieve cases for which one or more of the following activities were recorded:

- diagnostic testing had been performed.
- an etiological diagnosis had been made.
- treatment with an antimicrobial had been initiated.

Case definitions were developed for diagnostic testing and etiological diagnoses to classify cases using the text miner and also by an external reviewer. For classification purposes a diagnostic test was a laboratory test that could either be performed in the practice by the animal health technologist or sent to an external veterinary laboratory. A case was classified as positive for diagnostic testing if any of the following diagnostic tests were recorded within the variable 'Note':

- Fecal flotations and fecal smears and using light microscopy that provided a morphological diagnosis of helminths, protozoa or bacteria.
- Enzyme-linked immunosorbent (ELISA) assays to identify canine parvovirus or *Giardia* spp. infections from fecal samples.
- Real time PCR tests were performed to screen fecal samples for canine distemper virus, canine coronavirus, canine parvovirus, *Clostridium perfringens* enterotoxin A, *Cryptosporidium* spp. *Giardia* spp., *Salmonella* spp., feline coronavirus, feline panleukopenia, *Toxoplasma gondii*, and *Tritrichomonas foetus*.
- Fecal bacteria culture was performed.

A case was classified as positive for etiologic diagnosis if a positive outcome for any of the diagnostic tests described above was recorded. The positive classification included imprecise morphological diagnoses of bacterial infections such as bacterial overgrowth and *Campylobacter*-type spp. as recorded by a veterinarian or technician.

Positive antimicrobial use cases were defined as those diarrhea cases that were administered, dispensed or prescribed antimicrobials for the management of the diarrhea signs.

To calculate the number of diarrhea cases required to assess the ability of the text miner to accurately classify the cases by each management activity (diagnostic testing, etiological diagnosis and antimicrobial treatment), the assumptions of the precision-based sample size calculation were: i) significance level, 0.05, ii) *a priori* estimate of the proportion, conservatively = 0.5, iii) precision = 0.1. The calculated number of cases positive for each activity required in the sample was 96. To reach the target of 96 positive cases in the sample required an estimate of the proportion of cases that would be positive for each activity. This was unknown and was expected to differ for each activity so a proportion of 0.20 was selected. The number of controls required was calculated using, $N_{controls} = N_{Cases}(1-Prev/Prev) = 384$ controls +96 cases = 480 [23]. A sample of 500 records was randomly selected from the entire file of 15,928 diarrhea cases.

An experienced veterinarian clinician, blinded to the results of the text miner, reviewed all of the information contained in the extracted EMR's for the sample of 500 cases. The clinician reviewer classified each case as positive or negative for each of: i) laboratory diagnostics performed; ii) etiological diagnosis made; and iii) antimicrobial treatment. This served as the external standard.

We cross-tabulated the dichotomous results from the text miner and the external standard. The results for each case definition were summarized as the sensitivity and the specificity of the text miner's ability to correctly classify cases. The 95% confidence intervals for the sensitivity and specificity were also calculated (Exact method, Stata/IC 10.0, StataCorp, College Station, Tx). The cases that were improperly classified (false positives and false negatives) were reviewed to determine why they had been misclassified and if there were any opportunities to improve the text-mining classifier.

The sample of 500 diarrhea positive cases was categorized into three categories: i) no diagnostic testing performed, ii) diagnostic testing performed with a negative result or no result recorded; and iii) diagnostic testing performed with a positive diagnosis. Within each of the 3 categories the proportion of patients that were managed with antimicrobials was determined. Odds ratios (OR) and their 95% confidence intervals (CI) were used to quantify the difference between the odds of cases within each category receiving antimicrobials.

Antimicrobial use trends

The text miner's categorization dictionary for antimicrobial use (described above) was then applied to all of the 15,928 diarrhea cases to classify cases that had been administered, dispensed or prescribed antimicrobials. Antimicrobial use was described by the class of antimicrobial used and by Health Canada's categorization of antimicrobial drugs based on importance to human medicine [24]. Co-occurrences of antimicrobial use were identified by the text miner and the antimicrobials used in combination were described.

We examined the temporal trends of the Category I (very high importance in human medicine) and Category II (high importance in human medicine) antimicrobials [24] for the 4 years of the study. For each month of the study, we determined the proportion of cases that had been treated with any antimicrobial and the proportions treated with each class of antimicrobial. The temporal trend for all antimicrobials combined and for each antimicrobial was examined by fitting a linear regression model to the data. The number of antimicrobial treated cases, normalized by the total number of diarrhea cases for each month, was the dependent variable and the month/year was the independent variable. If the antimicrobial use data fit the slope estimated by the linear regression (p<0.05), the proportions of cases treated with this antimicrobial were plotted as a function of time [25]. Further exploratory data analysis included data smoothing by: i) pooling

the number of cases treated with each class of antimicrobial in each quarter of each year; and ii) plotting the results in scatterplots with quadratic overlays (Stata/IC 10.0).

Results

Text mining

Estimates of the text miner's ability to distinguish between cases that had diagnostic testing performed (sensitivity = 70% and specificity = 85.1%) and which had an etiological diagnosis made (sensitivity = 72.4% and specificity = 97.4), were relatively low. There were wide confidence intervals around sensitivity which indicated poor precision of the estimate (Table 1, Table 2). The primary reason the text miner performed poorly when classifying these cases was that the context was relevant to the classification of the case. For example, the word "parvo" was associated with a diagnosis, a differential diagnosis, a past diagnosis, a diagnostic test, a serological titer, a vaccine, and a recommendation or a warning to owners. Despite repeated efforts, it was not possible to improve the performance of the text miner to classify cases by the diagnostic test performed or their etiological diagnosis, so the text miner was not used for these purposes.

In contrast, text mining classified cases that had been treated with an antimicrobial with high sensitivity (92.3%) and specificity (85%) when compared to a human reviewer (Table 3). The text miner misclassified cases if the name of the antimicrobial was not provided or improperly spelled, if the record contained information about past treatment or future considerations for treatment or if the pet was receiving antimicrobials but they were being used to treat a co-morbidity (not dispensed for diarrhea). Given the high sensitivity and specificity of the text miner for classifying cases with respect to antimicrobial use, it was used for the remainder of the analysis.

Diagnostic testing, diagnoses and antimicrobial use

As the text miner did not accurately classify cases that had laboratory testing performed or a diagnosis made, the results presented are from the manual review of the sample of 500 diarrhea positive cases only. The remaining diarrhea cases were not described by their diagnostic testing or etiological diagnosis. There were 88 cases (17.6%) in the sample of 500 diarrhea positive cases tested to identify an etiological diagnosis (Figure 1, Table 4). Fecal examinations (smears and/or floats) were performed in 56 of the 88 (63.6%) cases that underwent diagnostic testing; ELISA assays were run on 58 (65.9%) cases to identify canine parvovirus or *Giardia* spp.; multiple testing using a combination of fecal exams and ELISA tests was documented in 29 (33%) of those tested. Fecal cultures or PCR tests were each ordered in 1 (1.1%) and 3 (3.4%) of the cases respectively; all of which were negative. Thirty-six cases (40.9% of those tested, 7.2% of all cases) had a

Table 1. From a random sample of 500 companion animal cases of diarrhea, the accuracy of the text miner for classifying the cases as positive or negative for *'had diagnostic testing'* when compared to a manual review of the medical records serving as the external standard.

	External standard +	External standard -	Sum
Text miner +	63	61	124
Text miner -	27	349	376
Sum	90	410	500
	Sensitivity = 70.0% (95%CI, 59.4% - 79.2%)	Specificity = 85.1% (95%CI, 81.3% - 88.4%)	

Table 2. From a random sample of 500 companion animal cases of diarrhea, the accuracy of the text miner for classifying the cases as positive or negative for *'had an etiological diagnosis made'* when compared to a manual review of the medical records serving as the external standard.

	External standard +	External standard -	Sum
Text miner +	21	17	38
Text miner -	8	454	462
Sum	29	466	500
	Sensitivity = 72.4% (95%CI, 52.8%–87.3%)	Specificity = 97.4% (95%CI, 95.5%–98.7%)	

stated etiologic diagnosis in the EMR; all were prescribed an antihelmintic or antimicrobial medication. We inferred that given the management of cases with a positive result, that the veterinarians considered the findings to be relevant.

Patients that had diagnostic procedures performed had more antimicrobials administered, dispensed or prescribed (72.7%) than patients that had no diagnostic testing performed (41%) (OR = 3.8; 95% CI 2.2–6.7). There was little difference in the proportion of patients that were treated with antimicrobials and had a positive diagnostic test and those treated with antimicrobials and a negative diagnostic test (OR = 1.2, 95% CI 0.4–3.6) (Figure 1). Two hundred and thirty-three of the 500 diarrhea cases (46.6%) received antimicrobials; none of the cases receiving antimicrobials were culture positive for bacteria (Figure 1, Table 4).

Text mining of the diarrhea cases (n = 15,928) identified 7400 (46.5%) cases that were administered, dispensed or prescribed antimicrobials. There were 8041 occurrences of AMU in the 7400 cases. The distribution of the antimicrobial classes used in the management of diarrhea positive cases is summarized in Table 5. Category 1 (very high importance to human health) antimicrobials were prescribed in most (87.1%) of the antimicrobial-treated diarrhea cases. Veterinarians prescribed more than one antimicrobial in 641 (8.7%) of all cases treated with an antimicrobial. Nitroimidazole plus a penicillin was the most frequent treatment combination (n = 346) followed by nitroimidazole together with first and second generation cephalosporins (n = 79), penicillins with fluorquinolones (n = 67), and nitroimidazoles in combination with fluorquinolones (n = 66).

Antimicrobial use temporal trends

The linear regression analyses of 'all antimicrobials' (n = 7400), 'nitroimidazole' (n = 5814) and 'penicillin' (n = 808) were significant (p<0.05) and these variables were plotted against time (Figure 2). The graph and the slope coefficients (0.0002 to 0.0004) indicate a very small statistically significant, upward trend in the proportions of diarrhea cases treated with any antimicrobial and

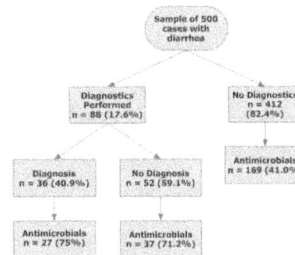

Figure 1. From a random sample of 500 companion animal cases with diarrhea, a flow diagram describing the proportion of cases that had laboratory diagnostics performed, had an etiological diagnosis made, and were administered, prescribed or dispensed antimicrobials.

treated with nitroimidazoles and penicillins. The regression analyses of the remaining antimicrobials were not statistically significant.

Smoothed scatterplots of the quarterly counts of cases treated with $3^{rd}/4^{th}$ generation cephalosporins and the penicillin β-lactamase inhibitor combinations showed patterns of antimicrobial use that were mirror images of each other (Figure 3). Scatterplots of the remaining antimicrobial class combinations did not show any recognizable patterns.

Discussion

Results of the text mining methods used in this study varied depending on the variable of interest. Text mining results for AMU were relatively accurate because the documentation of antimicrobial treatments by veterinarians was usually explicit and unambiguous; the meaning of the words did not depend upon the context in which they were used. However, the language used to

Table 3. From a random sample of 500 companion animal cases of diarrhea, the accuracy of the text miner for classifying the cases as positive or negative for *'had an antimicrobial administered, dispensed or prescribed'* when compared to a manual review of the medical records serving as the external standard.

	External standard +	External standard -	Sum
Text miner +	215	40	255
Text miner -	18	227	245
Sum	233	267	500
	Sensitivity = 92.3% (95%CI, 88.1%–95.4%)	Specificity = 85.0% (95%CI, 80.2%–89.1%)	

Table 4. Distribution of a sample of companion animal cases with diarrhea by the stated etiological diagnosis (n = 500).

Diagnosis	Number of cases (% of 500 cases)	% of diagnosed cases	Diagnostic test
All	36 (7.2)	-	
Helminths	1 (0.2)	2.7	Morphology
Coccidia	5 (1.0)	13.9	Morphology
Bacterial overgrowth	9 (1.8)	25	Morphology
Campylobacter-type	1 (0.2)	2.8	Morphology
Canine parvovirus	9 (1.8)	25.0	ELISA
Giardia spp.	11 (2.2)	30.6	Morphology or ELISA

record diagnostic procedures and diagnoses was highly context specific and the linguistic-based text mining approach used in this study was unable to discriminate between the various meanings. It is possible that trained or rule-based text-mining software could more accurately distinguish these cases and is an area for future study [26,27].

Most cases of acute (less than 14 days) diarrhea are mild and self-limiting and supportive treatment without a diagnosis is considered appropriate [2]. Therefore, it was not unexpected that less than 18% of the diarrhea cases in our study had diagnostic procedures performed. The recommended initial diagnostic approach to acute diarrhea is a fecal exam [28]. More than half of the diagnostic procedures in our study were fecal flotation and/or fecal smears. In animals with severe disease (febrile, dehydrated, hemorrhagic or persistent diarrhea) further efforts at establishing an etiological diagnosis are warranted [2,28]. Animals in this study that were subjected to diagnostic laboratory testing were more likely to be given antimicrobials than those that were not tested regardless of the test results. This may indicate an assessment of more severe disease by the veterinarian although this judgment was not often explicitly stated in the medical record. Despite efforts

to identify an etiological agent, a positive diagnosis was established in less than half of the cases undergoing diagnostic testing.

Giardiasis was the most frequent diagnosis in this study and antimicrobial treatment is usually recommended in *Giardia*-positive diarrheic animals [29]. However, *Giardia* spp. is commonly misdiagnosed in veterinary practice and most cases are self-limiting [30]. Antimicrobials are also recommended in the management of diarrhea in companion animals if there is a positive diagnosis of secondary bacterial overgrowth associated with inflammatory bowel disease or culture-confirmed primary bacterial infections of *Salmonella*, *Campylobacter*, *Clostridium* and enterotoxigenic *E. coli* [2,4,5,29], if there is evidence of a breach in the mucosal integrity of the intestines (hemorrhagic diarrhea), or to manage the immunosuppressive effects of parvovirus [2,4,5,28,29]. Other authors argue that while antimicrobials are commonly used in cases with a confirmed culture or if there is evidence of hematochezia, there is little objective information as to whether they are needed in all cases [3,5].

Our findings indicated that veterinarians commonly prescribed antimicrobials for diarrhea without any documentation that the

Table 5. Distribution of antimicrobials used by the veterinary practices in the treatment of companion animal diarrhea cases (n = 15,928) in 2007, 2008, 2009 and 2010.

Health Canada Category [24]	Antibiotic class	Number of cases (% of 15,928 diarrhea cases)	% antimicrobial treated cases (n = 7400)
Category 1 (Very High Importance)	3rd/4th Generation Cephalosporins	124 (0.8)	1.7
	Fluorquinolones	200 (1.3)	2.7
	Nitroimidazoles	5814 (36.5)	78.6
	Penicillin β – lactam inhibitors	310 (1.9)	4.2
	Total for Category I	**6448 (40.5)**	**87.1**
Category II (High Importance)	1st/2nd Generation Cephalosporins	426 (2.7)	5.8
	Lincosamides	76 (0.5)	1.0
	Macrolides	124 (0.8)	1.7
	Penicillins	808 (5.1)	10.9
	Timethoprim-Sulpha	84 (0.5)	1.1
	Total for Category II	**1518 (9.5)**	**20.5**
Category III (Medium Importance)	Choramphenicol	5 (0.0)	0.1
	Sulphonamides	62 (0.4)	0.8
	Tetracycline	8 (0.1)	0.1
	Total for Category III	**75 (0.5)**	**1.0**

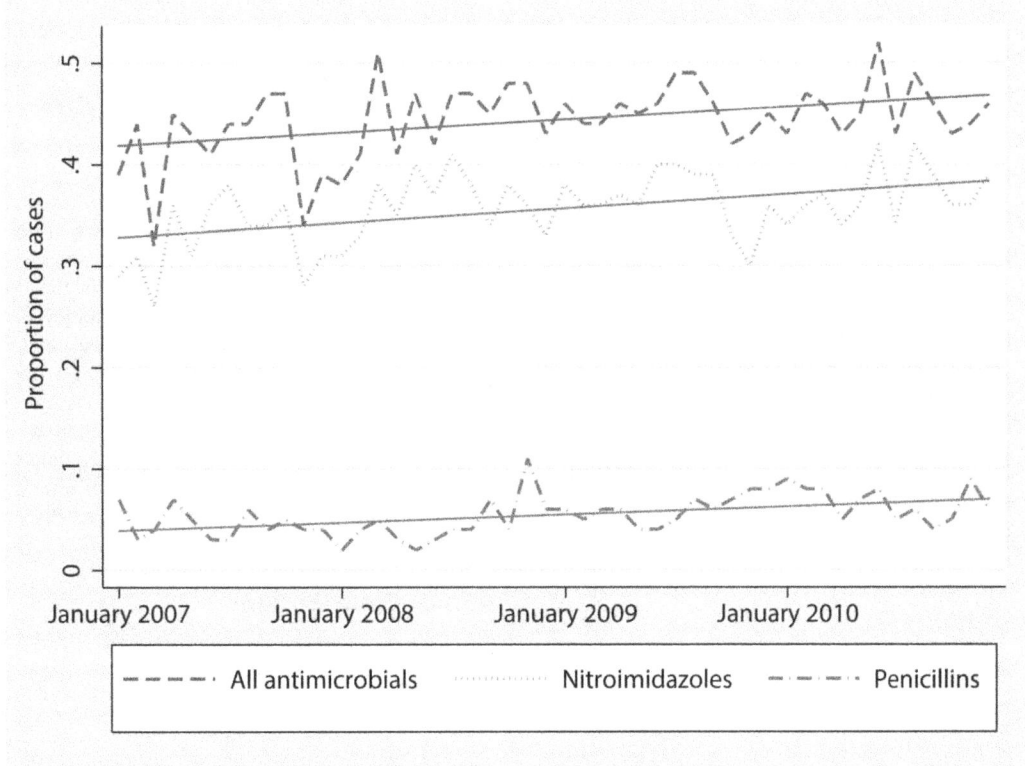

Figure 2. Changes in the proportion of companion animal diarrhea cases (n = 15,928) treated with any antimicrobial, nitroimidazole class and penicillin class from January 1, 2007 to December 31, 2010.

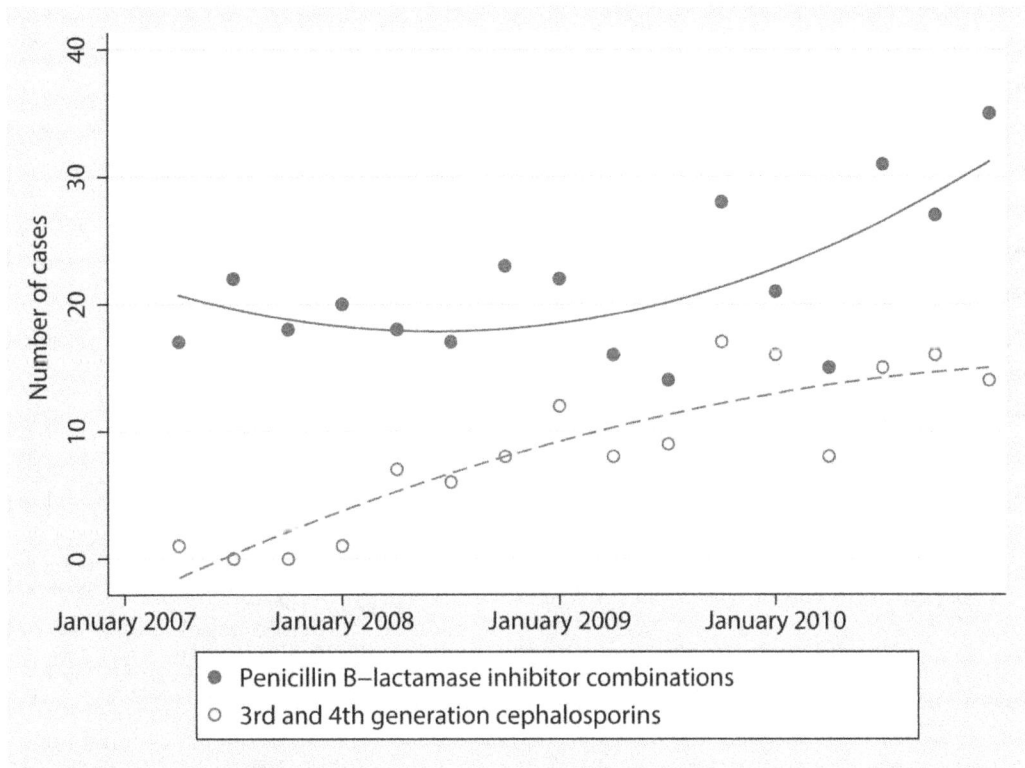

Figure 3. From 15,928 cases of companion animals with diarrhea, scattergrams of the counts of cases treated with B-lactam inhibitors and cephalosporins in each yearly quarter from January 1, 2007 to December 31, 2010.

animal's diarrhea had an infectious etiology. Empirical combinations of antimicrobial treatments was also common. Empirical antimicrobial use may lead to treatment failures and antimicrobial resistance [3,4,28,29]. We found no post-prescription, pharmacoepidemiological studies evaluating empirical antimicrobial management of diarrhea in pets in the refereed literature.

Using the data extracted from medical records it was possible to detect changing trends in AMU. Despite increased AMR concerns [4,6] there was evidence that nitroimidazole and penicillin use for the management of diarrhea in companion animals was increasing. Metronidazole (a drug of the Nitroimidazoles Class) was the most frequently prescribed antimicrobial and its use increased over the 4 years of the study. It is the drug of choice for anaerobic and microaerophilic bacteria (*Bacteroides* and *Clostridia*) and parasites (*Giardia* spp.) in animals [4]. In people it is important in the management of these pathogens and *Helicobacter pylori* [31,32]. There are few therapeutic alternatives for these infections in people and so it is classified as a Category I antimicrobial [24]. Sensitivity testing for anaerobes is not routinely performed but treatment failures have been documented [32,33] and the molecular basis for resistance has been established [31]. We found no papers documenting the transmission of metronidazole-resistant bacteria from pets to people.

The increase in the number of cases treated with 3rd and 4th generation cephalosporins in early 2008 coincided with the Canadian approval on May 30, 2007 and subsequent distribution of Convenia (Pfizer Animal Health, Kirkland, QC) later in 2007 [34]. Convenia is the trade name for cefovecin, a third generation cephalosporin. The increase in cefovecin use corresponded to a decrease in the use of penicillin β-lactamase inhibitor combinations. The indications for use are similar for the 2 classes of drugs so it is possible that one class was being used as an alternative to the other. Starting in the middle of 2009, the relationship appeared to be inverted and this trend continued until the end of 2010, the reason for which is unknown.

The results from this study suggest that informatics and EMR's could be useful for supporting evidence-based practice, and for monitoring trends in AMU and changes in veterinary prescription behavior following interventions to modify their use. Temporal trends and regional differences could prompt further investigations to explore why the observed trends were developing. Interventions such as confidential benchmarking by comparing AMU among veterinarians may serve to help veterinarians recognize problems and reduce AMU [35]. Analytical studies to see if there is an association between AMU in companion animals with diarrhea and the development of AMR in fecal microorganisms are indicated and informatics could provide the exposure data necessary to interpret AMR results.

Author Contributions

Conceived and designed the experiments: RMA JB CS. Performed the experiments: RMA. Analyzed the data: RMA. Contributed reagents/materials/analysis tools: RMA JB CR MR CS. Contributed to the writing of the manuscript: RMA JB CR MR CS.

References

1. Lidbury JA Turpin I, Suchodolski JS (2008) Gastrointestinal disease in a population of insured dogs and cats from the United Kingdome (2006–2007); 18th ECVIM-CA Congress; Ghent, Belgium. pp. 219.

2. Hall EJ, German AJ (2010) Diseases of the small intestine. In: Ettinger SJ, Feldman EC, editors. Textbook of Veterinary Internal Medicine, Diseases of the Dog and Cat. 7th ed. St. Lois, Missouri: Sanders Elsvier. pp. 1527–1572.

3. Weese JS (2011) Bacterial enteritis in dogs and cats: diagnosis, therapy, and zoonotic potential. Vet Clin North Am Small Anim Pract 41: 287.

4. Boothe DM (2012) Principles of antimicrobial therapy. In: Boothe DM, editor. Small Animal Clinical Pharmacology and Therapeutics. 2nd ed. St. Louis, Missouri: Elsevier Saunders.

5. Guerrant RL, Van Gilder T, Steiner TS, Thielman NM, Slutsker L, et al. (2001) Practice guidelines for the management of infectious diarrhea. Clin Infect Dis 32: 331–351.

6. Center for Disease Control Website. Interagency Task Force on Antimicrobial Resistance (2011) A public health action plan to combat antimicrobial resistance. Available: www.cdc.gov/./pdf/public-health-action-plan-combat-antimicrobial-resistance.pdf. Accessed 2013 February 2.

7. Morley PS, Apley MD, Besser TE, Burney DP, Fedorka-Cray PJ, et al. (2005) Antimicrobial drug use in veterinary medicine. J Vet Intern Med 19: 617–629.

8. Coffman JR (Chairman) National National Research Council (1999) The use of drugs in food animals: Benefits and risks. Washington, DC: Institute of Medicine.

9. Weese JS (2008) Antimicrobial resistance in companion animals. Anim Health Res Rev/Conf Res Workers Anim Dis 9: 169–176.

10. Guardabassi L, Schwarz S, Lloyd DH (2004) Pet animals as reservoirs of antimicrobial-resistant bacteria Review. J Antimicrob Chemother 54: 321–332.

11. Prescott JF, Hanna WJ, Reid-Smith R, Drost K (2002) Antimicrobial drug use and resistance in dogs. Can Vet J 43: 107–116.

12. Singer RS, Reid-Smith R, Sischo WM (2006) Stakeholder position paper: epidemiological perspectives on antibiotic use in animals. Prev Vet Med 73: 153–161.

13. Greco PJ, Eisenberg JM (1993) Changing physicians' practices. N Engl J Med 329: 1271–1274.

14. Meyer E, Schwab F, Jonas D, Rueden H, Gastmeier P, et al. (2004) Surveillance of antimicrobial use and antimicrobial resistance in intensive care units (SARI): 1. Antimicrobial use in German intensive care units. Intensive Care Med 30: 1089–1096.

15. Vlahović-Palc???evski V, Dumpis U, Mitt P, Gulbinovic J, Struwe J, et al. (2007) Benchmarking antimicrobial drug use at university hospitals in five European countries. Clin Microbiol Infect 13: 277–283.

16. Goossens H, Ferech M, Vander Stichele R, Elseviers M (2005) Outpatient antibiotic use in Europe and association with resistance: a cross-national database study. Lancet 365: 579–587.

17. Monnet D, López-Lozano JM, Campillos P, Burgos A, Yagüe A, et al. (2001) Making sense of antimicrobial use and resistance surveillance data: application of ARIMA and transfer function models. Clin Microbiol Infect 7: 29–36.

18. Public Health Agency of Canada website. Canadian Integrated Program for Antimicrobial Resistance Surveillance (2008) 2008 Annual Report. Available: http://www.phac-aspc.gc.ca/cipars-picra/2008/index-eng.php. Accessed 2012 November 29.

19. Friede A, Blum HL, McDonald M (1995) Public health informatics: how information-age technology can strengthen public health. Annu Rev Public Health 16: 239–252.

20. Chen ES, Hripcsak G, Xu H, Markatou M, Friedman C (2008) Automated acquisition of disease–drug knowledge from biomedical and clinical documents: an initial study. J Am Med Inform Assoc 15: 87–98.

21. Anholt RM, Berezowski J, MacLean K, Russel M, Jamal I, Stephen C (2014) The application of medical informatics to the veterinary management programs at companion animal practices in Alberta, Canada: A case study. Prev Vet Med 113: 165–174.

22. Anholt R, Berezowski J, Jamal I, Ribble C, Stephen C (2014) Mining free-text medical records for companion animal enteric syndrome surveillance. Prev Vet Med 113: 417–422.

23. Guyatt G SD, Haynes B. (2006) Evaluating diagnostic tests. In: Haynes BSD, Guyatt G., Tugwell P., editor. Clinical Epidemiology; How to do Clinical Practice Research. Third edition. Philadelphia: Lippincott William and Wilkins.

24. Health Canada website. Veterinary Drug Directorate (2009) Categorization of antimicrobial drugs based on importance to human medicine. Available: http://www.hc-sc.gc.ca/dhp-mps/vet/antimicrob/amr_ram_hum-med-rev-eng.php. Accessed 2012 November 29.

25. Jump RLP, Olds DM, Seifi N, Kypriotakis G, Jury LA, et al. (2012) Effective Antimicrobial Stewardship in a Long-Term Care Facility through an Infectious Disease Consultation Service: Keeping a LID on Antibiotic Use. Infect Control Hosp Epidemiol 33: 1185–1192.

26. Mooney RJ, Bunescu R (2005) Mining knowledge from text using information extraction. ACM SIGKDD Explorations newsl 7: 3–10.

27. Meystre SM, Savova GK, Kipper-Schuler KC, Hurdle JF (2008) Extracting information from textual documents in the electronic health record: a review of recent research. Yearbook Med Inform: 128–144.

28. Sherding RG, Johnson SE (2006) Diseases of the intestines. In: Birchard SJ, Sherding, RG, editor. Saunders Manual of Small Animal Practice. 3rd ed. St. Louis, Missouri: Saunders Elsevier.

29. Eddlestone SM (2002) Drug Therapies Used in Gastrointestinal Disease. Compendium: Small animal/exotics 24: 452–468.

30. Payne PA, Artzer M (2009) Biology and control of Giardia spp. and Tritrichomonas foetus. Vet Clin North Am Small Anim Pract 39: 993–1007.

31. Dhand A, Snydman DR (2009) Mechanism of Resistance in Metronidazole. Antimicrob Drug Resist: 223–227.

32. Megraud F, Lamouliatte H (2003) Review article: the treatment of refractory Helicobacter pylori infection. Aliment Pharmacol Ther 17: 1333–1343.

33. Fang H, Edlund C, Hedberg M, Nord CE (2002) New findings in beta-lactam and metronidazole resistant Bacteroides fragilis group. Int J Antimicrob Agents 19: 361.

34. Health Canada website. Veterinary Drug Directorate (2007) Notice of Compliance. Available: http://www.hc-sc.gc.ca/dhp-mps/prodpharma/notices-avis/index-eng.php. Accessed 2012 November 29.

35. Ibrahim OM, Polk RE (2012) Benchmarking antimicrobial drug use in hospitals. Expert Rev Anti Infect Ther 10: 445–457.

7

The Effect of Badger Culling on Breakdown Prolongation and Recurrence of Bovine Tuberculosis in Cattle Herds in Great Britain

Katerina Karolemeas[1], Christl A. Donnelly[2], Andrew J. K. Conlan[1], Andrew P. Mitchell[3], Richard S. Clifton-Hadley[3], Paul Upton[3], James L. N. Wood[1], Trevelyan J. McKinley[1]*

1 Disease Dynamics Unit, Department of Veterinary Medicine. University of Cambridge, Cambridge, United Kingdom, 2 MRC Centre for Outbreak Analysis and Modelling, Department of Infectious Disease Epidemiology, Imperial College, London, United Kingdom, 3 Animal Health and Veterinary Laboratories Agency, Weybridge, Surrey, United Kingdom

Abstract

Bovine tuberculosis is endemic in cattle herds in Great Britain, with a substantial economic impact. A reservoir of *Mycobacterium bovis* within the Eurasian badger (*Meles meles*) population is thought to have hindered disease control. Cattle herd incidents, termed breakdowns, that are either 'prolonged' (lasting ≥240 days) or 'recurrent' (with another breakdown within a specified time period) may be important foci for onward spread of infection. They drain veterinary resources and can be demoralising for farmers. Randomised Badger Culling Trial (RBCT) data were re-analysed to examine the effects of two culling strategies on breakdown prolongation and recurrence, *during* and *after* culling, using a Bayesian hierarchical model. Separate effect estimates were obtained for the 'core' trial areas (where culling occurred) and the 'buffer' zones (up to 2 km outside of the core areas). For breakdowns that started during the culling period, 'reactive' (localised) culling was associated with marginally increased odds of prolongation, with an odds ratio (OR) of 1.7 (95% credible interval [CI] 1.1–2.4) within the core areas. This effect was not present after the culling ceased. There was no notable effect of 'proactive' culling on prolongation. In contrast, reactive culling had no effect on breakdown recurrence, though there was evidence of a reduced risk of recurrence in proactive core areas during the culling period (ORs and 95% CIs: 0.82 (0.64–1.0) and 0.69 (0.54–0.86) for 24- and 36-month recurrence respectively). Again these effects were not present after the culling ceased. There seemed to be no effect of culling on breakdown prolongation or recurrence in the buffer zones. These results suggest that the RBCT badger culling strategies are unlikely to reduce either the prolongation or recurrence of breakdowns in the long term, and that reactive strategies (such as employed during the RBCT) are, if anything, likely to impact detrimentally on breakdown persistence.

Editor: Jean Louis Herrmann, Hopital Raymond Poincare - Universite Versailles St. Quentin, France

Funding: KK, TJM and JLNW were supported by grant VT0105 from the Department for Environment, Food and Rural Affairs (Defra) and Hefce. TJM is also supported by BBSRC grant (BB/I012192/1). JLNW is also supported by the Alborada Trust and the RAPIDD program of the Science & Technology Directorate, Department of Homeland Security. AJKC was funded by Defra grant SE3230 Cambridge reference PU/T/WL/07/46), sponsored by the Veterinary Laboratories Agency. The work was also funded by Defra, United Kingdom, under contract SE3230. CAD thanks the MRC for Centre funding. The funders had no role in study design, data collection and analysis, decision to publish, or preparation of the manuscript.

Competing Interests: The authors have declared that no competing interests exist.

* E-mail: tjm44@cam.ac.uk

Introduction

Bovine tuberculosis (bTB), caused by *Mycobacterium bovis*, is endemic in Great Britain (GB). A routine surveillance programme to slaughter cattle classified as infected has been unsuccessful, with incidence of herd 'breakdowns' (movement restrictions associated with detection of infection in cattle) increasing over the last 25 years [1]. Failure to eradicate bTB from GB has been complicated by the existence of a wildlife reservoir, namely the Eurasian badger (*Meles meles*) [2–4].

Nationally, around 30% of herd breakdowns are '*prolonged*' (≥240 days) [5], and around 23% and 38% are '*recurrent*' within 12 and 24 months respectively [6]. These persistent breakdowns are important as they are demanding on resources, and may additionally be acting as foci of infection, fuelling the increase in incidence. Furthermore, they can have a substantially detrimental

effect on the well-being of farmers [7]. Breakdowns may become persistent from the presence of underlying and undetected infection within the herd, or by transmission and re-infection into the herd from other herds or environmental reservoirs of infection. The relative contribution of the badger reservoir to these empirical measures of persistence is not clear.

Due to a lack of detailed data on badger densities and infection status (which is not routinely collected), many previous studies have focussed on measuring associations between proxies for badger risk and incidence of bTB. For example, in the Republic of Ireland (ROI) [8] there was found to be an association between the presence of badgers on farms and breakdowns that were either over 12 months in duration, or recurrent within a four-year period. In another study [9] there was found to be no association with the presence of badgers and recurrence at the test conducted six months after the end of a breakdown. In GB, an association between the relative density of badgers and breakdowns over six months duration has been reported [10]. Although the aforementioned studies were similar in that they all used bTB test-negative herds as controls, differences in their case definitions for persistence makes comparisons between the findings challenging.

Previous studies in GB that examined risk factors for breakdown prolongation and recurrence, in which a range of farm-level factors were considered, included examination of information on the presence or absence of badgers, and whether or not badger control policies were performed at the farm level [5,6]. Although no association was found between the badger variables examined and breakdown persistence, it is possible that this lack of association may have been due to confounding in measured or unmeasured variables, or that some of the variables identified in the model represented proxies for increased potential for transmission from badgers.

Further insight into the role that badgers play in infecting cattle herds can be gained from examining the effect of badger culling. Since 1971, when a dead badger infected with *M. bovis* was first discovered on a farm affected by bTB in GB, badgers have been strongly implicated in the transmission of *M. bovis* to cattle, prompting a number of badger culling strategies that occurred between 1973 and 1998. However, these culling operations [11], and those conducted in the ROI [12,13] lacked randomised control areas where no culling was conducted, making conclusions difficult to interpret.

The Randomised Badger Culling Trial (RBCT) was set up in 1998 to examine the effect of badger culling on bTB incidence in cattle herds in GB, and specifically included randomly selected matched control areas where no culling was undertaken [14]. The RBCT was designed and conducted by the Independent Scientific Group on Cattle TB (ISG; [14]). The data are a valuable resource, and various analyses have been conducted. Analyses to date have measured the effect of culling on *overall confirmed* and *total* (confirmed and unconfirmed) *incidence*, both during and subsequent to the trial [15–17], and more recently have examined individual herd risk factors for breakdowns [18,19]. Nonetheless, the effect of badger culling on *persistent* breakdowns within individual cattle herds has yet to be examined.

Widespread badger culling remains illegal in GB and is an ongoing subject of political debate [4,14,20]. However, in December 2011 Defra ministers announced a cull of badgers in two pilot areas, originally due to commence in 2012 [21], but now delayed until 2013 [22]. Farmers and landowners in these areas will be able to apply for licences to reduce badger populations at their own expense, and the humaneness of the culling will be judged by a panel of independent experts at the end of the period. The results from the pilot areas will inform policy decisions on whether this approach will be more widely adopted in the future. As an alternative, the vaccination of badgers is currently being trialled in one area of Gloucester [23], which is planned to continue until 2015, and in June 2012 the Welsh Assembly Government announced that a badger vaccination trial had begun as part of their bTB eradication strategy [24].

The perceived failure to address the wildlife reservoir has led to much distress and unrest in farming communities. Farmers are often reluctant to implement increased cattle controls when re-infection by badgers is perceived to be inevitable. Knowledge of the role of badgers in the re-infection of cattle herds is critical to inform those developing control policies. In this study we quantify the effects of the two badger culling strategies (proactive and reactive) conducted during the RBCT, on breakdown prolongation and recurrence in individual herds in areas of high cattle bTB incidence in GB.

Materials and Methods

Summary of RBCT Trial Areas and Culling Treatments

The RBCT was conducted in 30 trial areas, located in areas of high bTB incidence, mainly in the West and South-west of England [14,15]. Trial areas were grouped into triplets of three core areas (each approximately 100 km²), surrounded by buffers to ensure that the trial area boundaries were at least 3 km apart [14,15]. Within each triplet, each core area received one of three treatments.

Proactive culling was conducted across all accessible land with the aim of using annual culling to reduce badger density to the greatest extent possible within the constraints of welfare and logistical considerations. The first proactive culls occurred between 1998 and 2002 (depending on the triplet) and culling was repeated approximately once yearly (the total number of culls ranged from 4 to 7 across the ten triplets) to maintain the badger population at as low a level as possible. The last proactive cull in each triplet was in 2005.

Reactive culling was conducted in response to a confirmed breakdown (evidence of visible bTB lesions post-mortem or *M. bovis* cultured in at least one slaughtered animal) with the aim to remove all badger social groups in a localised area that might have access to the breakdown farm. The first reactive cull occurred between 1999 and 2003 (depending on the triplet). Reactive culling was suspended in November 2003 due to evidence of increased incidence of bTB in cattle herds in these areas observed at a planned interim analysis [15].

In *survey-only* areas badger activity was documented but no culling was conducted as part of the trial. These areas acted as control areas for the proactive and reactive areas. For both proactive and reactive culling treatments badgers were caught in cage traps and killed by gunshot [14].

Data and Study Design

Data recorded in VetNet (the national GB surveillance database for bTB) were provided by the Animal Health and Veterinary Laboratories Agency, and consisted of all *breakdowns* that occurred in herds located within the RBCT core and buffer areas for the periods prior to, during and subsequent to the RBCT. In addition, we also obtained all the VetNet testing data for these herds over the same period (the last recorded test for one of these herds was 23rd September 2011).

For proactively and reactively culled treatment areas, breakdowns were eligible for inclusion if they started after the end of the first proactive or reactive cull, respectively, in each triplet. For the survey-only areas, breakdowns were eligible for inclusion in the study if they started after the end of the first proactive cull in the corresponding triplet. Full details of the timings of these events have been previously published [2,25]. Also, only herds in the proactive and survey-only groups were included for Triplet J, since no reactive culling took place in this triplet.

To examine the effect of badger culling on breakdown *prolongation*, breakdowns of duration ≥240 days were classified as cases ('prolonged') and those <240 days as controls ('non-prolonged'), as justified in a previous study [5]. Where no end date was recorded in the data (indicative of an ongoing breakdown), breakdowns were excluded if the breakdown began <240 days before the last available test date (specified above), and classified as prolonged if it started at least 240 days before this date.

For the *recurrence* analysis, each breakdown was followed prospectively from its end date and classified as a case ('recurrent') if the herd experienced a further breakdown within a specified

Table 1. Numbers of cases (prolonged) and controls (non-prolonged), and the proportion prolonged, for the different treatment areas aggregated across the core and buffer zones.

Treatment	Core				Buffer			
	Cases	Controls	Total	Proportion	Cases	Controls	Total	Proportion
Proactive	460	893	1353	0.34	371	650	1021	0.36
Reactive	437	750	1187	0.37	298	535	833	0.36
Survey	686	1214	1900	0.36	399	796	1195	0.33

follow-up period (12, 24 or 36 months). Alternatively, a herd was classified as a control ('non-recurrent') if the herd experienced at least one herd-level test but did not suffer a further breakdown within the follow-up period. Breakdowns with insufficient follow-up (e.g. such as those that ended within 12 months of the last recorded test date for the 12 month analysis) were excluded. Full discussion of these definitions can be found in a previous study [6].

Statistical Methods

The effect of proactive and reactive culling on breakdown prolongation and recurrence was evaluated using logistic regression models. Although all triplets were located in areas of high cattle bTB incidence, a triplet-level effect was included to account for potential between-triplet heterogeneity. In addition, since it was possible that individual herds could be included in the dataset more than once (if they had multiple breakdowns during the time period examined), an individual herd-level effect was incorporated to account for potential herd-level correlation, such that:

$$\ln\left(\frac{p_i}{1-p_i}\right) = \alpha^T z_i + \beta^T x_i + \gamma_{A_i} + \theta_{H_i},$$

where $\alpha^T = (\alpha_1, \ldots, \alpha_q)$ is a vector of regression parameters relating to a set of nuisance variables $z_i = (z_{i1}, \ldots, z_{iq})$ for breakdown i. Similarly, $\beta^T = (\beta_0, \ldots, \beta_m)$ is a vector of regression parameters corresponding to a set of trial-specific variables $x_i = (x_{1i}, \ldots, x_{mi})$. A triplet-level effect is represented by γ_{A_i}, where $A_i = 1, \ldots, n_A$ corresponds to the triplet containing breakdown i; and θ_{H_i} represents a herd-level effect where $H_i = 1, \ldots, n_H$ corresponds to the herd containing breakdown i.

The nuisance variables, z_i, varied between the prolonged and recurrent analyses, and were chosen based on results from previous papers [5,6]. For prolongation, the estimates were

adjusted for the confirmation status of the breakdown, which had previously been identified to be by far the strongest variable associated with this measure of persistence [5]. By contrast, a combination of variables were identified as being associated with breakdown recurrence [6], and thus for the recurrence analyses, the estimates were adjusted for herd size (maximum herd size during the breakdown), recent breakdown history (a binary variable, taking the value 1 if the herd had experienced a breakdown in the previous three years, and 0 otherwise), and the total number of reactors during the breakdown. In order to linearise the relationship between the non-categorical confounding variables (herd size and total number of reactors) and the response variable, a log transformation was performed. To account for zeros in the data, and thus minimize bias in the covariates, 0.5 was added prior to the log transformation [26].

In each case the trial-specific variables were T_i^R, T_i^P, B_i and t_i, where T_i^R is a binary variable taking the value 1 if breakdown i was in a *reactive* area, and 0 otherwise; T_i^P is likewise for *proactive* areas; B_i is a binary variable taking the value 1 if breakdown i is located in a *buffer* zone, and 0 if it is located in one of the core areas, and t_i is a binary variable taking the value 1 if the breakdown started in the period *after* the cull, and 0 if it began *during* the cull. (Note here that $t_i = 0$ always in the survey-only areas, since no culling occurred.).

Therefore, the trial-specific component of the model is:

$$\beta^T x_i = \beta_0 + \beta_1 T_i^R + \beta_2 T_i^P + \beta_3 B_i + \beta_4 B_i T_i^R + \beta_5 B_i T_i^P$$
$$+ \beta_6 t_i T_i^R + \beta_7 t_i T_i^P + \beta_8 B_i t_i T_i^R + \beta_9 B_i t_i T_i^P,$$

and the marginal log-odds ratios for the different comparisons were extracted through examining different combinations of the β parameters.

The binary time variable was included in the model to adjust for the fact that the effect of culling on breakdown prolongation and recurrence may have differed in the periods *during* and *after* the culling treatments. The cut-offs for these classifications were derived from the known end dates of the cull in each triplet [25]. The interaction effects were included to assess the impact of each type of culling in the core and buffers zones during each of the two time periods.

The model was fitted to the data in a Bayesian framework using Markov chain Monte Carlo. The α and β parameters were given vague $N(0,1000)$ prior distributions (for the prolonged breakdown analysis) and $N(0,100)$ prior distributions (for the recurrent breakdown analysis). The triplet-level effects, γ, were given $N(0,1/\tau)$ prior distributions with precision $\tau \sim G(1,1)$, and the herd-level effects, θ, were given $N(0,1/\tau_\theta)$ prior distributions and precision $\tau_\theta \sim G(1,1)$. This Bayesian hierarchical framework

Table 2. Odds Ratios and 95% credible intervals– relative to a baseline of survey-only core areas–for prolongation in the different treatment areas in the periods during and after the culling; adjusted for breakdown confirmation status.

	Core		Buffer	
	During	After	During	After
Survey			0.95 (0.76–1.1)	
Reactive	1.7 (1.1–2.4)	0.97 (0.79–1.2)	1.2 (0.69–2.1)	1.2 (0.92–1.5)
Proactive	1.1 (0.87–1.4)	0.98 (0.79–1.2)	1.3 (0.94–1.7)	1.0 (0.79–1.4)

Results are further stratified into core and buffer zones.

Table 3. Numbers of cases (recurrent) and controls (non-recurrent), and the proportion recurrent, for the different treatment areas aggregated across the core and buffer zones and stratified by follow-up.

Follow-up	Treatment	Core				Buffer			
		Cases	Controls	Total	Proportion	Cases	Controls	Total	Proportion
	Proactive	309	676	985	0.31	209	505	714	0.29
12 months	Reactive	338	616	954	0.35	251	427	678	0.37
	Survey	479	900	1379	0.35	266	571	837	0.32
	Proactive	458	513	971	0.47	351	373	724	0.48
24 months	Reactive	498	442	940	0.53	336	316	652	0.52
	Survey	698	697	1395	0.50	436	439	875	0.50
	Proactive	475	360	835	0.57	370	262	632	0.59
36 months	Reactive	524	283	807	0.65	342	210	552	0.62
	Survey	768	477	1245	0.62	458	328	786	0.58

is analogous to a random intercepts model in a frequentist framework (though we avoid the use of this terminology since in the Bayesian framework all parameters are considered to be random variables).

In each case a burn-in of 5,000 iterations was used, followed by 20,000 updates and the posterior distributions were thinned to return 1000 samples. Convergence was assessed by running multiple chains from different starting values (from overdispersed initial values) and examining the trace plots. In addition to this visual assessment, we checked that the Gelman-Rubin statistic $(\hat{R})$ values were close to 1.0 [27].

Results are presented as odds ratios (ORs), with posterior means and 95% credible intervals (CI) reported to 2 significant figures. All analyses were carried out using the open-source R statistical package [28], except the fitting of the Bayesian model which was conducted in WinBUGS [29] using the R2WinBUGS package [30].

Results

Full model results for the α and β parameters are provided in Table S1.

Breakdown Prolongation

A total of 7489 breakdowns were analysed in the model, comprising of 4440 in the core areas and 3049 in the buffer zones. The proportion of breakdowns that were prolonged was similar between each of the treatment areas in both the core and buffer zones (Table 1).

The marginal posterior mean OR and 95% CI for the impact of confirmation status on breakdown prolongation–obtained from the model fit–is 9.4 (7.9–11); consistent with previous results [5]. The marginal posterior mean ORs for the treatment effects (adjusted for the confirmation status of the breakdown) are shown in Table 2. There is some evidence of an increase in the odds of prolongation in the core reactive areas in the period during the cull (OR: 1.7; 95% C.I. [1.1–2.4]), though the effect size is slight

Table 4. Odds Ratios and 95% credible intervals (in parentheses)–relative to a baseline of survey-only core areas–for recurrence in the different treatment areas in the periods during and after the culling; adjusted for herd size, number of reactors, and breakdown history in the previous three years.

Follow-up	Treatment	Core		Buffer	
		During	After	During	After
	Survey			0.89 (0.71–1.1)	
12 months	Reactive	1.1 (0.73–1.6)	0.92 (0.74–1.1)	1.3 (0.77–2.0)	1.2 (0.93–1.6)
	Proactive	0.86 (0.66–1.1)	0.85 (0.66–1.1)	0.85 (0.60–1.2)	0.89 (0.65–1.2)
	Survey			1.0 (0.84–1.2)	
24 months	Reactive	1.1 (0.76–1.5)	1 (0.84–1.3)	0.86 (0.54–1.3)	1.1 (0.85–1.4)
	Proactive	0.82 (0.64–1.0)	0.99 (0.77–1.3)	0.88 (0.67–1.1)	0.96 (0.72–1.3)
	Survey			0.89 (0.72–1.1)	
36 months	Reactive	0.99 (0.70–1.4)	1.1 (0.86–1.4)	0.78 (0.48–1.2)	1.3 (0.99–1.7)
	Proactive	0.69 (0.54–0.86)	1.2 (0.84–1.5)	1.0 (0.75–1.3)	1.0 (0.72–1.5)

Models are fitted to each follow-up period (12, 24 and 36 months) separately. Results are further stratified into core and buffer zones.

Table 5. Odds Ratios (ORs) and 95% credible intervals (in parentheses) of recurrence for the nuisance variables in the recurrent breakdown analyses.

Follow-up	Breakdown history	Max. herd size	Total no. of reactors
12 months	1.5 (1.3–1.7)	1 (0.97–1.1)	1.1 (1.1–1.2)
24 months	1.4 (1.2–1.6)	1 (0.93–1.1)	1.1 (1.1–1.2)
36 months	1.5 (1.3–1.8)	1 (0.97–1.1)	1.1 (1.1–1.2)

The OR for breakdown history is defined relative to having no breakdowns in the previous three years; the OR for the maximum herd size is per unit log-increase in herd size, and likewise for the total number of reactors. Models are fitted to each follow-up period (12, 24 and 36 months) separately.

(especially when compared to the effect of confirmation status), and it disappears after the culling period ends. There is no notable impact of either of the treatments on prolongation in the buffer zones.

Breakdown Recurrence

A summary of the number of breakdowns included in each of the recurrence analyses (i.e. at 12, 24 and 36 months) is shown in Table 3. The overall sample size is similar for each of the three analyses, constituting 3318, 3306 and 2887 breakdowns in the core areas, for 12, 24 and 36 months respectively; and likewise 2229, 2251 and 1970 breakdowns in the buffer zones. However, the overall proportions of recurrent breakdowns increases as the follow-up period increases, with similar increases observed in each of the treatment areas for each follow-up period (Table 3).

Table 4 provides the marginal posterior mean ORs and 95% CIs for the treatment effects (adjusted for herd size, number of reactors, and breakdown history in the previous three years). There is no notable impact of culling treatment in the buffer zones, but there is a decrease in the odds of recurrence in the proactively culled core areas during the culling period, for both the 24 month (OR: 0.82; 95% CI [0.64–1.0]), and 36 month (OR: 0.69; 95% CI [0.54–0.86]) follow-up periods.

The marginal posterior mean ORs and 95% CIs for the adjusted variables are shown in Table 5 and herds that have experienced a breakdown in the previous three years, as well as those that have a larger number of reactors during the breakdown, are at increased risk of recurrence, consistent with previous findings [6]. Herd size is deemed less important here, which contrasts against other studies looking at different definitions of recurrence [31–33], but is consistent with previous results using the same definitions [6].

Discussion

In this study we have quantified the effect of two badger culling strategies (proactive and reactive) on breakdown prolongation and recurrence in individual cattle herds in both the core areas and in the adjoining (and un-culled) buffer zones. We also explored the impacts of the culling treatment on persistence in two time periods: during the cull and after the cull.

In terms of breakdown prolongation, we found marginal evidence of an increase in the odds of prolongation in the core reactive areas in the period during the cull (OR: 1.7; 95% C.I. [1.1–2.4]). However, this detrimental effect did not persist in the period after the cull. There was no notable impact of culling treatment on prolongation in the buffer zones.

The mechanisms underlying these results are unclear. Both reactive and proactive culling have been shown to result in an increased prevalence of bTB infection in badger populations [34], most likely due to social and territorial disruption in mixing patterns in the badger populations as a result of the cull [35] and potentially leading to an increase in mixing and transmission between badgers and cattle [36,37]. It is possible that these behaviours could result in an increase in the force-of-infection acting on an already infected cattle herd, and hence potentially increase the degree of within-herd spread of the disease.

In proactively culled areas, any increase in prevalence in badgers was likely to have been offset by a large reduction in badger density, which was not observed to anywhere near the same magnitude in the reactively culled areas [38]. Coupled with the fact that reactive culling was conducted over small, localised areas surrounding *confirmed* breakdowns, this may have resulted in increased contact between cattle and badgers in localised regions (i.e. herds) that were already experiencing above-average levels of underlying infection. This mechanism would also be consistent with the effect disappearing in the period after the culling ended, since there is evidence to suggest that re-colonisation (and hence stabilisation) of the badger populations was quick in the reactive areas [35,37].

The perturbation effect hypothesis has been questioned by some who suggest a lag period is necessary before any effect might be expected to be seen [39]. The Godfray report [40], published in 2004, concluded that there was insufficient information in the reactive areas to support the perturbation effect hypothesis, questioning whether firm conclusions can be drawn from the reactively-culled areas due to the low numbers of badgers removed from relatively small areas. A similar consideration is whether reactive culling, on the scale conducted in the RBCT, would be able to influence breakdown prolongation and recurrence as measured in our study. However, subsequent analysis of cattle TB in and around proactively culled RBCT areas found a 29% increase in bTB risk observed among cattle herds living close to (but outside) proactive trial areas [17], consistent with the earlier finding in reactive areas. Our findings, albeit marginal, suggest that reactive culling, as practiced in the RBCT, is associated with a detrimental effect in the shorter term. This complements the results of a recent study [25], which examined the change in bTB risk in nearby cattle herds as a direct result of reactive culling over different time periods up to January 2007, concluding that the risk of having a confirmed breakdown was increased in the period during the reactive cull, even after adjusting for other important local risk factors.

Disruption to testing caused by the 2001 foot-and-mouth disease (FMD) epidemic is likely to have a more pronounced impact on the data obtained from reactive areas due to the timing of the culling periods with respect to the FMD outbreak. Reactive culling was stopped at a much earlier stage than the proactive cull, with all reactive areas experiencing their last cull in 2003, compared to 2005 for the proactive culls. In the model, the definition of the time period during the cull is centred around these earlier years in the reactive areas, which span the FMD epidemic. Figure 1A shows the proportions of prolonged breakdowns that started in each year, stratified by treatment. It can be seen that there was a spike in the levels of prolongation in each of the treatment regions in 2001, however the proportions of prolonged breakdowns were already higher in 2000 in the reactive areas compared to the proactive and survey-only areas, which carried through to higher levels in 2001. It is these patterns that are reflected in the increased OR for prolongation in the reactive areas during the culling period. However, there is no clear systematic or mechanistic

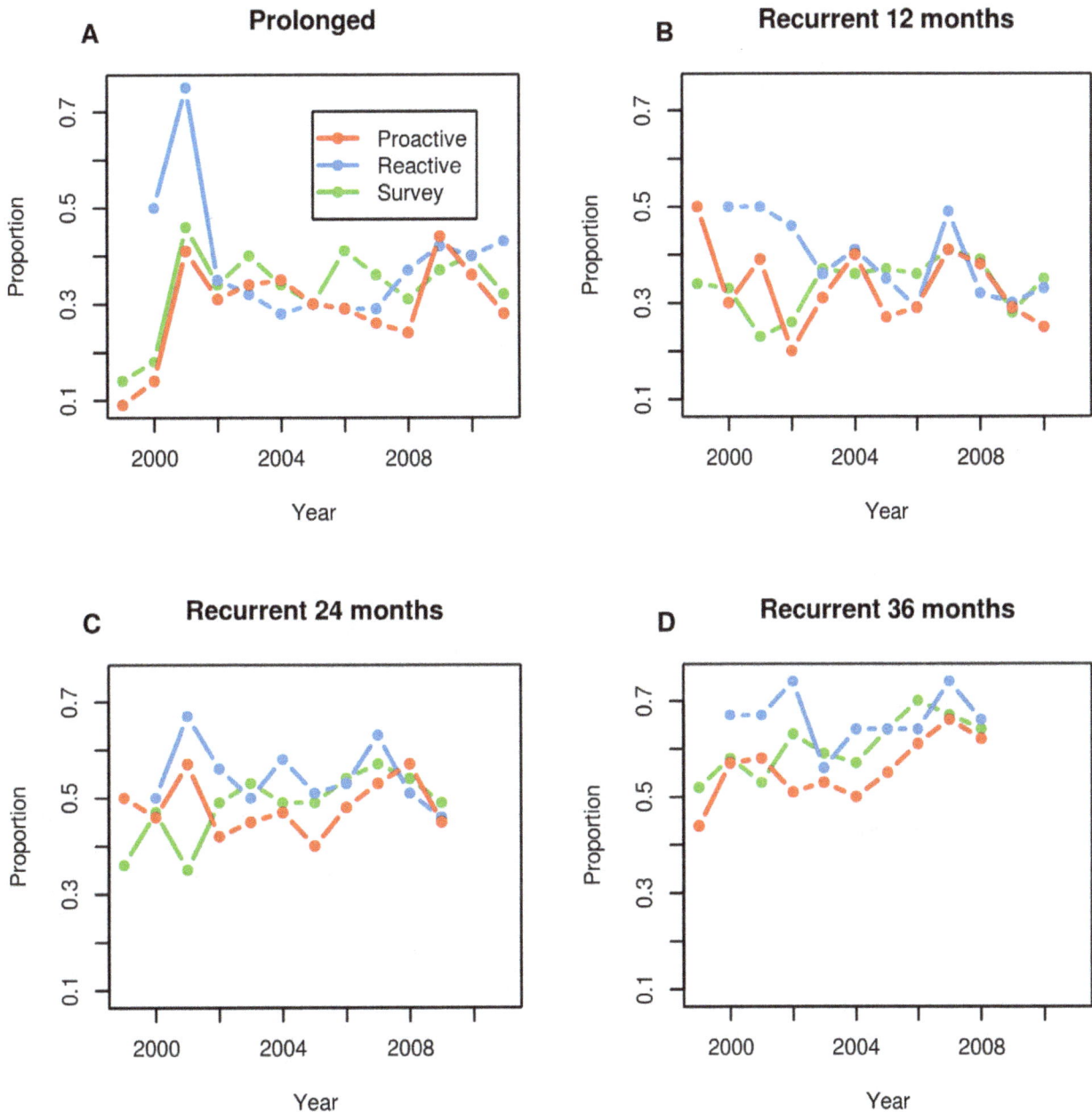

Figure 1. Plot showing the proportions of breakdowns starting in each year for each persistence category, stratified by culling treatment. Panels show prolonged breakdowns (**A**), recurrent breakdowns at 12 months (**B**), recurrent breakdowns at 24 months (**C**) and recurrent breakdowns at 36 months (**D**).

reason why the reactive areas should have been disproportionately affected by FMD compared to the other areas. It is also worth noting that the sample sizes at these earlier time points is much smaller than at later time points (Table S2), and it is possible that the observed effect may simply be due to an artefact of the small sample size. However, we note that this should also be reflected in the uncertainty in the parameter estimates.

In terms of breakdown recurrence, we found a small decrease in the odds of recurrence at 24 and 36 months (ORs and 96% C.I.s of 0.82 [0.64–1.0] and 0.69 [0.54–0.86] respectively) in the proactively culled core areas in the period during the culling. These beneficial effects consequently reduced in the period subsequent to the cull. No notable impact of culling on recurrence

was observed in the buffer zones. Recent work on the mechanisms of recurrence [41] suggest that due to the testing regime imposed upon a herd as a result of a breakdown, it is likely that re-introduction of infection (rather than persistence of infection within a herd) is the main driver of recurrence. To this end a large reduction in badger density, such as was observed in the proactively culled areas [38], would be consistent with a reduced risk of re-introduction of infection by badgers into cattle herds. However, re-infection by badgers is only one possible source of re-introduction of infection into a herd, with cattle movements being the other main potential source.

Some work has been conducted exploring the relative impacts of cattle movements and localised sources on between-herd transmission of bTB [42], however the relative contributions of cattle-to-cattle and badger-to-cattle transmission have not yet been accurately quantified, though work has been done towards modelling these interactions [43]. Certainly if cattle-to-cattle transmission was responsible for a larger degree of cattle infection than badger-to-cattle transmission, then this would be consistent with the observation that proactive culling reduces the risk of recurrence by a relatively small degree in the first instance, before the beneficial effects tail off.

The optimal control policies directed at an individual farm to reduce breakdown prolongation and recurrence, for which an individual farmer will have a vested interest, might be quite different to the optimal policies aimed at reducing incidence across a wider area. Since it is likely that future culling would be at the farmer's expense (the Government wildlife unit that performed the culling during the RBCT has since been disbanded), the financial cost, as well as the time that farmers would have to outlay for culling operations, should be weighed against any potential beneficial/detrimental effects of the culling.

This work could be extended to examine the spatial relationships of whether localised (reactive) culling leads to prolongation or recurrence on the farm itself, and/or on contiguous farms. This might give further insight for policymakers regarding the spatial scale of effects of localised culling on persistence, and may shed more light on potential biological mechanisms regarding the interaction between badger culling and persistence.

Conclusions

Our results suggest that a future culling policy that mirrored the proactive strategy used in the RBCT may have a marginal effect on reducing the degree of recurrence in the short-term, but this benefit is unlikely to extend much further beyond the end of the culling period. In contrast, a reactive strategy, such as that used in the RBCT, would most likely increase the average duration of breakdowns in the short-term, with little impact on reducing recurrence. These detrimental effects are unlikely to last in the long-term. In order to have any beneficial impact on recurrence, albeit most likely marginal, any culling strategy would have to mirror more closely the proactive treatment. These findings should be considered alongside those from other studies if badger culling is to form part of the future bTB control programme for cattle in GB.

Supporting Information

Table S1 Parameter estimates and 95% credible intervals from Bayesian model fits.

Table S2 Counts of breakdowns in each persistence category, starting in each year and stratified by treatment group.

Author Contributions

Conceived and designed the experiments: KK AJKC AM RSC-H CAD JLNW TJM. Performed the experiments: KK AJKC JLNW TJM. Analyzed the data: KK AJKC JLNW TJM. Wrote the paper: KK AJKC AM RSC-H PU CAD JLNW TJM. Instrumental in collating and providing the data: AM PU.

References

1. Defra (2005) Government strategic framework for the sustainable control of bovine tuberculosis (bTB) in Great Britain. Available:http://www.archive.defra.gov.uk/foodfarm/farmanimal/diseases/atoz/tb/documents/tb-strategicframework.pdf. Accessed: 7 April 2011.
2. Defra (2005) Report by the Independent Scientific Review Group on TB in cattle and badgers. Available:http://www.archive.defra.gov.uk/foodfarm/farmanimal/diseases/atoz/tb/publications/krebs.htm. Accessed: 7 April 2011.
3. Corner LA, Murphy D, Gormley E (2010) *Mycobacterium bovis* infection in the Eurasian Badger (*Meles meles*): the disease, pathogenesis, epidemiology and control. J Comp Pathol 144: 1–24.
4. Defra (2010) Bovine Tuberculosis: The Government's approach to tackling the disease and consultation on a badger control policy. Available:http://archive.defra.gov.uk/corporate/consult/tb-control-measures/100915-tb-control-measures-condoc.pdf. Accessed 1 April 2011.
5. Karolemeas K, McKinley TJ, Clifton-Hadley RS, Goodchild AV, Mitchell A, et al. (2010) Predicting prolonged bovine tuberculosis breakdowns in Great Britain as an aid to control. Preventive Veterinary Medicine 97: 183–190. doi:10.1016/j.prevetmed.2010.09.007.
6. Karolemeas K, McKinley TJ, Clifton-Hadley RS, Goodchild AV, Mitchell A, et al. (2010) Recurrence of bovine tuberculosis breakdowns in Great Britain: risk factors and prediction. Preventive Veterinary Medicine: 22–29. doi:10.1016/j.prevetmed.2011.06.004.
7. Farm Crisis Network (2009) Stress and Loss: A report on the impact of TB on farming families. Available:www.farmcrisisnetwork.co.uk/file_download/60. Accessed: 1 April 2011.
8. Griffin JM, Hahesy T, Lynch K, Salman MD, McCarthy J, et al. (1993) The association of cattle husbandry practices, environmental factors and farmer characteristics with the occurrence of chronic bovine tuberculosis in dairy herds in the Republic of Ireland. Preventive Veterinary Medicine 17: 145–160.
9. Christiansen KH, O'Keefe JO, Harrington BP, McDonald EP, Duggan MJ, et al. (1992) A case-control study of herds which fail the tuberculin test six months after being derestricted for tuberculosis. Tuberculosis Investigation Unit, University College, Dublin. p45–48.
10. Reilly LA, Courtenay O (2007) Husbandry practices, badger sett density and habitat composition as risk factors for transient and persistent bovine tuberculosis on UK cattle farms. Preventive Veterinary Medicine 80: 129–142.
11. Defra (2005) Bovine TB: History of badger controls. Available:http://archive.defra.gov.uk/foodfarm/farmanimal/diseases/atoz/tb/abouttb/atbreview.htm. Accessed 7 April 2011.
12. Eves JA (1999) Impact of badger removal on bovine tuberculosis in east County Offaly. Irish Veterinary Journal 52: 199–203.
13. Griffin JM, Williams DH, Kelly GE, Clegg TA, O'Boyle I, et al. (2005) The impact of badger removal on the control of tuberculosis in cattle herds in Ireland. Preventive Veterinary Medicine 67: 237–266.
14. Bourne J, Donnelly C, Cox D, Gettinby G, McInerney J, et al. (2007) Bovine TB: the scientific evidence. Independent Scientific Group on Cattle TB. Available:http://www.defra.gov.uk/foodfarm/farmanimal/diseases/atoz/tb/isg/report/final_report.pdf. Accessed: 1 April 2011.
15. Donnelly CA, Woodroffe R, Cox DR, Bourne J, Gettinby G, et al. (2003) Impact of localized badger culling on tuberculosis incidence in British cattle. Nature 426: 834–837.
16. Donnelly, C A., Wei G, Johnston WT, Cox DR, Woodroffe R, et al. (2007) Impacts of widespread badger culling on cattle tuberculosis: concluding analyses from a large-scale field trial. Int J Infect Dis 11: 300–308.
17. Jenkins HE, Woodroffe R, Donnelly CA (2010) The duration of the effects of repeated widespread badger culling on cattle tuberculosis following the cessation of culling. PLoS One 5: e9090.
18. Vial F, Johnston WT, Donnelly CA (2011) Local cattle and badger populations affect the risk of confirmed tuberculosis in British cattle herds. PLoS One 6: e18058. doi:10.1371/journal.pone.0018058.
19. W.T Johnston, G Gettinby, D.R Cox, C.A Donnelly, J Bourne, et al. (2005) Herd-level risk factors associated with tuberculosis breakdowns among cattle herds in England before the 2001 foot-and-mouth disease epidemic. Biology Letters 1: 53–56. doi:10.1098/rsbl.2004.0249.
20. King D (2007) Bovine Tuberculosis in Cattle and Badgers: A Report by the Chief Scientific Adviser. Available:http://www.bis.gov.uk/assets/biscore/corporate/migratedD/ec_group/44-07-S_I_on. Accessed: 1 April 2011.
21. Defra (2012) Bovine TB: Pilot areas confirmed. Available:http://www.defra.gov.uk/news/2012/01/19/pilot-areas-confirmed/. Accessed: 31 May 2012.
22. Badger cull postponed (2012). Veterinary Record 171: 413. doi:10.1136/vr.e7175.
23. Defra (2010) Bovine TB: Badger Vaccine Deployment Project. Available:http://www.defra.gov.uk/news/2010/06/24/tbbadger-vaccine/. Accessed: 31 May 2012.
24. Welsh Assembly Government (2012) Badger vaccination in North Pembrokeshire is under way. Available:wales.gov.uk/topics/environmentcountryside/ahw/disease/bovinetuberculosis/?lang=en. Accessed: 5 September 2012.
25. Flavie Vial, Christl A Donnelly (2012) Localized reactive badger culling increases risk of bovine tuberculosis in nearby cattle herds. Biology Letters 8: 50–53. doi:10.1098/rsbl.2011.0554.
26. Cox DR (1955) Some statistical methods connected with a series of events. Journal of the Royal Statistical Society, Series B 17: 129–164.

27. Gelman A, Rubin DB (1992) Inference from iterated simulation using multiple sequences. Statistical Science 7: 457–511.
28. R Core Development Team (2011) R: A Language and Environment for Statistical Computing. Vienna, Austria. p. Available:http://www.R-project.org.
29. Spiegelhalter D, Thomas A, Best N, Lunn D (2003) WinBUGS User Manual, Version 1.4. Available:http://www.mrc-bsu.cam.ac.uk/bugs/welcome.shtml.
30. Sturtz S, Ligges U, Gelman A (2005) R2WinBUGS: A Package for Running WinBUGS from R. Journal of Statistical Software 12: 1–16.
31. Olea-Popelka FJ, White PW, Collins JD, O'Keeffe J, Kelton DF, et al. (2004) Breakdown severity during a bovine tuberculosis episode as a predictor of future herd breakdowns in Ireland. Preventive Veterinary Medicine 63: 163–172. doi:10.1016/j.prevetmed.2004.03.001.
32. Abernethy DA, Graham D, Skuce R, Gordon A, Menzies F, et al. (2010) The Bovine Tuberculosis Eradication Scheme. In Proceedings of Society for Veterinary Epidemiology and Preventive Medicine, Nantes, France: 167–173.
33. Wolfe DM, Berke O, Kelton DF, White PW, More SJ, et al. (2010) From explanation to prediction: A model for recurrent bovine tuberculosis in Irish cattle herds. Preventive Veterinary Medicine 94: 170–177. doi:10.1016/j.prevetmed.2010.02.010.
34. Woodroffe R, Donnelly CA, Jenkins HE, Johnston WT, Cox DR, et al. (2006) Culling and cattle controls influence tuberculosis risk for badgers. Proceedings of the National Academy of Sciences 103: 14713–14717.
35. Woodroffe R, Donnelly CA, Cox DR, Bourne FJ, Cheeseman CL, et al. (2006) Effects of culling on badger (*Meles meles*) spatial organization: implications for the control of bovine tuberculosis. Journal of Applied Ecology 43: 1–10.
36. Jenkins HE, Woodroffe R, Donnelly CA, Cox DR, Johnston WT, et al. (2007) Effects of culling on spatial associations of *Mycobacterium bovis* infections in badgers and cattle. Journal of Applied Ecology 44: 897–908.
37. Woodroffe R, Donnelly CA, Cox DR, Gilks P, Jenkins HE, et al. (2009) Bovine tuberculosis in cattle and badgers in localized culling areas. Journal of Wildlife Diseases 45: 128–143.
38. Woodroffe R, Gilks P, Johnston WT, Le Fevre AM, Cox DR, et al. (2008) Effects of culling on badger abundance: implications for tuberculosis control. Journal of Zoology 274: 28–37.
39. More SJ, Clegg TA, McGrath G, Collins JD, Corner LA, et al. (2007) Does reactive badger culling lead to an increase in tuberculosis? Veterinary Record 161: 208–209.
40. CJ Godfray, RN Curnow, C Dye, D Pfeiffer, WJ Sutherland, et al. (2004) Independent scientific review of the randomised badger culling trial and associated epidemiological research.
41. Conlan AJK, McKinley TJ, Karolemeas K, Brooks Pollock E, Goodchild AV, et al. (2012) Estimating the hidden burden of bovine tuberculosis in Great Britain. PLoS Computational Biology 8: e1002730. doi:10.1371/journal.pcbi.1002730.
42. Green DM, Kiss IZ, Mitchell AP, Kao RR (2008) Estimates for local and movement-based transmission of bovine tuberculosis in British cattle. Proceedings of the Royal Society B: Biological Sciences 275: 1001–1005. doi:10.1098/rspb.2007.1601.
43. Cox DR, Donnelly CA, Bourne FJ, Gettinby G, McInerney JP, et al. (2005) Simple model for tuberculosis in cattle and badgers. Proceedings of the National Academy of Sciences of the United States of America 102: 17588–17593.

8

Canine Lipomas Treated with Steroid Injections: Clinical Findings

Barbara Lamagna[1], Adelaide Greco[2,3,4]*, Anna Guardascione[1], Luigi Navas[1], Manuela Ragozzino[1], Orlando Paciello[5], Arturo Brunetti[2,3,4], Leonardo Meomartino[6]

1 Department of Veterinary Clinical Sciences, Unit of Surgery, University of Naples Federico II, Naples, Italy, 2 Department of Biomorphological and Functional Science, University of Naples Federico II, Naples, Italy, 3 Ceinge, Biotecnologie Avanzate, scarl, Naples, Italy, 4 Institute of Biostructure and Bioimaging, CNR, Naples, Italy, 5 Department of Pathology and Animal Health, Unit of Pathology, University of Naples Federico II, Naples, Italy, 6 Interdepartmental Veterinary Radiology Centre, University of Naples Federico II, Naples, Italy

Abstract

Lipomas are common benign tumours of fat cells. In most cases, surgical excision is curative and simple to perform; however, such a procedure requires general anaesthesia and may be associated with delayed wound healing, seroma formation and nerve injury in deep and intramuscular tumours. The objective of this study was to evaluate treatment of subcutaneous, subfascial or intermuscular lipomas using intralesional steroid injections in dogs. Fifteen dogs presenting with lipomas were selected for treatment with ultrasound-guided intralesional injection of triamcinolone acetonide at a dose of 40 mg/mL. Nine subcutaneous and subfascial tumours showed a complete regression. The other lipomas decreased in diameter, achieving, in some cases, remission of discomfort and regression of lameness. Steroid injection was a relatively safe and effective treatment for lipomas in dogs; only six dogs experienced polyuria/polydipsia for about 2 weeks post-treatment.

Editor: Waldemar Debinski, Wake Forest University, School of Medicine, United States of America

Funding: The authors have no support or funding to report.

Competing Interests: The authors have declared that no competing interests exist.

* E-mail: adegreco@unina.it

Introduction

Lipomas occur approximately in about 16% of dogs [1]. They are benign tumors of fat cells, most common in adult female or elderly obese dogs [2].

Lipomas usually occur as solitary masses, but multiple lipomas can also occur in dogs. These tumours are frequently localised in the subcutaneous tissues but may extend intramuscularly or along deep fascial planes; a non-infiltrative lipoma has been described that can occur intermuscularly in the caudal thigh region [3] or in the thoracic limb, almost in the axilla [4]. Deep lipomas often have a paratesticular location [5]. They have occasionally been described within the thorax and the abdomen, causing clinical signs associated with organ compression [6–8]. The occurrence of a thymolipoma has been reported in one dog [9] and of thymofibrolipomas in two dogs [10]. Infiltrative lipomas have also been recognised in dogs, appearing histologically as benign adipocytes invading the muscle, the fascia, and occasionally the bone [11–14]. Diagnosis of lipoma is provided only by cytology or biopsy with histological evaluation [1].

Many lipomas are asymptomatic, can be diagnosed with cytological examination and do not require any treatment; however, some tumours may elicit discomfort in dogs due to nerve compression, or, especially if they become large enough, cause functional difficulties [1]. One report described a case of a dog exhibiting lameness secondary to the carpal canal compression [15]. Usually, owners concerned about the growth and appearance

of tumours and discomfort to their animals request to have lipomas removed.

In most cases, surgical excision is curative and simple to perform; however, it requires general anaesthesia and may be associated with the risk of delayed wound healing, seroma formation and nerve injury in deep and intermuscular lesions. It has been reported that intralesional injections of 10% calcium chloride solution cause lipoma regression, but this treatment is not recommended because irritation and skin necrosis can occur [16]. Minimally invasive liposuction of a giant lipoma in one dog [17], and irradiation of infiltrative lipomas in 13 dogs have been reported [18]; however, these procedures require general anaesthesia and special devices. In a recent retrospective study of 20 dogs, dry liposuction was effective in preventive the growth of existing lipomas less than 15 cm in diameter, while giant lipomas associated with fibrous trabeculae could not be easily removed and attempts at removal resulted in a high risk of bruising, hematoma and seroma; furthermore, regrowth of tumours was observed in 28% of lipomas treated with liposuction at follow-up between 9 and 36 months [19].

Recent clinical experiences indicate that the use of subcutaneous deoxycholate injections may be a relatively safe and effective treatment for small lipomas, although controlled clinical trials are necessary to substantiate these observations [20]. Recently, the use of a subdermal 1064-nm Nd: YAG laser resulted in complete or almost complete removal of lipoma in 100% of patients [21]. In human patients, there is only about one report that describes intralesional injection of steroids to treat lipomas non invasively

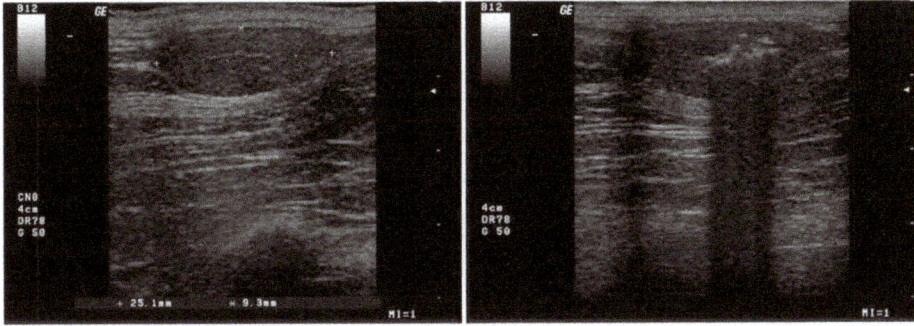

Figure 1. Ultrasound images of an untreated and a treated lipoma. A - An oval sub-fascial lipoma in the right axillary region. A well defined hyperechoic capsule is visible; a hypoechoic homogeneous echostructure interrupted by thin stripes is observed. **B** – The lipoma after infiltration of the steroid solution.

[22]. The present study was designed to evaluate the results of treatment of subcutaneous, subfascial, intermuscular or infiltrative lipoma in dogs using steroidal intralesional injections.

Methods

Our study was reviewed by the committee for experimental animal health at the University of Naples Federico II. The committee stated that the protocol was configured as a Veterinary Medical Diagnostic clinical trial as described in paragraph 3 of article 7 of DL 116/92, which refers to legal obligations of the investigators. Therefore, it was not submitted to the Ministry of Health that normally accompanies each experimental protocol but it was presented as summary activity to the Public Local Health Utility Napoli 1 Center. We confirmed that all animal procedures in this study were conducted by a veterinarian and conformed to all regulations protecting animals used for research purposes, including national guidelines (DL 116/92) as well as the protocols recommended by Workman, et al. (1998).

We enrolled dogs not treated previously for lipoma whose owners sought an alternative treatment to surgery. All dogs underwent laboratory tests to determine their general medical condition. No dogs selected presented with major clinical signs of illness. Written informed consent was obtained from each owner. No anaesthesia or sedation was necessary during the procedures, and no signs of discomfort were observed in dogs during the treatment.

Fifteen dogs referred with subcutaneous, subfascial or inter-muscular lipomas and one infiltrative lipoma were selected for this study.

The diagnosis of lipoma was made in all cases on the basis of a physical examination (superficial, well-circumscribed soft mass), ultrasonographic features of the mass (oval or irregularly pedunculated shape, generally with a defined capsule, and with a homogeneous thin striped echo-pattern) and confirmed with Fine Needle Aspiration cytology (FNAC).

For the cytological examination, the samples were spread on glass slides, air-dried and stained with a May-Gruwald Quick stain (Bio-Optica, Milano). The slides were observed with an optical microscope (Nikon, E600) at different magnifications. Ultrasound examination was performed with an 11-MHz linear transducer with a footprint of 4 cm and a scan depth of 6 cm (Logiq MD400, General Electric).

Lipomas were injected with triamcinolone acetonide 40 mg/ml (kenacort®; Bristol-Myers Squibb). A 1-mL or 2-mL syringe with a 22-gauge needle was used to inject the solution transcutaneously at the centre of the lipoma guided by ultrasound. The volume of the steroid injection depended on the size of the lesion: 0.5 mL for small lipomas (<3 cm in diameter); 1 mL for large lipomas (>3 cm in diameter). When the lipoma measured more than 3 cm, two injections of 0.5 mL were made in two sites along the major axis of the lesion. If there were no signs of lipoma regression, the procedure was repeated one month later.

Measurements of tumours were performed by ultrasound before treatment, and 1 and 6 months later. If complications occurred after treatment, they were recorded by the owners and reported at the subsequent visit.

Results

A total of 15 lipomas (9 subcutaneous, 3 subfascial, 2 intermuscular, 1 infiltrative) in 15 dogs (9 mixed, 6 purebred dogs, mean age 8 year, 4 male, 11 female) were injected with 0.5 mL (10 cases) or 1 mL (5 cases) of triamcinolone acetonide (Tab 1).

For all cases, diagnoses of lipomas originally identified by clinical evaluation and ultrasound were confirmed by cytological examination; lipomas showed histological evidence of normal

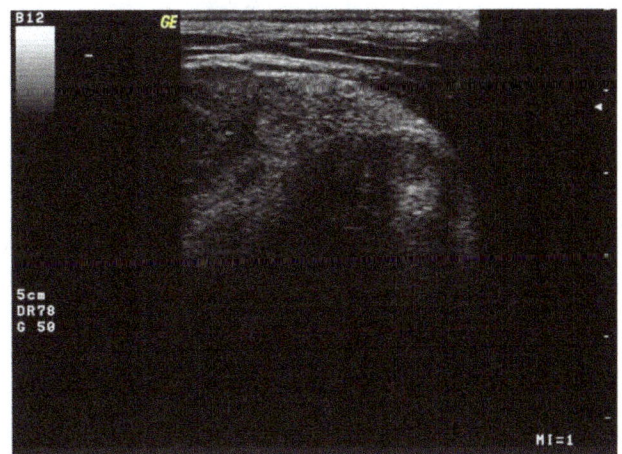

Figure 2. Ultrasound image of an intermuscolar lipoma. An intermuscular lipoma of the caudal region, ultrasonographically appearing hyperechoic and heterogeneous; the capsule is clearly appreciable.

Table 1. Steroid injections in 15 dogs.

Dog No Breed	Weight Kg, sex	Age years	Site (clinical signs)	Pre-treatment major diameter (mm)	First injection Triamcinolone (mg)	Posttreatment major diameter (mm) after 1 month	Second injection Triamcinolone (mg)	Side Effects
1 Mixed	15 obese, F	7	Right Flank Subcutaneus	25.5	20 mg	Regressed after 1 week	No	Polyuria/polydipsia
2 Schnautzer	35, F	14	Ventral Neck Subcutaneous	49.9	40 mg	4.9×28.5	40 mg	None
3 Pit bull	37 obese, M	8	Right Axillary Subfascial	25.1	20 mg	Regressed after 1 week	No	Polyuria/polydipsia
4 Yorkshire	5, F	10	Left Perineal Infiltrative (discomfort)	70.3	40 mg (in two sites)	62 (more soft after 1 week resolution of discomfort)	20 mg (in two sites)	Polyuria/polydipsia
5 German Shepherd	24, F	3	Right Lumbar Subfascial	43	40 mg	Regressed after 1 week	No	None
6 Mixed	17 obese, F	14	Left rump intermuscular Gluteal MM (Lameness)	45.5	40 mg (in two sites)	Regressed for 9 months then recurred more soft (resolution of lameness)	No	None
7 Dalmatian	20, Mn	13	Xiphoid Subcutaneous	29.7	20 mg	Regressed after 1 week	No	None
8 Mixed	18 obese, Fn	6	Xiphoid Subcutaneous	45	20 mg	27 (Unchanged after 1 year)	No (Owners refused)	Polyuria/polydipsia
9 Mixed	15, Fn	10	Inguinal Subcutaneous	38.5	20 mg	19	No (Owners refused)	Polyuria/polydipsia
10 Rottweiler	45, M	6	Right Flank Subcutaneous	25	20 mg	Regressed after 1 week		None
11 Mixed	25, Fn	7	Left Lumbar Subfascial	30	20 mg	Regressed after 1 week		None
12 Mixed	15 obese, F	7	Rigt rump Intermuscolar Gluteal MM (Lameness)	50.5	40 mg (in two sites)	30.3 (More soft. After 1 week resolution of lameness)	20 mg (in two sites)	Polyuria/polydipsia
13 Mixed	15 obese, Fn	8	Right Flank Subcutaneous	24.8	20 mg	Regressed after 1 week	No	Polyuria/polydipsia
14 Mixed	28, M	8	Ventral Neck Subcutaneous	28.2	20 mg	Regressed after 1 week	No	None
15 Mixed	23, M	10	Left Flank Subcutaneous	27.4	20 mg	Regressed after 1 week	No	None

Note: (F = female, Fn = neutered female, M = male, Mn = neutered male).

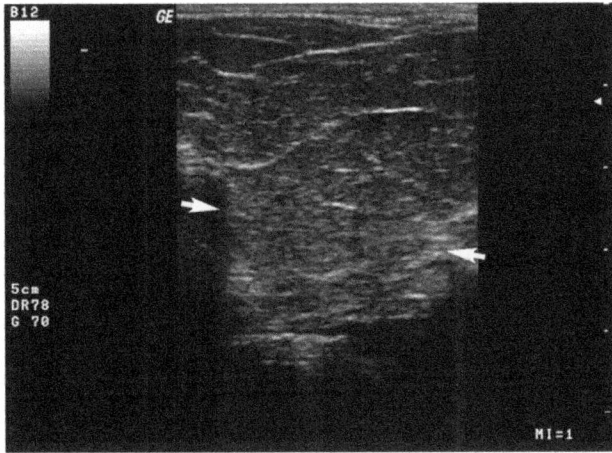

Figure 3. Ultrasound image of perineal lipoma. An infiltrative perineal lipoma, ultrasonographically appearing hypoechoic and multi-lobulated because of thin hyperechoic lines; a thin limiting capsule is visible (arrows).

adipocities on a proteinaceous, bluish background, and, in some cases, aggregated around a blood vessel.

After one injection, nine lipomas (six subcutaneous and three subfascial) regressed completely by 6 months follow up. Before the steroid injection, the above-mentioned lipomas showed the following ultrasound features: a hyperechoic capsule, a poorly vascularised hypoechoic or isoechoic echotexture (1 case) with thin hyperechoic stripes homogeneously distributed throughout (fig. 1).

One intermuscular lipoma (dog no. 6) regressed completely after one steroid injection, but, after nine months, recurred, although softer and without any lameness (Table 1). Sonograph-ically, this lipoma appeared hyperechoic, moderately dishomoge-neous with a well defined capsule (fig. 2).

Another intermuscular lipoma (dog no. 12) after the first injection partially reduced its size and consistence, with regression of lameness, while a second steroid injection produced further reduction (to less than 50% of the original size).This lipoma was sonographically characterized by a poor vascularized hypoechoic (in comparison with muscles) echotexture, and it appeared to be lobulated.

Larger tumors (subcutaneous tumors located on the neck, on the xiphoid region and on the inguinal region) were partially reduced in size and consistency after the first injection. In the lipoma located on the neck the second steroid injection produced further reduction (to less than 50% of the original size), but after one year, the lipoma returned to its original size. Upon ultrasound examination, the mass appeared isoechoic to the surroundings fat tissues, capsulated, and with a homogeneous thin hyperechoic striped echotexture interrupted by a hypoechoic core showing a mild peripheral vascularity. After 2 years, the lipoma exhibited no alterations in its consistency or size.

An infiltrative perineal lipoma was reduced in size by 70% and in firmness after a second steroid injection, but exhibited a mild increase in size after 10 months. According to the owners, the dog was finally treated with surgical excision of the mass. At surgery, an infiltration of the lipoma into the surrounding tissues was evident. After 2 years post-surgery, the lipoma recurred, but at this time the owners refused further treatment. Upon ultrasound examination, the infiltrative lipoma appeared to be hypoechoic and multilobulated due to the presence of hyperechoic intrale-

sional lines; the tumour displayed a thin capsule poorly defined due to deep pedunculations (fig. 3).

After the first injection of triamcinolone, only six dogs showed secondary effects of polyuria/polydipsia for about 15 days. We observed temporary polyuria/polydipsia in one dog with a weight of less than 8 Kg (small sized dogs) and in five dogs with weights between 8 Kg and 20 Kg (medium sized dogs). No side effects were observed in dogs with weights greater than 20 Kg (large sized dogs) using the described dosage. Treated dogs showed no signs of discomfort.

Discussion

Steroid injections have the potential to be a safe and effective treatment for small lipomas in dogs. We demonstrated that small lipomas (<3 cm in diameter) and also one of the larger lipomas (>3 cm in diameter) regressed completely after the treatment. The remaining large lipomas (3 subcutaneous, 1 infiltrative, and 2 intermuscular) became less firm and decreased in size. Larger tumours in this study responded less successfully to treatment than smaller tumours, most likely due to the inability of the drug to be distributed throughout the tumour. We recommend that patients with this type of larger tumour undergo surgery. When comparing various available treatments, surgery is generally considered the gold standard, but it has disadvantages, such as the requirement of general anaesthesia.

In our experience, local steroid injection guided by ultrasound achieves reduction of discomfort in dogs with large lipomas and never requires sedation. This treatment could be considered an alternative to surgical excision in older animals that are not candidates for general anaesthesia or deep sedation, and for animals presenting at shows. Previous descriptions of the ultrasonographic appearance of superficial lipomas in dogs [5,23,24] are in accordance with our findings. Usually, the ultrasonographic appearance of a lipoma is quite characteristic and easily recognisable as a homogeneous, hypo-isoechoic, capsulated mass, possibly lobulated by thin hyperechoic septa. However, in our sample, one of the intermuscular lipomas displayed a hyperechoic heterogeneous echotexture not common in lipomas. In a report of five cases of infiltrative lipomas in dogs, the masses displayed different echogenicities and echotextures [11], and authors stated that ultrasound was not able to diagnose and visualise the full extent of infiltrative lipomas. Therefore, we conclude that ultrasound examination may have a lower specificity in diagnosing infiltrative and intermuscular lipomas.

It is well known that other drugs such as insulin, antibiotics and methothrexate could also cause localised lipodystrophy in the injection site [25]. The exact mechanism behind the regression of tumours after steroid injections is still unknown. Certain authors reported on the cases of two patients with localised involutional lipoatrophy [26]. These patients received intramuscular steroid injections and immunohistochemical studies with anti-macrophage antibodies (anti-CD68 antigen) showed positive cells scattered around blood vessels and shrunken lipocytes in subcutaneous tissues. Yamamoto T et al (2002) reported on the cases of six patients with localised lipoatrophy characterised by a depressed plaque at the injection sites of corticosteroids [27]. In another report, a case of involutional lipoatrophy was observed post-steroid injection in a 53-year-old woman. Ultrastructural evidence of macrophages in close proximity to altered adipocytes was observed; in addition, macrophages displayed an activated phenotype and were observed engulfing segments of altered adipose and stromal tissue [28].

On the basis of the aforementioned studies, we postulated that steroid injection in the canine lipoma could stimulate an inflammatory response with secondary macrophage activation and production of cytokines. However, to assess the exact mechanism of canine lipid atrophy, it could be useful to perform serial biopsies during the treatment.

Our investigation was conducted choosing an average dosage of triamcinolone acetonide related to the dosage recommended in human patients and derived based on the size of the lipoma [22]. It would be useful to identify the minimum effective dose of steroids on the basis of body weight or body surface area units to prevent side effects in small-breed dogs. Perhaps, in order to reduce complications in dogs with weights less than 20 Kg, several monthly injections of smaller volumes of steroid could be safer than a single injection of steroid as we tested in our protocol.

Conclusions

Although the exact mechanism of action is still unclear, it appears that steroidal intra-lesional injections may constitute a safe and effective treatment for small collections of fat in dogs.

To prevent any complications, it would be useful to calculate the volume of drug based on the size of dogs and the size of the lipoma.

Author Contributions

Conceived and designed the experiments: LM BL. Performed the experiments: BL LM OP. Analyzed the data: LM BL A. Guardascione. Contributed reagents/materials/analysis tools: ML LN MR A. Greco. Wrote the paper: LM A. Greco AB.

References

1. Randall C, Fox T, Fox LE (1998) Tumors of the skin and subcutis. In: Wallace B M editor. Cancer in Dogs and Cats, medical and surgical management. Philadelphia: Lippincott Williams & Wilkins. pp. 489–510.
2. Goldsmith MH, Hendrick MJ (2003) Tumors of the skin and soft tissues. In: Meuten DJ editor: Tumors in domestic animals, Lowa State Press: Blackwell. pp. 45–117.
3. Thomson MJ, Withrow SJ, Dernell WS, Powers BE (1999) Intermuscular lipomas of the thigh region in dogs: 11 cases. J Am Anim Hosp Assoc. 35 (2): 165–7
4. Case JB, MacPhail CM, Withrow SJ (2012) Anatomic distribution and clinical findings of intermuscular lipomas in 17 dogs (2005–2010). J Am Anim Hosp Assoc 48 (4): 245–9.
5. Volta A, Bonazzi M, Gnudi G, Gazzola M, Bertoni G (2006) Ultrasonographic features of canine lipoma. Veterinary Radiology & Ultrasound 47(6): 589–591.
6. Mc Laughlin R, Kuzma AB (1991) Intestinal strangulation caused by intra-abdominal lipoma in a dog. J Am Vet Med Assoc 199: 1610–1.
7. Mayhew PD, Brockman DJ (2002) Body cavity lipoma in six dogs. J Small Anim Pract 43: 177–181.
8. Miles J, Clarke D (2001) Intrathoracic lipoma in a Labrador retriever. J Small Anim Pract 42: 26–28.
9. Ramìrez GA, Spattini G, Altimira J, Garcìa B, Vilafranca M (2008) Clinical and histopathological features of a thymolipoma in a dog. J Vet Diagn Invest 20 (3): 360–4.
10. Morini M, Bettini G, Diana A, Spadai A, Casadio Tozzi A, et al. (2009) Thymofibrolipoma in two dogs. J Comp Pathos 141 (1): 74–7.
11. McChesney AE, Stephens LC, Lebel J, Snyder S, Ferguson HR (1980) Infiltrative lipoma in dogs. Vet Pathol 17: 316–322.
12. Bergman PJ, Withrow SJ, Straw RC, Powers BE (1994) Infiltrative lipoma in dogs: 16 cases (1981–1992). J Am Vet Med Assoc 205: 322–4.
13. Kramek BA, Spackman CJA, Hayden DW (1985). Infiltrative lipoma in three dogs. J Am Vet Med Assoc 186: 81–3.
14. Frazier KS, Herron AJ, Dee JF, Altman NH (1993) Infiltrative lipoma in a canine stifle joint. J Am Anim Hosp Assoc 29: 81–3.
15. Szabo D, Ryan T, Scott HW (2011) Carpal canal lipoma causing lameness in a dog. Vet Comp Orthop Traumatol 4: 299–302.
16. Albers GW, Theilen GH (1985) Calcium chloride for treatment of subcutaneous lipoma in dogs. JAVMA 186: 492–494.
17. Böttcher P, Klüter S, Krastel D, Grevel V (2007) Liposuction-removal of giant lipomas for weight loss in a dog with severe hip osteoarthritis. JSAP, 48: 46–48
18. McEntee MC, Page RL, Mauldin GN, Thrall DE (2000) Results of irradiation of infiltrative lipoma in 13 dogs. Vet Radiol Ultrasound 41: 554–556.
19. Hunt GB, Wong J, Kuan S. (2011) Liposuction for removal of lipomas in 20 dogs. J Small Anim Practice 52: 419–425.
20. Rotunda AM, Ablon G, Kolodney MS (2005) Lipoma treated with subcutaneous deoxycholate injections. J Am Acad Dermatol 53: 973–8.
21. Goldman A, Wollina U (2009) Lipoma treatment with a subdermal Nd:YAG laser technique. Int J Dermatol 48: 1228–1232.
22. Salam. Gohar A (2002) Lipoma Excision. American Family Physician 65 (5): 901–905.
23. Samii VF, Long CD (2002) Muskoloskeletal system. In: Nyland TG, Mattoon JS editors. Small animal diagnostic ultrasound. Philadelphia: WB Saunders Company. pp. 267–284.
24. Nyman HT, Kristensen AT, Lee MH, Martinussen T, Mcevoy FJ (2006) Characterization of canine superficial tumors using gray-scale B mode, color flow mapping, and spectral doppler ultrasonography- A multivariate study. Vet Radiol Ultrasound 47(2):192–8.
25. Herranz P, De Lucas R, Pérez E, Mayor M (2008) Lipodystrophy Syndromes. Dermatol Clin 26: 569–578.
26. Hisamichi K, Suga Y, Hashimoto Y, Matsuba S, Mizoguchi M, et al. (2002) Two Japanese cases of localized involutional lipoatrophy. Int J Dermatol 41 (3): 176–7.
27. Yamamoto T, Yokozeki H, Nishioka K (2002) Localized involutional lipoatrophy: report of six cases. J Dermatol 29 (10):638–43.
28. Iftikhar A (2006) Post-Injection Involutional Lipoatrophy: Ultrastructural Evidence for an activated Macrophage Phenotype and Macrophage Related Involution of Adipocytes. Am J Dermatopathol (4):334–337.

9

How Does Reviewing the Evidence Change Veterinary Surgeons' Beliefs Regarding the Treatment of Ovine Footrot? A Quantitative and Qualitative Study

Helen M. Higgins[1]*, Laura E. Green[2], Martin J. Green[1], Jasmeet Kaler[1]

1 School of Veterinary Medicine and Science, University of Nottingham, Sutton Bonington, Leicestershire, United Kingdom, 2 School of Life Sciences, University of Warwick, Coventry, West Midlands, United Kingdom

Abstract

Footrot is a widespread, infectious cause of lameness in sheep, with major economic and welfare costs. The aims of this research were: (i) to quantify how veterinary surgeons' beliefs regarding the efficacy of two treatments for footrot changed following a review of the evidence (ii) to obtain a consensus opinion following group discussions (iii) to capture complementary qualitative data to place their beliefs within a broader clinical context. Grounded in a Bayesian statistical framework, probabilistic elicitation (roulette method) was used to quantify the beliefs of eleven veterinary surgeons during two one-day workshops. There was considerable heterogeneity in veterinary surgeons' beliefs before they listened to a review of the evidence. After hearing the evidence, seven participants quantifiably changed their beliefs. In particular, two participants who initially believed that foot trimming with topical oxytetracycline was the better treatment, changed to entirely favour systemic and topical oxytetracycline instead. The results suggest that a substantial amount of the variation in beliefs related to differences in veterinary surgeons' knowledge of the evidence. Although considerable differences in opinion still remained after the evidence review, with several participants having non-overlapping 95% credible intervals, both groups did achieve a consensus opinion. Two key findings from the qualitative data were: (i) veterinary surgeons believed that farmers are unlikely to actively seek advice on lameness, suggesting a proactive veterinary approach is required (ii) more attention could be given to improving the way in which veterinary advice is delivered to farmers. In summary this study has: (i) demonstrated a practical method for probabilistically quantifying how veterinary surgeons' beliefs change (ii) revealed that the evidence that currently exists is capable of changing veterinary opinion (iii) suggested that improved transfer of research knowledge into veterinary practice is needed (iv) identified some potential obstacles to the implementation of veterinary advice by farmers.

Editor: Bernhard Kaltenboeck, Auburn University, United States of America

Funding: HMH is funded by a Wellcome Trust clinical research training fellowship [087797/Z/08/Z] (http://www.wellcome.ac.uk). The School of Veterinary Medicine and Science, University of Nottingham, United Kingdom provided additional funding (http://www.nottingham.ac.uk/vet/index.aspx). The funders had no role in study design, data collection and analysis, decision to publish, or preparation of the manuscript.

Competing Interests: Some of co-authors own published work (JK, LEG) was included in the review of the evidence that was presented to the veterinary surgeons in this study. To minimize any impact, including the possibility of inhibiting participants from critically appraising and debating the evidence presented, the power point containing the evidence was delivered to participants by HMH, in the absence of either JK or LEG. Similarly, the group discussions were facilitated by HMH, in the absence of either JK/LEG. HMH took no part in producing any of the evidence presented in the review.

* E-mail: helen.higgins@nottingham.ac.uk

Introduction

The UK national flock comprises 14 million breeding ewes and the mean prevalence of lameness in ewe flocks has been estimated to be 8–10% [1,2]. Lameness costs the UK sheep industry 24 million pounds per annum [3], and is a welfare problem. Footrot is a contagious bacterial disease caused by *Dichelobacter nodosus* and it is responsible for over 80% of lameness in sheep. In the UK, farmers have traditionally treated footrot by paring the hoof horn (foot trimming) [2] and spraying the foot with a topical antibacterial. However, evidence from recent studies suggest that treatment with a parenteral long acting antibacterial cures over 90% of cases of footrot in 3 to 10 days [4–6]; in contrast, only 30% of sheep treated by foot trimming recovered within 10 days [4]. Prompt treatment with systemic antibacterial therapy can reduce the flock prevalence of lameness from 6%–8% to 2% [6].

Assuming the results from this study [6] are generalizable, then if this treatment were adopted by all sheep farmers the national prevalence of lameness would fall and the welfare of sheep would be improved. The Farm Animal Welfare Council published a recommendation in 2011 that 'the prevalence of lameness in flocks farmed in Great Britain should be reduced to 5% or less within 5 years as an interim target, and to 2% or less, (which is already possible with best practice) within 10 years' [7].

Veterinary surgeons working in private practice are ideally placed to advise and help farmers reduce lameness in sheep. A Bayesian approach was used to assess the current diversity and strength of beliefs amongst veterinary surgeons, and to quantify how presenting a review of the current evidence base influenced their opinions. In this statistical framework, probability is defined subjectively as a personal degree of belief [8]. Specifically, we used probabilistic elicitation to capture veterinary surgeons' clinical beliefs numerically as probability distributions. An extensive literature exists on probabilistic elicitation; it is integral to Bayesian statistics and has been applied in a wide variety of fields [9], although only a few studies have used this technique in a veterinary context. Furthermore, to the authors' knowledge, there are currently no peer-reviewed papers that have used this method to probabilistically assess how veterinary surgeons' beliefs change in light of a review of the evidence base.

To understand why veterinary surgeons' beliefs alter (or why they do not) requires qualitative information to augment the quantitative methodology. Qualitative information also helps to place veterinary beliefs regarding treatment efficacy in a broader clinical context and facilitates the identification of possible obstacles to the implementation of recommendations to farmers, from a veterinary perspective. Knowing these obstacles is useful so that veterinary advice can be offered to farmers in a way that they are likely to adopt; farmers will have their own beliefs regarding treatment outcomes and are faced with the practical challenges of implementing any treatment.

The aims of this research were: (i) to use probabilistic elicitation to quantify how veterinary beliefs regarding the efficacy of two treatments for footrot changed following a review of the current evidence (ii) to obtain a consensus opinion following group discussions (iii) to capture complementary qualitative data, including advice regarding treatments for footrot in general, and approaches to the delivery of advice to farmers.

Methods

1. Ethics Statement

This study was approved by the Research and Ethics Committee at the School of Veterinary Medicine and Science, University of Nottingham, UK. An information sheet was provided to each participant that detailed the research objectives and requirements, and explained that the information gathered would be anonymized and published in the peer reviewed literature. It also explained that participants could stop the task at any point without giving reason; subsequently, voluntary signed consent was obtained from each participant.

2. Identification and Recruitment of Veterinary Surgeons

A selection of 12 veterinary surgeons was made with the following inclusion criteria: (i) at least 2 years and less than 35 years qualified, and (ii) within 4 hours driving distance of Nottingham. Of these 12 veterinary surgeons, 6 were selected using a random number generator (software program R, version 2.10.1, [10]) from the 68 who hold the Royal College of Veterinary Surgeons (RCVS) post-graduate Certificate in Sheep Health and Production (CertSHP). These are subsequently referred to as 'certificate holders'. The remaining 6 veterinary surgeons did not hold a CertSHP, but were acknowledged within the veterinary practice in which they worked to have a demonstrable involvement with the delivery of healthcare to sheep clients, and are referred to as 'non-certificate holders'. To identify these subjects, a random number generator was used to select veterinary practices registered as treating sheep from the RCVS database. Selected practices were contacted by telephone and the project explained; subsequently written details of the study objectives and eligibility criteria were sent by e-mail and practices were asked to confirm if an eligible veterinary surgeon was willing to attend. Potential exclusion criteria for all participants were: (i) unavailable to attend on the relevant date (ii) unwilling/unable to travel to Nottingham (iii) uncomfortable with any aspect of the task: given the nature of the exercise, full engagement and enthusiasm for the process was important for success [9].

3. Definitions of Treatments for Footrot

Our hypothesis was that a diverse spectrum of clinical beliefs currently exists with respect to the efficacy of two treatments for footrot in lame ewes, both of which are currently used in practice. The first treatment we considered was intra-muscular injection of long-acting oxytetracycline antibiotic (correctly dosed for the weight of animal) and topical oxytetracycline spray, with no foot paring performed. This treatment is subsequently referred to as 'systemic and topical oxytetracycline'. The second treatment was foot paring to remove under run horn (by a proficient and experienced person) and topical oxytetracycline spray. This treatment is subsequently referred to as 'foot trimming and topical oxytetracycline'.

4. Data Collection Synopsis

The non-certificate holders attended a workshop held at the University of Nottingham on the 2nd July 2012, and certificate holders attended an analogous event on the 5th July 2012. We ran separate workshops for certificate and non-certificate holders to avoid the possibility that some participants might be inhibited from expressing their opinions in the group discussions if they knew that other members of the group held a CertSHP, when they themselves did not. Both workshops lasted six hours and participants were provided with an inconvenience allowance of £100 per hour (pro-rata) in recognition of the time and travel required to attend the event. Participants were met on arrival and accompanied during the day by an assistant, to avoid debate until the facilitated group discussion. During the workshops, data were collected as follows.

Each veterinary surgeon was interviewed separately for one hour by either HMH or JK. The interview was recorded. The first half of the interview captured qualitative data using a standard script, concerning: (i) characteristics of the veterinary surgeons themselves, including their current clinical ovine workload and their recent appraisal of the evidence regarding footrot (ii) their current clinical approaches to treating footrot in ewes and how it compared to their perceptions of gold standard care (iii) their approaches to monitoring clinical outcomes, and how they deliver their advice to farmers. The second half of the interview captured their beliefs concerning the difference in cure rates between the two treatments for footrot (see Section 3) as probability distributions using probabilistic elicitation. This required the participant to place chips on a laminated sheet to create a histogram that quantified their current belief (see Section 5 for details).

Once all participants had completed their individual interviews, the group listened to a 30 minute power point presented using a standard script. This provided a summary of the current peer-reviewed evidence regarding the treatment of footrot and was written by LEG/JK; selection of the content included is described in Section 6. It should be noted that some of co-authors own research (JK, LEG) was included in the review of the evidence. In recognition of a potential conflict of interest, and to avoid any possibility of inhibiting participants from critically appraising and debating the evidence presented, the power point was delivered to participants by HMH, in the absence of JK and LEG, who were also not present for the remainder of the workshop.

Immediately after this, without any discussion, each participant was presented with their own laminated sheet showing the probability distribution that they had created earlier, during their interview. Participants were asked to re-consider their clinical opinions regarding the two treatments for footrot, in light of the review of the evidence, and to express their beliefs for a second time, in the same format as previously (by placing another set of chips on a new laminated sheet) to quantify their belief after hearing the review of the evidence; if their opinions had not altered, they were asked to simply replicate their original answer. A total of 45 minutes were devoted to this task, and an information sheet summarising the content of the power point presentation and copies of the four key peer-reviewed papers it described were provided to each participant, to enable participants to further appraise the information themselves. An additional sheet was also completed; this captured qualitative information relating to why participants' beliefs had, or had not, changed. This task was completed individually, and participants were not shown the beliefs of other members of their group.

A recorded group discussion between participants followed, lasting approximately 1.5 hours. This was facilitated by HMH using a standard script, and the group were guided to discuss, in the context of the treatment of lame ewes with footrot, their views on the following: (i) the review of the evidence base (ii) foot trimming (iii) systemic antibiotics (iv) which of the two treatments had greater efficacy. Finally, the group were asked to try and achieve a consensus opinion and to express this probabilistically (in the same format as previously), such that the final probability distribution was a reflection of the knowledge, experience and beliefs of the whole group. It was recognised that to achieve a group consensus would almost inevitably involve some degree of compromise for at least some individuals, but nevertheless it was important that all participants agreed with the group distribution. This was made clear in the standard script, and in particular participants were told: 'If necessary we can have two or more final answers which reflect real differences in opinion within the group that cannot be resolved by simply discussing and sharing current knowledge and experience.'

The method (excluding the facilitated group discussion/ elicitation) was piloted on three veterinary surgeons to ensure it was tenable, and revisions made as appropriate. Data analysis is described in Section 7.

5. Probabilistic Elicitation

5.1 Clinical context and elicited parameter. The clinical context concerned commercial flocks containing ewes lame with footrot, uncomplicated by other conditions, and affecting one foot only. The binary outcome of interest was lame (yes/no), where lame was defined as an observable limp (of any severity) and head flicking, equivalent to a locomotion score of ≥ 2 on the scale most commonly employed by researchers in this field [11].

The question of interest was: which treatment (as defined in Section 3) is more effective at curing footrot, in terms of the rate of recovery from lameness? There were therefore two unknown parameters: θ_1 which was defined as the probability of cure in 5 days or less with systemic and topical oxytetracycline, $\theta_1 \in [0,1]$, and θ_2 which was defined as the probability of cure in 5 days or less with foot trimming and topical oxytetracycline, $\theta_2 \in [0,1]$. The question concerned a contrast between these two cure rates.

The time period of 5 days was chosen for two reasons. Firstly, it is likely that the recovery rate within 5 days is important with regard to limiting contagious spread and therefore has important implications for flock level control [6]. Secondly, rapid recovery is positively associated with improved ewe body condition score and lamb growth rates [12].

To quantify veterinary surgeons' beliefs, a probability distribution was elicited for the difference in cure rates, $\theta_d = \theta_2 - \theta_1$, where $\theta_d \in [-1, +1]$, because this is a clinically intuitive scale for veterinary surgeons to use. To quantify beliefs in full regarding

two unknown variables requires elicitation of the joint probability distribution however for dependent variables, as was the case here, this is a considerably more complex task [9], and was not necessary for this context.

5.2 Method employed to elicit the difference in cure rates (θ_d). A variety of different methods have been reported in the literature to elicit beliefs probabilistically [13]. This study employed the roulette method (also called 'chip and bins') because it has been shown to be feasible, valid and reliable in a clinical setting [14]. Current best practice for elicitation was followed [9,14], which included: (i) a face-to-face interview (ii) providing examples as a training exercise (iii) use of a standardized script (see Appendix S1), (iv) a design that avoided heuristics, which are mental strategies people use to make numerical assessments in the face of uncertainty, but can introduce bias [15] (v) provision of feedback (vi) the opportunity for participants to revise their response (vii) use of simple graphical methods.

Following the general methodology of Johnson *et al* [14], participants were asked to express their belief probabilistically by indicating the weight of their belief for θ_d using chips each worth 0.05 probability, and placing them in discrete 5% difference intervals (the 'bins') across the range of θ_d. Coins, specifically 5 pence pieces, were used for the chips. Participants were given 20 chips to place, making the total probability sum to 1. Adhesive putty (Blu-Tack®, Bostik) was used to make the coins adhesive to, but easily detachable from, a laminated sheet; this is important to allow participants to revise their answers easily.

For the training exercise, 6 examples were shown to participants, each demonstrating a different belief, and the meaning of each example was explained using the standard script. The examples made abstract reference to a 'treatment 1' and a 'treatment 2' and no context was provided in order to avoid anchoring heuristics by giving a specific clinical scenario. To create familiarity with the task, the examples were created with 5 pence pieces on an almost identical laminated sheet to the one that the participants subsequently used; the only difference being that the words 'treatment 1' and 'treatment 2' were replaced by descriptions of the actual treatments.

To further minimise anchoring heuristics, the 6 examples were balanced, such that the first 2 examples illustrated beliefs that treatment 2 was definitely superior, the second 2 examples that treatment 1 was definitely superior, and the final 2 examples displayed uncertainty over which treatment was superior. Between the examples, different levels of confidence, centres of location and shapes of distribution, were illustrated. The examples are shown schematically in Appendix S2. Participants were encouraged to ask questions during this exercise. Once training was completed, the examples were placed out of sight, to avoid anchoring the participant to any of the example beliefs when considering their own answer.

The first part of the actual task involved a clarification discussion to ensure the correct clinical condition was understood by use of the term footrot. This included describing the clinical condition, and providing photographs of the clinical presentation. Clarification was also given with respect to other factors that could influence the cure rates in the first 5 days, such as the initial severity of lameness, vaccination status, and breed of ewe. Of interest was the true difference between the two treatments, i.e. any difference that is attributable to which treatment was given, once appropriate adjustments for the influence of any other factors have been made; this was made clear in the elicitation script.

Once the task was completed, the facilitator fed back to the participant the meaning of the distribution they had created in words. Participants were also encouraged to reflect upon the shape and distributions of their coins, and revise them as required. This was necessary to ensure that the distribution was a fair reflection of the participants beliefs and how much uncertainty they had in their answer.

To gather some information regarding the actual (marginal) values for θ_1 and θ_2 (as opposed to the difference between them), participants were also asked for an expected value and an upper and lower boundary for each parameter separately, such that they believed there was very little chance that the cure rate could fall outside of this range.

6. Review of the Evidence Provided during the Workshops

The details of the literature search and its results, as summarised here, were reported to the participants during the 30 minute power point presentation. In order to gather the published scientific evidence relevant to the study question, 2 databases were searched: Scopus (http://www.scopus/home.url) and MEDLINE (http://www.ncbi.nlm.nih.gov/pubmed), using a combination of one or more of the following terms: footrot, sheep, ovine, antibiotics, antibacterials, foot trimming, paring, treatment, Dichelobacter, clinical trial, randomised. This resulted in 15 primary research articles, 5 of which were discarded, either because there was no clear information regarding when sheep were monitored post treatment [16], or because they were not relevant to the treatments of interest (e.g. if the efficacy of foot trimming was only assessed when used in combination with treatments other than topical antibacterial spray) [17–20]. Of the remaining 10 articles, 5 were clinical trials based in Australia that assessed clinical outcome 4 to 6 weeks after treatment with systemic antibacterials [21–25]; these trials reported cure rates of between 80% and 99% but they did not assess foot trimming as a treatment. There were 2 UK studies that monitored the clinical outcome after 5 to 6 weeks following initial treatment with systemic antibacterials and reported cure rates above 80% but they did not assess foot trimming as a treatment [26,27]. The remaining 3 research papers [4–6] were judged to be the key evidence of relevance to the question of interest, because unlike the other 7 articles, the clinical outcome was monitored at daily to weekly intervals after treatment. Furthermore, one of these papers provided information on foot trimming and topical oxytetracycline as a treatment [4]; this randomised clinical trial conducted in England, UK, involved 53 sheep in total, and reported that sheep receiving systemic antibacterials recovered faster from lameness than positive controls (odds ratio 4.92, 95% confidence interval 1.2–20.1), whereas sheep foot trimmed recovered more slowly than positive controls (odds ratio 0.05, 95% confidence interval 0.005–0.51). They also estimated the cure rate in ewes treated with long acting systemic oxytetracycline in combination with topical oxytetracycline to be 72% within 5 days, compared with a cure rate of 11% in ewes treated with foot trimming in combination with topical oxytetracycline; hence this paper supported a difference in cure rate between these two treatments in the region of 61%.

7. Data Analysis

7.1 Quantitative data derived from probabilistic elicitation. The raw data were entered into Microsoft Excel (Version 2007, Microsoft Corp). All subsequent analysis was carried out using the software program R. It is common practice to fit parametric distributions to data originating from probabilistic elicitations, although it is widely acknowledged that this inevitably introduces some degree of imprecision, particularly as the shape inferred by the raw data may not be exactly replicated when constrained to a parametric form [15]. However as Garthwaite *et al.* [15] highlighted, 'often a reasonable goal for elicitation is to capture the "big message" in the expert's opinion', and in the context of this study the precise shape of participants distributions was not a primary concern; however, the raw data overlaid with the fitted distributions are provided in Appendix S3, so the interested reader can visualise both.

Due to the scale involved, a suitable choice for the raw data was the Gaussian family, and probability density functions were fitted using numerical optimisation based on the simplex algorithm [28]_ENREF_2 to select the best fitting hyperparameters (mean and variance) by minimising the sum of the squared differences between the fitted cumulative distribution and the elicited cumulative distribution. Differences in the fitted hyperparameters before and after the review of the evidence were calculated to quantify for each participant the change in their clinical belief, whereby the mean was used as a measure of the change in central location, and the standard deviation as a change in clinical confidence. In addition, 95% Bayesian credible intervals were calculated from the fitted distributions, and used as an approximation for the interval such that participants would have assigned a 95% probability that the difference in cure rates would fall within the interval.

7.2 Qualitative data from the individual interviews and facilitated group discussions. The qualitative data were transcribed and analysis involved a thematic approach [29] using NVivo qualitative data analysis software; QSR International Pty Ltd. Version 10, 2012. Transcripts were read and coded into different categories and the categories were then arranged into themes. To ensure reliability of the data the transcripts were double coded by HMH and JK. Themes were redefined where necessary after discussion to ensure there was coherence with the coded data. All the analysis of the qualitative data was inductive and was guided by the collected data.

Results

1. Response Rates

For the non-certificate holders, 14 veterinary practices were contacted in total because 8 declined, giving a 43% initial response rate. Reasons given for declining were: (i) lack of enthusiasm for the task (1 practice), (ii) only a newly qualified veterinary surgeon prepared to travel to attend the workshop, but they failed the inclusion criteria with respect to years qualified (1 practice) (iii) only a newly qualified veterinary surgeon involved with delivering healthcare to sheep clients (2 practices) (iv) eligible veterinary surgeons working in the practice, but unavailable to attend on the day (four practices). For the certificate holders, 8 veterinary surgeons were contacted in total because 2 declined; in both cases, the reason given for declining was unavailable to attend on the day. For the non-certificate holders, one veterinary surgeon who confirmed their attendance, cancelled with short notice due to unpredicted clinical workload; hence this group contained only 5 veterinary surgeons, not 6.

2. Characteristics of Participants

Table 1 provides background information regarding the 11 participants including their current ovine workload and their appraisal of the recent evidence base with respect to footrot. All participants worked in private veterinary practice, in either England or Wales, except one veterinary surgeon who was employed by government. Numerical identifiers are subsequently used to refer to participants: non-certificate holders (1–5), certificate holders (6–11). For non-certificate holders, the median number of years qualified was 6 (range 2–20 years) compared with 22.5 years for the certificate holders (range 12–31 years). For non-certificate holders the percentage of current time spent working with sheep had a median value of 25% (range 10–25%) versus 7.5% (range 1–50%) for certificate holders. Thus, although certificate holders had more clinical experience overall, currently as a group, they reported that they were spending less of their time with sheep compared with the non-certificate holders.

3. Qualitative Results from the Individual Interviews

3.1 Current veterinary advice regarding the treatment of footrot in lame ewes. An open question invited participants to describe the advice they have most commonly given to commercial sheep farmers regarding treatment(s) for ewes lame with footrot, uncomplicated by other conditions of the feet. A total of 8 different pieces of advice/treatments were cited. Table 2 (column 2) gives the frequency with which each piece of advice was reported. Table 2 also contains information regarding gold standard care (see next section for details).

Of the 4 participants who stated that they would usually advise foot trimming, one made reference to potential negative consequences of over-trimming and suggested that a minimal approach should be taken. Another stated that they would, if practical, advise delaying foot trimming for a few days until the infection was resolving and only trim then, if required.

An open question explored if (and how) this veterinary advice may differ, depending on the reproductive cycle. The majority of participants placed extra emphasis on minimising handling stress during very late gestation, whilst at the same time acknowledging that even heavily pregnant lame sheep must be treated promptly. One participant commented that their advice involved actively encouraging farmers to regularly monitor the flock at all times throughout the year, inferring that otherwise, in some instances, problems may only be noticed when farmers gather the flock out of necessity for key events (e.g. tupping). Another advised against footrot vaccination during the summer months to avoid the potential complication of myiasis; they also advised the use of analgesia when treating heavily pregnant lame ewes at risk of twin-

lamb disease, but questioned the economic viability of analgesics at other times of the year.

Most participants stated that their advice would normally involve specifically bringing up with the farmer the question of how quickly the lame ewes need to be treated, and that they would advise treating as quickly as possible, citing limiting the spread of infection as a key reason for doing so. However some participants also suggested that treatment may be delayed in reality because of practical difficulties, and in particular identified problems associated with catching lame sheep; this issue was further explored during the group discussions (see Results Section 6.3). A minority of participants stated that they would not specifically raise the question of speed of treatment, based on an assumption that the farmer would know that treatment should be instigated immediately.

3.2 Gold standard care for treating a single lame ewe. A theoretical categorical question invited participants to tick from a list of nine options the advice/treatment(s) they would consider as the initial gold standard approach to treating footrot in a *single* lame ewe, in the sense that there are no barriers to treatment such as money, or practical considerations; the frequency with which participants selected the different pieces of advice/treatments is presented in Table 2 (column 3). By comparing column 2 with column 3 (Table 2) it can be seen that the largest discrepancies between the advice usually given to commercial farmers and gold standard care for a single lame ewe were: (i) non-steroidal anti-inflammatory pain relief (ii) isolate from non-lame sheep, and (iii) removal from current environment. The most commonly cited reasons for these differences were: cost, time, labour, and/or practical considerations.

With respect to foot trimming, more participants would advise proficient trimming as part of gold standard care for a single ewe, in comparison to the advice they would usually give to commercial farmers (Table 2). A comment here was:

"OK, with this one I think there's a danger if you tell the farmer to trim the feet that he'll trim it too much. So in leaving it he's not going to do any harm. I know what I'm doing, I don't necessarily know he knows what he's doing, so I think it's safer for him just to jab them and spray them, because I think that will make them better. But if I'm doing it, I know I'm not going to over trim it".

Table 1. Characteristics of participating veterinary surgeons (n = 11).

Gender	Years qualified	Holder of the CertSHP?[+]	% of current working time spent dealing with sheep?	Attended CPD[++] events on footrot within 3 years?	Read peer-reviewed papers on footrot within 3 years?	Read non peer-reviewed material on footrot within 3 years?
Male	20	No	25	No	No	No
Female	2	No	25	No	Yes	Yes
Female	5	No	10–40	Yes	Yes	No
Male	6	No	10	Yes	No	No
Male	7	No	5–30	No	No	No
Male	14	Yes	50	Yes	Yes	Yes
Male	26	Yes	10	Yes	No	Yes
Female	12	Yes	5	No	No	Yes
Male	24	Yes	<1	Yes	Yes	Yes
Female	21	Yes	5	No	Yes	Yes
Male	31	Yes	5–25	Yes	Yes	Yes

[+]Certificate in Sheep Health and Production (a post-graduate qualification).
[++]continuing professional development (i.e. training).

Table 2. Tally of treatments/advice recommended for footrot in lame ewes by veterinary surgeons, (n = 11).

Treatment/advice for footrot	Most commonly given advice for lame ewes in a commercial flock	Gold standard care for a single lame ewe
Proficient foot trimming	4[+]	8*
Topical antibacterial spray	8	10*
Systemic antibacterials	10	11
Antibacterial foot bath	0	1
Non-antibacterial foot bath	2	1
Non-steroidal anti-inflammatory pain relief	1	11
Footrot vaccination	3[+]	3
Remove from or improve current environment	2	8
Isolate from non-lame sheep	2	10

[+]2 vets stated they would only use vaccination as a treatment if >5% of the flock are lame.
*2–3 vets inferred that this was case dependent.

3.3 Veterinary approaches to monitoring the clinical outcome in lame ewes. Participants were asked 'Do you usually assume that the ewes have got better following the initial treatment, if you don't hear anything to the contrary?' A diversity of views was expressed. Several participants referred to trusting the farmer to report back to them if there was a poor clinical response, and this was also perceived by some to be typical practice:

"Yes, it's a standard vet thing, isn't it? We just assume animals get better until you happen to see the farmer again. It's rare that you will do a follow-up visit because the farmer won't pay for that follow-up visit."

All the participants who said they would not assume a clinical recovery in the absence of any information, stressed the importance of actively establishing outcomes, and reference was also made to the need for diplomacy, as exemplified by this participant:

"I think that the most important thing you can do with farmers is actually continue to probe them really, without being offensive or without accusing them of things, because you find that they don't always do what you expect them to do. I find that's very common, you can't just trust them to… and this is in all walks of life, you can't trust people to do what you tell them to do and I think if you can audit it in some way without offending them, then I think you pick up a lot of discrepancies in what you think has happened and then you can mould that into what you really want to happen".

One participant alluded to the fact that trusting farmers to report clinical outcomes was entirely dependent on the individual farmer:

"There are some farmers that can be relied on to give you feedback if things aren't going according to plan, there are some farmers that can be relied on not to. So you have to know who you're talking to".

3.4 Veterinary approaches to delivering advice to farmers. There were 2 open questions that explored how participants deliver their advice to farmers. All the participants agreed that they tailor the advice they give according to the action they think the farmer is likely to take in reality and the facilities and/or labour they know are available on the farm. Between them, participants provided several examples of very different situations where they would tailor their advice in the context of managing footrot (Appendix S4). Several participants acknowledged that tailoring their advice may have some negative consequences, but they also emphasised the importance of offering practical advice; some referred to perceived concerns that no action would be taken at all, if one piece of the advice they offered was considered to be impractical to the farmer, for example:

[Vet] *"So there's no point advising stuff that you know somebody's never going to do".*

[Facilitator] *"And how do you make sure that you definitely know that?".*

[Vet] *"You know the client, you get a feeling, but also you've potentially given that advice before and you've had a response….You know if you say isolate them they're going to go pff! So you say 'in an ideal world I would have you isolate them, I know that's going to be difficult for you, it would be better if you could, but if you can't…' Which maybe gives them a get out clause…But they won't listen to the rest of it if you add in a bit that's so unrealistic without taking into account that you understand their system, if that makes sense".*

4. The Individual and Group Elicited Probability Distributions

Recall that θ_d was defined as the % difference in cure rates, in ewes lame with footrot, within 5 days of receiving either (i) systemic and topical oxytetracycline or (ii) foot trimming and topical oxytetracycline. Figure 1 presents the fitted probability distributions for θ_d, elicited individually from participants, both before and after the review of the evidence base; Table 3 details the hyperparameters of the fitted distributions and quantifies how they altered. When appraising Figure 1, it is worth recalling that the current published evidence supports a difference in cure rates in the region of 60% in favour of systemic and topical oxytetracycline [4]. Figure 1 reveals that for both groups, substantial heterogeneity existed in the beliefs of participants before the review of the evidence base, both in terms of central location and confidence. For non-certificate holders, participants' 95% Bayesian credible intervals (together) covered a range from 83% in favour of systemic and topical oxytetracycline, to 70% in favour of foot trimming and topical oxytetracycline. For certificate holders this range was narrower, spanning 88% in favour of systemic and topical oxytetracycline to 33% favouring foot trimming and topical oxytetracycline. Furthermore, both groups contained one participant who entirely favoured foot trimming and topical oxytetracycline, in the sense that they assigned negligible probability to systemic and topical oxytetracycline offering a superior cure rate.

Table 4 presents the elicited values for θ_1 and θ_2, before the evidence review. It reveals that most participants expected cure rates with systemic and topical oxytetracycline to be in excess of 70%, with one notable outlier having an expectation of 20%; however there was considerably more diversity apparent over the expected cure rate with foot trimming and topical oxytetracycline.

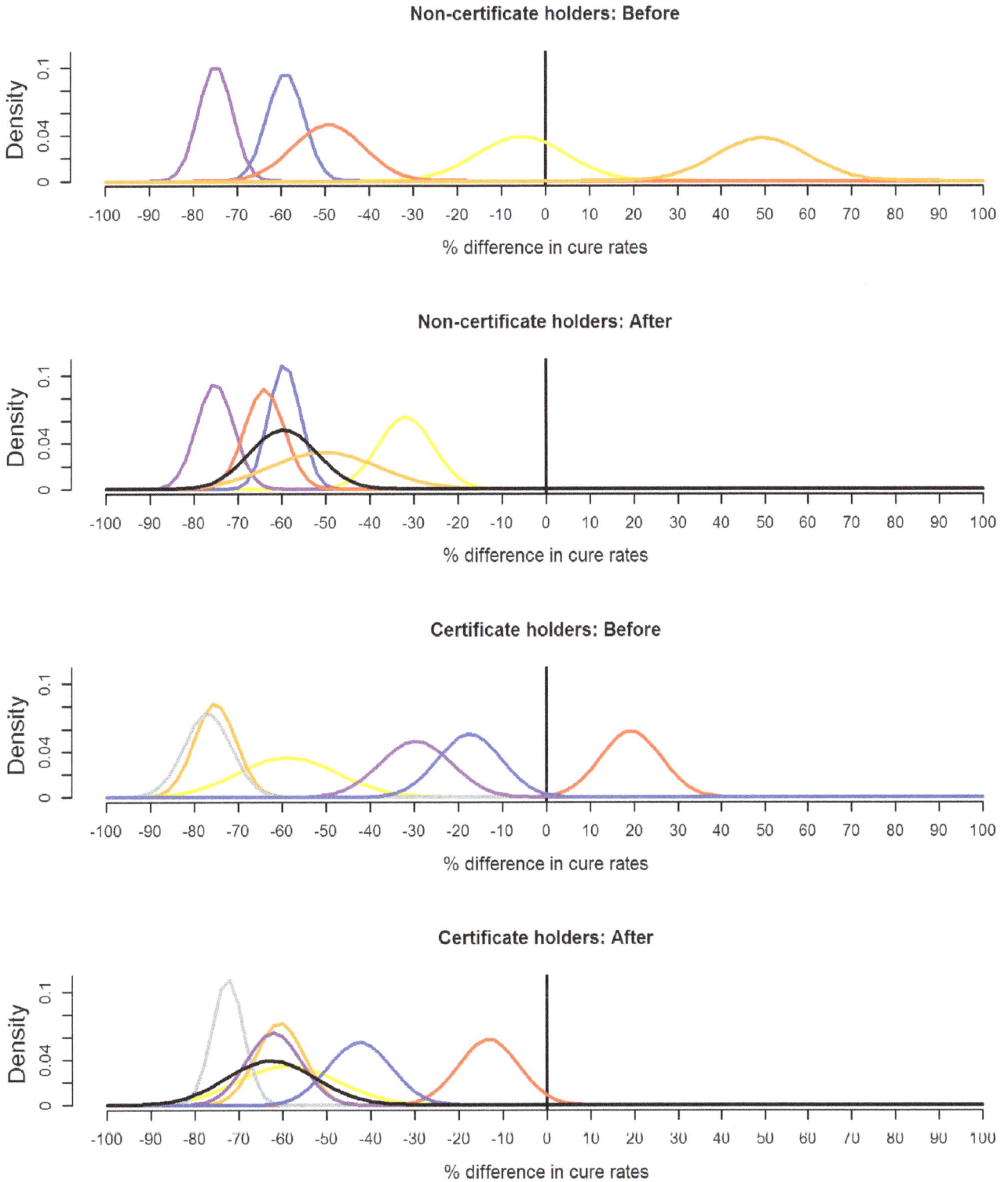

Figure 1. The fitted probability distributions, before and after a review of the evidence. Gaussian probability density functions fitted to the raw data for each veterinary surgeon individually, before and after a presentation of a review of the current evidence. The % difference in cure rates refers to ewes, lame with footrot, within five days of receiving either (i) systemic and topical oxytetracycline or (ii) foot trimming and topical oxytetracycline. Positive differences favour foot trimming and topical oxytetracycline, negative differences favour systemic and topical oxytetracycline. Non-certificate holders: vet 1 = yellow, vet 2 = blue, vet 3 = purple, vet 4 = red, vet 5 = orange. Certificate holders: vet 6 = yellow, vet 7 = orange, vet 8 = red, vet 9 = grey, vet 10 = purple, vet 11 = blue. The fitted probability density function to the group consensus raw data is shown in black. Values for the fitted hyperparameters (mean and variance) are listed in Table 3. The current published evidence supports a difference in cure rates of 60% in favour of systemic and topical oxytetracycline [4].

Table 3. Hyperparameters for the fitted Gaussian probability distributions.

Vet ID**	Fitted probability distribution, before evidence review*			Fitted probability distribution, after evidence review			Difference in fitted parameters (after-before)	
	Mean	Standard deviation	95% credible interval	Mean	Standard deviation	95% credible interval	Mean	Standard deviation
1	−5.5	10.2	−26,15	−32.0	6.2	−44, −20	−26.5	−4.0
2	−59.0	4.2	−67, −51	−59.3	3.6	−66, −52	−0.3	−0.6
3	−75.0	3.9	−83, −67	−75.2	4.3	−84, −67	−0.2	0.4
4	−49.3	8.0	−65, −34	−63.9	4.5	−73, −55	−14.6	−3.5
5	+49.3	10.6	29,70	−50.4	12.3	−75, −26	−99.7	1.7
6	−58.8	11.4	−81, −37	−58.8	11.4	−81, −37	0.0	0.0
7	−75.3	4.8	−85, −66	−60.6	5.5	−71, −50	14.7	0.7
8	+19.2	6.8	6,33	−13.3	6.8	−27,0	−32.5	0.0
9	−77.0	5.4	−88, −66	−72.5	3.6	−80, −66	4.5	−1.8
10	−29.7	8.0	−45, −14	−62.0	6.2	−74, −50	−32.3	−1.8
11	−17.5	7.2	−32, −4	−42.5	7.2	−57, −28	−25.0	0.0
Non-certificate holder group consensus	NA	NA	NA	−59.6	7.7	−75, −45	NA	NA
Certificate holder group consensus	NA	NA	NA	−62.6	10.2	−83, −43	NA	NA

*Positive differences favour foot trimming and topical oxytetracycline, negative differences favour systemic and topical oxytetracycline.

**Numbers 1–5 denote non-certificate holders, numbers 6–11 certificate holders.

Table 4. Elicited values for the cure rate with systemic and topical oxytetracycline (θ_1) and foot trimming and topical oxytetracycline (θ_2).

Vet ID*	Expected value, $E[\theta_1]$	θ_1 Lower to upper values	Expected value, $E[\theta_2]$	θ_2 Lower to upper values	Expected difference: $E[\theta_2]$–$E[\theta_1]$
1	0.75	0.55–0.85	0.65	0.50–0.75	−0.10
2	0.70	0.40–0.90	0.10	0.00–0.25	−0.60
3	0.90	0.80–0.99	0.10	0.00–0.25	−0.80
4	0.80	0.60–1.00	0.30	0.10–0.50	−0.50
5	0.20	0.00–0.50	0.50	0.30–0.60	+0.30
6	1.00	0.95–1.00	0.30	0.25–0.50	−0.70
7	0.80	0.75–0.85	0.08	0.05–0.10	+0.72
8	0.60	0.50–0.80	0.80	0.50–0.90	+0.20
9	0.80	0.60–1.00	0.05	0.00–0.10	−0.75
10	0.80	0.70–0.85	0.50	0.30–0.60	−0.30
11	0.80	0.60–1.00	0.70	0.5–0.90	−0.10

*Numbers 1–5 denote non-certificate holders, numbers 6–11 certificate holders.

Table 4 also shows that the two participants who entirely favoured foot trimming and topical oxytetracycline initially (vet 5 and 8, Figure 1) had very different beliefs with regard to the cure rates achievable with each treatment.

Figure 1 also shows that following a review of the evidence base the heterogeneity in beliefs was demonstrably reduced, and in particular all participants now entirely favoured systemic and topical oxytetracycline. Furthermore, although the variation was greater for the non-certificate holders initially, reviewing the evidence reduced this heterogeneity relatively more in this group compared to the certificate holders. Thus for the non-certificate holders, participants' 95% credible intervals subsequently covered a range from 20% to 84% in favour of systemic and topical oxytetracycline, whereas for certificate holders this range was wider at 0% to 81%. This was mainly due to differences in the magnitude of the change that occurred between the two participants who entirely favoured foot trimming and topical oxytetracycline at the outset; in terms of central location, vet 5 alter their belief by nearly 100% whereas vet 8 altered by 32% (Table 3).

Although three participants made only very minor adjustments to their distributions following the evidence review, only one participant (vet 6, certificate holder) did not alter their belief at all (Table 3), and interestingly the consensus for the certificate holder group was very similar to this participant's belief.

However, even after the evidence review considerable heterogeneity remained, such that within both groups, several pairs of participants still had completely non-overlapping 95% credible intervals. Despite this, following group discussions, both groups did achieve a consensus for the difference in cure rates (Figure 1, black curves). The group consensus represents a considerable reconciliation for two participants (one in each group, vet 1 and 8), in the sense that the group 95% credible interval is non-overlapping with that of their previously expressed individual belief. The two group distributions express a very similar belief in terms of central location (means of 59.6%, versus 62.6%, Table 3), that is in keeping with the current published evidence. However the non-certificate holders expressed their consensus with slightly more confidence than the certificate holders (standard deviations of 7.7 versus 10.2, Table 3), perhaps reflecting the reduced heterogeneity

amongst non-certificate holders relative to certificate holders following the evidence review.

5. Participants Explanations for Any Change in their Beliefs

There were 4 participants who stated that reviewing the evidence had not altered their clinical beliefs and this was reflected quantitatively (Table 3, vets 2,3,6,9). Of these, 2 confirmed that they had not changed their beliefs because they were already aware of all of the evidence provided, whilst the other 2 revealed that at least some of the information presented was new, but it concurred with their existing clinical experiences and beliefs and hence did not alter them. The remaining 7 participants stated that reviewing the evidence had altered their clinical beliefs, and again this was reflected quantitatively; of these, 2 acknowledged that they had not been previously aware of any of the evidence provided, whilst the other 5 reported to being previously aware of at least some of it. All confirmed that it was the review of the evidence base that had altered their beliefs.

6. Facilitated Group Discussions

Thematic analysis identified the following themes: (i) the role of foot trimming in the treatment of ewes lame with footrot (ii) veterinary involvement with lameness in sheep (iii) the practical challenges of prompt treatment (iv) elimination of footrot from some UK flocks. The debate and concepts associated with each theme are summarised below.

6.1 The role of foot trimming for the treatment of lame ewes. During both group meetings, the advantages and disadvantages of foot trimming for the treatment of footrot were contested, and a diversity of views expressed; whilst some participants believed that foot trimming has no role to play in the treatment of footrot, others believed that it did, but for different reasons and to varying extents. The following extract from the certificate holders group discussion, demonstrates some of the debate:

"I think over-paring of sheep's feet has been proven to have disadvantages, and it does extend recovery time for lameness, but I think if trimmed carefully to expose the lesions and get air to them, it can help in recovery".

"No, [be]cause that paper shows that quite clearly, even if they're trimmed on day 6, that it makes no difference or in fact slows it down. I don't think it has any place in the treatment of footrot".

"I would disagree because when you've got a lot of under-running you get a situation where you have instability in the hoof and rubbing of the hoof on underlying tissue, and then I think foot trimming is very, very important, not for curing the footrot, but for stopping collateral damage if you like. I think it does matter and I think it is worth, if you can, inspecting feet sometime after they've been treated to see if you've got that problem".

Overall, the following arguments were put forward in favour of trimming: (i) necessitates turning the sheep over and examining the foot, and hence facilitates establishing the correct diagnosis in every individual animal (ii) it opens the lesion to the air which facilitates healing (iii) under-run or loose horn can cause mechanical damage and foot instability and needs removing (iv) if the feet are over-grown or grossly deformed they need trimming. Arguments made against recommending trimming were: (i) they may be over-trimmed, causing tissue damage which may delay recovery and/or causes additional lesions/lameness (ii) infection may be spread on equipment/hands (iii) it constitutes more, unnecessary, work for shepherds (iv) pregnant lame sheep are more likely to be treated if foot trimming is not advised because whilst some farmers may be reluctant to foot trim heavily pregnant animals for fear of inducing parturition early, they will inject them with antibiotics which is less stressful.

On both days, and throughout the individual interviews and the group discussions, the majority of participants perceived that many farmers over–trim and by doing so cause accidental damage. However the point was also raised that veterinary surgeons may not know for certain whether commercial sheep farmers trim proficiently, unless they have specifically asked the shepherd to show them how they perform this task, whilst attending the farm for some other reason:

"You've clearly watched them. I have never watched. I've trained smallholders how to trim feet, but I've never watched my big [commercial] guys trimming feet."

One participant proposed time pressure as a reason why farmers may over-trim and also described asking farmers to demonstrate their foot trimming technique:

"I think often farmers who are pushed for time over-trim because they take too big a bit each time, and that's [be]cause generally I see them foot trimming… if we're discussing lameness or we're doing something else we grab a lame sheep, and I say, 'Look, how would you treat this normally' and pretty much without exception they make it bleed".

With respect to the concept that foot paring can facilitate the spread of infection, it was suggested that wearing gloves should be standard practice by farmers, with hands and shears disinfected between sheep, but there was general agreement that this was rarely carried out in practice:

"It's not rocket science, but does it happen in practice? I would say 99% of the time it doesn't."

The point was also made that not all veterinary surgeons may be giving this advice, or carrying it out themselves:

"..always have a bucket of disinfectant, disinfect your shears between every sheep, because I do not think anybody does that unless you tell them to…. Ever since I've started giving that advice, I've been doing it myself, but I'm sure I didn't do it before…we're probably as guilty as the farmers".

There was also debate over when foot trimming should be performed; some participants agreed that a few days following initial treatment with systemic antibiotics the lesions are markedly less painful and that if foot trimming is required this is the preferred time to conduct it, both for welfare reasons and because the task is easier; however it was also acknowledged that this protocol has practical implications.

An interesting comment was that veterinary support for foot trimming as a treatment for lameness in sheep may have been influenced to some degree by the fact that foot trimming plays a major role in treating lameness in dairy cattle. However it was also noted that the aetiologies of lameness in the two species are very different; a substantial proportion of lameness in cattle is related to claw horn disease whereas the majority in sheep is infectious in origin. Other issues raised during the workshops were: (i) whilst para-professional cattle foot trimmers are now recognised in the UK through a national association, with competence established by obtaining qualifications, the equivalent does not exist for sheep farmers and their para-professionals and there is scope for development in this area (ii) some farmers who have traditionally treated footrot by trimming may be difficult to convince to change this habit; settling on a compromise whereby they trim only very loose horn may be required, at least in the short term (iii) some participants commented that their advice regarding the treatment of footrot had changed in recent years towards either recommending not to foot trim, or only to trim very loose horn (iv) there was general agreement amongst certificate holders that their advice on *routine* foot trimming has changed in recent years, with a move towards not advising this practice.

6.2 Veterinary involvement with lameness in sheep. During discussions, regular references were made to how much work and anxiety is created by lame sheep for farmers, as well as how widespread the problem is:

"The problem of footrot in ewes specifically is not a small problem in clinical practice and in sheep farming, it's an absolutely massive problem, it costs a lot of resources on a lot of sheep farms, it causes a lot of welfare problems. I think it's a big target to aim for and that makes it doubly worth trying to improve anything to do with the treatment and control and possible eradication."

It was also suggested that reducing the prevalence of lameness is a key priority for many farmers. In spite of this, however, an important theme concerned how uncommon it is for veterinary surgeons to be specifically asked by farmers for lameness advice; indeed some participants reported that they usually only become involved when a member of the public has observed lame sheep and reported the farmer to an external organisation, such as the Royal Society for the Prevention of Cruelty to Animals (R.S.P.C.A). It was suggested that this is because lameness becomes tolerated by farmers, who may believe they are taking all possible action to tackle a disease that they perceive to be an inevitable constant problem. Thus farmers may only seek advice when the prevalence escalates demonstrably beyond the level they have traditionally experienced, and hence have come to accept, on their farm:

"..but they wouldn't necessarily bring it up, because it's a problem that's always there, grumbling along, and they don't see it as a big problem unless it, I guess, balloons out of control and gets significantly worse than it was. [But that is not to say].whether or not it was a good or bad [prevalence] in the first place."

The point was also made that the perceived 'acceptable' prevalence could vary considerably between farms. Several participants emphasised the importance of taking a proactive approach, and volunteered some examples of how they themselves have done this, which included: (i) by making enquiries regarding lameness when called to attend the farm for other reasons (ii) during flock health visits (iii) through hosting farmers meetings. It was proposed that there is considerably more scope for veterinary involvement, but that without proactivity on behalf of participants, it was suggested that this was unlikely to occur:

"I think a lot of the time you have to be proactive and when you're on the farm or dealing with a different problem you have to be proactive and ask

what's happening, 'How many lame sheep have you got today? Isn't that dreadful, you're going to have to get them all in again!' And if you're not proactive and if you don't start the conversation it often doesn't happen."

However, the importance of farmer levy boards (such as EBLEX in England) and the farming press, for promoting farmer awareness that lameness is a problem that should not be tolerated was highlighted and it was acknowledged that awareness is increasing. The following participant emphasised the advantages of early veterinary input:

"I don't think probably vets are going in until there's a lot lame, whereas really you need to be getting in and talking to farmers preferably when there's none lame! But you know...when there are just a few lame...the time to get in is when you can fix it, rather than trying to fix a shattered vase!".

In this context, several participants referred to farmers purchasing treatments for lameness from the veterinary practice without their knowledge, for example:

"I think it would be really interesting to see how many treatments per sheep or per farm are going out to animals under our care without us knowing....people come in and buy however many bottles of Oxytet [antibiotic] and the receptionist doesn't question it, they've always had however many bottles of that and they've had a few more this year, and we have no idea really what level of treatment is going on in terms of lameness in sheep in our practice."

In terms of ways to overcome this, both groups mentioned the usefulness of setting up an in-house practice monitoring system, whereby the number of treatments purchased that are likely to be deployed to treat lame sheep is regularly checked to facilitate veterinary intervention:

"... put a note on the computer that next time they want Oxytet [antibiotic] spray they'll need to speak to someone. We've done that for a few [farmers]– you try and catch them in the car park as they're leaving with another box".

6.3 The practical challenges of prompt treatment. During both the individual and the group discussions, several references were made to the considerable practical challenge of catching lame ewes in order to provide prompt treatment, especially for large commercial flocks with several thousand ewes grazing several hundred acres of land. In this situation, highly skilled shepherds with excellent working sheepdogs to separate individuals from the main flock along with mobile pens are a necessity, or alternatively the whole flock must be gathered. It was emphasised that gathering the entire flock can constitute a considerable amount of work, and consequently many sheep farmers only gather the flock to carry out several tasks simultaneously:

"People rarely gather sheep to do this one thing to them; they gather sheep because they've got to do ...gotta tail the lambs and give them their first vaccine and give them the first drench and all that lot....They try very much to group stuff like that because they haven't got time, particularly with a big number of sheep, to go gathering them...which makes it even more difficult for treating individual lame sheep, if you say, 'Oh that should be treated now.' But it's a lot of work to gather a lot of sheep to treat a couple of lame ones, and time is precious on farms, very precious."

Gathering the flock also carries subsequent identification difficulties, with lame sheep extremely difficult to detect; once gathered and penned, their acute stress (adrenaline) response masks their clinical signs. With the flock in close contact, the point was also made that the potential to facilitate spread of infection is increased, depending on the handling facilitates. In this context, labour was mentioned, and reported by some participants to be typically equivalent to one full-time stockperson per one thousand ewes. Thus, whilst it was acknowledged that spot treating individual lame ewes promptly is very important and is a preventive measure (by minimising spread) it was clear that for some participants the major challenge of prompt treatment for

some commercial flocks made them inclined to attach extra importance to the combined use of several control measures, particularly routine vaccination, as this participant explained:

"We've had issues with one large client who has 3,000 ewes and they run in open park fields of 100 or 200 acres, so unless the shepherd has a very good dog at catching things, he can't catch individual sheep and so although the goal might be to treat them within three or four days, practically it depends on how easy it is to catch the animal, so that's why I would advise them to vaccinate in the first place - to get the initial incidents down."

It was noted that this carries additional advantages in terms of the reduced use of systemic antibiotics. However it was agreed that when the flock are housed, prompt treat should not be under the influence of any practical considerations.

6.4 Elimination of footrot from some individual flocks in the UK. Some attention was given during both group discussions to the issue of eliminating footrot from some individual flocks in the UK. There were some marked differences in opinion between the two groups, with non-certificate holders appearing more pessimistic; indeed some considered elimination from any flock to be extremely unlikely to be successful in the UK, primarily due to (i) the wet weather conditions (favouring environmental persistence and spread of *D. nodosus*) and (ii) the poor levels of biosecurity on UK commercial sheep farms. However certificate holders were noticeably more optimistic, indeed some participants had attempted to eliminate footrot on some of their clients' farms, with reportedly some success; one participant reported to have eliminated footrot from approximately 40,000 sheep in total, with only a few breakdowns, usually in larger flocks (over 2,000 ewes).

There was debate over different protocols for elimination from individual flocks, including treating the entire flock once with systemic antibiotics (so called blanket use) justified on the basis that once eliminated, future use would fall to zero, versus a more conservative approach of proactively segregating and treating only lame sheep with systemic antibiotics. Irrespective of the protocol, the caveat was clearly that elimination of footrot from individual flocks should only be attempted with veterinary input and if excellent biosecurity measures are in place:

"... But that's because there's no point ... as number 6 says, going for the eradication if we use a lot of antibiotics and then the next week, or two weeks later, neighbour's sheep are on the hill, poorly fenced, straying in and re-infecting."

Moreover, with respect to biosecurity, the possibility that wildlife may act as mechanical vectors was also mentioned. Choice of antibiotic in this context was debated, including the lack of licensed products in sheep, and it was argued that programmes that are quick and simple to implement, such as a blanket approach, are considerably more likely to be successful, especially for large flocks. The following point was also made:

"All farmers want to eradicate lameness, but not all farmers are able to do it. I think that has to be spelled out to them".

Discussion

By demonstrating considerable heterogeneity in the clinical beliefs of veterinary surgeons before a review of the evidence base, these results provide support for the hypothesis that currently a diverse spectrum of clinical beliefs exist with respect to the efficacy of systemic and topical oxytetracycline versus foot trimming and topical oxytetracycline for treating footrot. The results also showed that 7 out of the 11 participants in this study quantifiably, and in some cases markedly, altered their clinical beliefs after hearing a review of the currently published evidence. This suggests that a considerable amount of the variation in participants' beliefs related to differences in their knowledge of the current evidence base.

These findings support the notion that keeping up-to-date with the latest research findings may be difficult in veterinary practice and there are several possible reasons for this. It is recognised that the information infra-structure that underpins the translation of research findings into veterinary practice, (which includes organizations that produce systematic reviews and point-of-care decision support) is significantly underdeveloped when compared to human medicine [30]. Furthermore, the teaching of evidence-based veterinary medicine to under-graduate veterinary students has only recently gained momentum [31], and hence it is possible that some veterinary surgeons may not have fully developed the skills to search and appraise the current evidence base as efficiently as possible. Other possible obstacles include time management issues, financial constraints with respect to attending professional training events and difficulties keeping fully informed across many species.

These results have demonstrated that the current published evidence was, in this instance, of sufficient strength to sway current clinical opinion to the extent that it did convince the two participants who previously considered foot trimming and topical oxytetracycline superior, to adjust their beliefs entirely in favour of systemic and topical oxytetracycline. This is notable because it has been recognised in human medicine that an important explanation for why research may fail to alter disease management is because clinical trial results are not sufficiently strong to alter doctors' current clinical opinions [8].

The quantitative results showed that even after a review of the evidence, considerable heterogeneity still existed amongst veterinary surgeons, both in terms of central location and confidence. The qualitative results revealed a diversity of clinical opinion concerning the role of foot trimming in the treatment of footrot, which supported the quantitative results and provided further insight. Possible reasons for the remaining heterogeneity in clinical beliefs include: (i) differences in clinical experiences per se, and how compatible the current evidence base was with a participants original beliefs (ii) differences in how the evidence base was interpreted, i.e. how 'convincing' it appeared (iii) differences in the perceived biological plausibility of the two treatments; given footrot is an infectious condition, systemic antibacterials as a treatment method has pharmacological credibility, whereas the biological rational for foot trimming is based on knowledge that *Dichelobacter nodosus* is an anaerobic pathogen and that paring the foot 'lets the air in' (iv) differences in knowledge of the non-peer reviewed literature (v) differences in personality types; in particular, some veterinary surgeons may be inherently more likely to give confident answers (narrower distributions) compared to others.

Whilst caution should be taken when attempting to make inferences to the wider veterinary community, the implications of these findings are that currently veterinary approaches to treating ovine footrot may be markedly inconsistent in practice, with potentially very different advice being given to farmers. It is proposed that more consistent advice could be achieved by improving the transfer of the latest research findings to veterinary surgeons; we suggest that far more should be done to facilitate the practice of evidence-based veterinary medicine, and research to identify the most appropriate mechanisms for rapidly disseminating species-specific research results, in an easily interpretable manner, to the relevant majority of the practising veterinary community is warranted. It should also be noted that the key research papers pertaining to the clinical question were published within the last two years, and this may explain some of the variation observed currently; eventually over time, it is likely that these findings will pervade more widely into clinical practice. However, our results also support the view that considerable

heterogeneity would still be likely to remain amongst practitioners, even if knowledge transfer is improved; hence more evidence, for example in the form of a larger clinical trial, would be useful.

In terms of methodology, this study has demonstrated that using the roulette (chip and bins) elicitation approach is a practical way to quantitatively assess how veterinary surgeons' beliefs change, in this case following a review of the current evidence, although the method could be used in any situation where formally quantifying a change in a person's belief is required. The diversity in the elicited distributions provides support for the argument that anchoring bias was minimised; if all (or most) participants had produced very similar distributions, it would have aroused suspicion that they had been inadvertently anchored. Furthermore, the authors' subjective perception was that veterinary surgeons found this method of elicitation straightforward, in the sense that they all appeared to quickly grasp the nature of the task and seemed comfortable with it; this was particularly important in this instance, because they had to repeat the task three times. We emphasize the usefulness of the training exercise.

In addition, the use of a combined qualitative and quantitative methodology proved fruitful to contextualize the quantitative data and identify some potential obstacles to the implementation of veterinary advice by the farming community. Perhaps most importantly, our results support the notion that despite the fact that lameness is a considerable problem, sheep farmers are unlikely to actively seek veterinary advice on this issue; hence whilst there appears to be considerably more scope for veterinary surgeons to have a positive impact, this is likely to require a proactive approach on their behalf. An important point raised by the veterinary surgeons in our sample related to the monitoring of treatments being dispensed to farmers to treat lame sheep, and the suggestion that this may be lacking in some instances. Any activity that serves to enhance veterinary involvement in lameness control would be worthwhile.

These results also support the view that more attention could usefully be given to understanding and improving veterinary approaches to *the way in which* advice is delivered to farmers. As Procter et al [32] commented, veterinary surgeons do not merely transfer research findings to farmers, rather they combine that information with their own field knowledge, in order to 'tailor the knowledge to the circumstances of the individual farmer' [32]. However, whilst it is clearly essential that veterinary surgeons tailor their advice to the individual farmer, nevertheless our results support the view that there may be some negative consequences of doing so, particularly if advice is tailored by veterinary surgeons' perceived assumptions, or judgements based on failed attempts to implement control measures in the past. As Results Section 3.4 revealed, veterinary perceptions of how difficult it will be for a farmer to implement a control measure, and their concern that if they fail to acknowledge this, then no action will be taken at all, may hinder the uptake of good advice, dependent upon *how* the advice is consequently delivered. Considering alternative ways to deliver veterinary advice that do not negate the need to demonstrate an understanding of the practical challenges a farmer faces, may be useful. For example, rather than telling a farmer that it is going to be difficult for him to catch lame sheep promptly and immediately offering a (sub-optimal) alternative, broaching the issue from a positive angle at the outset could be considered. This might include beginning the conversation by highlighting the major advantages of promptly treating lame sheep and re-counting an example of another farmer who has successfully managed to do so; this could be followed by asking open questions to elicit the farmer's thoughts on how this is will be achieved on their farm, and implicitly bringing to the discussion the supportive notion that and that *we believe* this is achievable for them. Recently, more attention has been given to the area of veterinary communication and ways to facilitate changes on farms, particularly in relation to dairy cattle [33,34], however the same concepts apply in the context of ovine medicine.

Conclusions

The practical importance of this study is that it has: (i) explored the current heterogeneity in veterinary beliefs regarding treatments for footrot in sheep from a sample of veterinary surgeons (ii) demonstrated a practical method for probabilistically assessing how clinical beliefs changed following a review of the evidence (iii) revealed that the current evidence that exists on the use of systemic and topical antibiotics to treat footrot in sheep is capable of changing veterinary opinion (iv) provides support for the notion that more needs to be done to improve the transfer of new evidence into clinical veterinary practice (v) identified, from a veterinary perspective, some potential obstacles to the implementation of veterinary advice by the farming community.

Supporting Information

Appendix S1 Standard probabilistic elicitation script.

References

1. Grogono-Thomas R, Johnston KM (1997) A study of ovine lameness. MAFF Open Contract OC59 45K. MAFF final report. MAFF publications.
2. Kaler J, Green LE (2009) Farmers' practices and factors associated with the prevalence of all lameness and lameness attributed to interdigital dermatitis and footrot in sheep flocks in England in 2004. Prev Vet Med 92: 52–59.
3. Nieuwhof GJ, Bishop SC (2005) Costs of the major endemic diseases of sheep in Great Britain and the potential benefits of reduction in disease impact. Anim Sci 81: 23–29.
4. Kaler J, Daniels SLS, Wright JL, Green LE (2010) Randomized clinical trial of long-acting oxytetracycline, foot trimming, and flunixine meglumine on time to recovery in sheep with footrot. J Vet Intern Med 24: 420–425.
5. Kaler J, Wani SA, Hussain I, Beg SA, Makhdoomi M, et al. (2012) A clinical trial comparing parenteral oxytetracyline and enrofloxacin on time to recovery in sheep lame with acute or chronic footrot in Kashmir, India. BMC Vet Res 8: 12.
6. Wassink GJ, King EM, Grogono-Thomas R, Brown JC, Moore LJ, et al. (2010) A within farm clinical trial to compare two treatments (parenteral antibacterials and hoof trimming) for sheep lame with footrot. Prev Vet Med 96: 93–103.
7. Farm Animal Welfare Council (2011) Report to governement: opinion on lameness in sheep. Farm Animal Welfare Council website. Available: http://www.fawc.org.uk/pdf/sheep-lameness-opinion-110328.pdf. Accessed 2013 Mar 16.
8. Spiegelhalter DJ, Abrams KR, Myles JP (2004) Bayesian approaches to clinical trials and health-care evaluation. Wiley, England.
9. O'Hagan A, Buck CE, Daneshkhah A, Eiser, JR, Garthwaite PH, et al. (2006) Uncertain judgements: eliciting experts' probabilites. Wiley, England.
10. R Development Core Team (2009) R: A language and environment for statistical computing. R foundation for statistical computing,Vienna, Austria. Available: http://wwwR-projectorg/.
11. Kaler J, Wassink GJ, Green LE (2009) The inter- and intra-observer reliability of a locomotion scoring scale for sheep. Vet J 180: 189–194.
12. Green LE, Kaler J, Wassink GJ, King EM, Grogono-Thomas R (2012) Impact of rapid treatment of sheep lame with footrot on welfare and economics and farmer attitudes to lameness in sheep. Anim Welf 21: 65–71.
13. Johnson SR, Tomlinson GA, Hawker GA, Granton JT, Feldman BM (2010) Methods to elicit beliefs for Bayesian priors: a systematic review. J Clin Epidemiol 63: 355–369.
14. Johnson SR, Tomlinson GA, Hawker GA, Granton JT, Grosbein HA, et al. (2010) A valid and reliable belief elicitation method for Bayesian priors. J Clin Epidemiol 63: 370–383.
15. Garthwaite PH, Kadane JB, O'Hagan A (2005) Statistical methods for eliciting prior distributions. J Am Stat Assoc 100: 680–701.
16. Sagliyan A, Gunay C, Han MC (2008) Comparison of the effects of oxytetracycline and penicillin-streptomycin in the treatment of footrot in sheep. J Anim Vet Adv 7: 986–990.
17. Casey RH, Martin PAJ (1988) Effect of foot paring of sheep affected with footrot on response to zinc-sulfate sodium lauryl sulfate foot bathing treatment. Aust Vet J 65: 258–259.
18. Bulgin MS, Lincoln SD, Lane VM, Matlock M (1986) Comparison of treatment methods for the control of contagious ovine foot rot. J Am Vet Med Assoc 189: 194–196.
19. Bagley CV, Healey MC, Hurst RL (1987) Comparison of treatments for ovine foot rot. J Am Vet Med Assoc 191: 541–546.
20. Malecki JC, Coffey L (1987) Treatment of ovine virulent footrot with zinc-sulfate sodium lauryl sulfate footbathing. Aust Vet J 64: 301–304.
21. Egerton JR, Parsonson IM, Graham NPH (1968) Parenteral chemotherapy of ovine foot-rot. Aust Vet J 44: 275–283.
22. Venning CM, Curtis MA, Egerton JR (1990) Treatment of virulent footrot with lincomycin and spectinomycin. Aust Vet J 67: 258–260.
23. Ware JKW, Scrivener CJ, Vizard AL (1994) Efficacy of erythromycin compared with penicillin streptomycin for the treatment of virulent footrot in sheep. Aust Vet J 71: 88–89.
24. Jordan D, Plant JW, Nicol HI, Jessep TM, Scrivener CJ (1996) Factors associated with the effectiveness of antibiotic treatment for ovine virulent footrot. Aust Vet J 73: 211–215.
25. Rendell DK, Callinan APL (1997) Comparison of erythromycin and oxytetracycline for the treatment of virulent footrot in grazing sheep. Aust Vet J 75: 354–354.
26. Grogono-Thomas R, Wilsmore AJ, Simon AJ, Izzard KA (1994) The use of long-acting oxytetracycline for the treatment of ovine footrot. Br Vet J 150: 561–568.
27. Duncan JS, Grove-White D, Moks E, Carroll D, Oultram JW, et al. (2012) Impact of footrot vaccination and antibiotic therapy on footrot and contagious ovine digital dermatitis. Vet Rec 170: 462–U461.
28. Nelder JA, Mead R (1965) A simplex algorithm for function minimization. Comput J 7: 308–313.
29. Braun V, Clarke V (2006) Using thematic analysis in psychology. Qual Res Psychol 3: 77–101.
30. Toews L (2011) The information infrastructure that supports evidence-based veterinary medicine: a comparison with human medicine. J Vet Med Educ 38: 123–134.
31. Hardin LE, Robertson S (2006) Learning evidence-based veterinary medicine through development of a critically appraised topic. J Vet Med Educ 33: 474–478.
32. Proctor A, Lowe P, Phillipson J, Donaldson A (2011) Veterinary field expertise: using knowledge gained on the job. Vet Rec 169: 408–410.
33. Jansen J, Steuten CDM, Renes RJ, Aarts N, Lam TJGM (2010) Debunking the myth of the hard-to-reach farmer: effective communication on udder health. J Dairy Sci 93: 1296–1306.
34. Whay HR, Main DCJ (2009) Improving animal welfare: practical approaches for achieving change. In: Grandin T, editor. Improving animal welfare: a Practical Approach: CABI Publishing.

Appendix S2 Schematic illustration of the 6 training examples provided.

Appendix S3 Gaussian probability distributions fitted to the raw elicitation data.

Appendix S4 Examples given by veterinary surgeons of tailoring their veterinary advice.

Acknowledgments

Our thanks go to the veterinary surgeons who piloted the method, all those who assisted and participated in the two workshops, and the reviewers for their helpful comments.

Author Contributions

Conceived and designed the experiments: HMH LEG MJG JK. Performed the experiments: HMH JK. Analyzed the data: HMH JK. Wrote the paper: HMH LEG MJG JK.

10

Comparable High Rates of Extended-Spectrum-Beta-Lactamase-Producing *Escherichia coli* in Birds of Prey from Germany and Mongolia

Sebastian Guenther[1]*, Katja Aschenbrenner[1], Ivonne Stamm[2], Astrid Bethe[1], Torsten Semmler[1], Annegret Stubbe[3], Michael Stubbe[3], Nyamsuren Batsajkhan[4], Youri Glupczynski[5], Lothar H. Wieler[1], Christa Ewers[1,6]

1 Institute of Microbiology and Epizootics, Veterinary Faculty, Freie Universität Berlin, Berlin, Germany, 2 Vet Med Labor GmbH, Ludwigsburg, Germany, 3 Department of Zoology, Institute of Biology, Martin Luther Universität Halle-Wittenberg, Halle, Germany, 4 Department of Zoology, National University of Mongolia, Ulan-Bator, Mongolia, 5 National Reference Laboratory for Antimicrobial Resistance in Gram-negative bacteria, Centre Hospitalier Universitaire de Mont-Godinne, Université Catholique de Louvain, Yvoir, Belgium, 6 Institute of Hygiene and Infectious Diseases of Animals, Veterinary Faculty, Justus-Liebig-Universität Giessen, Giessen, Germany

Abstract

Frequent contact with human waste and liquid manure from intensive livestock breeding, and the increased loads of antibiotic-resistant bacteria that result, are believed to be responsible for the high carriage rates of ESBL-producing *E. coli* found in birds of prey (raptors) in Central Europe. To test this hypothesis against the influence of avian migration, we initiated a comparative analysis of faecal samples from wild birds found in Saxony-Anhalt in Germany and the Gobi-Desert in Mongolia, regions of dissimilar human and livestock population characteristics and agricultural practices. We sampled a total of 281 wild birds, mostly raptors with primarily north-to-south migration routes. We determined antimicrobial resistance, focusing on ESBL production, and unravelled the phylogenetic and clonal relatedness of identified ESBL-producing *E. coli* isolates using multi-locus sequence typing (MLST) and macrorestriction analyses. Surprisingly, the overall carriage rates (approximately 5%) and the proportion of ESBL-producers among *E. coli* (Germany: 13.8%, Mongolia: 10.8%) were similar in both regions. Whereas $bla_{CTX-M-1}$ predominated among German isolates (100%), $bla_{CTX-M-9}$ was the most prevalent in Mongolian isolates (75%). We identified sequence types (STs) that are well known in human and veterinary clinical ESBL-producing *E. coli* (ST12, ST117, ST167, ST648) and observed clonal relatedness between a Mongolian avian ESBL-*E. coli* (ST167) and a clinical isolate of the same ST that originated in a hospitalised patient in Europe. Our data suggest the influence of avian migratory species in the transmission of ESBL-producing *E. coli* and challenge the prevailing assumption that reducing human influence alone invariably leads to lower rates of antimicrobial resistance.

Editor: Christopher James Johnson, USGS National Wildlife Health Center, United States of America

Funding: This work was supported by the Federal Ministry of Education (BMBF) and Research Network Zoonosis (FBI-Zoo, Grant no. 01KI1012A) and the German Research Foundation (DFG) funded Indo-German Research Training Group (Grant GRK1673). The funders had no role in study design, data collection and analysis, decision to publish, or preparation of the manuscript.

* E-mail: guenther.sebastian@fu-berlin.de

Introduction

Previous studies have demonstrated high carriage rates of Extended-spectrum beta-Lactamase- producing *E. coli* (ESBL-*E. coli*) in faecal excreta of various wild avian hosts, including birds of prey and waterfowl [1–4] Most of these studies conducted in Central Europe, a region with high human and livestock densities [5,6],facilitating interactions between wild birds and human-influenced habitats like urban environments, wastewater treatment facilities, landfills, and land used for intensive agricultural and livestock farming. It has been suggested that such interactions increase the probability for wildlife to acquire antibiotic-resistant bacteria [7,8]and preliminary evidence shows that birds of prey carry more of these resistant bacteria when they live in an area with intensive livestock production [9]. Certain ESBL-*E. coli* isolates from wild avian hosts belong to phylogenetic lineages that are closely related to those found in human and veterinary clinical

settings, presumably explaining the frequent observation of ESBL-*E. coli* in wild birds [10,11]Thus, an indirect transmission of ESBL-*E. coli* from humans or domestic animals to wild animals, including wild birds, and vice versa, is plausible. However, the frequencies of such events and the routes of transmission are largely unknown, leaving several unanswered questions; namely whether (a) higher detection rates of ESBL-*E. coli* in avian hosts could be related to spatially linked higher human density, and/or whether (b) prolonged shedding of ESBL-*E. coli* in the birds excreta might compensate for infrequent transmission events.

To begin answering these questions, there is a clear need for studies comparing the microbiota of avian hosts in areas with contrasted exposure to human antimicrobial "practice" (use). This study therefore aimed to (i) assess the rate of ESBL-*E. coli* carriage by birds of prey in remote areas compared to those in Central Europe, (ii) characterize these ESBL-*E. coli* genotypically, and ultimately, (iii) provide preliminary data that might help assess the possible role of migrating avian hosts in the spread of ESBL-*E. coli* into remote environments.

The selection of both the sampling areas and the avian species to be sampled was crucial. Beyond enabling factors like legal access to avian samples from remote areas, it was important to select two sampling sites decidedly different in their human and livestock densities and agricultural practices, but still with comparable avian populations; different groups of avian species seem to differ largely in their carriage rates of ESBL-*E. coli* [11].

We therefore chose sampling spots in semi-desert areas of the South Gobi in Mongolia, among the least densely human populated areas in the world. Besides extensive pasture farming of ruminants, Mongolia features relatively low livestock indices for pigs, cattle and poultry due to the absence of industrial animal breeding. However, as overgrazing by free-ranging livestock, including camels, horses, sheep, goats and cattle, has become a problem in some parts of Mongolia, we were careful not to select these areas. Manure spread on the fields is estimated to be of minor relevance as only a marginal area of the country is arable [5,6,12]. By contrast, we selected the sampling area in Saxony-Anhalt, Germany, because it represents typical Central European conditions, e.g. high human densities and industrial animal breeding. High livestock indices for pigs, cattle and poultry presumably lead to increased therapeutic use of antimicrobial substances in livestock farming and intensive liquid manuring [5,6,12].

The host-side sampling of birds of prey were considered since (i) there is growing evidence that these may carry ESBL-*E. coli* at a high frequency and (ii) in both of the sampling areas some of the same species were present. Furthermore, the German and Mongolian raptor populations were not connected by migration; the main avian migration routes for raptors in both locations are north-south [1–4,13]. Although we sampled different species of raptors in the two areas to reach a minimum acceptable sample size, it should be stressed that raptors demonstrate common feeding behaviours, distinct from other groups of birds.

Methods

Ethics Statement

We carried out the sampling of nestlings in Germany and Mongolia during bird ringing and the animals were released afterward in accordance with the Ornithological Council's guidelines on the use of wild birds in research [14]. We conducted sampling in Mongolia with the approval and in cooperation with the National University of Mongolia in Ulaan-Baatar, Mongolia. Sampling in Germany was performed under the approval of the State Office of Environmental Protection of Saxony-Anhalt, which also granted M. Stubbe the general permission to ring birds.

According to the IUCN Red List of Threatened species, the conservation status of nearly all animals of this study was of "least concern" (LC), with the exceptions of *M. milvus*, *A. monachus* (both nearly threatened; NT) and *F. cherrug* (endangered, EN).

Sampling of Birds

In spring 2010, while ringing the nestlings of sixteen wild avian species, we obtained cloacal swabs in both Germany and Mongolia; most of the avian hosts sampled were birds of prey. We sampled four non-raptor species in Mongolia, but the isolates originating from these birds were excluded from the calculation of the number of ESBL-*E. coli* (Tab.1).

We carried out sampling in Central Germany, Saxony-Anhalt, in the Northern region of the Harz-mountains, (around the Hakel-Woodland) in an area of 30 km^2 around N 51°56′24.5″; E 11°13′13.2″ (human density: 116 n/km^2, livestock densities: cattle/swine 50–100 n/km^2, small ruminants 10 n/km^2, poultry 1.000–2.500 n/km^2) [12] and at several sampling spots in the South-Mongolian semi-desert and in West Mongolia during the Mongolian-German Biological Expedition 2010 by M. and A. Stubbe (detailed geographic origin: Tab. 1, human density: 1–2 n/km^2, livestock densities: swine <1 n/km^2, cattle 1–5 n/km^2, small ruminants 5–10 n/km^2, poultry <10 n/km^2) [12,13]. We sampled animals once and shipped cloacal swabs (MASTASWAB containing Amies Medium with charcoal, Mast Diagnostics Reinfeld, Germany) to the lab in Berlin.

Isolation of *E. coli*

Cloacal swabs were streaked out on CHROMagar orientation (with and without 4 µg/ml cefotaxime; Mast Diagnostica, Reinfeld, Germany) and incubated overnight to isolate *E. coli* and to preselect for cefotaxime-resistant *E. coli*. One colony per sample with coliform appearance on CHROMagar was processed further and bacterial species identification was carried out using the automated VITEK®2 system (BioMérieux, Germany).

Phenotypic Characterization of ESBL-*E. coli*

E. coli isolates showing growth on CHROMagar containing cefotaxime were confirmed as ESBL producers using the phenotypic confirmatory test for ESBL production, performed and interpreted according to CLSI guideline M31-A3 [15].[Using the VITEK®2 system (BioMérieux, Germany) minimal inhibitory concentration testing for antimicrobials was performed according to the guidelines given by the CLSI.

Genotypic Characterization of ESBL-*E. coli*

The genomic make-up of the confirmed ESBL-*E. coli* was characterised using established PCR protocols with amplification and subsequent sequencing for the most prevalent beta lactam resistance genes (bla_{CTX-M}, bla_{SHV}, bla_{TEM} and bla_{OXA}) and non-beta-lactam resistance genes ($tet(A)$, $tet(B)$, $tet(C)$, $sul1$, $sul2$, $sul3$, $strA$, $strB$, $aadA1$-like, $aacC4$, $acc(6')$-Ib $qnrA$, $qnrB$, and $qnrS$) [16–26] The presence of the $intI1$ and $intI2$ genes, encoding class 1 and 2 integrases, was also determined by PCR [23].

MLST and Phylogenetic Grouping by Structure Analysis

Multi-locus sequence type (MLST) determination was carried out as described previously [27,28]. Gene amplification and sequencing were performed by using primers specified on the *E. coli* MLST web site (University of Cork website, http://mlst.ucc.ie/mlst/mlst/dbs/Ecoli, accessed 2012 November 29th). Sequences were analysed by the software package Ridom SeqSphere 0.9.39 (Ridom website, http://www3.ridom.de/seqsphere, accessed 2012 November 29th) and sequence types were computed automatically. The phylogenetic group of the *E. coli* strains was determined using the software Structure 2.3.X based on the concatenated sequences of the seven housekeeping genes used for MLST (University of Chicago website http://pritch.bsd.uchicago.edu/structure.html, accessed 2012 November 29th).

Macrorestriction Analyses by Pulsed Field Gel Electrophoresis (PFGE)

To asses possible clonal relatedness of ESBL-producing *E. coli* isolates, macrorestriction analysis was performed as previously described using a CHEF DRIII System (BioRad, Munich, Germany) [27]. PFGE profiles generated by restriction of chromosomal DNA with *Xba*I were compared digitally using

Table 1. Wild bird species sampled and number of *E. coli* and ESBL-producing *E. coli* isolated from respective host species.

Origin	Total number of birds and avian species	No. of *E. coli* isolated (% avian hosts)	No. ESBL-*E. coli* (% of all *E. coli*)	Strain name ESBL-*E. coli*	Sampling site of ESBL-*E. coli*
Germany	Total 171	65 (38.0)	9 (13.8)		
	13 Black Kites (*Milvus migrans*)	9 (69.2)	2 (22.0)	IMT21743 IMT21823	all within 30 km² around N51°56′24.5″, E 11°13′13.2″
	73 Red Kites (*Milvus milvus*)	32 (43.8)	6 (18.8)	IMT21774 IMT21783 IMT21790 IMT21810 IMT21818 IMT21829	
	68 Buzzards (*Buteo buteo*)	15 (22.0)	1 (6.6)	IMT21813	
	2 Sea Eagles (*Haliaeetus albicilla*)	1 (50.0)	–	–	–
	1 Spotted Eagle (*Aquila pomarina*)	1 (100.0)	–	–	–
	14 Goshawks (*Accicepter gentilis*)	7 (50.0)	–	–	–
Mongolia	Total 91	37 (40.7)	4 (10.8)		
	19 Black Kites (*Milvus migrans*)	13 (68.4)	1 (7.6)	IMT23464	N 44°24′03.6″, E 105°21′17.9″
	9 Buzzards (*Buteo hemilasius*)	3 (33.3)	–		
	30 Black Vultures (*Aegypius monachus*)	11 (36.6)	3 (27.3)	IMT21913	N 47°40′22.4″, E 105°56′51.9″
				IMT23462	N 45°48′05.4″, E 107°15′07.9″
				IMT23463	N 45°46′53.6″, E 107°15′23.7″
	4 Steppe Eagles (*Aquila nipalensis*)	2 (50.0)	–	–	–
	1 Golden Eagle (*Aquila chrysaetos*)	0 (0)	–	–	–
	1 Short-toed Eagle (*Circaetus gallicus*)	0 (0)	–	–	–
	3 Eurasian Hobbys (*Falco subbuteo*)	0 (0)	–	–	–
	14 Kestrels (*Falco tinnunculus*)	4 (28.7)	–	–	–
	8 Saker Falcons (*Falco cherrug*)	2 (25.0)	–	–	–
	2 Lesser Kestrels (*Falco naumanni*)	2 (100.0)	–	–	–
	15 Demoiselle Cranes (*Anthropoides virgo*)*	6 (40.0)	1 (16.6)	IMT23465	N 46°41′32.6″, E 106°31′02.0″
	2 Sandpipers (*Actitis hypoleucos*)*	0 (0)	–	–	–
	1 Nightjar (*Caprimulgus europaeus*)*	0 (0)	–	–	–
	1 Hoepoe (*Upupa epops*)*	0 (0)	–	–	–

*Non-birds of prey species, not included in the calculations;
–=no ESBL identified.

BioNumerics software (Version 6.6, Applied Maths, Belgium). Cluster analysis of Dice similarity indices based on the unweighted pair group method with arithmetic mean (UPGMA) was applied to generate dendrograms depicting the relationships among PFGE profiles. Isolates were considered to belong to a group of clonally related strains if the Dice similarity index of the PFGE pattern was ≥85% [29].

Results and Discussion

We isolated comparable rates of *E. coli* from birds sampled in the two sampling areas; 38% of the German and 41% of the Mongolian birds carried *E. coli* (Tab. 1). We confirmed ESBL-production in 13.8% (n = 9) of the sixty-five German and in 10.8% (n = 4) of the thirty-seven Mongolian *E. coli* isolates. Although we detected an ESBL-*E. coli*, originating from a Demoiselle Crane, the strain was excluded from the calculations as it represented a non-raptor bird, but we have provided the typing results of the strain in the manuscript. All ESBL-*E. coli* from this study originated from different individual raptors in different nests, thus precluding a possible bias caused by inter-sibling transfer in the nest. By including all birds of the study –even those who did not

carry *E. coli*, 5.2% of the wild birds from Germany and 4.5% of those from Mongolia carried ESBL-*E. coli*.

The detection rate of ESBL-*E. coli* observed for the German isolates (13.8%) correlates with data from other studies on raptors from Central Europe where detection rates from 10–20% have been observed [11]. Although based on a limited number of studies available on raptors, high carriage rates seem to be present in Europe independently from the origin of the birds, whether from natural preserves or land used for agricultural production [11]. There is no data on the occurrence of ESBL-*E. coli* in raptors from remote areas, but the detection rates of ESBL-*E. coli* for other avian species (Glaucus Winged Gull) were only about 1%. In this regard, the carriage rates of ESBL-*E. coli* detected in this study among Mongolian raptors (10.8%) is surprisingly high. Furthermore, the ESBL-*E. coli* detected by Hernandez et al. (2010) [30] was typed as O25b:H4-ST131-CTX-15, presenting an anthropogenic clinically important zoonotic pathogen and no commensal *E. coli* [31]. The mere detection of antimicrobial resistant commensal *E. coli* in the Mongolian samples, which has been described for wild birds or rodents in remote areas [32,33] could have been anticipated, but high rates of clinically important multi-resistant ESBL-*E. coli* like ST648 and ST167 have, to the best of our knowledge, not been yet detected in remote areas. As described in detail in the following, large proportions of the Mongolian ESBL-*E. coli* in this study displayed a high similarity to relevant clinical pathogenic strains from Europe, clearly indicating their zoonotic potential. Thus our data underline that the previous finding of O25b:H4-ST131-CTX-15 in a wild bird was not by chance [30], but that besides commensal *E. coli* displaying antimicrobial resistance, clinical zoonotic pathogens have also reached remote areas in significant numbers.

Genotypic characterisation of the isolates revealed that all ESBL-*E. coli* harboured bla_{CTX-M} genes, with $bla_{CTX-M-1}$ predominating among German (100%) and $bla_{CTX-M-9}$ amongst Mongolian isolates (80%) (Tab. 2). $bla_{CTX-M-1}$ represents the predominant ESBL type in poultry, pigs and cattle in Europe, but not in human clinical samples where $bla_{CTX-M-1}$ counts for only about 7%, as revealed by a meta-analysis recently published by our group [26]. The high prevalence of $bla_{CTX-M-1}$ in the German birds suggests transmission from livestock breeding into the environment, and subsequently, to wild birds, rather than from human sources. To our knowledge, clinical data on ESBL-*E. coli* from Mongolia are not available, but as for the rest of Asia, the major type found in the Mongolian birds ($bla_{CTX-M-9}$) only plays a minor role in human clinical samples [34]. $bla_{CTX-M-9}$ has also been found less frequently in livestock in Asia, underlining the highly complex spread of ESBL-*E. coli* [34].

Moreover, we detected several other resistance determinants for both sampling areas along with the beta-lactamase encoding genes (Tab. 2); the phenotypic resistance patterns these strains displayed confirmed these results (Tab. S1). Besides the production of ESBLs we also found concomitant resistance to tetracycline, sulphonamide/trimethoprim, and, to a lesser extent, fluoroquinolones. These results confirm recent data on common resistance in wild birds [35]. Ancestral group B2 strains (Sequence type ST12, ST2346), which are believed to be of high extra-intestinal virulence (ExPEC; extra-intestinal pathogenic *E. coli*), were present in one bird from Mongolia and one from Germany. Hybrid group ABD ESBL-*E. coli* strains (ST117, ST648) which are also believed

to be of extra-intestinal virulence, predominated in Mongolian birds (60%). Thus several isolates from both sampling areas combined multiresistance with a certain extra-intestinal virulence potential resembling a trend that has been observed in ESBL isolates worldwide and is highlighted by the intercontinental spread of O25b:H4-ST131-CTX-15 which represents an ESBL-producing ExPEC [31].

Overall, ten different STs were detected among the avian ESBL-*E. coli*; several of these, including ST12 (ancestral group B2), ST847 (B1), ST167 (A), and ST117 (ABD) have already been reported from human and veterinary clinical ESBL-producing isolates [34,36–39]. Interestingly, ST167 belongs to STs that have been associated with the global carriage of ESBL-*E. coli* in humans [34,38–41]. Recently, we found that this phylogenetic lineage was highly prevalent in ESBL-*E. coli* from companion animals (own unpublished data), while to the best of our knowledge, this is the first report of ST167 ESBL-*E. coli* in wildlife. In a previously published study on the epidemiology of ESBL-producing *Enterobacteriaceae* in Belgian hospitals [37] an ESBL-producing ST167 *E. coli* isolate (BICS2006/5510/1) was detected in a clinical sample from a 67-yr old patient with urinary tract infection. Indeed, a comparative macrorestriction analysis of this strain with the Mongolian ST167 Black vulture ESBL-*E. coli* isolate IMT23462 confirmed the clonal relatedness of both isolates (dice similarity index >90%) (Fig. 1 A). This finding is in line with recent data indicating that wildlife principally carries strains from the same phylogenetic background as clinical strains or even identical ESBL strains [11].

Interestingly, four of the isolates collected from wild birds in Germany were all assigned to ST744 and were subsequently found to belong to a single and identical PFGE clone (Fig. 1 B), although they originated from individuals (belonging to three avian species) sampled at different locations within an area of 30 square kilometres. A possible explanation for this could be either the existence of one single environmental origin or a yet unidentified non-point source, thus implying the general occurrence of this particular clone in that area to that time point.

Table 2. Molecular characteristics of ESBL-producing *E. coli* obtained from wild avian hosts according to phylogenetic background and resistance profile.

Strain	Host	Origin	Ances-tral group	ST	STC	ESBL type	Non extended spectrum beta-lactam resistance genes and integron cassettes
IMT21743	Milvus migrans	Ger	A	744	10	$bla_{CTX-M-1}$	$bla_{TEM-1-like}$, tet(B), sul2, strA, strB, aac(6')-IB-cr, integron class I
IMT21774	Milvus milvus	Ger	A	744	10	$bla_{CTX-M-1}$	$bla_{TEM-1-like}$, tet(B), sul2, strA, strB, aac(6')-IB-cr, integron class I
IMT21783	Milvus milvus	Ger	A	744	10	$bla_{CTX-M-1}$	$bla_{TEM-1-like}$, tet(B), sul2, strA, strB, aac(6')-IB-cr, integron class I
IMT21790	Milvus milvus	Ger	B2	12	12	$bla_{CTX-M-1}$	$bla_{TEM-1-like}$, tet(A), integron class I
IMT21810	Milvus milvus	Ger	B1	847	none	$bla_{CTX-M-1}$	$bla_{TEM-1-like}$, bla_{OXA-1}, tet(A), sul2, strA, strB, integron class I
IMT21813	Buteo buteo	Ger	A	744	10	$bla_{CTX-M-1}$	$bla_{TEM-1-like}$, tet(B), sul2, strA, strB, aac(6')-IB-cr, integron class I
IMI21818	Milvus milvus	Ger	A	2199	155	$bla_{CTX-M-1}$	tet(B), sul2, strA, strB, integron class I
IMT21823	Milvus migrans	Ger	D	2198	none	$bla_{CTX-M-1}$	$bla_{TEM-1-like}$, sul2, strA, strB, integron class I
IMT21829	Milvus milvus	Ger	AxB1	1640	350	$bla_{CTX-M-1}$	sul2, strA, strB, aac(6')-IB-cr, integron class I
IMT21913	Aegypius monachus	Mon	ABD	117	117	$bla_{CTX-M-55}$	$bla_{TEM-1-like}$, sul2, strA, strB, aac(3)-IV
IMT23462	Aegypius monachus	Mon	A	167	10	$bla_{CTX-M-9}$	sul2, strA, strB, integron class I
IMT23463	Aegypius monachus	Mon	ABD	648	648	$bla_{CTX-M-9}$	$bla_{TEM-1-like}$, bla_{OXA-1}, tet(A), sul2, strA,strB, aac (6')-IB-cr, integron class I
IMT23464	Milvus migrans	Mon	ABD	648	648	$bla_{CTX-M-9}$	$bla_{TEM-1-like}$, bla_{OXA-1}, tet(A), sul2,strA, strB, aac (6')-IB-cr, integron class I
IMT23465	Anthropoides virgo*	Mon	B2	2346	none	$bla_{CTX-M-9}$	$bla_{TEM-1-like}$, bla_{OXA-1}, tet(A), sul1, integron class I

Abbreviations: ST = sequence type; STC = ST complex; Ger = Germany; Mon = Mongolia,
*Non-birds of prey species.

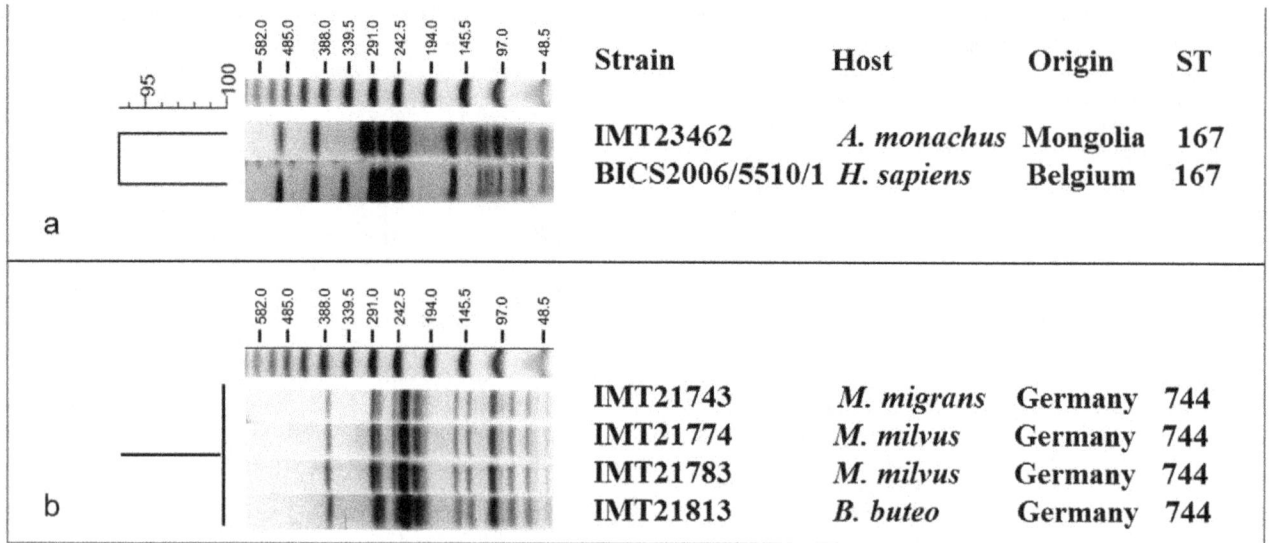

Figure 1. Dendrogram showing (A) the relationship of one avian ESBL-*E. coli* isolate and a human clinical isolate [39], both of ST167, and (B) PFGE profiles of four avian ST744 ESBL-*E. coli* isolates based on *Xba*I restriction calculated with Bionumerics 6.6 (Applied Maths, Belgium). ST = sequence type; *A.* = *Aegypius*; *B.* = *Buteo*; *H.* = *Homo*; *M.* = *Milvus*, A size marker (Lambda Ladder PFG Marker; New England Biolabs GmbH, Frankfurt a. M., Germany) with respective fragment sizes (kb) is given on top of the agarose gel.

The low-level prevalence of ESBL-*E. coli* that has been reported previously in wild birds from remote areas [30] contrasts with the findings in the present study. This is surprising since it has been recently shown that proximity to human-influenced settings was associated with an increase in antimicrobial-resistant bacteria [42]. The occurrence of ESBL-*E. coli* seems to be species dependent and this may have influenced the high rates obtained in this study [11]. Nevertheless the southward migration of Mongolian Birds to areas with higher human influence and the possible spill-over of multi-resistant bacteria from a spatially segregated, polluted environment might be the reason for the frequent occurrence of ESBL-*E. coli* in the avian hosts in remote areas. This would also contradict previous assumptions that multi-resistant bacterial contaminations should be low in remote environments that lack constant antibiotic pressure [43].

relevant ESBL-*E. coli* are present in remote environments as well. The contribution of international human travel to the spread of multi-resistant *E. coli* has only recently garnered attentions [49] and avian migration follows essentially the same principles. Its importance is often neglected although the number of migrating birds worldwide has been estimated to be five billion a year [50]. We would encourage additional studies focusing on carriage rates, persistence and duration of shedding/excretion of ESBL-*E. coli* in migratory birds on a larger scale. Studies on the necessary frequency of antibiotic exposure to generate significant resistance in wildlife are needed. Such data could help to estimate the potential influence of avian hosts on the pandemic spread of ESBL-*E. coli* into the environment, the community and ultimately, human and veterinary clinical settings.

Conclusions

The possible contribution of avian migration to the transmission of multi-resistant bacteria has been discussed previously [11,44]. In this study, we found that ESBL-*E. coli* from wild birds originating from Germany and from remote regions of Mongolia differed in their resistance genes and phylogenetic background. This is not unexpected, since the examined avian species do not migrate between Mongolia and Central Europe. Nonetheless, all Mongolian avian hosts sampled in this study undergo southward migration, namely on the Korean Peninsula (Black vulture), to China (Buzzards), and to India (Demoiselle Crane), connecting remote areas to the globalised world with high frequencies of ESBL-*E. coli* in human and livestock [13,45–47].

Although we acknowledge that the presented data are based on a limited number of samples, they clearly suggest the equation "no man, no resistance" is an over simplification [48], as clinically

Acknowledgments

We would like to thank Michael F.C. Moreland for careful proofreading of the manuscript.

Author Contributions

Conceived and designed the experiments: SG AS MS NB LHW CE. Performed the experiments: SG KA IS AB TS AS MS YG CE. Analyzed the data: SG AB TS AS MS NB YG LHW CE. Wrote the paper: SG LHW CE.

References

1. Pinto L, Radhouani H, Coelho C, Martins da Costa P, Simoes R, et al. (2010) Genetic detection of extended-spectrum beta-lactamase-containing *Escherichia coli* isolates from birds of prey from Serra da Estrela Natural Reserve in Portugal. Appl Environ Microbiol 76: 4118–4120.

2. Costa D, Poeta P, Saenz Y, Vinue L, Rojo-Bezares B, et al. (2006) Detection of *Escherichia coli* harbouring extended-spectrum beta-lactamases of the CTX-M, TEM and SHV classes in faecal samples of wild animals in Portugal. J Antimicrob Chemother 58: 1311–1312.

3. Radhouani H, Pinto L, Coelho C, Goncalves A, Sargo R, et al. (2010) Detection of *Escherichia coli* harbouring extended-spectrum beta-lactamases of the CTX-M classes in faecal samples of common buzzards (*Buteo buteo*). J Antimicrob Chemother 65: 171–173.

4. Literak I, Dolejska M, Janoszowska D, Hrusakova J, Meissner W, et al. (2010) Antibiotic-resistant *Escherichia coli* bacteria, including strains with genes encoding the extended-spectrum beta-lactamase and QnrS, in waterbirds on the Baltic Sea Coast of Poland. Appl Environ Microbiol 76: 8126–8134.

5. Bloom DE (2011) 7 billion and counting. Science 333: 562–569.

6. Eds. Steinfeld H, Mooney HA, Schneider F, Neville LE (2010) Livestock in a Changing Landscape, Drivers, Consequences and Responses. Island Press.

7. Allen HK, Donato J, Wang HH, Cloud-Hansen KA, Davies J, et al. (2010) Call of the wild: antibiotic resistance genes in natural environments. Nat Rev Microbiol 8: 251–259.

8. Nelson M, Jones SH, Edwards C, Ellis JC (2008) Characterization of *Escherichia coli* populations from gulls, landfill trash, and wastewater using ribotyping. Dis Aquat Organ 81: 53–63.

9. Blanco G, Lemus JA, Grande J, Gangoso L, Grande JM, et al. (2007) Geographical variation in cloacal microflora and bacterial antibiotic resistance in a threatened avian scavenger in relation to diet and livestock farming practices. Environ Microbiol 9: 1738–1749.

10. Wieler LH, Ewers C, Guenther S, Walther B, Lubke-Becker A (2011) Methicillin-resistant staphylococci (MRS) and extended-spectrum beta-lactamases (ESBL)-producing *Enterobacteriaceae* in companion animals: nosocomial infections as one reason for the rising prevalence of these potential zoonotic pathogens in clinical samples. Int J Med Microbiol 301: 635–641.

11. Guenther S, Ewers C, Wieler LH (2011) Extended-spectrum beta-lactamases producing *E. coli* in wildlife, yet another form of environmental pollution? Front Microbio 2:246.

12. Wint W, Robinson T (2007) Gridded Livestock of the World 2007. FAO, Rome: 131.

13. Stubbe M, Stubbe A, Batsajchan N (2010) Grid mapping and breeding ecology of raptors in Mongolia. Erforsch biol Ress Mongolei (Halle/Saale) 11: 23–175.

14. The Ornithological Counsil website. Available: http://oacu.od.nih.gov/WildBirdGuide.pdf. Accessed 2012 Nov 28.

15. CLSI (2008) Performance standards for antimicrobial disk and dilution susceptibility tests for bacteria isolated from animals; approved standard - Third Edition CLSI document M31-A3. Wayne, PA, U.S.A.: Clinical and laboratory standards institute, 2008.

16. Rodriguez I, Barownick W, Helmuth R, Mendoza MC, Rodicio MR, et al. (2009) Extended-spectrum beta-lactamases and AmpC beta-lactamases in ceftiofur-resistant *Salmonella enterica* isolates from food and livestock obtained in Germany during 2003–07. J Antimicrob Chemother 64: 301–309.

17. Carattoli A, Bertini A, Villa L, Falbo V, Hopkins KL, et al. (2005) Identification of plasmids by PCR-based replicon typing. J Microbiol Methods 63: 219–228.

18. Bertrand S, Weill FX, Cloeckaert A, Vrints M, Mairiaux E, et al. (2006) Clonal emergence of extended-spectrum beta-lactamase (CTX-M-2)-producing *Salmonella enterica* serovar Virchow isolates with reduced susceptibilities to ciprofloxacin among poultry and humans in Belgium and France (2000 to 2003). J Clin Microbiol 44: 2897–2903.

19. Robicsek A, Strahilevitz J, Jacoby GA, Macielag M, Abbanat D, et al. (2006) Fluoroquinolone-modifying enzyme: a new adaptation of a common aminoglycoside acetyltransferase. Nature medicine 12: 83–88.

20. Park YJ, Yu JK, Lee S, Oh EJ, Woo GJ (2007) Prevalence and diversity of qnr alleles in AmpC-producing *Enterobacter cloacae*, *Enterobacter aerogenes*, *Citrobacter freundii* and *Serratia marcescens*: a multicentre study from Korea. J Antimicrob Chemother 60: 868–871.

21. Grimm V, Ezaki S, Susa M, Knabbe C, Schmid RD (2004) Use of DNA microarrays for rapid genotyping of TEM beta-lactamases that confer resistance. J Clin Microbiol 42: 3766–3774.

22. Jouini A, Vinué L, Slama KB, Sáenz Y, Klibi N, et al. (2007) Characterization of CTX-M and SHV extended-spectrum beta-lactamases and associated resistance genes in *Escherichia coli* strains of food samples in Tunisia. J Antimicrob Chemother 60: 1137–1141.

23. Skurnik D, Le Menac'h A, Zurakowski D, Mazel D, Courvalin P, et al. (2005) Integron-associated antibiotic resistance and phylogenetic grouping of *Escherichia coli* isolates from healthy subjects free of recent antibiotic exposure. Antimicrobial agents and chemotherapy 49: 3062–3065.

24. Maguire AJ, Brown DF, Gray JJ, Desselberger U (2001) Rapid screening technique for class 1 integrons in *Enterobacteriaceae* and nonfermenting gram-negative bacteria and its use in molecular epidemiology. Antimicrob Agents Chemother 45: 1022–1029.

25. Martinez-Martinez L, Pascual A, Jacoby GA (1998) Quinolone resistance from a transferable plasmid. Lancet 351: 797–799.

26. Ewers C, Grobbel M, Stamm I, Kopp PA, Diehl I, et al. (2010) Emergence of human pandemic O25:H4-ST131 CTX-M-15 extended-spectrum beta-lactamase-producing *Escherichia coli* among companion animals. J Antimicrob Chemother 65: 651–660.

27. Ewers C, Janssen T, Kiessling S, Philipp HC, Wieler LH (2004) Molecular epidemiology of avian pathogenic *Escherichia coli* (APEC) isolated from colisepticemia in poultry. Vet Microbiol 104: 91–101.

28. Wirth T, Falush D, Lan R, Colles F, Mensa P, et al. (2006) Sex and virulence in *Escherichia coli*: an evolutionary perspective. Mol Microbiol 60: 1136–1151.

29. Carrico JA, Pinto FR, Simas C, Nunes S, Sousa NG, et al. (2005) Assessment of band-based similarity coefficients for automatic type and subtype classification of microbial isolates analyzed by pulsed-field gel electrophoresis. J Clin Microbiol 43: 5483–5490.

30. Hernandez J, Bonnedahl J, Eliasson I, Wallensten A, Comstedt P, et al. (2010) Globally disseminated human pathogenic *Escherichia coli* of O25b-ST131 clone, harbouring *bla*CTX-M-15, found in Glaucous-winged gull at remote Commander Islands, Russia. Environ Microbiol Rep 2: 329–332.

31. Nicolas-Chanoine MH, Blanco J, Leflon-Guibout V, Demarty R, Alonso MP, et al. (2008) Intercontinental emergence of *Escherichia coli* clone O25:H4-ST131 producing CTX-M-15. J Antimicrob Chemother 61: 273–281.

32. Gilliver MA, Bennett M, Begon M, Hazel SM, Hart CA (1999) Antibiotic resistance found in wild rodents. Nature 401: 233–234.

33. Williams NJ, Sherlock C, Jones TR, Clough HE, Telfer SE, et al. (2011) The prevalence of antimicrobial-resistant *Escherichia coli* in sympatric wild rodents varies by season and host. J Appl Microbiol.

34. Ewers C, Bethe A, Semmler T, Guenther S, Wieler LH (2012) Extended-spectrum ß-lactamase-producing and AmpC-producing *Escherichia coli* from livestock and companion animals, and their putative impact on public health: a global perspective. Clinical Microbiology and Infection 18: 646–655.

35. Guenther S, Grobbel M, Lubke-Becker A, Goedecke A, Friedrich ND, et al. (2010) Antimicrobial resistance profiles of *Escherichia coli* from common European wild bird species. Vet Microbiol 144: 219–225.

36. Nemoy LL, Kotetishvili M, Tigno J, Keefer-Norris A, Harris AD, et al. (2005) Multilocus sequence typing versus pulsed-field gel electrophoresis for characterization of extended-spectrum beta-lactamase-producing *Escherichia coli* isolates. J Clin Microbiol 43: 1776–1781.

37. Rodriguez-Villalobos H, Bogaerts P, Berhin C, Bauraing C, Deplano A, et al. (2011) Trends in production of extended-spectrum beta-lactamases among *Enterobacteriaceae* of clinical interest: results of a nationwide survey in Belgian hospitals. J Antimicrob Chemother 66: 37–47.

38. Leverstein-van Hall MA, Dierikx CM, Cohen Stuart J, Voets GM, van den Munckhof MP, et al. (2011) Dutch patients, retail chicken meat and poultry share the same ESBL genes, plasmids and strains. Clin Microbiol Infect 17: 873–880.

39. Oteo J, Diestra K, Juan C, Bautista V, Novais A, et al. (2009) Extended-spectrum beta-lactamase-producing *Escherichia coli* in Spain belong to a large variety of multilocus sequence typing types, including ST10 complex/A, ST23 complex/A and ST131/B2. Int J Antimicrob Agents 34: 173–176.

40. Naseer U, Haldorsen B, Tofteland S, Hegstad K, Scheutz F, et al. (2009) Molecular characterization of CTX-M-15-producing clinical isolates of *Escherichia coli* reveals the spread of multidrug-resistant ST131 (O25:H4) and ST964 (O102:H6) strains in Norway. APMIS 117: 526–536.

41. Valverde A, Canton R, Garcillan-Barcia MP, Novais A, Galan JC, et al. (2009) Spread of bla$_{CTX-M-14}$ is driven mainly by IncK plasmids disseminated among *Escherichia coli* phylogroups A, B1, and D in Spain. Antimicrob Agents Chemother 53: 5204–5212.

42. Skurnik D, Ruimy R, Andremont A, Amorin C, Rouquet P, et al. (2006) Effect of human vicinity on antimicrobial resistance and integrons in animal faecal *Escherichia coli*. J Antimicrob Chemother 57: 1215–1219.

43. Sjölund M, Bonnedahl J, Hernandez J, Bengtsson S, Cederbrant G, et al. (2008) Dissemination of multidrug-resistant bacteria into the Arctic. Emerg Infect Dis 14: 70–72.

44. Bonnedahl J (2011) Antibiotic resistance in *Enterobacteriaceae* from Wild birds. Acta Universitatis Upsaliensis Uppsala.

45. Woodford N, Turton JF, Livermore DM (2011) Multiresistant Gram-negative bacteria: the role of high-risk clones in the dissemination of antibiotic resistance. FEMS microbiology reviews 35: 736–755.

46. Naseer U, Sundsfjord A (2011) The CTX-M conundrum: dissemination of plasmids and *Escherichia coli* clones. Microb Drug Resist 17: 83–97.

47. Peirano G, Pitout JD (2010) Molecular epidemiology of *Escherichia coli* producing CTX M beta lactamases: the worldwide emergence of clone ST131 O25:H4. Int J Antimicrob Agents 35: 316–321.

48. Thaller MC, Migliore L, Marquez C, Tapia W, Cedeno V, et al. (2010) Tracking acquired antibiotic resistance in commensal bacteria of Galapagos land iguanas: no man, no resistance. PloS one 5: e8989.

49. Peirano G, Laupland KB, Gregson DB, Pitout JDD (2011) Colonization of Returning Travelers With CTX-M-Producing *Escherichia coli*. J Travel Med 18: 299–303.

50. Berthold P (2001) Bird migration. A general survey. Oxford ornithological series 2nd ed. Oxford Univ. Press Oxford, Great Britain.

11

Serial Non-Invasive Measurements of Dermal Carotenoid Concentrations in Dairy Cows following Recovery from Abomasal Displacement

Julia Klein[1,2], Maxim E. Darvin[2]*, Kerstin E. Müller[1], Juergen Lademann[2]

1 Clinic for Ruminants and Swine, Faculty of Veterinary Medicine, Freie Universität Berlin, Berlin, Germany, 2 Center of Experimental and Applied Cutaneous Physiology, Department of Dermatology, Venerology and Allergology, Charité – Universitätsmedizin Berlin, Berlin, Germany

Abstract

Maintaining the health of farm animals forms the basis for a sustainable and profitable production of food from animal origin. Recently, the effects of carotenoids on the oxidative status as well as on reproductive and immune functions in cattle have been demonstrated. The present study aimed at investigating dermal carotenoid levels in cattle recovering from abomasal displacement. For this purpose, serial *in vivo* measurements were undertaken using a miniaturized scanner system that relies on reflection spectroscopy (Opsolution GmbH, Kassel, Germany). In a first trial, repeated measurements of dermal carotenoid concentrations were performed on the udder skin of healthy non-lactating cattle (n = 6) for one month in weekly intervals. In a second trial, *in vivo* dermal carotenoid concentrations were determined in intervals in 23 cows following surgical treatment of abomasal displacement. The results show that dermal carotenoid concentrations, determined on a weekly basis over a period of one month, showed variations of up to 18% in the healthy individuals kept under constant conditions with respect to housing and nutrition. Repeated measurements during the recovery period following surgical treatment of abomasal displacement resulted in an increase in dermal carotenoid concentrations in 18 of 20 animals with a favourable outcome when compared with results obtained within 12 hours following surgery. The mean increase in dermal carotenoid concentrations in subsequent measurements was 53±44%, whereas levels decreased (mean 31±27%) in cattle with a fatal outcome. These results indicate potential applications for reflection spectroscopy for non-invasive early detection of changes in the dermal carotenoid concentrations as a reflection of the antioxidant status in an animal.

Editor: Corinne Ida Lasmezas, The Scripps Research Institute Scripps Florida, United States of America

Funding: The authors have no support or funding to report.

Competing Interests: The authors have declared that no competing interests exist.

* E-mail: maxim.darvin@charite.de

Introduction

As herd sizes increase, the early detection of metabolic diseases is becoming more and more important. A suitable method for the surveillance of the health status in food producing animals should be simple to use, inexpensive and reliable, and should allow the detection of diseases or deficiencies at an early stage.

Recent studies in humans demonstrate that various kinds of stress, including an unhealthy lifestyle as well as metabolic disorders and tumorgenesis, have an effect on the oxidative status [1,2,3,4,5,6]. The latter disorders have been demonstrated to result in the generation of free radicals that cause the destruction of antioxidants. Carotenoids take part of the chain of antioxidants in the body. To this end a decrease in the carotenoid levels in blood and various tissues is regarded an indicator for antioxidant reduction [7,8,9,10]. Recent investigations have shown that dermal carotenoids could serve as marker substances for the entire antioxidant status of human skin [11,12].

Until recently, the determination of the oxidative status in humans and animals demanded the sampling of blood or biopsy materials [13,14]. Innovative technologies such as reflection spectroscopy have been applied to determine dermal carotenoid concentrations in order to evaluate the effects of stress conditions on the oxidative status of humans. A hand-held miniaturized spectroscopic system (Opsolution GmbH, Kassel, Germany) is available, which allows serial non-invasive measurements of the dermal carotenoid concentrations in real-time on humans or animals [15,16].

In the present study, dermal carotenoid concentrations were determined once weekly over a period of one month on six healthy cattle that were kept under the same environmental conditions and received the same diet. In addition, repeated measurements of dermal carotenoid concentrations were performed on 23 dairy cows during the recovery period following surgical treatment of abomasal displacement. The decision for abomasal displacement was taken considering the importance of this disease on the one hand as well as the absence of the influence on metabolism of carotenoids in the body, the relatively short recovery phase and the good comparability of the animals after surgery on the other.

Materials and Methods

Miniaturized spectroscopic system (MSS)

A LED-based compact scanner system (Opsolution GmbH, Kassel, Germany) was used for non-invasive determination of the dermal carotenoid concentration by reflection spectroscopy. The pattern of the light reflected from the skin is mainly based on the presence of chromophores in the skin which contain carotenoids that absorb light at certain wavelengths. Taking into consideration the absorption spectrum of carotenoids, which is located in the blue-green range of the optical spectrum, the blue LED-emitted bright spectrum in the range between 440 nm and 490 nm was used as a source of excitation. The small dip in the reflected spectrum is based on the absorption by dermal carotenoids. The dermal carotenoid concentrations are determined by calculating the difference in intensity between the emitted and reflected spectra, and are expressed in arbitrary units. Prior to its application on bovine udder skin, the system was calibrated using Resonance Raman Spectroscopy [17]. A strong correlation was found (R = 0.81). Stability of the measurements was determined by the standard deviation of the measured values, which normally do not exceed 10% [15].

Measurement protocol

Measurements of dermal carotenoid concentrations took place once weekly over a period of one month as follows: The measurements were performed on the left body side on three pre-determined sites on the surface of the udder skin. The different sites were located 10 cm proximal to the basis of the teat. Two sites were located perpendicularly above the teats, while the third site was located halfway between these points. Prior to the measurements, the udder skin was carefully shaved without injuring the stratum corneum, using a single-use shaver, and the homogeneously pigmented skin sites of approx. 0.8 cm^2 were marked (Figure 1). The MSS was placed on marked sites of the udder skin. Each site was subjected to three subsequent measurements. Measurements were performed in triplicate on each marked site. To this end, the MSS was removed from the skin between measurements and then positioned on the same skin area again. The time interval between the measurements was only a few seconds. This procedure has previously been described in detail by Klein et al. [16]. The median and the standard deviation were calculated from the triploid measurements at three different sites in close proximity.

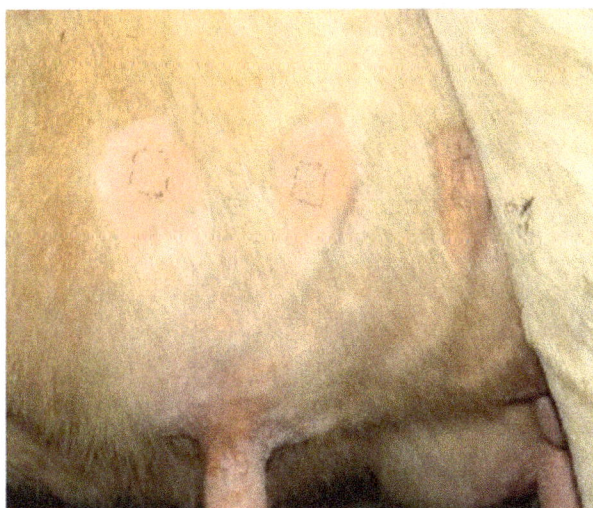

Figure 1. Measuring sites on the udder skin of a cow.

Serial determinations of the dermal carotenoid concentrations in six healthy cows (Trial 1)

In a first trial, six healthy non-lactating female cows belonging to the breeds German Holstein (n = 4), Uckermaerker (n = 1) and Simmentaler (n = 1) aged between two and 15 years were investigated. All animals were kept in tied stalls on straw bedding under the same environmental conditions, and received the same diet consisting of hay and grass silage ad libitum. In addition, each animal received 0.5 kg of Hendrix Illesch concentrate per day. None of the animals had calved in the six preceding months, was gravid or received any medical treatment. The carotenoid concentration was determined weekly over a period of four weeks.

Course of dermal carotenoid levels following surgical treatment of abomasal displacement (Trial 2)

In a second trial, the dermal carotenoid levels were determined in 23 German Holstein dairy cows aged two to nine years (mean 4.37 years) that had been submitted to the Clinic for Ruminants in the period from January to April 2011 by local veterinarians due to abomasal displacement (DA). The animals originated from eight different dairy farms in the Brandenburg region and underwent surgery for DA either by endoscopical abomasopexy (Janowitz) or by celiotomy in the right flank followed by omentopexy (method according to Dirksen, Hanover, Germany). The first measurement took place within 12 hours after surgical intervention and was followed by repeated measurements during hospitalization. The last measurement was performed after dismissal at the farm of origin (between 20 and 60 days after surgery). In cases with a fatal outcome, the last measurement prior to euthanasia or death was considered for evaluation.

Statistical Analysis

The software program SPSS 18.00 for Windows was used for the statistical analysis, with p<0.05 being considered statistically significant and p<0.001 being considered statistically highly significant. As part of the data was not normally distributed, the median was used for representation. The calculation was performed using non-parametric tests. While more than two dependent samples were subjected to Friedman's test, the Wilcoxon test was applied to compare two dependent samples.

Ethics Statement

In the present study, all measurements were performed non-invasively according to §7 of the German Animal Welfare Act, which clarifies the necessity of ethical approval in the case of interventions or treatments involving pain, suffering or damage to the animals. Taking this definition into account, no application for ethical approval of animal experiments was filed, because it had been very clear already prior to commencement of the measurements that the animals would not be exposed to any pain, suffering or damage.

Both animal care and experimental procedures were approved and conducted under established standard of the Clinic for Ruminants and Swine, Faculty of Veterinary Medicine, Freie Universität Berlin and Charité - Universitätsmedizin Berlin, Germany.

Results

Repeated measurements on healthy cattle (Trial 1)

The median of dermal carotenoid concentrations, as determined by reflection spectroscopy applied to three adjacent sites of the udder skin of six healthy cattle, ranged from 0.91 to 1.79 as

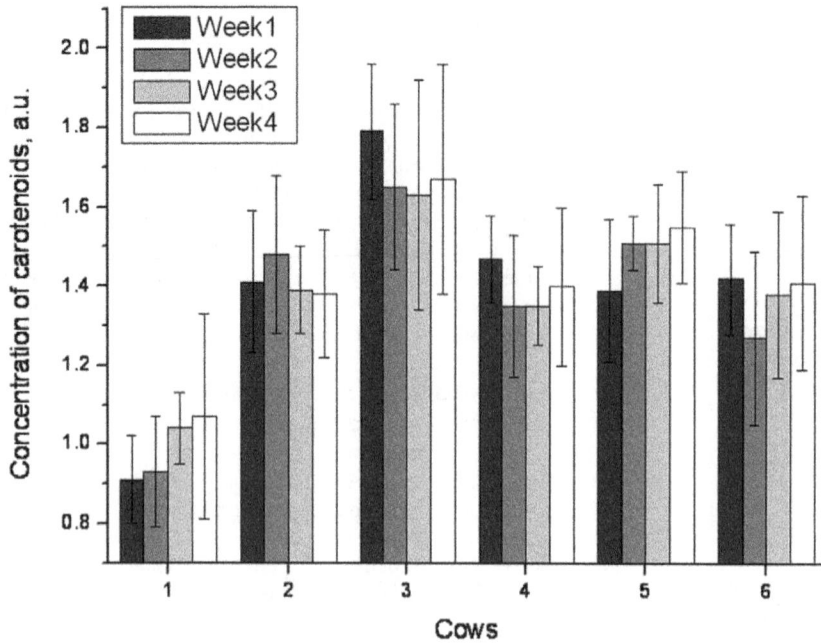

Figure 2. Course of dermal carotenoid concentrations expressed in arbitrary units in six healthy cows measured weekly over a period of one month.

expressed in arbitrary units (Figure 2). Significant differences were observed between individual animals kept under the same conditions. Serial measurements performed on single animals at weekly intervals over a period of one month delivered results that ranged from 0.99 to 1.66 as expressed in arbitrary units. No significant differences (p = 0.44) were observed when the results of repeated measurements in individual animals with time were compared (Figure 2 and Table 1). Mean deviations determined for individual cows within the time frame of one month amounted to ≤18%.

Results of repeated determinations of dermal carotenoid concentrations in cows following surgical treatment of left abomasal displacement

The results obtained from 23 cows which underwent surgery due to left displaced abomasum ranged from 0.41 to 1.30 arbitrary units in the perioperative phase (<12 hours post operationem). Six

cows underwent surgery for DA by endoscopic abomasopexy (Janowitz) and 17 cows by celiotomy in the right flank followed by omentopexy (method according to Dirksen, Hanover, Germany). 3 cows (number 21, 22 and 23 in the Table 2) died or were euthanized, respectively, on day 3, 14 and 15 post operationem, they were measured at the farm of origin before their death. 18 of the 20 animals that recovered from left DA showed an increase in dermal carotenoid concentrations compared to the results of initial measurements, when examined after their dismissal on the farm of origin between day 20 and 60 post operationem (Table 2). Decreases were observed in two of the 20 cows (Figure 3). The mean increase in the 20 recovered cows was 53±44% compared to the initial value. Figure 4 illustrates the increase in the dermal carotenoid concentrations in two cows post operationem. The course of the dermal carotenoid concentrations was not consistent, but depended on the reconvalescence of the individual cow. Cow 8 was discharged from the clinic two days post operationem due to the favourable development of its condition. Its values kept

Table 1. Median and standard deviation (SD) of the nine individual values of the dermal carotenoid concentration as expressed in arbitrary units over a period of one month.

	week 1		week 2		week 3		week 4	
	median	SD	median	SD	median	SD	median	SD
cow 1	0,91	0.11	0.93	0.14	1.04	0.09	1.07	0.26
cow 2	1.41	0.18	1.48	0.2	1.39	0.11	1.38	0.16
cow 3	1.79	0.17	1.65	0.21	1.63	0.29	1.67	0.29
cow 4	1.47	0.11	1.35	0.18	1.35	0.1	1.4	0.2
cow 5	1.39	0.18	1.51	0.07	1.51	0.15	1.55	0.14
cow 6	1.42	0.14	1.27	0.22	1.38	0.21	1.41	0.22
Mean values	1.40	0.28	1.37	0.25	1.38	0.20	1.41	0.20

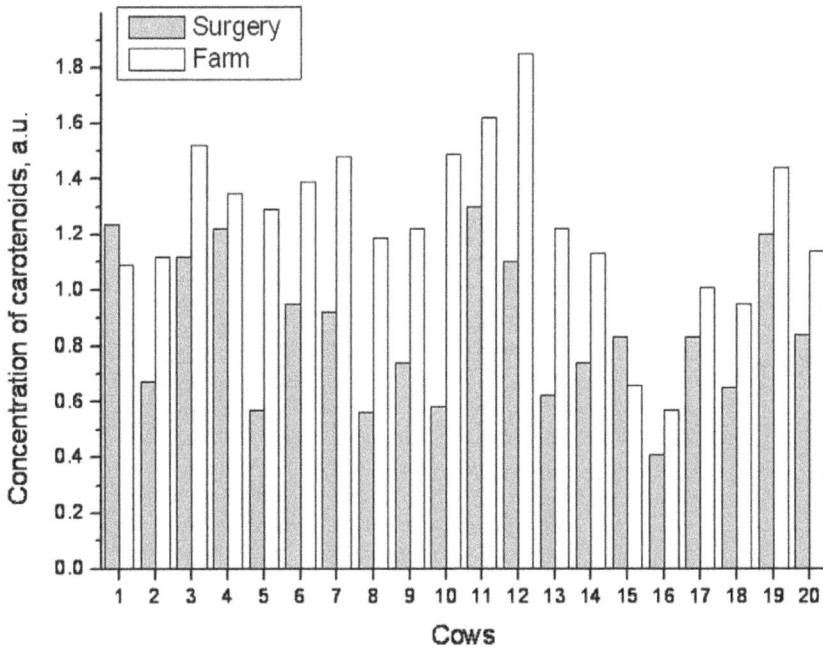

Figure 3. Course of the dermal carotenoid concentrations in 20 dairy cows treated surgically for abomasal displacement. Measurements were taken by reflection spectroscopy within 12 hours following surgery and at the farm of origin.

increasing. Cow 2 stayed in the clinic until day 16 post operationem due to insufficient progress of its condition. Its dermal carotenoid concentration increased with considerable delay (Figure 4).

20 days post operationem, the average median dermal carotenoid concentration of the 20 cows that had recovered exhibited a difference which was statistically highly significant ($p<0.001$) compared to the initial value.

In contrast the levels decreased (mean $31\pm27\%$) in the three cattle in which the outcome was fatal (Figure 5).

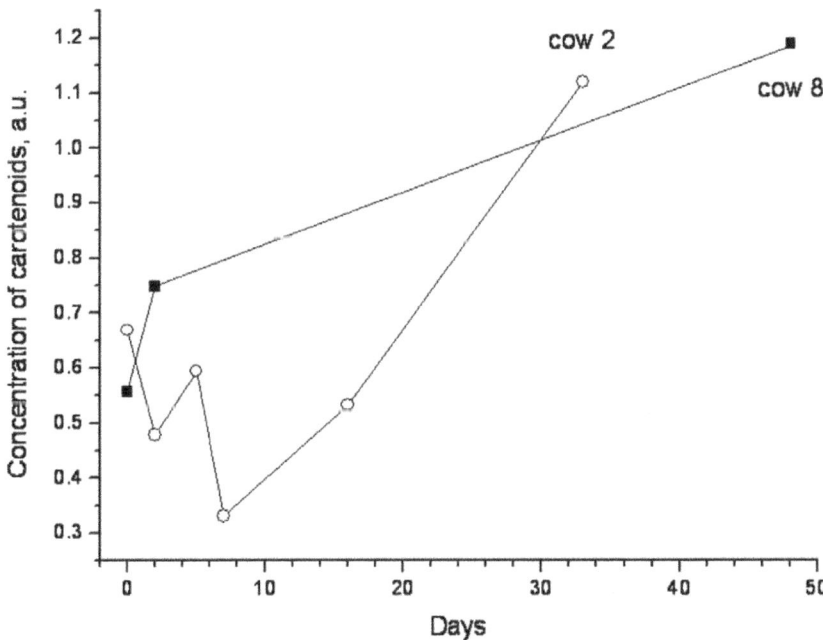

Figure 4. Course of recovery of cutaneous carotenoid concentrations in two cows from the day of surgery to the last measurement at the farm of origin. Cow 2 was discharged from the clinic two days post operationem due to the favourable development of its condition, while cow 8 stayed in the clinic until day 16 post operationem due to insufficient progress of its condition.

Table 2. Median and standard deviation (SD) of the dermal carotenoid concentrations in all 23 cows during their convalescence from DA involved in the study in the perioperative phase and at the farm of origin.

cow	day of surgery		at farm of origin	
	median	SD	median	SD
1	1.24	0.24	1.09	0.11
2	0.67	0.19	1.12	0.02
3	1.12	0.13	1.52	0.17
4	1.22	0.07	1.35	0.02
5	0.57	0.08	1.29	0.1
6	0.95	0.05	1.39	0.05
7	0.92	0.09	1.48	0.17
8	0.56	0.14	1.19	0.1
9	0.74	0.12	1.22	0.33
10	0.58	0.07	1.49	0.08
11	1.3	0.11	1.62	0.11
12	1.1	0.26	1.85	0.26
13	0.62	0.09	1.22	0.1
14	0.74	0.39	1.13	0.24
15	0.83	0.06	0.66	0.11
16	0.41	0.04	0.57	0.08
17	0.83	0.03	1.01	0.13
18	0.65	0.08	0.95	0.02
19	1.2	0.05	1.44	0.05
20	0.84	0.24	1,14	0.1
21	0.55	0.07	0.39	0.05
22	0.67	0.1	0.52	0.09
23	0.79	0.05	0.47	0.18
mean values	0.83	0.12	1.14	0.12

Cows 21–23 died after the surgery and were measured before the death at farm of origin.

Discussion

Repeated measurements in healthy cattle (Trial 1)

Measurements of the dermal carotenoid concentrations in six healthy cows kept under the same conditions rendered substantial interindividual differences. The latter findings are in accordance with earlier observations in healthy dairy cows that were examined at their farm of origin and that were kept under the same conditions and received the same diet [16]. When measuring isolated perfused cow udders ex vivo using reflection spectroscopy, Niedorf et al. also established a strong heterogeneity of the samples in terms of the β-carotene concentration in the skin [18]. Large interindividual differences regarding the β-carotene concentrations in the blood were also detected by both Lotthammer et al. and Noziere et al. [19,20,21]. Moreover, the dermal carotenoid concentrations in human volunteers covered a wide range of levels [22,23,24]. These findings were related to differences in the eating habits, lifestyles and, possibly, different stress conditions [1,25,26].

Repeated measurements in the same animal and the same skin area in weekly intervals revealed deviations of ≤18% which were not significant. Also the measurements taken within four days yielded no significant differences [16].

The udder skin was chosen as it can be easily accessed in cows and the light-coloured hair coat is only sparse in this region compared to the rest of the body. Measurements in humans have shown that the carotenoid concentration also depends on the side of the body on which the measurement is conducted [27,28]. Contrary to the measurements reported by Niedorf et al. on an isolated perfused cow udder [18,29], the data measured in this study were not influenced by absorption spectra of other chromophores due to the design of MSS [15]. The thickness of the epidermis of cow udder skin does usually not exceed 200 μm [30]. Taking into consideration the penetration depth of blue light into the skin, which is approximately 150–200 μm, as well as a design of MSS, the influence of dermal chromophores, such as melanin, haemoglobin, bilirubin, etc., is negligible [15]. Comparing β-carotene concentrations in the blood with dermal carotenoid concentrations in the same animal delivered significant correlations between the results of the two techniques for cattle with a moderate to obese body condition (unpublished data).

Using reflection spectroscopic measurements, a dose-dependent distribution of β-carotene in the skin and a decrease of the cutaneous β-carotene concentrations under UV irradiation could be demonstrated in an isolated perfused cow udder model [31]. Experiments in which β-carotene was administered to the model showed a satiety phenomenon with increasing concentrations and individually strongly varying increases in the cutaneous β-carotene concentrations. None of the β-carotene concentrations applied led to a plateau [18]. In human skin, the exposition to UV and IR radiation also induces a carotenoid reduction [32,33,34]. The cows subjected to the study were measured between January and early May, so that the cutaneous carotenoid concentration was not significantly affected by the varying influence of UV or IR radiation at the farms of origin.

Course of dermal carotenoid concentrations following surgical treatment of DA (Trial 2)

DA is a common disease occurring in post partum dairy cattle. For this reason, dairy cows with DA that underwent surgery at a large animal hospital were chosen as probands to exemplify a disease condition in order to follow the course of dermal carotenoid concentrations over time until complete recovery. Reflection spectroscopy as performed in the present study does not provide absolute values but expresses dermal carotenoid concentrations in arbitrary units. As in healthy animals, significant differences were observed in the dermal carotenoid concentrations of cows with DA. When evaluating repeated measurements in single cows over time, those cows that recovered from DA showed an increase in their dermal carotenoid concentrations. Most likely this increase is a consequence of an increased appetite and the uptake of carotenoids with the feed as well as reduced consumption of dermal carotenoids due to decreased oxidative stress with the body functions returning to normal following reposition and fixation of the abomasum.

Hummel et al. [35] observed a highly significant improvement of the feed intake within the first seven days after abomasal surgery. Also, the ruminal activity, the characteristics of the excrements and the abdominal wall tension were normal to a large extent. The milk yield was also highly significantly increased in this period. In cows with left displaced abomasums, Gorber et al. could not detect wound swellings in any of the cows from day 20 post operationem [36]. Consequently, the animal is supposed to have completely recovered at day 20 post operationem and beyond. Due to the low number of cases, the significance was not calculated for the three cows that died or were euthanized.

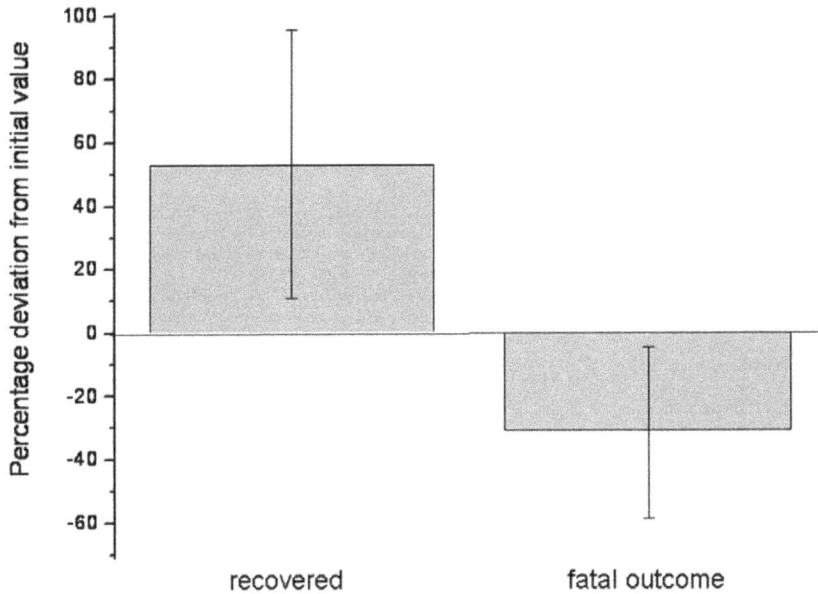

Figure 5. Percentage of increase and decrease in the cutaneous carotenoid concentration from the initial measurement to the final measurement at the farm of origin of the 20 recovered cows and to the last measurement prior to the death of 3 cows, respectively.

Darvin et al. [1] and Vierck et al. [37] could show that illness and extreme stress also reduce the concentration of dermal carotenoids in humans due to formation of free radicals and especially reactive oxygen species. Investigations undertaken by Sattler et al. confirm that the antioxidative status of cows with abomasal displacement, measured based on the activities of superoxide dismutase and glutathione peroxidase, is affected by oxidative stress, with the severity depending on the duration and intensity of such stress [38]. In addition, the TEAC (Trolox Equivalent Antioxidative Capacity) concentrations were lower in the diseased cows (hoof and claw diseases, mastitis, metritis, abomasal displacement) than in the animals of the control group, with the time lapse to the partus being considered for comparison [39].

Many other studies have shown that both the carotenoid concentration in the blood and the antioxidative status as a whole is lower in cattle in the course of various diseases and in the periparturient period [40,41,42,43]. It is supposed, therefore, that besides the stress that entailed the decrease in the carotenoid antioxidants, the reduced feed intake was the main reason for the reduced cutaneous carotenoid concentrations. As the general condition of the cows improved, they took in more feed and simultaneously their dermal carotenoid concentrations increased.

Reestablishment of hepatic functions is crucial for the recovery of cows with DA and the return to normal feed intake [44,45]. Precision farming is a recent development in agriculture that includes introduction of recent innovations on the farm that allow cheap and fast determinations of parameters related with health and welfare of farm animals. Among these are determination of ketone bodies and urea in milk at milking. Future studies have to show if this novel scanning technique might be suitable for serial determinations of the oxidative status in farm animals in order to

detect disorders that could cause harm to the health status of the animals at an early phase.

Conclusions

Different cows show differences in the concentration of dermal carotenoids even if they are kept under identical conditions.

Under constant conditions, no significant differences were observed in median dermal carotenoid concentrations as determined in single animals by serial measurements over a period of one month.

In cows in which the recovery followed after abomasal displacement surgery, the average median dermal carotenoid concentration increased to a statistically highly significant value ($p<0.001$) when compared to the concentrations at initial measurements. In cows with fatal outcome, a decline of $31\pm27\%$ in the dermal carotenoid concentration was detected during hospitalization.

Further studies are needed to test whether the scanner system is suitable for use in the concept of precision farming.

Acknowledgments

We would like to thank Dr. Köcher of Opsolution GmbH, Kassel, Germany for making the sensor systems available, as well as for the technical supervision and for the highly helpful discussions.

Author Contributions

Conceived and designed the experiments: JK MED KEM JL. Performed the experiments: JK. Analyzed the data: JK MED KEM JL. Contributed reagents/materials/analysis tools: MED KEM JL. Wrote the paper: JK MED KEM JL.

References

1. Darvin ME, Patzelt A, Knorr F, Blume-Peytavi U, Sterry W, et al. (2008) One-year study on the variation of carotenoid antioxidant substances in living human skin: influence of dietary supplementation and stress factors. Journal of Biomedical Optics 13: 0440281–0440289.

2. Gecit I, Aslan M, Gunes M, Pirincci N, Esen R, et al. (2012) Serum prolidase activity, oxidative stress, and nitric oxide levels in patients with bladder cancer. J Cancer Res Clin Oncol 138: 739–743.

3. Lima XT, Kimball AB (2011) Skin carotenoid levels in adult patients with psoriasis. J Eur Acad Dermatol Venereol 25: 945–949.

4. Maeda H, Akaike T (1998) Nitric oxide and oxygen radicals in infection, inflammation, and cancer. Biochemistry-Moscow 63: 854–865.

5. Stone V, Johnston H, Clift MJ (2007) Air pollution, ultrafine and nanoparticle toxicology: cellular and molecular interactions. IEEE Trans Nanobioscience 6: 331–340.

6. Mudron P, Rehage J, Qualmann K, Sallmann HP, Scholz H (1999) A study of lipid peroxidation and vitamin E in dairy cows with hepatic insufficiency. Journal of Veterinary Medicine Series a-Physiology Pathology Clinical Medicine 46: 219–224.

7. Meinke MC, Darvin ME, Vollert H, Lademann J (2010) Bioavailability of natural carotenoids in human skin compared to blood. European Journal of Pharmaceutics and Biopharmaceutics 76: 269–274.

8. Valko M, Leibfritz D, Moncol J, Cronin MT, Mazur M, et al. (2007) Free radicals and antioxidants in normal physiological functions and human disease. Int J Biochem Cell Biol 39: 44–84.

9. Bickers DR, Athar M (2006) Oxidative stress in the pathogenesis of skin disease. Journal of Investigative Dermatology 126: 2565–2575.

10. Lademann J, Schanzer S, Meinke M, Sterry W, Darvin ME (2011) Interaction between Carotenoids and Free Radicals in Human Skin. Skin Pharmacology and Physiology 24: 238–244.

11. Haag SF, Taskoparan B, Darvin ME, Groth N, Lademann J, et al. (2011) Determination of the antioxidative capacity of the skin in vivo using resonance Raman and electron paramagnetic resonance spectroscopy. Experimental Dermatology 20: 483–487.

12. Darvin ME, Sterry W, Lademann J, Vergou T (2011) The Role of Carotenoids in Human Skin. Molecules 16: 10491–10506.

13. Lykkesfeldt J, Svendsen O (2007) Oxidants and antioxidants in disease: Oxidative stress in farm animals. Veterinary Journal 173: 502–511.

14. Calderon F, Chauveau-Duriot B, Pradel P, Martin B, Graulet B, et al. (2007) Variations in carotenoids, vitamins A and E, and color in cow's plasma and milk following a shift from hay diet to diets containing increasing levels of Carotenoids and vitamin E. Journal of Dairy Science 90: 5651–5664.

15. Darvin ME, Sandhagen C, Koecher W, Sterry W, Lademann J, et al. (2012) Comparison of two methods for noninvasive determination of carotenoids in human and animal skin: Raman spectroscopy versus reflection spectroscopy. Journal of Biophotonics doi:10.1002/jbio.201100080

16. Klein J, Darvin ME, Müller KE, Lademann J (2012) Non-invasive reflection spectroscopic measurements of carotenoids in bovine udder skin. Journal of Biomedical Optics 17: 101514.

17. Darvin ME, Gersonde I, Meinke M, Sterry W, Lademann J (2005) Non-invasive in vivo determination of the carotenoids beta-carotene and lycopene concentrations in the human skin using the Raman spectroscopic method. Journal of Physics D-Applied Physics 38: 2696–2700.

18. Niedorf F (2001) Entwicklung eines Verfahrens zur quantitativen Auswertung nicht-invasiver reflexionsspektroskopischer Messungen von Beta-Carotin in der Haut. Hannover. 109 p.

19. Lotthammer KH, Ahlswede L (1977) Vitamin-a Independent Effect of Beta-Carotene on Bovine Fertility .3. Deutsche Tierarztliche Wochenschrift 84: 220–226.

20. Noziere P, Grolier P, Durand D, Ferlay A, Pradel P, et al. (2006) Variations in carotenoids, fat-soluble micronutrients, and color in cows' plasma and milk following changes in forage and feeding level. Journal of Dairy Science 89: 2634–2648.

21. Noziere P, Graulet B, Lucas A, Martin B, Grolier P, et al. (2006) Carotenoids for ruminants: From forages to dairy products. Animal Feed Science and Technology 131: 418–450.

22. Meinke MC, Lauer A, Taskoparan B, Gersonde I, Lademann J, et al. (2011) Influence on the carotenoid levels of skin arising from age, gender, body mass index in smoking/non-smoking individuals. Free Radicals and Antioxidants 1: 15–20.

23. Darvin ME, Gersonde I, Albrecht H, Gonchukov SA, Sterry W, et al. (2005) Determination of beta carotene and lycopene concentrations in human skin using resonance Raman spectroscopy. Laser Physics 15: 295–299.

24. De Spirt S, Sies H, Tronnier H, Heinrich U (2012) An encapsulated fruit and vegetable juice concentrate increases skin microcirculation in healthy women. Skin Pharmacol Physiol 25: 2–8.

25. Scarmo S, Henebery K, Peracchio H, Cartmel B, Lin H, et al. (2012) Skin carotenoid status measured by resonance Raman spectroscopy as a biomarker of fruit and vegetable intake in preschool children. Eur J Clin Nutr 66: 555–560.

26. Whitehead RD, Re D, Xiao D, Ozakinci G, Perrett DI (2012) You are what you eat: within-subject increases in fruit and vegetable consumption confer beneficial skin-color changes. PLoS One 7: e32988.

27. Stahl W, Heinrich U, Jungmann H, von Laar J, Schietzel M, et al. (1998) Increased dermal carotenoid levels assessed by noninvasive reflection spectrophotometry correlate with serum levels in women ingesting Betatene. J Nutr 128: 903–907.

28. Darvin ME, Fluhr JW, Caspers P, van der Pool A, Richter H, et al. (2009) In vivo distribution of carotenoids in different anatomical locations of human skin: comparative assessment with two different Raman spectroscopy methods. Experimental Dermatology 18: 1060–1063.

29. Niedorf F, Jungmann H, Kietzmann M (2003) Non-invasive spectroscopy in experimental pharmacology: Evaluation of tissue chromophore concentrations and their spatial distribution. Naunyn-Schmiedebergs Archives of Pharmacology 367: R110–R110.

30. Ludewig T (1996) Light and electron-microscopic investigation of the blood-milk-barrier in lactating cow udders. Anatomia Histologia Embryologia-Journal of Veterinary Medicine Series C-Zentralblatt Fur Veterinarmedizin Reihe C 25: 121–126.

31. Haag SF, Bechtel A, Darvin ME, Klein F, Groth N, et al. (2010) Comparative study of carotenoids, catalase and radical formation in human and animal skin. Skin Pharmacol Physiol 23: 306–312.

32. Darvin ME, Gersonde I, Albrecht H, Sterry W, Lademann J (2006) In vivo Raman spectroscopic analysis of the influence of UV radiation on carotenoid antioxidant substance degradation of the human skin. Laser Physics 16: 833–837.

33. Darvin ME, Haag S, Meinke M, Zastrow L, Sterry W, et al. (2010) Radical production by infrared A irradiation in human tissue. Skin Pharmacol Physiol 23: 40–46.

34. Zastrow L, Groth N, Klein F, Kockott D, Lademann J, et al. (2009) The missing link–light-induced (280–1,600 nm) free radical formation in human skin. Skin Pharmacol Physiol 22: 31–44.

35. Hummel M (2005) Elektromyographische Verlaufsuntersuchungen bei Kühen nach operativer Reposition einer linksseitigen Labmagenverlagerung. Gießen: Justus-Liebig-Universität Gießen, Klinik für Wiederkäuer und Schweine. 165 p.

36. Gorber J (2009) Sonographische Überwachung der Wundheilung bei Kühen im Anschluss an eine Laparotomie. Zürich: Vetsuisse-Fakultät Universität Zürich, Departement für Nutztiere. 33 p.

37. Vierck HB, Darvin ME, Lademann J, Reisshauer A, Baack A, et al. (2012) The influence of endurance exercise on the antioxidative status of human skin. Eur J Appl Physiol 112(9): 3361–3367.

38. Sattler T (2001) Untersuchungen zum antioxidativen Status von Kühen mit Labmagenverlagerungen. Leipzig: Veterinärmedizinische Fakultät der Universität Leipzig, Medizinische Tierklinik. 86 p.

39. Dinges G (2004) Untersuchungen zum antioxidativen Status bei verschiedenen Formen der Dislocatio abomasi des Rindes im Blut der V. jugularis und der V. epigastrica. Leipzig: Veterinärmedizinische Fakultät der Universität Leipzig, Medizinische Tierklinik. pp. 66–77, 93–96.

40. Heinrichs AJ, Costello SS, Jones CM (2009) Control of heifer mastitis by nutrition. Veterinary Microbiology 134: 172–176.

41. Ranjan R, Swarup D, Naresh R, Patra RC (2005) Enhanced erythrocytic lipid peroxides and reduced plasma ascorbic acid, and alteration in blood trace elements level in dairy cows with mastitis. Veterinary Research Communications 29: 27–34.

42. Kankofer M (2001) Non-enzymatic antioxidative defence mechanisms against reactive oxygen species in bovine-retained and not-retained placenta: Vitamin C and glutathione. Reproduction in Domestic Animals 36: 203–206.

43. Batra TR, Singh K, Ho SK, Hidiroglou M (1992) Concentration of Plasma and Milk Vitamin-E and Plasma Beta-Carotene of Mastitic and Healthy Cows. International Journal for Vitamin and Nutrition Research 62: 233–237.

44. Rehage J, Mertens M, StockhofeZurwieden N, Kaske M, Scholz H (1996) Post surgical convalescence of dairy cows with left abomasal displacement in relation to fatty liver. Schweizer Archiv Fur Tierheilkunde 138: 361–368.

45. Martens H (1998) Beziehungen zwischen Fütterung, Physiologie der Vormägen und der Pathogenese der Dislocatio abomasi. In: Fürll M, editor. Leipzig. Proc. Internat. Workshop. pp. 81–101.

12

Lack of Evidence for a Role of Islet Autoimmunity in the Aetiology of Canine Diabetes Mellitus

Kerstin M. Ahlgren[1,9], Tove Fall[2*,9], Nils Landegren[1], Lars Grimelius[3], Henrik von Euler[4], Katarina Sundberg[5], Kerstin Lindblad-Toh[6,7], Anna Lobell[1], Åke Hedhammar[4], Göran Andersson[5], Helene Hansson-Hamlin[4], Åke Lernmark[8], Olle Kämpe[1]

1 Department of Medical Sciences, Science for Life Laboratory, Uppsala University, Uppsala, Sweden, 2 Department of Medical Sciences, Molecular Epidemiology and Science for Life Laboratory, Uppsala University, Uppsala, Sweden, 3 Department of Immunology, Genetics and Pathology, Uppsala University, Sweden, 4 Department of Clinical Sciences, Swedish University of Agricultural Sciences, Uppsala, Sweden, 5 Department of Animal Breeding and Genetics, Swedish University of Agricultural Sciences, Uppsala, Sweden, 6 Broad Institute of Harvard and MIT, Cambridge, Massachusetts, United States of America, 7 Science for Life Laboratory, Department of Medical Biochemistry and Microbiology, Uppsala University, Uppsala, Sweden, 8 Diabetes and Celiac Disease Unit, Department of Clinical Sciences, Lund University, Malmö, Sweden

Abstract

Aims/Hypothesis: Diabetes mellitus is one of the most common endocrine disorders in dogs and is commonly proposed to be of autoimmune origin. Although the clinical presentation of human type 1 diabetes (T1D) and canine diabetes are similar, the aetiologies may differ. The aim of this study was to investigate if autoimmune aetiology resembling human T1D is as prevalent in dogs as previously reported.

Methods: Sera from 121 diabetic dogs representing 40 different breeds were tested for islet cell antibodies (ICA) and GAD65 autoantibodies (GADA) and compared with sera from 133 healthy dogs. ICA was detected by indirect immunofluorescence using both canine and human frozen sections. GADA was detected by *in vitro* transcription and translation (ITT) of human and canine GAD65, followed by immune precipitation. Sections of pancreata from five diabetic dogs and two control dogs were examined histopathologically including immunostaining for insulin, glucagon, somatostatin and pancreas polypeptide.

Results: None of the canine sera analysed tested positive for ICA on sections of frozen canine or human ICA pancreas. However, serum from one diabetic dog was weakly positive in the canine GADA assay and serum from one healthy dog was weakly positive in the human GADA assay. Histopathology showed marked degenerative changes in endocrine islets, including vacuolisation and variable loss of immune-staining for insulin. No sign of inflammation was noted.

Conclusions/Interpretations: Contrary to previous observations, based on results from tests for humoral autoreactivity towards islet proteins using four different assays, and histopathological examinations, we do not find any support for an islet autoimmune aetiology in canine diabetes mellitus.

Editor: Thomas W.H. Kay, St. Vincent's Institute, Australia

Funding: This work was supported by the European Commission (FP7-LUPA, GA-201370), the Swedish Research Council, the Torsten and Ragnar Söderberg Foundation, The NovoNordisk Foundation and Agria Djurförsäkringar Research Foundation. KLT is the recipient of EURYI award from the ESF. The funders had no role in study design, data collection and analysis, decision to publish, or preparation of the manuscript.

* Email: tove.fall@medsci.uu.se

9 These authors contributed equally to this work.

Introduction

Diabetes mellitus occurs in dogs in Sweden with an incidence of 13 cases per 10,000 years-at-risk and a mean age of onset at 8.6 years [1]. The domestic dog shares its environment and lifestyle with its owner and has a breed structure that is highly suitable for genetic analysis [2]. A prerequisite for comparative genetic studies is, however, a common aetiology of disease.

There is no internationally accepted classification system for canine diabetes mellitus but the aetiology has been broadly divided into primary insulin resistance or primary insulin deficiency diabetes. According to this classification, canine insulin resistance is not depicting a primary cellular peripheral insulin resistance, but can occur as a consequence of diverse hormonal disturbances. Furthermore, canine insulin deficiency diabetes, universally claimed to resemble latent autoimmune diabetes in the adult, has suggested to be a result of autoimmunity or in some cases,

Table 1. Breed and disease status of dogs analysed in the study.

Breed	Diabetic	Healthy	Lymphocytic Thyroiditis	Adrenal insufficiency
Afghan hound		1		
Airedale terrier		1		
Australian cattle dog	1			
Australian terrier	6			
Basenji		1		
Basset artesian normand		2		
Beagle		17		
Bearded collie				1
Border collie	9	2		
Border terrier	2	1		
Borzoi	1			
Boxer		6		1
Bullmastiff	1	1		
Cairn terrier	3			
Cavalier king charles spaniel	1			
Cocker spaniel	1	1		
Collie		2		
Dachshund	9			
Danish/Swedish farm dog	1			
Doberman pinscher	1			
Drever (Swedish dachsbracke)	2			
English springer spaniel	1	3		
Finnish hound		2		
Finnish lapphound	1			
Finnish spitz		1		
Flat-coated retriever		2		
Fox terrier		2		
German shepherd dog	1	5		
Giant schnauzer	1	9	13	
Golden retriever		8		
Hollandse herder (Dutch shepherd)	1			
Hovawart		1		
Irish setter	1	1		
Irish wolfhound		3		
Jack Russell terrier		4		
Labrador retriever	5	2		
Laika		1		
Lapp hound	2			
Medium poodle		2		
Miniature poodle	2			
Mixed breed	9	4		
Norwegian elkhound		7		
Nova Scotia duck tolling retriever		3		3
Papillion		1		
Petit brabancon	1			
Polski owczarek nizinny	6	2		
Poodle	2			
Portuguese waterdog	1			
Rhodesian ridgeback		1		
Rottweiler	5	2		

Table 1. Cont.

Breed	Diabetic	Healthy	Lymphocytic Thyroiditis	Adrenal insufficiency
Saluki	1			
Samoyed	2			
English Setter	1	1		
Schipperke	2	1		
Staffordshire bull terrier	1			
Standard poodle		1		
Swedish elkhound	26	22		
Swedish spitz (västgötaspets)	1			
Swedish/Norwegian elkhound	1			
Tervueren		3		
Tibetan terrier	2			
Vorsteh		2		
West highland white terrier	7	2		
Sum	121	133	13	5

secondary to exocrine pancreatic disease [3,4]. Different breeds could be predisposed to different form of diabetes mellitus as shown for the Swedish and Norwegian elkhounds, which develop a reversible form of diabetes during pregnancy or pseudopregnancy, resembling human gestational diabetes mellitus [5].

Findings in pancreatic biopsy samples from diabetic dogs have been conflicting. Two fairly large studies of diabetic dogs [6,7] (n = 33, n = 30) have shown a reduced number or total absence of islets, together with degeneration, hyalinisation or vacuolisation. Pancreatic biopsy samples from dogs with diabetes mellitus secondary to hormonal disturbances also showed degeneration and vacuolisation of the beta cells [8] No lymphocytic infiltration was seen in any of these three studies. On the other hand, Alejandro et al reported that 6/13 diabetic dogs in their study had lymphocytic infiltration associated with islets (insulitis) and that 5/18 dogs displayed extensive exocrine pancreatic damage [9]. There were no control groups in any of these studies.

The occurrence of autoantibodies is a central characteristic of human T1D, and islet cell antibodies (ICA) and GAD65 autoantibodies are valuable diagnostic markers. The presence of autoantibodies in canine diabetes mellitus remains controversial, since both presence and absence of autoantibodies have been reported [5,9–12]. Insulitis is commonly reported in samples from recent onset human T1D subjects [13]. In this study we investigated sera from dogs with and without diabetes using four different assays in addition to histopathological examination of diabetic and control pancreata, with the aim to investigate if autoimmune aetiology resembling human T1D is prevalent in dogs.

Methods

Dogs

Serum samples were obtained from privately owned diabetic (n = 121) and healthy control (n = 133) dogs of 64 breeds in total (60% female) [14] (Table 1). In addition, sera from dogs diagnosed with adrenocortical insufficiency (n = 5) and lymphocytic thyroiditis (n = 13) were included. The diagnosis of diabetes mellitus in cases was based on the clinical picture and chronic fasting hyperglycaemia. The mean age at diagnosis of diabetes was 8.2 years (SD 1.9). Samples for analysis of autoantibodies were taken at a median of 88 days after diagnosis of DM (IQR 11-448 days).

In a subset (n = 51) of the dogs, a glucagon stimulation test with C-peptide measurements was performed [14], which turned out negative for the vast majority of dogs indicating an insulin deficiency-type of diabetes mellitus. Pancreata were available from five dogs of different breeds diagnosed with diabetes (4 females and 1 male). Dogs were euthanized at the time of diagnosis. Specimens from two normoglycemic dogs euthanized for other reasons than diabetes served as controls. The study was approved by the Uppsala animal ethics committee (C 267/5) and all dog owners gave informed written consent.

Pathology

Tissue specimens were fixated in 10% buffered neutral formalin at room temperature, followed by routine processing to paraffin wax. Approximately 4-μm thick sections were cut and attached to positively charged glass slides (IHC Microscopic Slides, Flex (DAKO, Glostrup, Denmark).The sections were microwave treated for 2×5 min at 700 W by using 50 mM Tris buffer saline, as retrieval solution and immunostained by using a polymer detection system, Dako Cytomation, EnVision+ System-HRP; K4010 for primary antibodies and K4006 for primary mouse antibodies. The incubation time was 30 min at room temperature. Diaminobenzidine was used as chromogen. The antibodies were diluted in Dako's antibody diluent. The following antibodies were used: Insulin (mouse monoclonal, diluted 1:2000, K36AC10, Sigma-Aldrich), Glucagon (mouse monoclonal, 1:10000, K79bB10, Abcam), Somatostatin (rabbit polyclonal, 1.4000, A0566, Dako), pancreas polypeptide (rabbit polyclonal, 1:10000, A0619, Dako). Meyer's hematoxylin from Histolab (Gothenburg, Sweden) was used for nuclear counterstain. Negative controls, excluding the primary antibody, were used.

Immunostainings for presence of anti-islet antibodies in sera

Pancreata were dissected from dogs euthanized for reasons other than endocrine and pancreatic disorders and snap frozen in liquid nitrogen. Six μm thick cryostat sections were placed on glass slides (Superfrost plus, Thermo Scientific, Braunschweig, Ger-

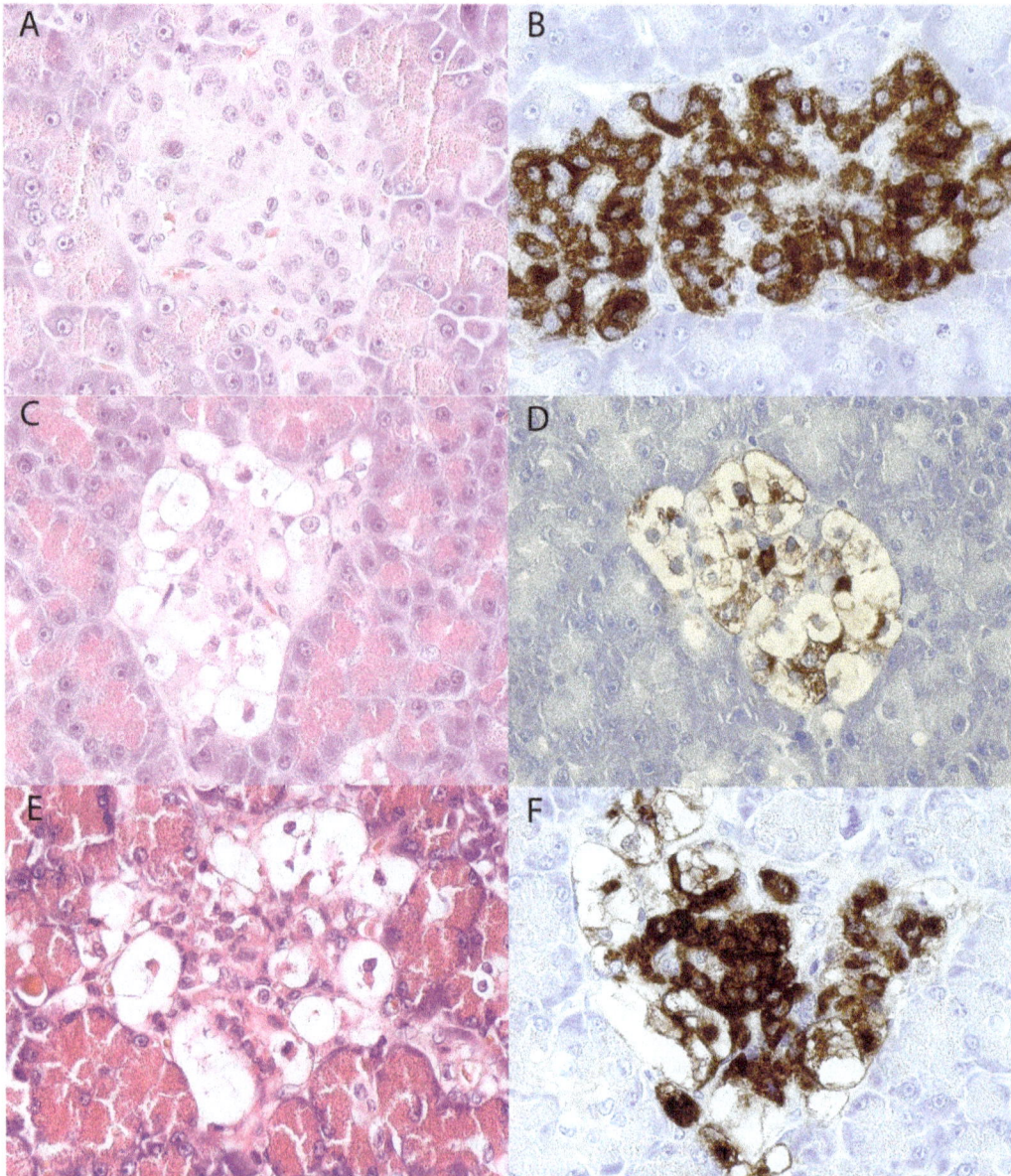

Figure 1. Pancreatic specimens stained with hematoxylin-eosin (A, C, E) and immunostained for insulin (B, D, F). The samples shown in A and B come from a non-diabetic male Swedish Elkhound, C and D come from a diabetic male Polish Owczarek Nizinny dog and E and F from a diabetic female English Setter. The islet in Fig D contains few insulin-immunoreactive cells except the vacuolated cells, while these normal-appearing insulin-stained cells are numerous in Fig F.

many), air-dried and blocked for unspecific binding for 30 min in room temperature using 10% normal goat sera (Dako, Glostrup, Denmark) in phosphate buffered saline (PBS) pH 7.4, containing 14% aprotinin (Trasylol, Bayer, Germany). The immunostainings were performed over night at +4°C, using 100 µl serum/glass from every diabetic and control dog individually –diluted in the range 1:16 to 1:64. Three positive controls were used, including sera from a human diabetes patient, sera from a patient with stiff person syndrome and a monoclonal mouse GAD antibody (BD Biosciences, San Jose, CA, USA) diluted to 1:200. The slides were rinsed three times in PBS and incubated with 100 µl of either secondary pre-adsorbed, FITC conjugated goat anti dog IgG (Santa Cruz Biotechnology, CA, USA), FITC conjugated goat anti human IgG (H+L) or Cy3 conjugated goat anti human IgG and

Cy3 conjugated goat anti mouse IgG (all three from Jackson Immuno Research, West Grove, PA, USA) in 1:200 dilutions. After one h incubation at room temperature the slides were rinsed five times in PBS and mounted with Vectashield (Vector Laboratories, Burlingame, CA, USA) with or without nuclear staining 4′,6-diamidino-2-phenylindole (DAPI). All incubations were performed in a covered humid chamber. The presence of Ab staining was assessed in a Nikon microphot–FXA fluorescence microscope. For documentation images were also taken using a Zeiss LSM 501 confocal microscope. The human ICA assay was performed by an accredited laboratory at Malmö Academic Hospital according to standard procedures.

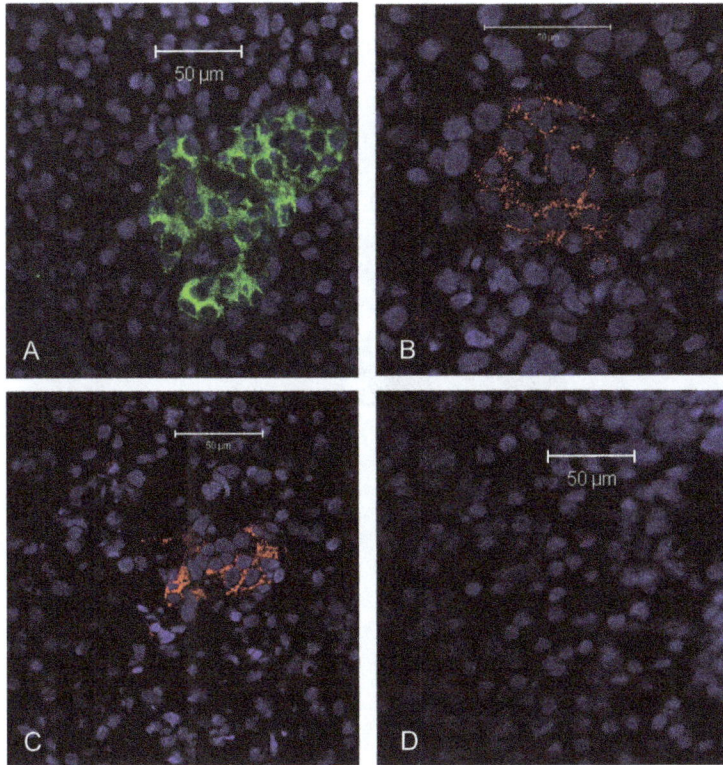

Figure 2. Canine pancreas stained by immunofluorescence. A) Stained with a mouse monoclonal Ab to human GAD65, B) stained using a GADA positive human serum and C) stained using a GADA positive serum from a patient with stiff person syndrome and D) canine serum from a dog with diabetes. Nuclear stain in blue (DAPI). Green is secondary anti rat Ig-FITC and anti-canine Ig-FITC used in A) and D). Red is anti-human Ig -Cy5 used in B) and D).

In-vitro transcription and translation with canine and human GAD65 followed by immunoprecipitations

In-vitro transcription and translation (ITT) of canine GAD65 was performed using the TNT-SP6 quick coupled transcription/translation system (Promega, Madison, WI, USA) with the addition of 0.5 mCi of [^{35}S]-methionine (10 µCi/µl, Perkin Elmer, Waltham, MA, USA) as previously described [5]. Approximately 20 000 cpm of the [^{35}S]-radio labelled ITT products were used for immunoprecipitation with 2.5 µl serum. Immunoprecipitations of the labelled protein with canine sera were performed using protein A Sepharose (GE Healthcare Biosciences, Uppsala, Sweden) followed by measurement of the radioactivity. Two GADA-positive human sera were used as positive controls. Furthermore, a clone encoding the human protein GAD65 was used as above. A human GADA-positive serum and BSA were used as positive and negative controls. The antibody reactivity was calculated as indices relative to a positive (human serum) and negative control (4% BSA) according to the following equation: Immunoreactivity index = ((cpm subject x-cpm negative standard)/(cpm positive standard -cpm negative standard) * 100). Sera with an immunoreactivity index exceeding the mean value for healthy dogs ($n = 133$) plus 4 standard deviations were regarded as positive.

Results

Pathology

The frequency and distributions of islets varied in the diabetic animals as well as in the non-diabetics. Generally the islet sizes in both groups were smaller compared to that observed in human pancreas. No inflammatory reaction was seen in any of the animal pancreata. There were no signs of degeneration or atrophy in the exocrine parenchyma. The islets in both animal groups contained all four endocrine cell types but a large fraction of the insulin-staining (beta) cells in the diabetic group were enlarged, vacuolated with no or only traces of insulin-immunoreactivity (Fig 1A–F). Non-vacuolated normal appearing insulin-stained cells were present in all diabetic pancreata with a varying frequency from rare to frequent. Images from all seven dogs with HE, insulin and glucagon staining is available in the Supplementary Material (Fig. S1).

Immunostainings for presence of anti-islet antibodies in sera

Using mouse monoclonal antibodies directed to rat GAD65, followed by fluorochrome-conjugated secondary antibodies directed to mouse IgG, the islets of Langerhans were visualized in pancreas from a healthy dog (Fig. 2a). Using sera from a GADA-positive human T1D patient (Fig. 2b) or a patient with stiff person syndrome (Fig. 2c) we were also able to stain the islets of Langerhans in the dog and human pancreata. Sera from dogs with diabetes mellitus and control dogs were in all cases unable to bind specifically (Fig. 2d). The level of unspecific binding was similar in samples from diabetic dogs and healthy control dogs. In addition, the certified human ICA assay was negative in all samples.

GAD65 immunoprecipitations

A strong titer of GAD65 autoantibodies was found in the human T1D serum used as a control, regardless whether canine or

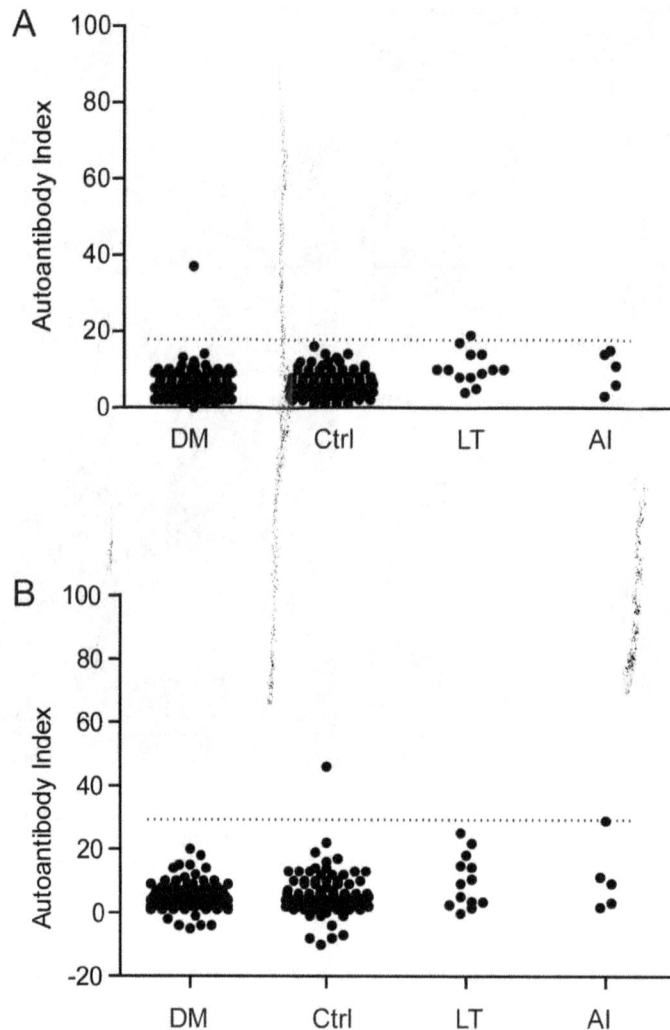

Figure 3. Immunoreactivity to A) Canine GAD65 and B) Human GAD65. DM = diabetes mellitus, *n* = 121, Ctrl = healthy control, *n* = 133, LT = lymphocytic thyroiditis, *n* = 13 and AI = adrenal insufficiency *n* = 5, Cut off index for positive vs. negative to GADA indicated by dotted line.

human GAD65 ITT products were used for immunoprecipita-tions. One diabetic Giant Schnauzer (0.8%) displayed weak reactivity against canine GAD65 (Fig. 2a) and one control Norwegian Elkhound (0.8%) was positive against human GAD65 (Fig. 2b). None of the dogs with lymphocytic thyroiditis or adrenal insufficiency were GADA-positive (Fig. 2a and 2b). The results are summarized in Fig. 3. Laboratory tests of the GADA-positive diabetic dog indicated a thyroid hormone deficiency, but the TSH level was normal (17 mIU/l). No further investigations of this dog were done as it was euthanized on request by the owner.

Discussion

It has previously been suggested that the majority of canine diabetes mellitus is due to autoimmune T1D or latent autoimmune diabetes of the adult. We first used the ICA assay, which visualizes islet reactivity regardless of molecular target of autoantibodies to assess this hypothesis. The results from nearly all assays were negative, which is in line with a previous study, which reported that in 18 examined dogs with spontaneous diabetes mellitus, no islet-directed humoral autoimmunity was present [9]. Our findings were also supported by histopathologic examinations on pancreata

obtained at the diagnosis of the disease and before start of insulin treatment, where no immune cells were seen in conjunction to the islets. The vacuolisation of some beta cells in combination with weak or absent insulin immune-staining may suggest that stress in the endoplasmic reticulum, so called ER-stress, due to a high demand for insulin and the consecutive protein misfolding [15]. There was a variety in the frequency of normal-appearing insulin-staining cells, even though time from onset of symptoms to euthanasia was similar among dogs. We speculate that the degree of insulin resistance in a dog will determine at what loss of beta cell mass the dog will go into a diabetic stage. Dogs are mainly carnivorous, and have fewer and smaller islets than humans. Even though some adaptation of the carbohydrate degradation path-ways has occurred since divergence from the wolf [16], it may be speculated that a carbohydrate-rich diet may induce an ER-stress response if demand for insulin supersedes production capacity and that protein misfolding is part of the pathological mechanism in the development of canine diabetes mellitus.

A variety of diabetes autoantigens has been described in humans, however GAD65 is the most prevalent and specific autoantigen in human T1D. Therefore a GAD65 ITT analysis followed by immunoprecipitation was employed to investigate whether also diabetic dogs produce such autoantibodies. Because of the lack of canine positive control serum a human sample was tested and proved useful. As a precaution we tested both a novel canine GADA assay as well as an established human GADA assay. Our results are in opposition to a previous study where 4 of 30 dogs were GADA-positive and 3 of 30 dogs IA–2A positive [11]. The GADA-positive dogs were mongrels and springer spaniels, a breed also included in the present study. Furthermore, later the same group also reported the presence of antibodies to proinsulin in diabetic and control dogs using a Western blot technique. The implications of proinsulin autoantibodies are, however, unclear since three out of 15 (20%) of the control dogs included in that study were positive compared to 8/15 (53%) of newly diagnosed and 6/15 insulin-treated dogs (40%) [10]. The Swedish dog population is somewhat different from those of other Western countries, where female dogs are spayed early in life. The high proportion of intact female dogs in Sweden is associated with a female predisposition to diabetes mellitus [1], shown to be caused by progesterone-related diabetes mellitus [5]. Hence, the study material is not fully comparable to that of the UK study [11], which could explain some of the differences in results, although breeds were overlapping.

Rodent models such as the NOD mouse have shown that the primary autoantigen may differ between species [17].In the present study, we used the ICA to screen for other autoantibodies against canine pancreata than GAD-65, but all findings were negative. We cannot rule out cell-mediated autoimmunity, even though the histological appearance is in favor of other etiologies. Future studies should preferably investigate possible T-cell responses to islet cell autoantigens.

Assessing genetic variation in the major histocompatibility complex might have been valuable to test similarities to human risk HLA-DQ2 as done for dogs in [18], but such candidate gene approaches in dogs are at high risk of false positive findings unless population stratification bias is ruled out. Future studies should preferably investigate possible T-cell responses to islet cell autoantigens. Another important aspect of diabetes aetiology research in dogs is that dogs seem sensitive to glucose toxicity, and hyperglycemic dogs not treated immediately after diagnosis are at severe risk of permanent diabetes irrespective of the cause of hyperglycaemia [5,19].

In conclusion, in this Swedish cohort of 121 diabetic dogs representing 40 different breeds, we find no ICA-positive canine sera, no insulitis and no differences between cases and controls in the GADA assay.

Acknowledgments

The authors thank the dog owners for participation in this study. We thank Dr. Anna-Stina Höglund for professional expertise on confocal microscopy. We also thank Åsa Hallgren and Ulrika M Gustavsson for excellent technical assistance and Sara Westberg for collection of dog sera.

Author Contributions

Conceived and designed the experiments: KMA TF LG HvE A. Lobell ÅH GA HHH Å. Lernmark KLT OK. Performed the experiments: KMA NL TF LG HvE KS HHH Å. Lernmark. Analyzed the data: KMA TF LG OK. Contributed reagents/materials/analysis tools: LG OK NL. Contributed to the writing of the manuscript: KMA TF NL LG HvE KS KLT A. Lobell ÅH GA HHH Å. Lernmark OK.

References

1. Fall T, Hamlin HH, Hedhammar A, Kampe O, Egenvall A (2007) Diabetes mellitus in a population of 180,000 insured dogs: incidence, survival, and breed distribution. J Vet Intern Med 21: 1209–1216.
2. Lindblad-Toh K, Wade CM, Mikkelsen TS, Karlsson EK, Jaffe DB, et al. (2005) Genome sequence, comparative analysis and haplotype structure of the domestic dog. Nature 438: 803–819.
3. Catchpole B, Ristic JM, Fleeman LM, Davison LJ (2005) Canine diabetes mellitus: can old dogs teach us new tricks? Diabetologia 48: 1948–1956.
4. Rand JS, Fleeman LM, Farrow HA, Appleton DJ, Lederer R (2004) Canine and feline diabetes mellitus: nature or nurture? J Nutr 134: 2072S–2080S.
5. Fall T, Hedhammar A, Wallberg A, Fall N, Ahlgren KM, et al. (2010) Diabetes mellitus in elkhounds is associated with diestrus and pregnancy. J Vet Intern Med 24: 1322–1328.
6. Ling GV, Lowenstine LJ, Pulley LT, Kaneko JJ (1977) Diabetes mellitus in dogs: a review of initial evaluation, immediate and long-term management, and outcome. J Am Vet Med Assoc 170: 521–530.
7. Gepts W, Toussaint D (1967) Spontaneous diabetes in dogs and cats. A pathological study. Diabetologia 3: 249–265.
8. Eigenmann JE, Eigenmann RY, Rijnberk A, van der Gaag I, Zapf J, et al. (1983) Progesterone-controlled growth hormone overproduction and naturally occurring canine diabetes and acromegaly. Acta Endocrinol (Copenh) 104: 167–176.
9. Alejandro R, Feldman EC, Shienvold FL, Mintz DH (1988) Advances in canine diabetes mellitus research: etiopathology and results of islet transplantation. J Am Vet Med Assoc 193: 1050–1055.
10. Davison LJ, Herrtage ME, Catchpole B (2011) Autoantibodies to recombinant canine proinsulin in canine diabetic patients. Res Vet Sci 91: 58–63.
11. Davison LJ, Weenink SM, Christie MR, Herrtage ME, Catchpole B (2008) Autoantibodies to GAD65 and IA-2 in canine diabetes mellitus. Vet Immunol Immunopathol 126: 83–90.
12. Hoenig M, Dawe DL (1992) A qualitative assay for beta cell antibodies. Preliminary results in dogs with diabetes mellitus. Vet Immunol Immunopathol 32: 195–203.
13. Foulis AK, Liddle CN, Farquharson MA, Richmond JA, Weir RS (1986) The histopathology of the pancreas in type 1 (insulin-dependent) diabetes mellitus: a 25-year review of deaths in patients under 20 years of age in the United Kingdom. Diabetologia 29: 267–274.
14. Fall T, Holm B, Karlsson A, Ahlgren KM, Kampe O, et al. (2008) Glucagon stimulation test for estimating endogenous insulin secretion in dogs. Vet Rec 163: 266 270.
15. Gardner BM, Pincus D, Gotthardt K, Gallagher CM, Walter P (2013) Endoplasmic reticulum stress sensing in the unfolded protein response. Cold Spring Harb Perspect Biol 5: a013169.
16. Axelsson E, Ratnakumar A, Arendt ML, Maqbool K, Webster MT, et al. (2013) The genomic signature of dog domestication reveals adaptation to a starch-rich diet. Nature 495: 360–364.
17. Nakayama M, Abiru N, Moriyama H, Babaya N, Liu E, et al. (2005) Prime role for an insulin epitope in the development of type 1 diabetes in NOD mice. Nature 435: 220–223.
18. Kennedy LJ, Davison LJ, Barnes A, Short AD, Fretwell N, et al. (2006) Identification of susceptibility and protective major histocompatibility complex haplotypes in canine diabetes mellitus. Tissue Antigens 68: 467–476.
19. Imamura T, Kofler M, Helderman JH, Prince D, Thirlby R, et al. (1988) Severe diabetes induced in subtotally depancreatized dogs by sustained hyperglycemia. Diabetes 37: 600–609.

13

Evaluating the Accuracy of Molecular Diagnostic Testing for Canine Visceral Leishmaniasis Using Latent Class Analysis

Manuela da Silva Solcà[1], **Leila Andrade Bastos**[1], **Carlos Eduardo Sampaio Guedes**[1], **Marcelo Bordoni**[1], **Lairton Souza Borja**[1], **Daniela Farias Larangeira**[1,2], **Pétala Gardênia da Silva Estrela Tuy**[3], **Leila Denise Alves Ferreira Amorim**[3], **Eliane Gomes Nascimento**[4], **Geraldo Gileno de Sá Oliveira**[1,5], **Washington Luis Conrado dos-Santos**[1], **Deborah Bittencourt Mothé Fraga**[1,2,5], **Patrícia Sampaio Tavares Veras**[1,5]*

1 Laboratório de Patologia e Biointervenção, Centro de Pesquisa Gonçalo Moniz–Fundação Oswaldo Cruz, Salvador, Bahia, Brazil, 2 Escola de Medicina Veterinária, Universidade Federal da Bahia, Salvador, Bahia, Brazil, 3 Instituto de Matemática –Departamento de Estatística, Universidade Federal da Bahia, Salvador, Bahia, Brazil, 4 Centro de Referência em Doenças Endêmicas Pirajá da Silva (PIEJ), Jequié, Bahia, Brazil, 5 Instituto Nacional de Ciência e Tecnologia em Doenças Tropicais (INCT - DT), Salvador, Bahia, Brazil

Abstract

Host tissues affected by *Leishmania infantum* have differing degrees of parasitism. Previously, the use of different biological tissues to detect *L. infantum* DNA in dogs has provided variable results. The present study was conducted to evaluate the accuracy of molecular diagnostic testing (qPCR) in dogs from an endemic area for canine visceral leishmaniasis (CVL) by determining which tissue type provided the highest rate of parasite DNA detection. Fifty-one symptomatic dogs were tested for CVL using serological, parasitological and molecular methods. Latent class analysis (LCA) was performed for accuracy evaluation of these methods. qPCR detected parasite DNA in 100% of these animals from at least one of the following tissues: splenic and bone marrow aspirates, lymph node and skin fragments, blood and conjunctival swabs. Using latent variable as gold standard, the qPCR achieved a sensitivity of 95.8% (CI 90.4–100) in splenic aspirate; 79.2% (CI 68–90.3) in lymph nodes; 77.3% (CI 64.5–90.1) in skin; 75% (CI 63.1–86.9) in blood; 50% (CI 30–70) in bone marrow; 37.5% (CI 24.2–50.8) in left-eye; and 29.2% (CI 16.7–41.6) in right-eye conjunctival swabs. The accuracy of qPCR using splenic aspirates was further evaluated in a random larger sample (n = 800), collected from dogs during a prevalence study. The specificity achieved by qPCR was 76.7% (CI 73.7–79.6) for splenic aspirates obtained from the greater sample. The sensitivity accomplished by this technique was 95% (CI 93.5–96.5) that was higher than those obtained for the other diagnostic tests and was similar to that observed in the smaller sampling study. This confirms that the splenic aspirate is the most effective type of tissue for detecting *L. infantum* infection. Additionally, we demonstrated that LCA could be used to generate a suitable gold standard for comparative CVL testing.

Editor: Yara M. Traub-Csekö, Instituto Oswaldo Cruz, Fiocruz, Brazil

Funding: This work was supported by grants and fellowships from INCT (Instituto Nacional de Ciência e Tecnologia em Doenças Tropicais - http://inctdt.cebio. org - Grant number: 576269/2008-5) and PPUS - FAPESB (Programa de Pesquisa para o Sistema Único de Saúde - Fundação de Amparo a Pesquisa no Estado da Bahia - http://www.fapesb.ba.gov.br - Grant number: SUS0011/2010). The funders had no role in study design, data collection and analysis, decision to publish, or preparation of the manuscript.

Competing Interests: The authors have declared that no competing interests exist.

* Email: pveras@bahia.fiocruz.br

Introduction

Visceral leishmaniasis (VL) is a disease with both medical and veterinary importance that is endemic in Brazil, and in many other countries throughout Latin America, Asia, and Europe [1]. One of the etiological agents of VL is *Leishmania infantum* (syn. *Leishmania chagasi*), which is transmitted to vertebrate hosts through the bites of female sand flies [2–5].

Dogs are considered the main domestic reservoir for this parasite because of their high rates of infection and the high frequency of parasites found in their skin [6–9]. Once infected with *L. infantum*, dogs have clinical manifestations that range from asymptomatic to systemic, including weight loss or cachexia; hypertrophy of the lymph nodes; and changes to the skin such as

onychogryphosis, footpad swelling, localized or generalized alopecia, skin ulcers, and nasal or periocular dermatitis. They can also present with pathological alterations such as anemia or hepatic and renal failure [10,11].

Canine visceral leishmaniasis (CVL) can be diagnosed using parasitological, serological, or molecular methods in conjunction with clinical and epidemiological parameters [12]. Serological tests to diagnose CVL are the most common procedures used worldwide [13], however they lack sensitivity and specificity, which makes diagnosing the disease difficult when animals present with low antibody titers or there is cross-reactivity [14–17]. Hence, additional tests could be advantageous for confirming the diagnosis of inconclusive cases. For use as a confirmatory test, the molecular detection of *Leishmania* spp. provides greater sensitivity and specificity than other diagnostic techniques [8,18].

Numerous studies have described highly sensitive detection of low parasitic loads using quantitative real-time PCR (qPCR) [19–21]. qPCR has also been used to monitor the tissue parasitic load in dogs following anti-*Leishmania* treatment in countries where this procedure is unrestricted [22,23].

Several invasive, and non-invasive, techniques have been used to obtain biological tissue samples to diagnose *Leishmania* infection using conventional PCR and qPCR. The biological samples most widely used for molecular diagnosis of *Leishmania* spp. infection in dogs are the spleen, bone marrow, lymph node, and skin [12,18,24]. However, molecular diagnostic tests in studies using these tissue types have produced variable, and sometimes conflicting, results, for identifying *Leishmania*-infected dogs [19,25,26]. This might be because culturing the parasite, which has been used as the gold standard assay [27,28], has a low sensitivity threshold for detecting dogs with a low parasite burden [29,30], which compromises the accuracy evaluation of diagnostic testing.

Therefore, the authors hypothesized that the lack of a reliable gold standard assay could account for the varying accuracy of the molecular diagnostic tests for *Leishmania* infection in different tissues. Latent class analysis (LCA) appraises tests with imperfect reference standards [31–33] using a statistical model to construct the latent class variable. Recently, LCA has been used to accurately evaluate the results of serological tests for diagnosing CVL [34].

The aim of the present study was to determine which type of canine tissue sample in an area with endemic VL provided the highest rate of *Leishmania* DNA detection by qPCR. In addition, qPCR results were compared to parasitological and serological diagnostic tests to determine which test provided the most accurate diagnosis of *L. infantum* infection.

Materials and Methods

1. Ethics Statement

Experimental procedures involving dogs were performed in accordance with Brazilian Federal Law on Animal Experimentation (Law no. 11794), the guidelines for animal research established by the Oswaldo Cruz Foundation [35], and the Brazilian Ministry of Health Manual for the Surveillance and Control of VL [36]. The CPqGM - FIOCRUZ Institutional Review Board for Animal Experimentation approved protocols for both animal euthanasia and sample collection procedures (Permit Number: 015/2009; Permit Number 017/2010).

2. Dogs

As previously described by Lima etal. (2014), over a one week period in July 2010, 51 stray dogs were taken from the streets of Jequié, a municipality located in the State of Bahia, Brazil, which is an area endemic for CVL. These dogs were selected as part of a surveillance and control program for VL that our group conducted in collaboration with the Endemic Diseases Surveillance Program of the State Health Service [37]. A CVL diagnosis was established based on the presence or absence of the following clinical signs: emaciation, alopecia, anemia, conjunctivitis, dehydration, dermatitis, erosion, ulcerations, lymphadenopathy, and onychogryphosis as previously detailed by Lima etal. (2014). Dogs from Jequié were clinically classified as having mild (stage I), moderate (stage II), and severe CVL (stage III) according to Solano-Gallego etal. (2009) [38].

3. Tissue Sampling

Tissue samples were obtained during necropsies as previously described by Lima etal. (2014). Briefly, the dogs were anesthetized and then euthanized by intracardiac injection of a supersaturated solution of potassium chloride (2 mL/kg). Immediately before the lethal injection, 50 mL of blood were collected by intracardiac puncture. Blood samples were preserved in EDTA-2Na tubes (Greiner bio-one, Kremsmünster, Austria) and in blood collection tubes (BD Vacutainer; Becton, Dickinson and Co). During the necropsy, splenic aspirate samples were collected by puncturing the central region of the spleen and bone marrow samples were obtained by puncturing the wing of the ilium, approaching from the dorsal crest. Conjunctival swabs of the right and left eyes were taken by rubbing the swab multiple times against the surface of the lower eyelid. A small fragment of the popliteal lymph node was cut from the whole organ and a skin fragment was collected using a sterile 5 mm punch (Kolplast, Brazil) from the medial portion of the pinna. Tissue samples were collected using sterile needles, swabs, and blades and all of the samples were stored in DNAase- and RNAase-free tubes at −70°C until DNA extraction.

4. Hematological and Biochemical Parameters

Hematological and biochemical parameters were evaluated on the day of the necropsy. Total red blood cell and white blood cell counts were determined using an automated cell counter (Pentra 80 counter, ABX Diagnostics, Montpellier, France). Micro-hematocrit tubes containing blood samples were centrifuged at 12,000 rpm for 5 min, and then the hematocrit levels were estimated. Serum was collected by centrifuging the Vacutainer tubes, and was used for the biochemical tests including total protein, globulin, albumin, blood urea nitrogen, and creatinine, using an enzymatic colorimetric method with an A15 auto-analyzer (BioSystems, Barcelona, Spain).

5. Serological and Parasitological Tests

The following serological tests were performed to detect anti-*Leishmania* antibodies: the DPP CVL rapid test which detects rk28-specific antibodies and the EIE CVL with crude *L. major* antigen diagnostic test provided by FIOCRUZ (Bio-Manguinhos Unit, Rio de Janeiro, Brazil). These serum tests were performed in accordance with manufacturer instructions. An in-house ELISA, with crude *L. infantum* antigen was also performed as previously described [39,40]. Parasitological evaluation was performed by culturing part of the splenic aspirate collected during necropsy in Novy–MacNeal–Nicolle (NNN) biphasic medium supplemented with 20% Fetal Bovine Serum (FBS – Gibco BRL, New York, USA) and 100 µg/mL gentamicin to avoid contamination (Sigma Chemical Co., St. Louis, MO) for four weeks at 24°C [41]. Parasites were detected using microscopy performed at weekly intervals for no less than four weeks. Each splenic culture was prepared in duplicate. All of the culture labels were double-checked to avoid misidentification.

Parasite isolates were randomly selected from five dogs and sent to the national reference laboratory for *Leishmania* typing at the Oswaldo Cruz Institute (CLIOC, Rio de Janeiro, RJ, Brazil). The isolates were typed using monoclonal antibodies and enzyme electrophoresis analysis in order to determine the *Leishmania* species.

6. Control Samples

Splenic aspirate samples from 20 dogs that had previously been identified as *Leishmania*-positive from an endemic area [18] were used as positive controls. Splenic aspirates of 20 healthy dogs from the municipality of Pelotas, Rio Grande do Sul, Brazil, an area without endemic CVL, were used as negative controls. All of the healthy dogs had no clinical signs of CVL, and tested negative for infection using the in-house ELISA, parasite culturing, and qPCR techniques.

7. Sample Handling and Decontamination Procedures

Due to the high degree of sensitivity inherent in qPCR, exceptional care was taken to avoid cross-contamination during not only the sample collection procedures, but also during DNA extraction and qPCR testing. As previously described [18], all procedures were carried out in an environment that was suitable for sample collection and qPCR procedures. All of the disposable surgical materials were used for a single animal, and the laminar flow hood was decontaminated by UV radiation before each procedure. Filter tips were routinely used throughout all DNA extraction steps and when performing the qPCR [42].

8. DNA Extraction

DNA was obtained from 200 µL of splenic and bone marrow aspirate, 200 µL of blood, 20 mg of lymph node, and 20 mg of a skin fragment using a DNeasy Blood & Tissue Kit (Qiagen, Hilden, Germany) in accordance with the manufacturer's protocols. DNA samples from the conjunctival swabs were purified using a phenol–chloroform method as previously described [42]. The DNA pellets were suspended in 30 µL of Tris–EDTA buffer (10 mmol/L Tris and 1 mmol/L EDTA, pH 8.0). Once extracted, the quality and concentration of each DNA sample were evaluated using a digital spectrophotometer (NanoDrop ND-1000, Thermo Scientific, Wilmington, USA) [43]. All of the DNA samples were adjusted to a final concentration of 30 ng/µL, aliquoted, and kept at −20°C until the qPCR assays were performed.

Parasite DNA was extracted from *L. infantum* (MHOM/BR2000/MERIVALDO), *Leishmania amazonensis* (MHOM/Br88/Ba-125), *Leishmania braziliensis* (MHOM/BR/94/H3456), and *Leishmania major* (MHOM/RI//WR-173) promastigotes cultivated at 24°C. For the DNA extraction, the parasites were counted and centrifuged. DNA was extracted from pellets corresponding to a known number of parasites in accordance with the Qiagen protocols.

9. Quantitative PCR (qPCR)

9.1 Inclusion and exclusion criteria. To assess positivity, DNA samples were only included in the analysis if they met the minimum quality criteria: i) the DNA sample concentration was above 30ng/µl; ii) DNA samples amplified with the same efficiency as the DNA curve; and iii) amplification of the 18s rRNA housekeeping gene was successful. Any samples that did not fulfill one or more of the above inclusion criteria were excluded, only 10 out of 51 for skin fragments and 26 out of 51 for bone marrow aspirate. To compare parasitic load in different tissue types, DNA samples were only included in the analysis if they met the minimum quality criteria for all tissue types (samples from 20 dogs out of 51).

9.2 Quantitative PCR Assay. qPCR was used to determine the amount of parasite DNA in canine tissue samples. qPCR assays were performed following an amplification protocol previously described by Francino etal. (2006). The qPCR technique targeted a conserved region of *L. infantum* kDNA to obtain a 120-bp amplicon. All of the reactions were performed in triplicate. The reaction was in a final volume of 25 µL containing: 5 µL (150 ng) of each DNA sample diluted in deionized water and 20 µL of the PCR mixture. The PCR mixture contained: 12.5 µL

of Universal Mastermix (Life Technology Corporation, Carlsbad, CA-USA), the forward primer 5′-AACTTTTCTGGTCCTCCG-GGTAG-3′ (LEISH-1) and the reverse primer 5′-ACCCCCA-GTTTCCCGCC-3′ (LEISH-2) both at a final concentration of 900 nM, and a fluorogenic probe 5′-AAAAATGGGTGCAGAA-AT-3′ with a FAM reporter molecule attached to the 5′ end and an MGB-NFQ quencher (200 nM final concentration) linked to the 3′-end (Life Technology Corporation). In order to overcome limitations caused by endogenous PCR inhibitors in the blood, skin fragment, and conjunctival swab samples, all of the steps leading up to DNA amplification were performed in the presence of bovine serum albumin (5 µg/each reaction) (Sigma Chemical) [44].

9.3 Quantification of *Leishmania* kDNA. Quantification of *Leishmania* kDNA was performed using an absolute method based on comparing the cycle threshold (Ct) values from the samples to a standard curve, which was constructed using serial 10-fold dilutions from 10^5 to 10^{-1} parasites performed in triplicate. Reactions were performed using the Applied Biosystems 7500 Fast Real-Time PCR System (Life Technology Corporation). The reaction was carried out under the following conditions: 1 cycle at 50°C for 2 min, 1 cycle at 95°C for 10 min, and 40 two-step cycles, first at 95°C for 15 s and then at 60°C for 1 min. In order to minimize variability between plates, the values from each plate were normalized using a common fluorescence detection baseline. Each sample's Ct value was calculated by determining the point at which its fluorescence signal was above the established detection baseline. The Ct cut-off value was determined using a Receiver-Operator Characteristic (ROC) curve. The optimal Ct cut-off value for the parasite kDNA qPCR assay was determined by calculating sensitivity and specificity for different Ct cut-off points and the ROC curve derived from the amplification values of *Leishmania*-negative samples and *Leishmania*-positive samples (see item 6). Tissue samples were considered positive when the Ct values were equal to or less than the Ct cut-off point determined using the ROC curve analysis. If the standard deviation between triplicates was >0.38, the sample set was reanalyzed by qPCR [45]. The efficiency of the qPCR protocol was evaluated by calculating the slope value of the standard curve for the parasite kDNA. This value, −3.657 (SD = 0.148), was obtained from the mean slope values of nine independent experiments with a correlation coefficient (R^2) of 0.998.

9.4 Assessment of qPCR Analytical Sensitivity and Specificity. Analytical sensitivity was evaluated by determining whether the presence of host tissue interferes with the amplification profiles when using qPCR to detect *L. infantum* DNA in infected dogs. First, a standard curve was constructed using ten-fold dilutions from reference strain *L. infantum* DNA (see item 9.3). Next, a ten-fold dilutions of reference strain *L. infantum* DNA was mixed with the splenic aspirate DNA from negative control animals (see item 6) and another standard curve was constructed from these dilutions. Finally, the amplification profiles of the two curves were compared. The analytical specificity of the qPCR analysis was assessed by comparing the amplification profiles of DNA samples from the *L. infantum* reference strain to profiles from several other *Leishmania* species, including the New World *L. amazonensis* and *L. braziliensis*, and the Old World *L. major*. As described in item 9.3, standard curves for each species were constructed from ten-fold serial dilutions ranging from 10^5 to 10^{-1} parasites performed in triplicate. Analytical specificity was further assessed by evaluating the amplification profiles of DNA obtained from other canine pathogens, such as *Ehrlichia canis* and *Babesia canis*. Briefly, 150 ng of DNA from each pathogen was amplified and compared to the *L. infantum* amplification profile.

9.5 Quantification of 18S rRNA Gene Expression. The expression of the canine housekeeping gene 18S rRNA was measured in order to normalize the concentration of input DNA for each sample and to obtain a reference amplification value to ensure the use of high-quality DNA samples [46]. TaqMan Pre-Developed Assay Reagents (Life Technology Corporation) were used to detect and quantify 18S rRNA gene expression. All of the reactions were performed at a final volume of 25 μL containing: 5 μL of DNA canine tissue sample diluted in deionized water and 20 μL of PCR mixture. The PCR mixture contained: 12.5 μL of Universal Mastermix (Life Technology Corporation), 1.25 μL of 18S GeneEx Assay primer and probe sets (Life Technology Corporation) at a concentration of 20x, and deionized water to obtain the final volume. The positive and negative controls for the housekeeping genes were plated in triplicate and the samples were plated in duplicate. Reactions were performed on an Applied Biosystems 7500 Fast Real-Time PCR System (Life Technology Corporation) using the following protocol: 1 cycle at 50°C for 2 min; 1 cycle at 95°C for 10 min; and 40 two-step cycles, first at 95°C for 15 s and then 50°C for 1 min. A seven point standard curve was constructed for the housekeeping gene ranging from 450–18.75 ng. The slope of the standard curve for the 18s rRNA gene was -3.399 (SD $= 0.296$), which represents the mean slope value of 11 independent experiments with the corresponding coefficient of determination (R^2) of 0.990.

9.6 Parasitic Load in DNA Samples. Samples from 20 of the 51 dogs were used to determine which tissue type harbored the highest parasitic load by comparing the splenic and bone marrow aspirates, blood, conjunctival swab of right and left eyes, lymph node and skin fragments. The parasitic load was expressed as the number of parasites normalized to the established reference amplification value for the 18S rRNA gene in 150 ng of DNA from each tissue sample [47]. Then the value obtained was calculated per 100 mg of host tissue DNA.

10. Evaluation of qPCR accuracy using splenic aspirate samples from a prevalence study

The accuracy of the qPCR assay was evaluated using splenic samples obtained from 800 dogs during a random prevalence study performed in Camaçari, BA, an endemic area for CVL in Brazil. All 800 dogs were clinically evaluated and classified as described in item 2. They were also tested using the following CVL diagnostic methods: DPP CVL rapid test, EIE CVL, our in-house ELISA, and parasite cultures from splenic aspirates as described in item 5. qPCR analysis of splenic aspirate samples was performed as described in item 9.

11. Statistical Analysis

In order to prevent bias, serological, parasitological and molecular techniques were performed and their results were judged without knowledge of the outcome of the other tests.

The ROC curve data analysis described in item 9.3 was performed using GraphPad Prism software v.5.0 (GraphPad Prism Inc., San Diego, CA). Differences in the parasitic load between each type of biological sample were assessed using the Friedman test followed by the Dunn's multiple comparison test. The relationship between parasitic load in the spleen and qPCR positivity in each infected tissue was assessed with the Spearman correlation test using log transformed values for the parasitic load ($p < 0.05$).

For the 800 dogs evaluated in the cross sectional study, the intensity of the parasitic load in the spleen (item 9.6) was categorized into three ranges: $<10^4$, $10^4 - 10^6$, and $>10^6$. The number of clinical signs in the dogs (item 2) was stratified into four

ranges: 0 (no clinical signs), 1–3, 4–6, and >6 clinical signs. Fisher's exact test was used to evaluate the association between the number of clinical signs and the splenic parasitic load ranges.

LCA was performed using a statistical model to define a latent variable that could be used as a gold standard. To define a latent variable that could accurately identify *L. infantum* infection, three indicators representing serologic (DPP CVL), parasitological (culture from splenic samples), and molecular (splenic aspirate qPCR) diagnostic techniques were included. Animals were grouped into two categories, 'infected dogs', and 'not-infected dogs'. The latent classes were estimated and characterized using two parameters: (a) item-response probabilities and (b) class prevalence, which is the probability of belonging to a latent class according to the response pattern. The estimate was performed using the maximum likelihood with expectation-maximization (EM) algorithm. The goodness of fit of the statistical model was evaluated using entropy, which varied between 0 and 1, with the value 1 indicating that the individuals are perfectly classified into the latent classes. Average probabilities for each latent class, which expresses the uncertainty of global classification, were also assessed *a posteriori*, considering a higher *a posteriori* probability to be a better goodness of fit for the statistical model. The Vuong-Lo-Mendell-Rubin likelihood ratio test was used to choose the number of classes in LCA [48]. The Akaike information criterion (AIC) and Bayes information criterion (BIC) were also evaluated for each model. LCA was performed using the software Mplus 5.2, the syntax for fitting LCA in MPlus program is reported in Appendix S1 [49]. Additionally, the conditional independence was checked by evaluation of significant bivariate residuals [50,51].

The sensitivity and 95% confidence interval (CI) were calculated for each diagnostic technique and each tissue type analyzed, using the LCA latent variable as gold standard. The accuracy (sensitivity and specificity) of the qPCR technique using splenic aspirates was further evaluated with the LCA in a random sample of 800 dogs. Sensitivity of each test was measured as the proportion of positive results, only among those identified as such by the gold standard, while specificity was measured as the proportion of negative results, which were correctly identified as such by the gold standard.

Results

1. Sample description

All 51 dogs from the endemic area of Jequié were mixed-breed, their estimated ages varied from 1–10 years old, the animals weighed 5 30 kg, 45% (23/51) were males, and 55% (28/51) were females. All of the dogs exhibited clinical signs that could be related to CVL including splenomegaly (33/51), emaciation (17/51), hypertrophy of the lymph nodes (46/51), alopecia (21/51), cutaneous alterations (41/51), onychogryphosis (29/51), and ocular alterations (10/51). With respect to clinical pathology, 73% of the dogs presented with anemia (35/48), 98% with hypergammaglobulinemia (49/50), and 98% with hypoalbuminemia (49/50). Using the scale published by Solano-Gallego etal. (2009), all of the dogs were classified as having moderate CVL (stage II), except one animal that also exhibited a creatinine value greater than 1.4 mg/dL and was considered to have severe CVL (stage III).

2. Standardization of the qPCR Protocol

The Ct cut-off value for parasite DNA detection was performed using a ROC analysis. This analysis showed an area under the curve of 1.0, indicating a high probability ($p < 0.001$) that a randomly chosen positive sample would be correctly classified.

The Ct cut-off value of 37.0 had prediction rates of 100% sensitivity (CI 83.16–100) and 95% specificity (CI 75.13–99.87) with a likelihood ratio of 20. The analytical sensitivity was then determined. We found that the amplification profile of the reference strain *L. infantum* DNA was similar to that of the reference strain mixed with splenic aspirate DNA from negative control animals. The lower limit of detection was then determined and corresponded to 0.016 parasites per reaction.

In terms of the analytical specificity, the Old World *L. major* parasite DNA samples were remarkably similar to those of *L. infantum* at all of the concentrations tested. In contrast, DNA from *L. amazonensis* and *L. braziliensis* could only be successfully amplified at concentrations of 10^4 and 10^5 parasites per reaction. This corresponded to the same number of cycles needed to amplify DNA from 0.02 parasites per reaction of the *L. infantum* reference strain (Figure S1). *E. canis* and *B. canis* DNA did not amplify using this qPCR protocol (data not shown). With respect to the housekeeping gene, attempts to amplify18S rRNA from DNA samples of *Leishmania* spp. resulted in no detectable qPCR amplification using the same primer set that successfully amplified the gene in canine DNA samples (data not shown).

3. Positivity of diagnostic techniques

Using qPCR, 100% of the dogs from Jequié (51/51) tested positive for parasite DNA in at least one of the tissue types analyzed. Among these, 98% (50/51) tested positive in the splenic aspirate samples; 80.4% (41/51) in blood samples; 68.3% (28/41) in skin fragments; 54.9% (28/51) in lymph node fragments; 35% (7/20) in bone marrow aspirate; 37.3% (19/51) in left eye conjunctival swabs, and 33.3% (17/51) in right eye conjunctival swabs.

Parasites were observed in 35.3% (18/51) of the parasite cultures from splenic aspirate and anti-*Leishmania* antibodies were detected in 43.8% (21/48), 47.1% (24/51), and 66.7% (34/51) of the canine serum samples using the EIE CVL, DPP CVL rapid test, and in-house ELISA, respectively.

4. Accuracy of the diagnostic tests

Latent class was used to provide a reliable estimate of sensitivity and specificity in order to select the tissue that provided the greatest accuracy for qPCR DNA detection. Serological, parasitological, and molecular techniques were used to determine prevalence of the latent classes and conditional probabilities in the LCA model for *L. infantum* infection in dogs. The probability that a dog from Jequié would be classified as infected using the LCA model was 47.1%. Among the animals considered infected by the LCA, the probability that a dog would test positive using qPCR of the splenic aspirate was 95.8%. The probability that a dog tested positive using either DPP CVL or by parasite culture from splenic aspirates was 100.0% or 54.2%, respectively (Table 1).

Entropy was then calculated to assess how well the animals were classified *a posteriori* by the model. The entropy of the Jequié samples was 1.0; indicating accuracy in the classification of dogs using LCA. Moreover, *a posteriori* average probabilities that animals were properly classified into the latent classes "Infected" and "Not Infected" were 100% in both cases in the Jequié animals. The Lo-Mendel-Rubin test indicated that the model with 2 classes was a better fit for the data obtained from the Jequié dogs ($p<0.01$) when compared with the model with only 1 class (data not shown). These results are supported by the analysis of the AIC and BIC (data not shown).

The sensitivity of the tests employed in Jequié to diagnose *L. infantum* infection was assessed employing the latent variable obtained by LCA as the gold standard (Figure 1). Splenic aspirates

Table 1. Prevalence of latent classes and conditional probabilities to the LCA model for *L. infantum* infection detection in dogs.

Technique	Result	Dogs from Jequié n = 51			Dogs from Camaçari n = 800		
		Result Frequency (%)	Latent Classes		Result Frequency (%)	Latent Classes	
			Infected n = 24 (47.1%)	Not Infected n = 27 (52.9%)		Infected n = 120 (14.5%)	Not Infected n = 680 (85.5%)
			Conditional Probabilities (%)			Conditional Probabilities (%)	
DPP CVL	Positive	47.1	100.0	0.0	16.6	82.9	5.5
	Negative	52.9	0.0	100.0	83.4	17.1	94.5
Splenic Aspirate Culturing	Positive	35.3	54.2	18.5	13.2	87.8	0.0
	Negative	64.7	45.8	81.5	86.8	12.2	100.0
Splenic Aspirate qPCR	Positive	98.0	95.8	100.0	34.2	93.3	24.1
	Negative	2.0	4.2	0.0	65.8	6.7	75.9

provided the highest sensitivity of the available tissues sampled achieving 95.8% (95%CI 90.4–100) of sensitivity. The sensitivity attained in other tissues ranged from 80% to 30% as follows: lymph node fragments 79.2% (95%CI 68–90.3), skin fragments 77.3% (95%CI 64.5–90.1), blood 75% (95%CI 63.1–86.9), bone marrow aspirates 50% (95%CI 30–70), left eye swab 37.5% (95%CI 24.2–50.8), and right eye swab 29.2% (95%CI 16.7–41.6). It was not possible to calculate splenic qPCR specificity since only one sample tested negative in this method. Specificity of the other tissues achieved 66.7% for lymph node fragments (95%CI 53.7–79.6) as well as for bone marrow aspirates (95%CI 47.8–85.6), 63% (95%CI 49.7–76.2) for right and left eye swabs, 42.1% (95%CI 27–57.2) for skin fragments and 14.8% (95%CI 5.1–24.6) for blood. Considering the other diagnostic tests, the sensitivity of the serological tests was 100% for the DPP CVL, followed by 79.2% (95%CI 68–90.3) for the in-house ELISA, 65.2% (95%CI 51.7–78.7) for EIE CVL, while sensitivity for the splenic aspirate culturing was 54.2% (95%CI 40.5–67.8). The specificity was highest for DPP CVL 100%, followed by splenic parasite cultures 81.5% (95%CI 70.8–92.1), EIE CVL 76% (95%CI 63.9–88.1), in-house ELISA 44.4% (95%CI 30.8–58.1).

5. Parasitic load in different tissue types

To further characterize tissue performance for the molecular diagnostic assay, parasitic loads were determined in the different tissues analyzed. As shown in Table 2 a considerable degree of variation was observed among the samples with values ranging from 120 parasites in a splenic aspirate sample up to 186 million parasites found in a bone marrow aspirate sample. However, the median parasitic load was higher in splenic aspirate samples than in the conjunctival swabs from either eye ($p<0.05$) or bone marrow aspirate ($p<0.05$). No statistically significant differences were observed when comparing parasitic loads in the splenic aspirate to the blood or skin tissue samples.

6. Distribution of parasitic load according to number of clinical signs

The distribution of parasitic load according to the number of clinical signs is displayed in Table 3. We observed a significant positive association between the intensity of parasitic load in the spleen and the number of clinical signs present in the dogs. Animals with no clinical signs ($p<0.01$) or those exhibiting 1–3 clinical signs ($p<0.001$) had lower parasitic loads in splenic tissue

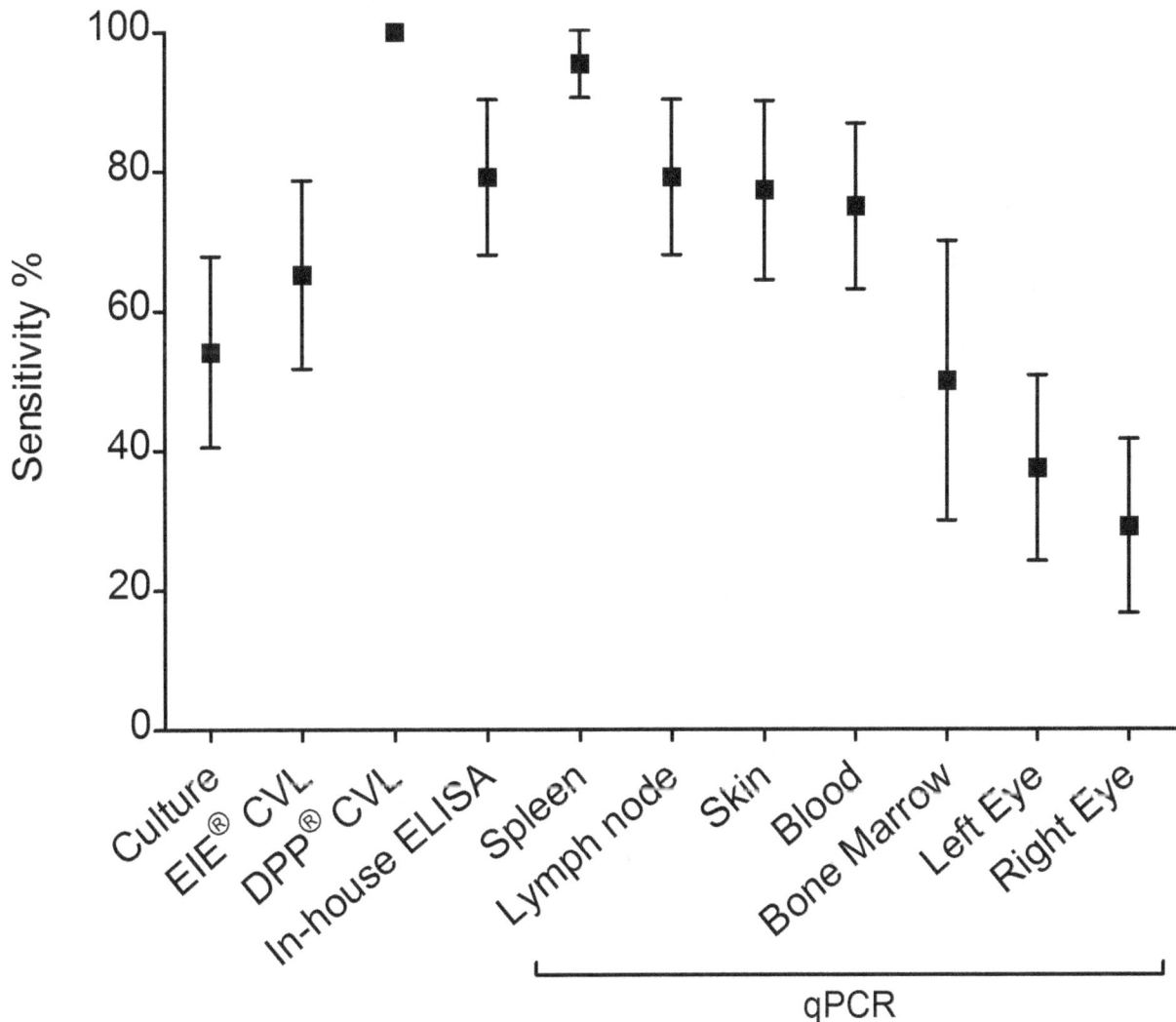

Figure 1. Sensitivity of the different diagnostic techniques employed in the biological samples obtained from Jequié animals (n = 51). Vertical bars represent the 95% confidence intervals. Sensitivity values were obtained using the latent variable as the gold standard.

Table 2. Parasitic loads detected in different canine tissue types from a total of 20 dogs from the endemic area of Jequié.

Tissue type	Positivity	Parasitic loads[a]				
		Minimum	25% Percentile	Median	75% Percentile	Maximum
Splenic Aspirate	100% (20/20)	120	1,088	4,365	14,325	74,000,000
Blood	70% (14/20)	0	0	7,960	19,800	228,000
Skin Fragment	60% (12/20)	0	0	1,870	21,500	32,400,000
Lymph node Fragment	60% (12/20)	0	0	830.5	9,288	7,800,000
Bone Marrow Aspirate	35% (07/20)	0	0	0.0*	28,275	186,000,000
Left Eye Swab	50% (10/20)	0	0	645.0*	2,073	240,000
Right Eye Swab	35% (07/20)	0	0	0.0*	3,141	147,000

[a]number of parasites normalized by the established reference amplification value for the housekeeping gene 18S rRNA in 100 mg of host tissue DNA.
*$p < 0.05$ Friedman's together with Dunn's multiple comparisons test of splenic aspirates and swab of right or left eye and splenic aspirates and bone marrow.

($<10^4$). In contrast, animals with >6 clinical signs ($p < 0.01$) showed relatively higher loads ($>10^6$). The dogs presenting with 4–6 clinical signs were homogeneously distributed throughout the three ranges.

7. Accuracy of qPCR using splenic aspirate samples from a prevalence study

Splenic aspirate samples collected from a random study conducted in the endemic area of Camaçari were used to evaluate the high sensitivity observed for the qPCR technique developed using convenience sampling from Jequié. Positive diagnoses in the samples from Camaçari varied according to diagnostic test. In this sample, 34.2% were positive using qPCR, 24.4% using EIE CVL, 19.8% using the in-house ELISA, and 16.6% using DPP CVL.

Similar to the samples from Jequié, LCA was used to analyze the results from the Camaçari samples. Reliability of the LCA model was evaluated and the probability of an animal being infected with *L. infantum* was calculated. The response patterns obtained from the latent class model that were used are listed in Table 4. Animals from Camaçari that had at least two positive test results were classified by the LCA model as 'Infected'. However, the presence of a positive result from the splenic aspirate parasite culture implied a 100% probability of being infected with *L. infantum*, regardless of the DPP CVL and splenic aspirate qPCR results. When dogs from this endemic area tested negative by all three diagnostic techniques, the probability that the animal was infected with *L. infantum* was 0%. Furthermore, the probability of animals being infected was still very low when only splenic aspirate qPCR (2.7%) or DPP CVL (1.4%) tested positive according to this LCA model.

The entropy of the Camaçari samples was 0.934, and the *a posteriori* average probabilities of being correctly classified as "Infected" and "Not Infected" were, respectively, 92.4% and 99.3%. Similar to the analysis performed with samples from Jequié, using random samples, the Lo-Mendel-Rubin test indicated that the model with 2 classes was optimal and was supported by the analysis of the AIC and BIC (data not shown).

Using LCA, the sensitivity of the splenic aspirate qPCR (95%; 95%CI 93.5–96.5) was higher than for the other diagnostic tests: DPP CVL (86.4%; 95%CI 84.1–88.8), splenic parasite cultures (83.5%; 95%CI 80.8–86.2), the in-house ELISA (78.3%; 95%CI 75.5–81.2), and EIE CVL (72.5%; 95% CI 69.4–75.6) (Figure 2A). However, the specificity was highest for splenic parasite cultures (100%), followed by DPP CVL (95.6%; 95%CI 94.2–97), the in-house ELISA (90.6%; 95%CI 88.6–92.6), EIE CVL (84.1%; 95%CI 81.6–86.6), and splenic aspirate qPCR (76.7%; 95%CI 73.7–79.6) (Figure 2B).

Discussion

The present study found that a qPCR protocol targeting *Leishmania* kDNA provided the highest diagnostic sensitivity in dogs from Jequié when compared to standard serological and parasitological methods. In this endemic area, the DPP CVL rapid test and EIE CVL were able to detect infection in 47.1% and 43.8%, respectively, of a population of symptomatic dogs. Interestingly, 100% of these dogs tested positive with respect to at least one of the tissue types analyzed using qPCR. Similar results have been obtained by other studies, in which high sensitivity was achieved using molecular techniques [14,16,52]. Together these results reinforce the notion that the number of

Table 3. Distribution of parasitic load according to number of clinical signs in dogs from the prevalence study.

Number of Clinical Signs	Splenic Parasitic Load Ranges			Fisher Exact Test
	$<10^4$	10^4–10^6	$>10^6$	
0	8 (57.1%)	5 (35.7%)	1 (7.1%)	$p < 0.01$
1–3	55 (42%)	49 (37.4%)	27 (20.6%)	$p < 0.001$
4–6	37 (39.4%)	27 (28.7%)	30 (31.9%)	$p = 0.11$
>6	5 (16.1%)	9 (29.0%)	17 (54.8%)	$p < 0.01$
Total	105	90	75	

Table 4. Response patterns[a] of Camaçari dogs for LCA model with 2 latent classes for diagnosis of CVL.

| Response pattern | | | | | |
DPP CVL	Splenic Aspirate Culturing	Splenic Aspirate qPCR	Frequency Observed % (n)	CVL Probability *a posteriori* (%)	Result Based on LCA
N	N	N	60.1 (429)	0.0	Not infected
N	N	P	20.5 (146)	1.4	Not infected
P	N	N	3.6 (26)	2.7	Not infected
N	P	N	0.1 (01)	100.0*	Infected
P	N	P	2.7 (19)	54.7	Infected
N	P	P	2.1 (15)	100.0	Infected
P	P	N	0.7 (05)	100.0	Infected
P	P	P	10.2 (73)	100.0	Infected

[a]Response patterns of all samples tested using the three techniques.
*Estimation based on only one animal sample presenting this pattern.
N: Negative; P: Positive.

infected dogs detected by serological surveys in endemic areas is severely underestimated [53,54].

Several methods have been recently developed for the molecular detection of *Leishmania* spp. [20,21,55], that provide divergent results when used in a variety of clinical canine samples [54]. Among the tissues analyzed, the authors observed that splenic aspirate samples provided the highest detection rate, successfully identifying 98% of the samples that tested positive. This result is supported by the fact that the spleen is a key site for parasite multiplication in naturally infected dogs [24,56]. Interestingly, following splenic aspirate samples, 80.4% of blood samples tested positive using qPCR. In addition, we found that the parasitic loads achieved were similar in the blood and splenic aspirate samples. These are promising results given that drawing blood is a much less invasive sampling technique to detect *Leishmania* infection in dogs than obtaining splenic aspirates. In contrast, several other studies have found that bone marrow and lymph node tissues offered a higher number of positive results than

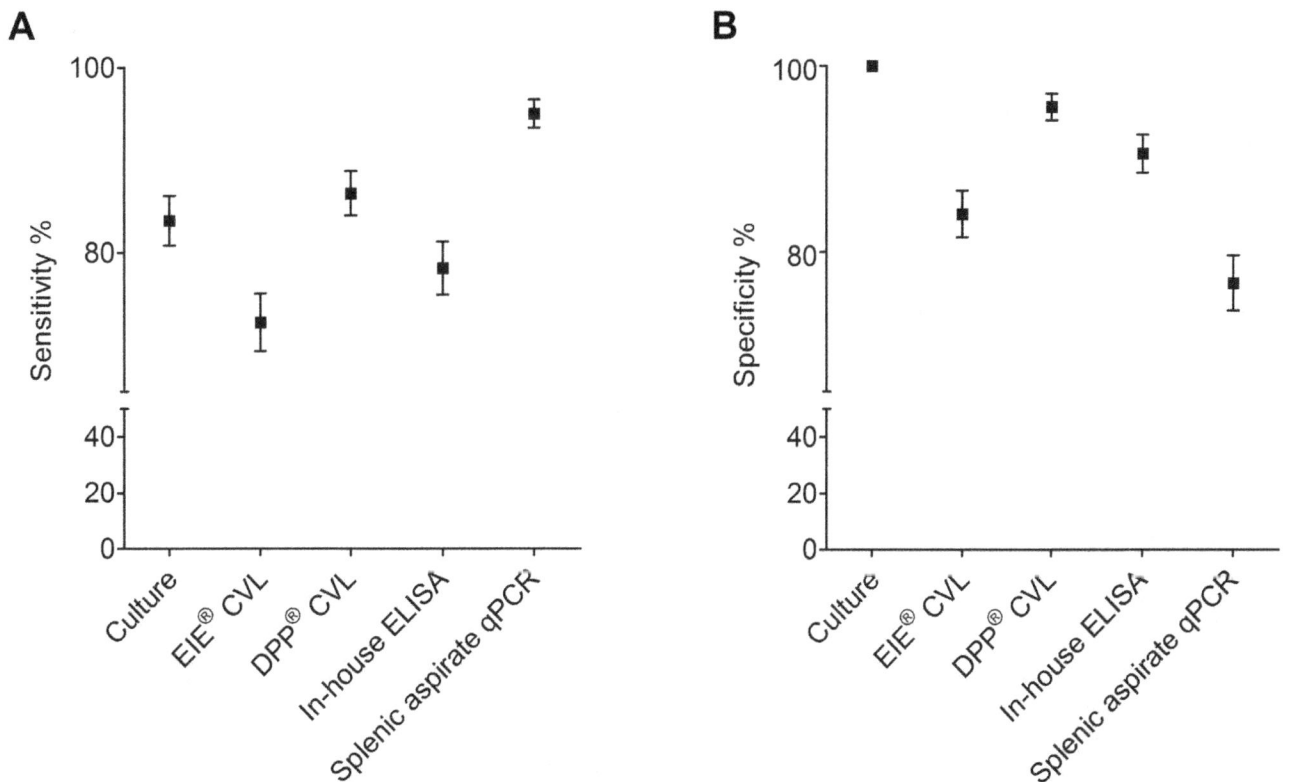

Figure 2. Sensitivity and specificity of the different diagnostic techniques employed in the biological samples obtained from Camaçari animals (n = 800). Vertical bars represent the 95% confidence intervals. **A)** Sensitivity and **B)** Specificity values obtained using the latent variable as the gold standard.

blood [46,55,57,58]. Francino etal. (2006) suggested that using qPCR to detect *Leishmania* parasites in blood samples might be sufficient to diagnose infection given the technique's ability to quantify extremely low parasitemia. However, other authors consider the blood to be a poor source of *Leishmania* DNA [59], mostly because blood samples do not have satisfactory detection rates using conventional PCR. The underlying cause of these poor results may be the high frequency of PCR inhibitors found in blood, in addition to low parasitic loads, which could lead to false negatives especially in asymptomatic dogs [52]. Serum albumin can be added to avoid any potential inhibiting effects in qPCR reaction [44]. In the present study we added serum albumin to blood, skin, and conjunctival swab samples. Our results demonstrate that splenic aspirates or blood can be effectively used to detect parasite DNA using qPCR [18,19].

The analytical specificity of the qPCR technique was also evaluated in the present study by comparing the amplification profiles of *L. infantum* DNA to other Old and New World *Leishmania* species. The amplification profile of the Old World species *L. major* was remarkably similar to that of *L. infantum* (Figure S1). This corroborates other studies that have shown a great deal of similarity between the genomes of these species [60]. To the best of our knowledge, *L. major* is not known to be a causative agent of CVL, nor have any cases linked to this parasite been reported in Latin America [61]. kDNA from New World parasites, such as *L. amazonensis* and *L. braziliensis*, was successfully amplified using this protocol, but only at high concentrations of 10^4 and 10^5 parasites per reaction (Figure S1). Protocols capable of distinguishing between *Leishmania* species are preferable in endemics areas for both cutaneous and visceral forms of the disease [62]. In this study, five *Leishmania* species isolated from the dogs were identified by multilocus enzyme electrophoresis as *L. infantum*. Nonetheless, the use of splenic aspirate samples can avoid misleading diagnostic results since visceralization of *L. braziliensis* has not been reported and visceralization of *L. amazonensis* is a relatively rare event both in humans or dogs [62–64].

Regrettably, an ideal gold standard is still lacking for CVL diagnosis [65]. Historically, parasite culturing and immunofluorescence antibody test (IFAT) have been abundantly used. However, culturing is shown to have low sensitivity, while IFAT low specificity [65]. An alternative to using a single technique as the gold standard is to utilize LCA, once this method defines a latent variable to be used as gold standard, considering all diagnostic tests impartially. Indeed, LCA has been proved to successfully estimate the sensitivities and specificities of different diagnostic tests for several diseases [34,66–69]. LCA has been an useful tool for validating serological diagnostic methods for VL, since this analysis provides more realistic estimates of diagnostic test performance [34,67]. In the scientific community still exist concerns regarding the high sensitivity of qPCR results, especially when this technique is able to detect very low parasitic loads. In addition, some authors state that is impossible for qPCR to differentiate between the DNA of a living parasite and a dead one. Otherwise, Prina etal. (2007) [70] were the only ones that proved that as soon as 1 h after exposure to a substance able to kill the parasites, only less than 1% of the initial *Leishmania* DNA could be detected by qPCR. No other group demonstrated these results, especially using invivo experiments. Thus, in the present study, we have decided not to consider all the dogs as infected, even if they displayed parasite in at least one tissue by the qPCR, and perform the qPCR accuracy evaluation using the latent variable.

Employing the latent class variable as the gold standard, we found that the sensitivity for splenic aspirate qPCR and DPP CVL

were 95.8% and 100% respectively, in a population of symptomatic dogs in Jequié. However, these results were limited since it was a small sample size. To address this, the results of the qPCR testing were evaluated using a larger random sampling of dogs that consisted of a population of positive and negative dogs, which are representative of the population of an endemic area for VL. In this random population survey using 800 dogs, the high sensitivity of splenic aspirate qPCR was confirmed achieving 95% of sensitivity, while the DPP CVL sensitivity was corrected to 83.5%. Despite the high sensitivity of the splenic aspirate qPCR, the specificity was relatively low (76.7%). This could be due to the large number of dogs from the randomly sampled population that tested positive only by splenic aspirate qPCR (20.5%) and were considered as 'Not infected' by the LCA. These animals were likely misclassified by LCA as false negatives, since the splenic aspirate qPCR is known to be the most sensitive diagnostic technique for CVL, most likely more sensitive than the variables used to define the variable latent class.

Several studies have demonstrated a positive correlation between clinical manifestations of CVL and parasitic load in the spleen, lymph nodes and skin using several techniques [20,41,56,71]. Using qPCR of splenic aspirate in dogs, we also found a positive association between parasitic load and clinical manifestations of CVL, reinforcing the notion that can be used not only for detection of infection but also to monitor disease severity in dogs.

Although splenic aspirate collection is considered an invasive procedure by many dog owners [27,72], Barrouin-Melo etal. (2006) noted that minor complications were observed in only three out of 257 dogs that underwent splenic aspiration. Complications can be further minimized by visualizing the spleen using an ultrasound device to guide splenic aspiration [72,73]. In our experience, during the prevalence study in the municipality of Camaçari, the splenic aspirate procedure assisted by ultrasonography was well tolerated in all 800 dogs without any reported complication.

In conclusion, the authors found that, the splenic aspirates and blood, provided the greatest sensitivity for detecting *Leishmania* DNA using qPCR. In addition, the results indicated that LCA could be used to create a suitable gold standard for diagnosis, since this technique offers a more comprehensive evaluation of the results obtained using different diagnostic testing methods for CVL.

Supporting Information

Figure S1   Amplification profiles of DNA samples from *Leishmania* spp. A) *L. infantum*; **B)** *L. major*; **C)** *L. amazonensis*; **D)** *L. braziliensis*. DNA samples derived from the *L. infantum* reference strain, and several other *Leishmania* species, including New World *L. amazonensis* and *L. braziliensis*, and Old World *L. major*. Standard curves were constructed using amplification patterns from ten-fold serial dilutions performed in triplicate ranging from 10^5 to 10^{-1} parasites per reaction.

Appendix S1   Syntax for fitting LCA in MPlus program.

Acknowledgments

The authors would like to thank Dr. Flávia W. Cruz McBride for support to obtain negative control samples in Pelotas, Dr. Virgínia Maria G. da Silva and Joselli S. Silva for the help in the endemic area. Additionally, the authors acknowledge Kyoshi Fukutani for help in the qPCR analysis. Finally, we are grateful to Andris K. Walter for providing English revision and consulting services and manuscript edition by native English-speaking experts from BioMed Proofreading LLC.

Author Contributions

Conceived and designed the experiments: MSS CESG DBMF PSTV. Performed the experiments: MSS LAB MB LSB DFL. Analyzed the data: MSS CESG PGSET LDAFA WLCS DBMF PSTV. Contributed reagents/materials/analysis tools: DFL GGSO EGN PGSET LDAFA. Wrote the paper: MSS CESG LDAFA DBMF PSTV.

References

1. Desjeux P (2004) Leishmaniasis. Nat Rev Microbiol 2: 692.
2. Killick-Kendrick R (1999) The biology and control of phlebotomine sand flies. Clin Dermatol 17: 279–289.
3. Kuhls K, Alam MZ, Cupolillo E, Ferreira GE, Mauricio IL, et al. (2011) Comparative microsatellite typing of new world Leishmania infantum reveals low heterogeneity among populations and its recent old world origin. PLoS Negl Trop Dis 5: e1155.
4. Lainson R, Shaw JJ (1978) Epidemiology and ecology of leishmaniasis in Latin-America. Nature 273: 595–600.
5. Mauricio IL, Stothard JR, Miles MA (2000) The strange case of Leishmania chagasi. Parasitol Today 16: 188–189.
6. Deane LM, Deane MP, Alencar JE (1955) [Control of Phlebotomus longipalpis by DDT house spraying endemic foci of kala-azar in Ceara]. Rev Bras Malariol Doencas Trop 7: 131–141.
7. Dye C (1996) The logic of visceral leishmaniasis control. Am J Trop Med Hyg 55: 125–130.
8. Gramiccia M, Gradoni L (2005) The current status of zoonotic leishmaniases and approaches to disease control. Int J Parasitol 35: 1169–1180.
9. Molina R, Amela C, Nieto J, San-Andres M, Gonzalez F, et al. (1994) Infectivity of dogs naturally infected with Leishmania infantum to colonized Phlebotomus perniciosus. Trans R Soc Trop Med Hyg 88: 491–493.
10. Ciaramella P, Oliva G, Luna RD, Gradoni L, Ambrosio R, et al. (1997) A retrospective clinical study of canine leishmaniasis in 150 dogs naturally infected by Leishmania infantum. Vet Rec 141: 539–543.
11. Koutinas AF, Polizopoulou ZS, Saridomichelakis MN, Argyriadis D, Fytianou A, et al. (1999) Clinical considerations on canine visceral leishmaniasis in Greece: a retrospective study of 158 cases (1989–1996). J Am Anim Hosp Assoc 35: 376–383.
12. Miro G, Cardoso L, Pennisi MG, Oliva G, Baneth G (2008) Canine leishmaniosis–new concepts and insights on an expanding zoonosis: part two. Trends Parasitol 24: 371–377.
13. Gomes YM, Paiva Cavalcanti M, Lira RA, Abath FG, Alves LC (2008) Diagnosis of canine visceral leishmaniasis: biotechnological advances. Vet J 175: 45–52.
14. Coura-Vital W, Marques MJ, Veloso VM, Roatt BM, Aguiar-Soares RD, et al. (2011) Prevalence and factors associated with Leishmania infantum infection of dogs from an urban area of Brazil as identified by molecular methods. PLoS Negl Trop Dis 5: e1291.
15. Ferreira Ede C, de Lana M, Carneiro M, Reis AB, Paes DV, et al. (2007) Comparison of serological assays for the diagnosis of canine visceral leishmaniasis in animals presenting different clinical manifestations. Vet Parasitol 146: 235–241.
16. Solano-Gallego L, Morell P, Arboix M, Alberola J, Ferrer L (2001) Prevalence of Leishmania infantum infection in dogs living in an area of canine leishmaniasis endemicity using PCR on several tissues and serology. J Clin Microbiol 39: 560–563.
17. Troncarelli MZ, Camargo JB, Machado JG, Lucheis SB, Langoni H (2009) Leishmania spp. and/or Trypanosoma cruzi diagnosis in dogs from endemic and nonendemic areas for canine visceral leishmaniasis. Vet Parasitol 164: 118–123.
18. Solca Mda S, Guedes CE, Nascimento EG, Oliveira GG, dos Santos WL, et al. (2012) Qualitative and quantitative polymerase chain reaction (PCR) for detection of Leishmania in spleen samples from naturally infected dogs. Vet Parasitol 184: 133–140.
19. Francino O, Altet L, Sanchez-Robert E, Rodriguez A, Solano-Gallego L, et al. (2006) Advantages of real-time PCR assay for diagnosis and monitoring of canine leishmaniosis. Vet Parasitol 137: 214–221.
20. Manna L, Reale S, Vitale F, Gravino AE (2009) Evidence for a relationship between Leishmania load and clinical manifestations. Res Vet Sci 82: 76–78.
21. Mary C, Faraut F, Lascombe L, Dumon H (2004) Quantification of Leishmania infantum DNA by a real-time PCR assay with high sensitivity. J Clin Microbiol 42: 5249–5255.
22. Maia C, Campino L (2008) Methods for diagnosis of canine leishmaniasis and immune response to infection. Vet Parasitol 158: 274–287.
23. Martinez V, Quilez J, Sanchez A, Roura X, Francino O, et al. (2011) Canine leishmaniasis: the key points for qPCR result interpretation. Parasit Vectors 4: 57.
24. Maia C, Ramada J, Cristovao JM, Goncalves L, Campino L (2009) Diagnosis of canine leishmaniasis: conventional and molecular techniques using different tissues. Vet J 179: 142–144.
25. Ferreira Sde A, Ituassu LT, de Melo MN, de Andrade AS (2008) Evaluation of the conjunctival swab for canine visceral leishmaniasis diagnosis by PCR-hybridization in Minas Gerais State, Brazil. Vet Parasitol 152: 257–263.
26. Lombardo G, Pennisi MG, Lupo T, Migliazzo A, Capri A, et al. (2012) Detection of Leishmania infantum DNA by real-time PCR in canine oral and conjunctival swabs and comparison with other diagnostic techniques. Vet Parasitol 184: 10–17.
27. Carvalho D, Oliveira TMFS, Baldani CD, Machado RZ (2009) An enzyme-linked immunosorbent assay (ELISA) for the detection of IgM antibodies against Leishmania chagasi in dogs. Pesquisa Veterinária Brasileira 29: 120–124.
28. Sundar S, Rai M (2002) Laboratory diagnosis of visceral leishmaniasis. Clin Diagn Lab Immunol 9: 951–958.
29. Moreira MA, Luvizotto MC, Garcia JF, Corbett CE, Laurenti MD (2007) Comparison of parasitological, immunological and molecular methods for the diagnosis of leishmaniasis in dogs with different clinical signs. Vet Parasitol 145: 245–252.
30. Ndao M (2009) Diagnosis of parasitic diseases: old and new approaches. Interdiscip Perspect Infect Dis 2009: 278246.
31. Baughman AL, Bisgard KM, Cortese MM, Thompson WW, Sanden GN, et al. (2008) Utility of composite reference standards and latent class analysis in evaluating the clinical accuracy of diagnostic tests for pertussis. Clin Vaccine Immunol 15: 106–114.
32. Butler JC, Bosshardt SC, Phelan M, Moroney SM, Tondella ML, et al. (2003) Classical and latent class analysis evaluation of sputum polymerase chain reaction and urine antigen testing for diagnosis of pneumococcal pneumonia in adults. J Infect Dis 187: 1416–1423.
33. Nascimento MC, de Souza VA, Sumita LM, Freire W, Munoz F, et al. (2007) Comparative study of Kaposi's sarcoma-associated herpesvirus serological assays using clinically and serologically defined reference standards and latent class analysis. J Clin Microbiol 45: 715–720.
34. Machado de Assis TS, Rabello A, Werneck GL (2012) Latent class analysis of diagnostic tests for visceral leishmaniasis in Brazil. Trop Med Int Health 17: 1202–1207.
35. Machado CJ, Filipecki AT, Teixeira MD, Klein HE (2010) Regulation of the use of animals in Brazil in the twentieth century and the process of forming the current regime applied to biomedical research. História, Ciências, Saúde-Manguinhos 17: 87–105.
36. Brasil MdSd (2006) Manual de vigilancia e controle da leishmaniose visceral: Ministerio da Saude - Secretaria de Vigilancia em Saude.
37. Lima IS, Silva JS, Almeida VA, Junior FG, Souza PA, et al. (2014) Severe clinical presentation of visceral leishmaniasis in naturally infected dogs with disruption of the splenic white pulp. PLoS One 9: e87742.
38. Solano-Gallego L, Koutinas A, Miro G, Cardoso L, Pennisi MG, et al. (2009) Directions for the diagnosis, clinical staging, treatment and prevention of canine leishmaniosis. Vet Parasitol 165: 1–18.
39. Baleeiro CO, Paranhos-Silva M, dos Santos JC, Oliveira GG, Nascimento EG, et al. (2006) Montenegro's skin reactions and antibodies against different Leishmania species in dogs from a visceral leishmaniosis endemic area. Vet Parasitol 139: 21–28.
40. Paranhos-Silva M, Freitas LA, Santos WC, Grimaldi GJ, Pontes-de-Carvalho LC, et al. (1996) A cross-sectional serodiagnostic survey of canine leishmaniasis due to Leishmania chagasi. Am J Trop Med Hyg 55: 39–44.
41. Barrouin-Melo SM, Larangeira DF, Trigo J, Aguiar PH, dos-Santos WL, et al. (2004) Comparison between splenic and lymph node aspirations as sampling methods for the parasitological detection of Leishmania chagasi infection in dogs. Mem Inst Oswaldo Cruz 99: 195–197.
42. Batista LF, Segatto M, Guedes CE, Sousa RS, Rodrigues CA, et al. (2012) An assessment of the genetic diversity of Leishmania infantum isolates from infected dogs in Brazil. Am J Trop Med Hyg 86: 799–806.
43. dos Santos Marques LH, Gomes LI, da Rocha IC, da Silva TA, Oliveira E, et al. (2012) Low parasite load estimated by qPCR in a cohort of children living in urban area endemic for visceral leishmaniasis in Brazil. PLoS Negl Trop Dis 6: e1955.
44. Giambernardi TA, Rodeck U, Klebe RJ (1998) Bovine serum albumin reverses inhibition of RT-PCR by melanin. Biotechniques 25: 564–566.
45. Naranjo C, Fondevila D, Altet L, Francino O, Rios J, et al. (2012) Evaluation of the presence of Leishmania spp. by real-time PCR in the lacrimal glands of dogs with leishmaniosis. Vet J 193: 168–173.
46. Solano-Gallego L, Rodriguez-Cortes A, Trotta M, Zampieron C, Razia L, et al. (2007) Detection of Leishmania infantum DNA by fret-based real-time PCR in urine from dogs with natural clinical leishmaniosis. Vet Parasitol 147: 315–319.
47. Manna L, Reale S, Viola E, Vitale F, Foglia Manzillo V, et al. (2006) Leishmania DNA load and cytokine expression levels in asymptomatic naturally infected dogs. Vet Parasitol 142: 271–280.
48. Muthen B, Asparouhov T (2012) Bayesian structural equation modeling: a more flexible representation of substantive theory. Psychol Methods 17: 313–335.

49. Muthen LK, Muthen BO (2007) Mplus - Statistical analysis with latent variable. Version 6.
50. Garrett ES, Zeger SL (2000) Latent class model diagnosis. Biometrics 56: 1055–1067.
51. Uebersax J (2009) A Practical Guide to Conditional Dependence in Latent Class Models. John Uebersax Enterprises LLC.
52. Lachaud L, Chabbert E, Dubessay P, Dereure J, Lamothe J, et al. (2002) Value of two PCR methods for the diagnosis of canine visceral leishmaniasis and the detection of asymptomatic carriers. Parasitology 125: 197–207.
53. Alvar J, Canavate C, Molina R, Moreno J, Nieto J (2004) Canine leishmaniasis. Adv Parasitol 57: 1–88.
54. Baneth G, Koutinas AF, Solano-Gallego L, Bourdeau P, Ferrer L (2008) Canine leishmaniosis - new concepts and insights on an expanding zoonosis: part one. Trends Parasitol 24: 324–330.
55. Maia C, Nunes M, Cristovao J, Campino L (2010) Experimental canine leishmaniasis: clinical, parasitological and serological follow-up. Acta Trop 116: 193–199.
56. Reis AB, Martins-Filho OA, Teixeira-Carvalho A, Carvalho MG, Mayrink W, et al. (2006) Parasite density and impaired biochemical/hematological status are associated with severe clinical aspects of canine visceral leishmaniasis. Res Vet Sci 81: 68–75.
57. de Almeida Ferreira S, Leite RS, Ituassu LT, Almeida GG, Souza DM, et al. (2012) Canine skin and conjunctival swab samples for the detection and quantification of Leishmania infantum DNA in an endemic urban area in Brazil. PLoS Negl Trop Dis 6: e1596.
58. Manna L, Reale S, Vitale F, Picillo E, Pavone LM, et al. (2008) Real-time PCR assay in Leishmania-infected dogs treated with meglumine antimoniate and allopurinol. Vet J 177: 279–282.
59. Reale S, Maxia L, Vitale F, Glorioso NS, Caracappa S, et al. (1999) Detection of Leishmania infantum in dogs by PCR with lymph node aspirates and blood. J Clin Microbiol 37: 2931–2935.
60. Peacock CS, Seeger K, Harris D, Murphy L, Ruiz JC, et al. (2007) Comparative genomic analysis of three Leishmania species that cause diverse human disease. Nat Genet 39: 839–847.
61. Alvar J, Velez ID, Bern C, Herrero M, Desjeux P, et al. (2012) Leishmaniasis worldwide and global estimates of its incidence. PLoS One 7: e35671.
62. Madeira MF, Schubach A, Schubach TM, Pacheco RS, Oliveira FS, et al. (2006) Mixed infection with Leishmania (Viannia) braziliensis and Leishmania (Leishmania) chagasi in a naturally infected dog from Rio de Janeiro, Brazil. Trans R Soc Trop Med Hyg 100: 442–445.

63. Barral A, Pedral-Sampaio D, Grimaldi Junior G, Momen H, McMahon-Pratt D, et al. (1991) Leishmaniasis in Bahia, Brazil: evidence that Leishmania amazonensis produces a wide spectrum of clinical disease. Am J Trop Med Hyg 44: 536–546.
64. Tolezano JE, Uliana SR, Taniguchi HH, Araujo MF, Barbosa JA, et al. (2007) The first records of Leishmania (Leishmania) amazonensis in dogs (Canis familiaris) diagnosed clinically as having canine visceral leishmaniasis from Aracatuba County, Sao Paulo State, Brazil. Vet Parasitol 149: 280–284.
65. Rodriguez-Cortes A, Ojeda A, Francino O, Lopez-Fuertes L, Timon M, et al. (2010) Leishmania infection: laboratory diagnosing in the absence of a "gold standard". Am J Trop Med Hyg 82: 251–256.
66. Hartnack S, Budke CM, Craig PS, Jiamin Q, Boufana B, et al. (2013) Latent-class methods to evaluate diagnostics tests for Echinococcus infections in dogs. PLoS Negl Trop Dis 7: e2068.
67. Boelaert M, Rijal S, Regmi S, Singh R, Karki B, et al. (2004) A comparative study of the effectiveness of diagnostic tests for visceral leishmaniasis. Am J Trop Med Hyg 70: 72–77.
68. Pan-ngum W, Blacksell SD, Lubell Y, Pukrittayakamee S, Bailey MS, et al. (2013) Estimating the true accuracy of diagnostic tests for dengue infection using bayesian latent class models. PLoS One 8: e50765.
69. Wu X, Berkow K, Frank DN, Li E, Gulati AS, et al. (2013) Comparative analysis of microbiome measurement platforms using latent variable structural equation modeling. BMC Bioinformatics 14: 79.
70. Prina E, Roux E, Mattei D, Milon G (2007) Leishmania DNA is rapidly degraded following parasite death: an analysis by microscopy and real-time PCR. Microbes Infect 9: 1307–1315.
71. Sanchez MA, Diaz NL, Zerpa O, Negron E, Convit J, et al. (2004) Organ-specific immunity in canine visceral leishmaniasis: analysis of symptomatic and asymptomatic dogs naturally infected with Leishmania chagasi. Am J Trop Med Hyg 70: 618–624.
72. Watson AT, Penninck D, Knoll JS, Keating JH, Sutherland-Smith J (2011) Safety and correlation of test results of combined ultrasound-guided fine-needle aspiration and needle core biopsy of the canine spleen. Vet Radiol Ultrasound 52: 317–322.
73. Barrouin-Melo SM, Larangeira DF, de Andrade Filho FA, Trigo J, Juliao FS, et al. (2006) Can spleen aspirations be safely used for the parasitological diagnosis of canine visceral leishmaniosis? A study on assymptomatic and polysymptomatic animals. Vet J 171: 331–339.

14

A Focused Ethnographic Study of Alberta Cattle Veterinarians' Decision Making about Diagnostic Laboratory Submissions and Perceptions of Surveillance Programs

Kate Sawford[1,2,3]*, Ardene Robinson Vollman[4], Craig Stephen[2]

1 Farm Animal & Veterinary Public Health, Faculty of Veterinary Science, University of Sydney, Camden, New South Wales, Australia, **2** Department of Ecosystem and Public Health, Faculty of Veterinary Medicine, University of Calgary, Calgary, Alberta, Canada, **3** Department of Medical Sciences, Faculty of Medicine, University of Calgary, Calgary, Alberta, Canada, **4** Department of Community Health Sciences, Faculty of Medicine, University of Calgary, Calgary, Alberta, Canada

Abstract

The animal and public health communities need to address the challenge posed by zoonotic emerging infectious diseases. To minimize the impacts of future events, animal disease surveillance will need to enable prompt event detection and response. Diagnostic laboratory-based surveillance systems targeting domestic animals depend in large part on private veterinarians to submit samples from cases to a laboratory. In contexts where pre-diagnostic laboratory surveillance systems have been implemented, this group of veterinarians is often asked to input data. This scenario holds true in Alberta where private cattle veterinarians have been asked to participate in the Alberta Veterinary Surveillance Network-Veterinary Practice Surveillance, a platform to which pre-diagnostic disease and non-disease case data are submitted. Consequently, understanding the factors that influence these veterinarians to submit cases to a laboratory and the complex of factors that affect their participation in surveillance programs is foundational to interpreting disease patterns reported by laboratories and engaging veterinarians in surveillance. A focused ethnographic study was conducted with ten cattle veterinarians in Alberta. Individual in-depth interviews with participants were recorded and transcribed to enable thematic analysis. Laboratory submissions were biased toward outbreaks of unknown cause, cases with unusual mortality rates, and issues with potential herd-level implications. Decreasing cattle value and government support for laboratory testing have contributed to fewer submissions over time. Participants were willing participants in surveillance, though government support and collaboration were necessary. Changes in the beef industry and veterinary profession, as well as cattle producers themselves, present both challenges and opportunities in surveillance.

Editor: Pascale Chavatte-Palmer, INRA, France

Funding: This work was funded by a Strategic Project Grant from the Natural Sciences and Engineering Research Council of Canada. The funders had no role in study design, data collection and analysis, decision to publish, or preparation of the manuscript.

Competing Interests: The authors have declared that no competing interests exist.

* E-mail: kate.sawford@sydney.edu.au

Introduction

In recent years, the global public health community has seen an increase in the number of emerging infectious disease (EID) events [1], with the majority of infectious agents originating in animals [2–4]. Countries and communities have failed to predict specific EID events and in many cases have been ill equipped to respond once a disease has emerged, making it difficult to contain both the disease and the social and environmental impacts of the disease [5]. In response to the challenge posed by EIDs, surveillance of animal populations is changing rapidly [5]. It is strongly believed that preventing or controlling disease in animals is optimal for limiting the impact of zoonotic EIDs [6,7].

Traditional methods of infectious disease surveillance in animal health have revolved around laboratories to which samples are submitted for diagnostics, most often from clinical cases, in hopes that an etiologic diagnosis can be made [8]. Surveillance of submissions to diagnostic laboratories will continue to be an important component of any infectious disease surveillance system because for many infectious diseases laboratory tests are the only way to make an etiologic diagnosis. In addition, etiological diagnoses can inform control procedures and response policies. However, the contribution of diagnostic laboratory-based surveillance to early detection of EIDs is compromised by the time lag between the onset of clinical signs and when an etiologic diagnosis is made and the availability of diagnostic laboratory tests to identify the infectious disease agent [9]. In addition, submission biases restrict the type and number of potentially infectious cases that are submitted to a diagnostic laboratory [10,11]. Veterinarians play a critical role in determining which cases will be submitted for diagnostic laboratory testing. Their decisions, in combination with direction from animal owners, influence the types and amounts of samples that are assessed at the level of the diagnostic laboratory, introducing potential sampling biases that will affect disease patterns described by laboratory-based surveillance [12]. In order to understand this selection bias in diagnostic laboratory-based surveillance, submission patterns of veterinarians and the factors that influence their decision to submit samples must be better understood [11–13].

In Alberta, in response to the need for early detection of EID events in the animal population, the Ministry of Agriculture and Rural Development (ARD) has developed the Alberta Veterinary Surveillance Network (AVSN), a multifaceted surveillance program that enables producers, veterinarians in clinical practice, and animal health authorities to respond to disease issues in the domestic animal population [14]. One component of the program is the Alberta Veterinary Surveillance Network-Veterinary Practice Surveillance (AVSN-VPS), a secure internet-based platform that allows cattle veterinarians to submit pre-diagnostic disease and non-disease case data to a centralized system. The AVSN-VPS is considered integral to the AVSN as it informs the activities of other program components, including disease investigations by ARD pathologists, epidemiologists, and veterinarians.

The success of the AVSN-VPS is dependent upon ongoing participation by private cattle veterinarians in Alberta. It began in 2005 with approximately twenty five veterinarians, and at the time this research was undertaken the AVSN-VPS covered greater than fifty percent of Alberta dairy cattle, thirty-five percent of cattle on cow-calf operations, and twenty-five percent of feedlot cattle (J. Berezowski, personal communication). Veterinarians receive monetary compensation for submissions that are received by the AVSN in a timely fashion and participation is voluntary (J. Berezowski, personal communication). In order for methods that rely on data inputs from private veterinarians to improve, continued involvement by these individuals is essential. The factors that inspired these practitioners to become involved in the AVSN-VPS are unclear, as are the reasons for ongoing involvement.

Qualitative research provides insight into human decisions and behaviour [15]. Qualitative approaches, one of which is focused ethnography, are not intended to permit researchers to make any statistical inferences from their findings that are generalized to the wider population. Instead, they allow researchers to gain a deeper understanding of the role that beliefs, circumstances, motivations, and context play in a variety of human behaviours, including decision making [15]. In other words, the strength of qualitative research is its ability to help answer *why* particular behaviours occur or to describe processes as opposed to outcomes [15] and thus is well suited to providing insight into the human dimensions of surveillance. Utilization of qualitative research methods is becoming increasingly common in the animal health field [16–18]. They have also been employed in the human health field to explore the use of health data in public health practice, as well as factors that act to facilitate or hinder use of these data [19–21]. However, in the animal and human health fields, qualitative studies are rare in comparison to the frequency of quantitative studies. The value of employing qualitative methods in understanding the human dimensions of diagnostic laboratory case submissions and participation of government veterinarians in pre-diagnostic disease surveillance initiatives has been demonstrated in Sri Lanka, a lower resource setting where the risk of disease emergence is deemed high [22]. However, Canada's experience with highly pathogenic avian influenza, pandemic influenza virus (H1N1) 2009, bovine spongiform encephalopathy (BSE), and severe acute respiratory syndrome (SARS) highlights that EIDs are a global phenomenon [5] and understanding the ability of surveillance systems to detect and respond to EID risks in animals is necessary across a range of resource contexts.

In this paper we report the results from a focused ethnographic study that aimed to advance understanding of the factors that influence cattle veterinarians engaged in mixed-animal and exclusively cattle private veterinary practice in Alberta to submit cases to a diagnostic laboratory, and to describe the complex of factors that affect the willingness of cattle veterinarians engaged in mixed-animal and exclusively cattle private veterinary practice in Alberta who are also part of the AVSN-VPS to participate in surveillance programs.

Methods

Study Method

The term "focused ethnography" describes a qualitative research approach employed when what is sought is an explication of behaviour or beliefs pertaining to a specific area so that their meaning among a defined group of individuals might be understood [23]. In focused ethnography, research is not directed towards a culture but rather a particular subculture or group of participants that share some feature or features [23]. This method is used when research questions are best responded to through descriptive analysis and interpretation [23].

Study Participants

Eligible participants were linked by their experience as cattle veterinarians in private veterinary practice in Alberta and participants in the AVSN-VPS at the time the interviews were conducted (October to December 2009). The administrator of the AVSN-VPS within the ARD initially approached participants, giving them a brief description of the research project and format and asking if they would allow their contact information to be shared with the researcher (KES).

There were only eleven prompt responses to the request for sharing of contact information and therefore the decision was made for KES to contact eligible participants as responses were received that indicated a willingness to participate. Eligible participants were characterized by sex, number of years in practice, and practice location and type. In qualitative research data saturation is defined as the completion point of the data set and results when there is data replication or redundancy, when there are no new information or themes emerging from subsequent interviews, and when the categories, themes and relationships among them are thoroughly described [24]. In studies that ask questions similar to the ones posed in this study, six in-depth interviews usually allows for data saturation, while when twelve in-depth interviews are performed data saturation is almost always attained [25]. Therefore, from the final group of fourteen eligible participants that initially responded, ten were purposively selected to take part in in-depth interviews with the aim to assemble a group of participants with maximum demographic variation in the characteristics listed previously, with an additional two selected should further in-depth interviews be required to achieve data saturation. Descriptive statistics were used to summarize the characteristics of the study participants. In order to maintain participant confidentiality, practice locations were not detailed.

In-depth Interview Structure

The ten selected participants were contacted individually to schedule times for individual interviews. In-depth interviews were conducted at participants' locations of choice: most often this was in their veterinary practice. While ideally all interviews would have been conducted face-to-face, three interviews were conducted over the telephone because of the long distance between KES and the three participants.

The Conjoint Faculties Research Ethics Board at the University of Calgary approved the study proposal (file number 4530). Prior to the interview, each participant reviewed and signed an informed consent form. Participants were asked at the beginning of the interview to confirm orally that they had signed the consent form. Each in-depth interview, conducted by KES, was no longer than 2 hours in length. A semi-structured format consisting of a series of three leading open-ended questions was used (Table 1). An initial set of follow-up probes was drafted and employed where appropriate: the purpose of the probes was to delve into participants' individual responses and therefore probe inclusion and exclusion, specific wording, and order in which they were asked varied between interviews. The leading open-ended questions remained the same for each interview however the follow-up probes evolved as subsequent interviews were conducted (Table 1).

All in-depth interviews were recorded using two digital audio recorders. At the end of each interview the recordings were downloaded onto a password-protected laptop computer. Both audio files were reviewed to ensure the interview had been recorded in its entirety. One file was then sent to a professional transcriptionist who transcribed the interview verbatim. Personal identifiers were removed from the transcribed files to ensure participants' responses remained anonymous. One of the telephone interviews, the fifth interview in the series, failed to record. The error was noted immediately following the conclusion of the interview. KES immediately updated the field notes to document all data that could be recalled from the interview to enable revision

of the probes used in subsequent interviews. As a result of this occurrence only nine interview transcripts were available for analysis.

After transcription of the first two interview audio files, the data were coded by interview question using QSR International's NVivo 9 (N9), a qualitative analysis software suite that enables researchers to organize and retrieve qualitative data, including textual material. The probes were then reviewed and revised based on analysis of the first two interviews. After the third and fourth interviews this process was repeated. The probes were reviewed and revised a third time after the fifth interview. The remaining five interviews were conducted during a three-week time period during December 2009, which did not allow for transcription of the audio files between interviews. However, field notes were reviewed after each interview and therefore informed the probes in subsequent interviews. Collection of interview data concluded after the tenth interview.

Data accumulated in addition to the in-depth interview transcripts included: memos made by KES to document decisions made in the data collection and analysis process, day-to-day activities, and any comments concerning the methodological approach; a reflective journal kept by KES further describing the research process and the researcher's experience with participants; and field notes used to record any observational data. Memos and the reflective journal were captured directly in Microsoft Word while field notes were made directly onto the interview guide

Table 1. Leading open-ended questions and follow-up probes used during in-depth interviews.

Topics
Leading open-ended questions and follow-up probes
Decision making around laboratory submissions
Please describe the various factors that affect your decision to submit samples for laboratory diagnostics.
What do you see as the benefits of laboratory confirmation?
What are the costs, in addition to monetary, of sample submission?
Are there instances where laboratory testing is more warranted – or less warranted?
When it comes to sample submission, who is the primary decision maker in the process?
What kind of value does laboratory testing provide?
Are there types of cases in which you feel laboratory testing is more urgent?
Do you have particular 'flags', 'indicators', or scenarios that prompt you to consider laboratory testing more carefully?
Participation in disease monitoring and surveillance
Please talk to me about how willing you think veterinarians are or would be to participate in a disease monitoring and surveillance program.
Why have you chosen to participate in the AVSN? Similarly, the BSE surveillance program?
What are the obstacles to participation?
What are the potential benefits to participation?
Is there conflict between the different roles veterinarians are supposed to play and the interests they are compelled to adhere to or represent?
How could veterinarians be better engaged in disease monitoring and surveillance?
Do you think veterinarians have additional information to provide that may be missed by diagnostic laboratory based disease monitoring and surveillance?
Disease monitoring and surveillance and client interactions
Do you discuss disease monitoring and surveillance with your clients?
Please talk to me about the range of attitudes you encounter, using specific examples wherever possible.
How do you address concerns clients have about the consequences of infectious disease identification?
What do you see as the potential benefits to such conversations?
What do clients see as their role in disease monitoring and surveillance or do they see themselves as having a role at all?
How concerned about the potential for disease outbreaks do they appear?
How do you think clients could be better engaged in disease monitoring and surveillance?

during each interview and later transcribed. All raw data and material arising from the research activity were scanned into electronic files and the original documents destroyed. A single copy of the original interview audio files was transferred onto a password-protected DVD and the original files were removed from the laptop computer. The electronic version of these materials is being stored by Craig Stephen, Principal Investigator and Doctoral Supervisor, for seven years as required by the University of Calgary's Faculty of Medicine Research Policy Guidelines for Integrity in Scholarly Activity.

Data Analysis

The first step in data analysis involved reading through all of the transcripts to get a sense of the data set as a whole. Thematic analysis [26] was then performed on the transcripts. During this process data were systematically organized within NVivo 9 using codes that KES inductively derived from the records. In thematic analysis, concepts are basic units of analysis whose central meaning is described in a short statement, referred to as a code. These are grouped into categories, groups of content that share common features. Similarly, categories are organized around themes. Creating themes is a way of linking underlying meanings that reoccur within categories [26]. All data presented in the results section reflect the observations, insights, and opinions expressed by participants.

Results

Study Participants

Study participants were located in a variety of practice settings in all areas of the province of Alberta. Each participant came from a different veterinary practice; two participants were female (20%). Veterinarians had from two to 38 years (median, 24 years; mean, 22) of clinical experience. Nine (90%) veterinarians were in mixed-animal practices, while one was exclusively in beef cattle practice. Further details on the study participants are not provided to protect their identities.

Terminology

When the examples provided by participants during the interviews referred to a particular component of the cattle industry it was often the beef industry as opposed to the dairy industry. In Alberta, the beef industry consists primarily of three types of operations: cow-calf, backgrounding, and feedlot finishing. Typically calves are born at cow-calf operations and later sold to feedlot finishing operations to be fed to market weight. On some occasions, calves are sold to backgrounding operations where they are fed for lower growth rates before being moved to a finishing feedlot operation. Producers may either be individuals with a number of mother cows who they breed to produce calves that are then sold to backgrounding operations or feedlot finishing operations, or individuals who buy calves and feed them to a desired weight. They may also own combined operations that include cow-calf, backgrounding, and/or feedlot finishing operations. Participants used the terms 'farmer' and 'producer' interchangeably.

Overview of the Research Aims, Themes, and Categories

One theme and five categories emerged from data analysis that are linked to the aim to advance understanding of the factors that influence cattle veterinarians engaged in mixed-animal and exclusively cattle private veterinary practice in Alberta to submit cases to a diagnostic laboratory. Two themes and eight categories emerged from data analysis that are linked to the aim to describe

the complex of factors that affect the willingness of cattle veterinarians engaged in mixed-animal and exclusively cattle private veterinary practice in Alberta who are also part of the AVSN-VPS to participate in surveillance programs. Themes and categories are summarized in Table 2 and linked to the research aims of this study.

Theme One: Veterinarians and Diagnostic Laboratory Submissions

There were five categories identified that relate to cattle veterinarians in Alberta and their diagnostic laboratory submissions: factors that encouraged diagnostic laboratory submissions; benefits realized through diagnostic laboratory testing; limitations of diagnostic laboratory testing; economic considerations related to diagnostic laboratory submissions; and characteristics of diagnostic laboratory submissions (Table 2).

Factors that encouraged diagnostic laboratory submissions. Participants reported a range of factors that encouraged them to submit cases to a diagnostic laboratory. Herd-level promoters included: outbreaks where the participant was unsure of the cause; unusual rates of mortality; and potential herd-level implications of the problem. In many instances participants wished to confirm the clinical diagnosis or know the cause of the disease. Participants targeted: particular syndromes of interest; cases with poor response to treatment or pharmaceutical produce failure; cases where results from diagnostic laboratory testing would inform clinical practice; cases where there was no diagnosis from clinical or gross post mortem examination; cases where there was a suspicion of a notifiable or reportable disease; atypical case presentations; cases where the economic consequences of disease were potentially high; cases in which there was a potential public health risk; cases involving high-value animals; bizarre cases; and insurance cases. Participants also submitted samples to a diagnostic laboratory at the request of owners/producers and in instances where it was convenient. A case condition emphasized by all participants was the importance of multiple animals affected. Participants emphasized that the decision to submit samples depended on the management context:

> Some guys backgrounding cattle aren't doing anything, so if I've got five or six calves out of 50 that are dying, that's not unexpected. If I've got a well-vaccinated herd and good management and good mineral program and good nutrition program and I've got more than two or three that are sick out of 40 or 50, then I'm concerned... Better managed herds have less disease but usually those kind of people usually we do more diagnostic stuff because they want to know whereas the poorer managed ones save money on management costs so they can afford to have more losses. (Interview 6, Lines 40–47)

Participants stressed that they were more likely to pursue diagnostic laboratory testing when the results impacted case management, including one participant who stressed that diagnostic laboratory testing in beef cattle practice that did not change therapy was 'academic':

> It depends what I'm dealing with. If there's something that I can't answer the question without ...then I need to do this. If it's something that is academic again, it may have some benefit or it may not and the cost is significant, then it goes back to the client to decide. ... Ultimately it comes down to

Table 2. Research aims linked to the themes and categories that emerged during data analysis.

Research aims
Themes
Categories
Advance understanding of the factors that influence cattle veterinarians engaged in mixed-animal and exclusively cattle private veterinary practice in Alberta to submit cases to a diagnostic laboratory
Veterinarians and diagnostic laboratory submissions
Factors that encouraged diagnostic laboratory submissions
Benefits realized through diagnostic laboratory testing
Limitations of diagnostic laboratory testing
Economic considerations related to diagnostic laboratory submissions
Characteristics of diagnostic laboratory submissions
Describe the complex of factors that affect the willingness of cattle veterinarians engaged in mixed-animal and exclusively cattle private veterinary practice in Alberta who are also part of the AVSN-VPS to participate in surveillance programs
Veterinarians and surveillance
Willingness to participate in surveillance initiatives
Veterinarians ought to participate in surveillance
Drivers for involvement in surveillance initiatives
Gains from the involvement of veterinarians in surveillance
Participants' perception of the role for government in surveillance
Participants' perceptions of the role of surveillance
The veterinary perspective
Changes to the beef industry and the veterinary profession
Cattle producers

that, my reason for testing, is it going to change my therapy when it comes to beef. If it's not going to change my therapy then it's academic. (Interview 7, Lines 128–134)

Benefits realized through diagnostic laboratory testing. The benefits of diagnostic laboratory testing referenced by participants included: enabling a definitive or etiological diagnosis; facilitating participant learning; improving confidence; and informing cases where there were legal concerns. When participants talked generally about arriving at a definitive or etiological diagnosis, they most often referenced cases from which it would have been nice to submit samples, as opposed to particular cases from which samples were sent. On the subject of facilitating learning and building confidence, one said:

As a new grad coming out… you get a lot of that counter talk where it's "this is what's going on, what do I do about it" and you have no confidence because cows are hard to diagnose things in anyways… So you get talking to somebody and it could be four different things and… it would be nice to be able to confirm something… So even if you don't see that animal the second time … you've got it in your memory bank that you confirmed something on the last one, right? I think that in terms of developing a rural mixed animal practitioner that is actually going to stay in rural mixed animal practice, it's extraordinarily important to be able to have the confidence in your ability to figure out what's going on and I think that's a huge part of retaining vets in these types of practices. (Interview 8, Lines 71–86)

Limitations of diagnostic laboratory testing. Participants also talked about the limitations of diagnostic laboratory testing. They mentioned that in many cases unanswered questions remain even after diagnostic laboratory testing was completed and the time lag between when samples were sent to a diagnostic laboratory and when results were available was a limitation. Carcass and tissue sample degradation in the field presented a challenge such that by the time samples were collected they had degraded to a point where they were unsuitable for many diagnostic laboratory tests.

Economic considerations related to diagnostic laboratory submissions. All participants talked about economic considerations that impacted their decision to submit samples to a diagnostic laboratory, often at multiple points during the interview: diagnostic laboratory testing needed to be worthwhile from the perspective of producers; diagnostic laboratory testing was cost prohibitive for producers; and the economic reality of producers meant that in the majority of instances samples were not submitted to a diagnostic laboratory. The economics of the cattle industry made diagnostic laboratory testing cost prohibitive and translated into small numbers of diagnostic laboratory submissions.

People don't even want an exam let alone take lab samples to send away and it's harder and harder to get on those farms because then they're paying you for an exam and mileage…A lot of what you see is on farm looking at the rest of the herd… If you don't get to see what's going on on-farm, you're kind of treating individual animals when it [the disease] may have a herd basis… so I think we're probably missing a fair bit. (Interview 4, Lines 25–29)

When asked about costs in addition to the monetary costs of sending samples to diagnostic laboratories, one participant replied:

> There is… a social cost or a reputation cost associated with sending them. People take pride in their animals and take pride in their herds and they like to have a healthy strong vibrant herd. They don't want to have something in there that's going to be a concern to them, […] they don't want to have a herd that's going to decimate the industry and they don't want to have a herd that they're not proud of that they're always looking for illness or issues - I think those are the non-monetary costs. (Interview 9, Lines 9–10)

Characteristics of diagnostic laboratory submissions. Participants indicated that they were submitting fewer cases to diagnostic laboratories over time. They attributed this decline to a variety of factors: as you moved along in your career as a veterinarian there were fewer things you had not seen; the value of cattle has decreased, making it more difficult to submit samples; and decreases to government support for diagnostic laboratories and a decline in access to diagnostic laboratories meant that submission patterns had become increasingly selective. Some participants provided estimates of the frequency of submissions ranging from one case out of 10 to one case out of 100.

> Very, very rarely. I have not sent anything this year and we're most of the way through the fall run. I've talked to lots of guys about lots of sick calves this fall and have not sent one thing in, have not done one post-mortem. (Interview 8, Lines 35–40)

Participants referred to reductions in services provided by the provincial veterinary diagnostic laboratory system and a lack of large animal clinicians at private veterinary diagnostic laboratories that led to fewer submissions to diagnostic laboratories. Many participants reported that it was the producer who was the final decision maker when it came to submitting samples to a diagnostic laboratory. In contrast two participants stated that they (veterinarians) acted as the final decision maker. A number of participants discussed the ability of veterinarians to influence the decisions made by producers.

Theme Two: Veterinarians and Surveillance

Veterinarians and surveillance occurred as a theme in the data, around which were six categories: willingness to participate in surveillance initiatives; veterinarians ought to participate in surveillance; drivers for involvement in surveillance initiatives; gains from the involvement of veterinarians in surveillance; participants' perceptions of the role for government in surveillance; and participants' perceptions of the role of surveillance (Table 2).

Willingness to participate in surveillance initiatives. All participants expressed the belief that veterinarians were willing to participate in surveillance. However, attached to this willingness were a number of caveats: there needed to be feedback of information that had value in participants' clinical practice; data submission could not be too time consuming; participants needed to be compensated for the time they dedicated to collecting data; the data collection process needed to be convenient; and in order to motivate ongoing involvement administrators of surveillance programs should demonstrate the relevance of the data collected.

Participants cited time and effort as the costs of surveillance they incurred.

Veterinarians ought to participate in surveillance. Participants expressed frequently the opinion that veterinarians should take a more active role in surveillance. When asked if veterinarians should be more involved in disease monitoring and surveillance, one participant replied:

> You bet… I think again it comes back to a bit of a responsibility to you as a veterinarian. I think the idea of shoot, shovel, shut up type thing is just the wrong approach to take. You can only solve the issues if you know what the issues are and … find out what it is. (Interview 7, Lines 312–316)

Drivers for involvement in surveillance initiatives. When asked about why they opted to participate in surveillance initiatives, including the AVSN-VPS and the BSE surveillance program in Alberta, participants cited a number of drivers behind involvement including: monetary compensation; information generated and fed back through the program; interest in surveillance; perceived value of the program; and access to additional diagnostic laboratory services. The first two drivers came up frequently across interviews. A couple of participants emphasized that while monetary compensation was important to offset the time it takes to participate, it does not serve as a motivator in and of itself. Drivers behind participation varied among veterinarians.

> Money talks. […] The BSE program is a good example of that. If you pay people, the right people, the job will get done. I think you'll get a core group of preventers doing it out of the goodness of their heart because they're interested in it and they think it's a good program but if you want to get more people on board… reward them economically. (Interview 3, Lines 163–167)

When participants talked about information they received through surveillance initiatives, they discussed the importance of receiving that information but a few said they did not often access the outputs from the AVSN-VPS.

Gains from the involvement of veterinarians in surveillance. All participants talked about gains through the involvement of veterinarians in surveillance. Participants highlighted that: the AVSN-VPS could be used to inform diagnostic laboratory-based surveillance; the AVSN-VPS received a greater number of submissions compared to diagnostic laboratories; and the AVSN-VPS was timelier in comparison to laboratory-based surveillance. A couple of participants talked about past cases where the AVSN-VPS informed diagnostic laboratory-based surveillance, but more expressed the view that they would be more engaged, and the program could be improved, if there was more diagnostic laboratory support provided through the program.

> We could decide what types of animals we're interested in monitoring… We could probably decide what clinical signs we're interested in pursuing, whether they would be of value in helping predict zoonotic problems or whether it would just help to keep the health of the herd intact… I don't think it would be that difficult to sit down and come up with a list and maybe even a decision tree for diagnostics that the government would subsidize. (Interview 1, Lines 65–66)

Participants felt frontline pre-diagnostic disease surveillance was vital to understanding disease trends, was essential as a marketing tool, and assisted in identification of outbreaks. The AVSN-VPS made participants aware of the regional differences in infectious disease occurrence.

I think the other thing that we fail to realize […] is how different geographically, even in Alberta, certain diseases are. […] I had no idea that *Clostridium hemolyticum* was more of an issue down there. We never had it in our area. In fact, when they told me how many cases they got, I thought they were just spoofing me […] Now you take across Canada and it's huge, […] just the different geographic areas and what diseases they see. (Interview 2, Lines 64–68)

Participants described how surveillance influences the frequency of veterinary presence on farms, referencing the BSE surveillance program in particular.

With BSE surveillance, […] financially we benefit, but… where it's really benefited is where we were able to go out to [farms]. In the past, a farmer loses one, […] a cow dies… He thinks it incidental, drags it in the bush and that's the end of it. When BSE hit they wanted samples from these specific ones and the ones that died were included in that. We got out there to find out what's going on and I really felt that we learned a lot because we could go out… In numerous cases we found issues…. We never would have had that opportunity before. It got us on the farm in a non-confrontational way. It didn't cost the guy so he was happy to have us out. […] In some cases, okay, it's an incidental death, don't worry about it. He was happy because he could rest at ease… In some cases, I hate to admit this in a way, but when BSE testing came about, some of our worst clients became our best from a financial standpoint because they were the poor managers in there, the ones that lost the cows and traded cows and bought cows and did all these things but at least we were able to figure out what was going on. (Interview 2, Lines 235–236)

Participants' perceptions of the role for government in surveillance. On the subject of the role of government in surveillance, all participants advocated for further support for diagnostic laboratory-based surveillance from the government. Participants frequently drew attention to the costs borne by producers.

I think that there's a big difference in the information that we want to receive and the economics borne by the producer. […] Right now the producer pays for the investigation, he pays for the test, then he may well pay for any adverse effects on his herd, his life or his livelihood that the results may show. (Interview 9, Lines 139–141)

Participants expressed the opinion that surveillance needed to be government driven and frustration with the lack of attention and resources the government directed towards disease surveillance in the animal population.

Government is so intent on cutting costs that they're putting their animals, their industries… The billions of dollars lost with BSE is way higher than the cost of running some extra provincial government labs. […] Our government is looking at cutting costs and providing bare necessity services and moving costs onto individuals. The individuals do not have the ability to pay for the costs of testing… Those things are going to create havoc in the industry when one of these things emerges [diseases] because we do not have a proper surveillance network in place… They talk about globalization, well globalization also means the occurrence of diseases that we would never have seen before whether it's human diseases like SARS or whether it's animal diseases like BSE but we have to improve and have to increase our lab availability. (Interview 9, Lines 95–96)

Problems with the existing BSE surveillance program in Alberta were highlighted.

I think part of the problem with the whole program is that it got to be in people's heads that it was out there for compensating the farmer… for these old lame skinny cows […] They [farmers] looked at it like the government doing them a favour. Then when all these restrictions came in, it was very hard to explain to people what the actual purpose of the program was and always has been […] If [animals qualify] then great, we want to give you some compensation but that was really hard for people to take […] I'd go from doing dozens a month [BSE sample submissions] to like one every five or six months. Obviously, I understand how they [the government] want to make it appealing to the producer to participate … but I think the main purpose of the program was never brought to the forefront like it should have been and that made our jobs a lot harder when they put these restrictions in place because these people are yelling and cursing at us and you're just trying to explain what the whole point of it is. (Interview 4, Lines 92–100)

Participants discussed their perceptions of government. The Canadian Food Inspection Agency (CFIA) was not viewed favourably, though the provincial government fared better. One participant stressed that the AVSN-VPS added to their respect for the provincial veterinarians as they saw the AVSN-VPS as a collaborative effort between veterinary practices and the province. One participant articulated dissatisfaction with the CFIA and its handling of reportable disease cases,

Reportable diseases that occur in the area the CFIA picks up, do you think we're notified first on the list that one of our clients might have a certain problem? No. We're usually one of the last people to find out and usually it's from the producer. I think that's pretty terrible […] Yeah there was one in our area from one of our clients and I knew nothing about it until he came in having all these questions… He was given very little information by them and I ended up having to phone the CFIA and chase someone down to talk to and get the story… Something reportable is right here in our own backyard and we weren't even notified by them […] It was on a random screening sample at one of their plants and they picked it up […]

Not only is that very poor relations but it sends a bad message to us because veterinarians are proactive type "A" people that want to be involved and if I'm going to go out [...] and invest my time, my effort and I care about this and ... something comes back or you find something out about a herd in our area and then you don't even bother to contact me and let me know, I think it sends a really bad message out: "We don't want to work together. We don't want to involve you or help you" - so that makes it difficult too when they want us to do stuff for them or send a certain message. (Interview 4, Lines 137)

Participants stressed the importance of communication, emphasizing that problems could persist if information was not made available to veterinarians and producers for use in prevention and treatment.

Participants' perceptions of the role of surveillance. Participants talked about surveillance and the greater good or its value beyond infectious disease event detection. Several participants discussed surveillance outputs to inform clinical practice and increase awareness of regional differences in infectious disease burden. In contrast, one participant expressed the opinion that disease had not changed much over the past twenty years and pre-diagnostic disease surveillance programs did not help significantly in addressing infectious diseases, though such programs were great for the international reputation of the cattle industry in Alberta.

Participants cited frequently that surveillance benefitted the cattle industry, though a few expressed frustrations that producers were not deriving any benefit from increased surveillance.

I have been frustrated. With a variety of these programs we've done a lot of hoops and it's just not changing this industry. It's in a sad state and yet they've [producers] connected the dots that have been asked of us ... You just keep on plodding hoping that at some point it will be recognized. (Interview 7, Lines 365–367)

Participants also cited veterinarians, the industry, and the public as beneficiaries of surveillance. During a number of interviews surveillance for EIDs was mentioned in particular, including one participant who expressed scepticism about the ability of the AVSN-VPS to provide information that might be missed by diagnostic laboratory-based surveillance.

Theme Three: The Veterinary Perspective

There were two categories identified that related to the veterinary perspective: changes to the beef industry and the veterinary profession; and cattle producers (Table 2).

Changes to the beef industry and the veterinary profession. All participants discussed the dynamic nature of the beef industry, the veterinary profession, and the relationship between the two. Economics were often drawn into the discussion. Emphasis was placed on the need for financial compensation to motivate changes to the beef industry.

Unfortunately I think a lot of producers, they won't change unless they have to and there's two ways you can do that, you can force them to by saying that you have to put these tags in or you'll get fined or we can say you have to do it or you can't sell your product. I think probably the better way is you somehow make these subtle changes in the system...

We're starting to do that anyway but the problem is if you're going to make those changes, you have to make it economical for the producer... You can't continue to download [...] a lot of work ...and regulations on this producer and then expect him to do it and not be compensated. He'll just get out. (Interview 3, Lines 260–262)

Participants highlighted that the role played by veterinarians had historically been different and was bound to continue to change.

I support my family by doing a lot of technical stuff... pulling calves, pushing prolapses, preg[nancy] testing cows. [...]The connection between animal and human disease and looking at the big picture, that's incredibly important and that's going to be a sustainable aspect of our profession. I think it's unrealistic to think that [...] the next generation veterinarians are going to do what I do. I showed you rings in the back of the clinic. You know that guy obviously made a living doing a thousand Caesarians in the spring. [...] He made a significant portion of income by vaccinating heifers for brucellosis. I don't do that anymore and so why would I expect the next generation of veterinarians to do what I do for a living... What do we do as a profession to maintain our relevancy? (Interview 3, Lines 105–111)

One participant described how much the veterinary profession had changed during their career.

I mean I've had herds that when I first started here in '94 that were losing ten or fifteen percent of their calf crop just with scours and through better management and vaccine programs, we've reduced that to less than two percent. So absolutely we make them money. [...] We've gone past that though [...] Historically that was true because we could make some big changes [...] When I started 30 years ago, it was an astronomical problem with bulls and Caesarians. We were doing two to three hundred Caesarians every fall in a 5,000 mother cow practice. Now in a 5,000 mother cow practice, we might do four or five Caesarians because we've improved the mother cows. We've improved the bulls. We've improved the feeding programs. [...] It's much smaller [the gains that can be made] so for them to quit using veterinarians now doesn't make as big an impact as it did before. [...] With us going away, they can still buy all their vaccines... We don't have any control of that like they do in Europe and other countries where they have to be bought through a veterinarian. (Interview 6, Lines 172–197)

The same participant predicted that cattle veterinarians in small mixed practices would no longer exist once current veterinarians retired.

Cattle producers. During all of the interviews the circumstances of producers was touched upon, and perceived to be as dynamic as that of veterinarians.

I think they're in a similar position that we are, they have to change, they can't continue to raise cattle the way their grandfather did, just like we can't continue to practice veterinary medicine like three generations ago. Part of that education process is I can count on one hand young cow producers that want to produce cattle, the majority of guys are old or older. If you can target these young guys that are ambitious and want to do it, you have to convince them that they have to do it differently and that's part of the education process is "how can I help you do something different to be sustainable and make a living raising cattle instead of having to have two off-farm jobs to support the farm", and that's a challenge. (Interview 3, Lines 237–239)

Participants expressed the view that producers feared a reportable or notifiable disease, though in contrast one participant expressed the view that producers would love it if the government were to come in and compensate them for the loss of their herd due to a notifiable disease as it would be a way for the producer to exit the cattle industry.

In the opinion of participants the fear of a reportable or notifiable disease was in part attributable to producers fearing the stigma of being the person in the community with the affected herd.

They understand that the chances of them having a positive is extremely low. What they're scared of is being in the spotlight and all of a sudden the neighbours, you know it's a bad stigma. [...] You don't want to be the guy that's got a ... positive anything - so I guess it's education on our part that it's sort of like, you know they tell people with cancer, the one thing worse than finding it is not finding it right? So you tell them that that if you don't find it now, that you're going to find it eventually. (Interview 3, Lines 220–223)

Some participants discussed the importance of independence to producers along with the concern that once current producers got out of cattle farming there would be no one willing to farm cattle in Alberta.

The only reason you farm is a lifestyle. I shouldn't say the only reason. It's one of the biggest reasons that people farm. It's a great place to raise a family and you're outside, you're your own boss, nobody else telling you, you have to do this. I don't have to get up today if I don't want to or I can work all day if I want to, ... and that has appealed to most of the people that come from a rural environment and they want to come back to that. A big chunk of my clientele [...] grew up on a family farm... They work in the oil patch to support their farm, and on their holidays, they come home and make hay. Their kids resent the farm and they will not take over the farm. [...] So the father who grew up feeling the farm was part of him and liked that, he comes back, can't afford to farm but can live on a farm, have a bit of a hobby farm with oil patch industry and income. It dies with him. When he's out of the game, there's nobody taking it over and they're a big chunk of who's supplying the cattle right now. (Interview 7, Lines 406–412)

Finally, a number of participants raised confidentiality and privacy as of concern to producers. In relation to surveillance initiatives and producers, one participant said:

There's a lot of less open minded people out that are very anti-government and there's also just people that aren't necessarily anti-government but that value privacy... I think if there's a way that we could surveil more anonymously, that would be [ideal] and you know people are always more willing to accept that than if they have to put their name on something. For example, this [interview] right, if I'm going to talk ... give you all these examples, I don't want people to know I'm from {town name} or people will be like who in {town name} has this disease you know so I understand that ... And some people are just very private and think whatever goes on, on my farm, is my business. (Interview 4, Lines 143–147)

Another participant expressed a slightly different view:

I think most producers want these kind of [surveillance] programs. They want to know what the diseases are in their cattle and they want to participate in making our, or making their, product healthier and better and superior to other countries. [...] I don't think there's anybody that really wants to hide anything. I think there's openness in most of these people, they're not afraid to share their information with anybody. At least not my clients... I mean they don't want us sharing it with all their neighbours, but with the government, that's alright. (Interview 6, Lines 157–162)

Following analysis of the nine interview transcripts the codes, concepts, categories, relationships, and themes were reviewed. The authors observed that there was data redundancy and the categories, themes and relationships between them were thoroughly described. It was also noted that though the last few interviews enriched the data set, they led to no new information or themes. Therefore it was determined that data saturation had been achieved and there were no further interviews conducted.

Discussion

Veterinarians and Diagnostic Laboratory Submissions

Study participants detailed a variety of factors that encouraged diagnostic laboratory submissions, with multiple animals affected and the impact of results on case management common to a number of scenarios. Participants stressed that the decision to submit samples depended on the management context and the impact of results on case management. Participants detailed some of the benefits and limitations of diagnostic laboratory testing that also factored into their decision to submit samples to a laboratory. However they also reported low submission rates and submission of fewer cases to laboratories over time. Economic realities, including the high cost of diagnostics relative to the decline in value of individual beef cattle, as well as a decline in government support for laboratory diagnostics, had contributed to a decreasing frequency of laboratory submissions over time.

The results show that diagnostic laboratory submissions from participants were biased toward: outbreaks; outbreaks with unusual mortality rates; atypical case presentations; bizarre cases; and cases with poor response to treatment or produce failure. Assuming that participants' submission patterns reflected those of cattle veterinarians in Alberta and remain relatively unchanged over time, the patterns detected by diagnostic laboratory testing are unlikely to reflect disease burden in the Alberta cattle population. This finding is supported by quantitative studies looking at diagnostic laboratory test submissions [11,12]. Consequently the patterns of diagnoses based on diagnostic laboratory findings should not be assumed to reflect disease trends in the

Alberta cattle population and it may not be appropriate to rely solely on disease prevalence outputs reported by diagnostic laboratory-based surveillance to guide future research priorities.

We recently undertook a similar research project with government field veterinarians in Sri Lanka [22]. It is interesting to note that while the circumstances of veterinarians in Sri Lanka were different to those in Alberta, there were similarities in the challenges to diagnostic laboratory testing across contexts, namely the availability of sufficiently timely results to inform treatment and access to desired diagnostic laboratory infrastructure. The outcome in both contexts was that veterinarians have become accustomed to relying on other means to make a diagnosis and guide treatment. Changes to the veterinary diagnostic laboratory infrastructure that would significantly impact this challenge to diagnostic laboratory-based surveillance would require considerable investment and political will, and the time to realization of the benefits of such efforts could be lengthy in both the Alberta and Sri Lanka context, particularly if no emerging disease issues were immediately detected.

One way of examining the diagnostic laboratory submission behaviour of participants is through the lens of expectancy theory from the field of sociology. Expectancy theory is concerned with the process individuals go through in arriving at the decision to perform one behaviour over another or others [27,28]. At its foundation is the idea that individuals decide to act in certain ways because they are motivated to select particular behaviours out of a range of possible behaviours due to the results they expect to stem from them. There are three components of expectancy theory: expectancy, instrumentality, and valence [27,28]. These three components play an interactive role in motivation. A large part of expectancy theory is what individuals perceive: individuals' actions will not be motivated by what the results will be, but by what they *believe* the results will be. One of the primary goals of cattle veterinarians in private veterinary practice in Alberta is to achieve positive case outcomes for their clients. Application of expectancy theory in this context reveals that if a veterinarian perceives a strong correlation between performing diagnostic laboratory testing and case outcome then instrumentality (an individual's belief that the rewards acquired as the result of an action are closely related to level of performance) will be high and the veterinarian will be motivated to pursue laboratory diagnostics. This theory helps to explain why diagnostic laboratory testing that does not inform treatment was viewed as 'academic'. However, participants also cited suspicion of a reportable or notifiable disease or concern for a public health risk as case characteristics that encourage sample submission. In these instances the goal may be to confirm the absence of a reportable or notifiable disease or a public health risk. Though based on past experience the likelihood of a reportable or notifiable disease or public health risk is low, the valence (the degree to which an individual values a particular award) attached to identifying either event is high.

Participants reported that the time lag between when samples were submitted to a laboratory and when results were available had lengthened as the diagnostic laboratory infrastructure in Alberta has changed. Additionally, the decline in cattle value and government support for diagnostic laboratory testing meant that the financial burden of diagnostic laboratory testing borne by producers might have been too great a cost compared to the perceived benefits diagnostic laboratory testing provided. Participants reported getting onto farms less and less, presenting fewer opportunities to even consider submission of diagnostic laboratory samples as an option. These factors have impacted the number of opportunities for veterinarians to *perceive* the benefits of diagnostic laboratory submissions, and likely would have had the greatest

impact on recently graduated veterinarians for whom diagnostic laboratory testing also facilitated learning and built confidence.

There are strengths and limitations to relying on diagnostic laboratory submissions from cattle veterinarians in Alberta for EID event detection. EID events characterized by atypical case presentations or bizarre cases are likely to make it to the level of the diagnostic laboratory, though participants reported that it would be unlikely for the index case to be submitted. Submission to diagnostic laboratories would also necessitate veterinarians to recognize that a number of cases over time were sufficiently similar to have an underlying etiology. The ordered diagnostic laboratory test would have to be capable of detecting the agent or, in the event that histopathology or cytopathology were the test ordered, the pathologist would need to recognize that the case represented something out of the ordinary. Alternatively, the diagnostician reviewing the case history would need to come to the conclusion that additional diagnostic tests were warranted, and consult with the veterinarian about additional testing and cost coverage. Participants also indicated that samples were submitted when there were unusual outbreaks or in situations where there were large numbers of animals affected. Surveillance of diagnostic laboratory submissions may therefore be sufficient for detection of EID events characterized by these types of presentations, though it is difficult to determine if detection would be sufficiently prompt to mitigate their impact on animal and public health. In contrast, given the overall small number of sample submissions reported by participants, diagnostic laboratory-based surveillance is unlikely to detect slower-moving EID events that present more sporadically or changes in trends of known endemic problems as incomplete sampling is unlikely to generate a signal in the diagnostic laboratory data stream [29].

The AVSN is part of the Canadian Animal Health Surveillance Network (CAHSN), a network of provincial, federal, university, and private animal health diagnostic laboratories [30]. This newly established network aims to: increase diagnostic laboratory capacity to detect infectious animal diseases; permit implementation of common protocols, including use of common reagents; coordinate surveillance activities; enable the sharing of technical and scientific expertise; and enable collation and analysis of laboratory data from participating diagnostic laboratories [30]. The objective of the CAHSN is "early detection of animal disease threats to the food supply, food safety or public health originating through bio-terrorism or 'natural' causes, especially foreign and emerging animal diseases" [30]. While this integration effort helps to ensure there is sufficient diagnostic laboratory capacity in place to respond to EID events, and detect certain types of EID events, the results reported here suggest that such efforts alone will be insufficient to permit early detection of animal disease threats: diagnostic laboratory submission results are unlikely to signal the occurrence of an EID event in the Alberta cattle population early in the epidemic process [29].

Veterinarians and Surveillance

Participants expressed a willingness to participate in surveillance initiatives, though their involvement required support via monetary compensation, feedback of relevant data and information, demonstrated program value, and subsidized diagnostic laboratory support. Further, participants expressed the belief that veterinarians should take a more active role in surveillance. They cited information to guide laboratory-based surveillance, greater numbers of submissions, and more timely information as gains from veterinary involvement in pre-diagnostic surveillance. Participants advocated for increased government involvement in surveillance, though they stressed that efforts should be collaborative.

Animal health surveillance is undertaken by people in a wide range of contexts: the practice of surveillance is directly related to the environment in which it takes place and therefore a socio-ecological approach to analysis is warranted. There are a number of variations of the socio-ecological model that have been developed based on the work by Bronfenbrenner, 1979 [31]. They all identify levels of influence on human behaviour that overlap and taken together comprise the environment in which human behaviours take place. An assumption inherent to the socio-ecological approach generally is that assessment and approaches to intervention that operate at multiple levels are more effective in comparison to those that operate on a single level [32]. For the purpose of this paper, five levels of influence will be individually explored (individual, interpersonal, organizational, community, and societal) that are widely utilized when adopting a socio-ecological approach [31].

Individual-level influences on surveillance. The individual level in the socio-ecological model emphasizes the importance of characteristics of the individual to intervention strategies. Cattle veterinarians in Alberta are part of a private industry and therefore some form of compensation for time dedicated to surveillance initiatives is essential. However, animal health surveillance is not the only duty of these veterinarians: the results show that while monetary compensation was important, it was not sufficient to guarantee veterinary participation in surveillance. Participants emphasized that surveillance that relies on private clinical veterinarians to input data must generate information that is of value to veterinary clinical practice. One challenge to animal health surveillance programs is that they need to serve the interests and needs of a number of stakeholders including governments, consumers, industry stakeholders, and producers [33]. Surveillance that is dependent upon veterinarians in private practice to submit data has the additional responsibility to provide data submitters with information that is clinically relevant [33]. Future surveillance initiatives and modifications to existing programs must take this task into account during design, implementation, and evaluation to help ensure surveillance system sustainability.

Interpersonal-level influences on surveillance. The interpersonal level in the socio-ecological model emphasizes the importance of social norms and social influences to intervention strategies. Veterinarians have an ethical duty to promote public health defined in the veterinarian's oath [34]. Participants expressed a willingness to contribute to pre-diagnostic surveillance initiatives, the belief that veterinarians should take a more active role in surveillance, and the opinion that government needs to deliver surveillance programs. However, the results show that this approach needs to be one of collaboration and must take into account the relationship between producers and veterinarians. The success of private veterinarians is dependent upon their relationship with producers: it is imperative that surveillance initiatives reliant on the participation of private veterinarians respect this relationship and not serve to undermine it. For example, pre-diagnostic surveillance initiatives may need to include mechanisms that ensure specific farm locations are excluded from case submissions in order to protect the privacy of producers and gain support from veterinarians, as was done with the AVSN-VPS (John Berezowski, personal communication). In addition, the goals of surveillance initiatives need to be communicated to producers so that when changes are made that are deemed necessary producers understand the reasons behind them. An even better approach would be to include producers in the process of negotiating changes to existing surveillance initiatives so their comments and perspective are considered and they are not caught off guard when changes are made.

While it is common practice to calculate the economic consequences of EIDs [35] and investigate their impact more broadly [36], projecting the economic benefits realized through surveillance remains a challenge [37]. It is also impossible to pinpoint EID events that have been averted as a result of surveillance. The results show that the BSE surveillance program in Alberta that requires veterinarians to visit cattle operations to collect samples has had both direct and indirect consequences to the veterinary perspective on the cattle health situation. While it serves to satisfy many consumers and trading partners that the prevalence of BSE in Canada's cattle population is very low, and the risk of a BSE-positive cow entering the food chain is very small, it has also translated into more veterinary contact with the cattle population, in particular with segments of the population that previously had minimal contact with the veterinary profession. This increased contact could prove essential to recognition of future EID events. Creating circumstances for veterinarians to get onto cattle operations in the absence of a major problem, or in a 'non-confrontational way', has had the added benefit of improving the relationship between veterinarians and producers. This enhanced affiliation could prove invaluable during future EID events as producers might be more likely to bring animal health concerns to the attention of their veterinarian, creating more opportunities for event recognition, thereby enabling more timely EID event detection and response. It could also be critical to enabling veterinarians to influence the producer's final decision when it comes to submitting samples to a diagnostic laboratory, thereby enabling more cases to reach the level of the diagnostic laboratory and potentially improving this source of surveillance data. Previous work has also suggested that the trust of producers is critical to event reporting, surveillance, and adoption of biosecurity measures [38], all of which are critical to EID event detection and response.

Organizational-level influences on surveillance. The organizational level in the socio-ecological model recognizes that changing the policies and practices of a workplace can serve to support behavioural change. In Alberta, providing the ARD with additional resources to support the activities of cattle veterinarians, in particular further diagnostic laboratory capacity, is an incentive for surveillance system participation that was identified by participants as essential. As suggested by one participant, collaboration on a list or decision tree that would inform diagnostic laboratory testing supported by the government is one approach to future diagnostic laboratory-based surveillance by the ARD that had been unexplored at the time of the interviews. This type of approach could be particularly useful as it would enable targeted case presentations to reach the level of the diagnostic laboratory and it would heighten awareness to these case presentations among cattle veterinarians. Efforts to communicate with farmers about such programs would help to ensure cases are being brought to the attention of veterinarians.

Community-level influences on surveillance. The community level in the socio-ecological model recognizes that coordinating the efforts of members of a community, in this case cattle veterinarians in Alberta, is necessary to bring about change. The results demonstrate how the AVSN-VPS has served to provide cattle veterinarians in Alberta with a shared perspective on the burden of clinical disease in Alberta's cattle population, an essential first step in bringing together members of a community [39,40]. However, the results also indicate that the information produced from the AVSN-VPS has had limited utility in cattle veterinary practice. Administrators of the AVSN-VPS should consider consulting with veterinarians who input data to determine how to make the information provided more relevant to data providers, and if any further data types might be worth collecting. This consultation process would also serve to enhance the collaboration between the AVSN and cattle veterinarians.

Societal-level influences on surveillance. The societal level in the socio-ecological model recognizes that there are societal or cultural high-level factors that create a climate that encourages or discourages behaviours. Broadly speaking, governments and the animal and public health communities create a climate that impacts willingness to report EID events. This process is operating at the level of nations, veterinarians, animal health care workers, and producers. Surveillance programs can serve to improve the relationship between veterinarians and government regulatory bodies [39]. The AVSN-VPS has generated information concerning the perspective veterinarians have on health-related events in the cattle population. This information has been shared between private cattle veterinarians and veterinarians at the ARD and has created a knowledge base around which to dialogue. Participants highlighted opportunities to enhance this relationship, in particular the need for diagnostic laboratory support guided by the outputs of the AVSN-VPS. The needs of consumers, producers, veterinarians, and the provincial and federal government could be well served were the ARD to utilize the willingness of veterinarians to participate in surveillance and participants' recognition of the need for change within the veterinary profession. A collaborative effort between cattle veterinarians and veterinarians at the ARD to develop a government-supported diagnostic laboratory surveillance program that satisfied veterinarians' desire for further diagnostic laboratory support, the requirement of the provincial and federal government to surveil for and report potential EIDs events as part of Canada's membership in the OIE, and the public's need to be assured of a safe food supply could enhance the relationship between cattle veterinarians and the ARD. This type of endeavour could be invaluable during future EID events, particularly as control of past events has required cooperation among producers, veterinarians, and multiple government agencies [41]. The CFIA should explore means of improving their relationship with cattle veterinarians as they are integral to detection of outbreaks of OIE-listed diseases and evidence of a healthy working relationship between the two parties from the perspective of participants was lacking.

The Veterinary Perspective

Participants highlighted that at the time the interviews were conducted the beef industry and the cattle veterinary profession in Alberta were going through a period of significant change, and that the two are strongly linked. Previously, cattle veterinarians had an important role in performing technical procedures, such as caesareans, to treat animal disease conditions. They also had a role in implementing management programs that have decreased the burden of animal health conditions requiring veterinary intervention. Producers have learned alongside veterinarians and no longer require veterinarians to perform all the functions they did previously. Participants in this study identified this phenomenon and the need for the veterinary profession to change in response, though there were differences between participants in what those changes might need to be. From an EID standpoint, one avenue the cattle veterinary profession might consider exploring is increasing its emphasis on healthy animal populations, as opposed to animal populations that are simply free from disease: healthy animals are more resistant to infectious diseases [42,43] and could serve to help mitigate the risk of future EID events in animal populations. If the model of private veterinary services to food-producing animals is going to persist, changes to the services

provided by the veterinary profession are going to have to be economically relevant to producers.

Participants perceived that farming has historically attracted individuals that value independence and privacy. As a result there is inherent potential for conflict between producers and the need for improved government-driven EID surveillance. Future surveillance initiatives will need to consider this aspect of cattle production to encourage producer involvement and to help build an industry that attracts a future generation of farmers. Participants also highlighted that challenges to the beef industry in Alberta have made raising beef cattle less economically viable and that BSE in Canada has placed producers under considerable strain: producers fear not only a reportable or notifiable disease but the stigma that would come along with being 'the guy in the community that's got a positive'. Participants believed that producers were bearing much of the cost of surveillance and had yet to realize the benefits of surveillance programs initiated in part in response to the BSE crisis. These circumstances remain an ongoing challenge to surveillance: the negative consequences of an EID or reportable or notifiable disease are more tangible than the purported benefits associated with robust surveillance initiatives [36]. As surveillance serves the interests of producers, the food-producing industry, consumers, and the public [44], distributing the economic burden of surveillance among these parties is warranted. Though the cost of pathogen surveillance in animals is already distributed among these parties, the opinion expressed by participants suggests that further study is needed to ensure cost sharing is equitable.

The economic impact of delayed detection of future epidemics could be tremendous [45,46]. Though the damage caused by delayed detection has been clearly demonstrated through retrospective analysis of previous outbreaks [35], these observations have been insufficient to motivate a global effort sufficient for early EID event detection and response [47]. A component of this issue is the relative lack of attention that has been paid to the social elements of EID surveillance. In order to be more effective, future surveillance initiatives need to incorporate an enhanced understanding of the human dimension of surveillance to encourage people closest to EID events to recognize, report, and respond.

Conclusions

Diagnostic laboratory case submission by participants was biased toward cases in which multiple animals were affected and test results were of direct consequence to clinical case management. Participants also indicated that the expected level of disease varied between farms according to management practices. Broader economic factors, including the cost of diagnostics relative to the value of individual beef cattle and decreasing government support for laboratory diagnostics, limitations of diagnostic laboratory testing, and decreasing veterinary presence on farms, together translated into a decline in case submissions to diagnostic laboratories over time. Efforts to network diagnostic laboratories are unlikely to overcome this challenge to detection of animal disease threats, particularly if these threats occur sporadically or as a result of changes to trends in known endemic problems.

The responses from participants demonstrate that cattle veterinarians in Alberta are an underutilized resource in terms of EID surveillance: they have a perspective on cattle health and a relationship with producers that could prove critical to future EID event detection and response. In order for governments to realize this group's potential for surveillance purposes there needs to be: adequate compensation for time and effort invested; generation of information that is clinically relevant; collaboration on surveillance system design, implementation, and evaluation; and due respect shown to the importance of the relationship between veterinarians and cattle producers. Governments face the added challenge of assuring producers that they will not disproportionately bear the social and economic costs of future EID events.

Acknowledgments

This study was made possible by support from the staff at the Ministry of Agriculture and Rural Development within the Government of Alberta. The importance of the participants in this project cannot be overemphasized. We would like to extend a very big thank you to all of the veterinarians who took part in the interview process; your time, insights, and expertise were critical, invaluable, and essential to this project.

Author Contributions

Conceived and designed the experiments: KS ARV CS. Performed the experiments: KS. Analyzed the data: KS ARV. Contributed reagents/materials/analysis tools: KS CS. Wrote the paper: KES ARV CS.

References

1. Greger M (2007) The human/animal interface: Emergence and resurgence of zoonotic infectious diseases. Crit Rev Microbiol 33: 243–299.
2. Christou L (2011) The global burden of bacterial and viral zoonotic infections. Clin Microbiol Infect 17: 326–330.
3. Taylor LH, Latham SM, Woolhouse ME (2001) Risk factors for human disease emergence. Philos T Roy Soc B 356: 983–989.
4. Woolhouse ME, Gowtage-Sequeria S (2005) Host range and emerging and reemerging pathogens. Emerg Infect Dis 11: 1842–1847.
5. Wagner MM, Moore AW, Aryel RM, editors. (2006) Handbook of biosurveillance. Burlington: Elsevier. 624 p.
6. Keusch GT, Pappaioanou M, Gonzalez MC, Scott KA, Tsai P, editors. (2009) Sustaining global surveillance and response to emerging zoonotic diseases. Washington: The National Academies Press. 340 p.
7. World Health Organization (2006) Regional influenza pandemic preparedness plan (2006–2008) (No. SEA-CD-148). New Dehli: Regional Office for South-East Asia. Available: http://www.searo.who.int/LinkFiles/Avian_Flu_SEA-CD-148_A4.pdf via the Internet. Accessed 12 Mar 2012.
8. Hueston WD (1993) Assessment of national systems for the surveillance and monitoring of animal health. Rev Sci Tec OIE 12: 1187–1196.
9. Doherr MG, Audige L (2001) Monitoring and surveillance for rare health-related events: A review from the veterinary perspective. Philos T Roy Soc B 356: 1097–1106.
10. Gibbens JC, Robertson S, Willmington J, Milnes A, Ryan JB et al. (2008) Use of laboratory data to reduce the time taken to detect new diseases: VIDA to FarmFile. Vet Rec 162: 771–776.
11. Thobokwe G, Heuer C (2004) Incidence of abortion and association with putative causes in dairy herds in New Zealand. N Z Vet J 52: 90–94.
12. Thurmond MC., Blanchard PC, Anderson ML (1994) An example of selection bias in submissions of aborted bovine fetuses to a diagnostic laboratory. J Vet Diagn Invest 6: 269–271.
13. Watson EN, David GP, Cook AJ (2008) Review of diagnostic laboratory submissions of adult cattle 'found dead' in England and Wales in 2004. Vet Rec 163: 531–535.
14. Berezowski J, Checkley S, Clarke R, Clarke S, Dary C et al. (2011) The Alberta Veterinary Practice Surveillance Network: A Veterinary Practice Surveillance System for Cattle in Alberta, Canada. Épidémiol et Santé Anim 59–60: 32–34.
15. Given L (2006) Qualitative research in evidence-based practice: A valuable partnership. Library Hi Tech 24: 376–386.
16. Coe JB, Adams CL, Bonnett BN (2007) A focus group study of veterinarians' and pet owners' perceptions of the monetary aspects of veterinary care. JAVMA-J Am Vet Med A 231: 1510–1518.
17. Hektoen L (2004) Investigations of the motivation underlying Norwegian dairy farmers' use of homeopathy. Vet Rec 155: 701–707.
18. Vaarst M, Thamsborg SM, Bennedsgaard TW, Houe H, Enevoldsen C et al. (2003) Organic dairy farmers' decision making in the first 2 years after conversion in relation to mastitis treatments. Livest Pro Sci 80: 109–120.
19. Bloom Y, Figgs LW, Baker EA, Dugbatey K, Stanwyck CA et al. (2000) Data uses, benefits, and barriers for the behavioral risk factor surveillance system: A qualitative study of users. J Public Health Man 6: 78–86.
20. Pope J, Counahan M (2005) Evaluating the utility of surveillance data to decision makers in Victoria, Australia. Sexual Health 2: 97–102.
21. Wilkinson D, Michie S, McCarthy M (2007) The use and perceptions of routine health data: A qualitative study of four cancer network teams in England. Health Serv Manage Res 20: 211–219.
22. Sawford K, Vollman AR, Stephen C (2012) A focused ethnographic study of Sri Lankan government field veterinarians' decision making about diagnostic laboratory submissions and perceptions of surveillance. PloS One 7: e48035.
23. Morse JM, Richards L (2002) Readme first for a user's guide to qualitative methods. Thousand Oaks: Sage Publications, Inc. 280 p.
24. Bowen GA (2008) Naturalistic inquiry and the saturation concept: A research note. Qual Res 8: 137–151.
25. Guest G, Bunce A, Johnson L (2006) How many interviews are enough? Field Method 18: 59–82.
26. Graneheim UH, Lundman B (2004) Qualitative content analysis in nursing research: Concepts, procedures and measures to achieve trustworthiness. Nurse Educ Today 24: 105–112.
27. Fudge RS, Schlacter JL (1999) Motivating employees to act ethically: An expectancy theory approach. J Bus Ethics 18: 295–304.
28. Liccione WJ (2007) A framework for compensation plans with incentive value. Perf Improv 46: 16–21.
29. Wagner MM, Tsui F, Espino JU, Data VM, Sittig DF et al. (2001) The emerging science of very early detection of disease outbreaks. J Public Health Man 7: 51–59.
30. Kloeze H, Mukhi S, Kitching P, Lees VW, Alexandersen S (2010) Effective animal health disease surveillance using a network-enabled approach. Transbound Emerg Dis 57: 414–419.
31. Bronfenbrenner U (1979) The ecology of human development: Experiments by nature and design. USA: Harvard University Press. 352 p.
32. Green LW, Richard L, Potvin L (1996) Ecological foundations of health promotion. Am J Health Promot 10: 270–281.
33. Del Rocio Amezcua M, Pearl DL, Friendship RM, McNab WB (2010) Evaluation of a veterinary-based syndromic surveillance system implemented for swine. Can J Vet Res 74: 241–251.
34. Babcock S, Marsh AE, Lin J, Scott J (2008) Legal implications of zoonoses for clinical veterinarians. JAVMA-J Am Vet Med A 23: 1556–1562.
35. Newcomb J (2003) Biology and borders: SARS and the new economics of biosecurity. Cambridge: Bio Economic Research Associates. 28 p.
36. Rushton J, Upton M (2006) Investment in preventing and preparing for biological emergencies and disasters: Social and economic costs of disasters versus costs of surveillance and response preparedness. Rev Sci Tech OIE 25: 375–388.
37. Elbakidze L, McCarl BA (2006) Animal disease pre-event preparedness versus post-event response: When is it economic to protect? J Agr Appl Econ, 38.
38. Palmer S, Fozdar F, Sully M (2009) The effect of trust on West Australian farmers' responses to infectious livestock diseases. Social Ruralis, 49: 360–374.
39. Baker EL, Ross D (1996) Information and surveillance systems and community health: Building the public health information infrastructure. J Public Health Man 2: 58–60.
40. Ndiaye SM, Quick L, Sanda O, Niandou S (2003) The value of community participation in disease surveillance: A case study from Niger. Health Promot Int 18: 89–98.
41. Scudamore JM, Harris DM (2002) Control of foot and mouth disease: Lessons from the experience of the outbreak in Great Britain in 2001. Rev Sci Tech OIE 21: 699–710.
42. Coop RL, Kyriazakis I (2001) Influence of host nutrition on the development and consequences of nematode parasitism in ruminants. Trends Parasitol 17: 325–330.
43. Field CJ, Johnson IR, Schley PD (2002) Nutrients and their role in host resistance to infection. J Leukocyte Biol 71: 16–32.
44. Umali DL, Feder G, Haan CD (1994) Animal health services: Finding the balance between public and private delivery. The World Bank Res Obser 9: 71–96.
45. Carpenter TE, O'Brien JM, Hagerman AD, McCarl BA (2011) Epidemic and economic impacts of delayed detection of foot-and-mouth disease: A case study of a simulated outbreak in California. J Vet Diagn Invest 23: 26–33.
46. Kaufmann AF, Meltzer MI, Schmid GP (1997) The economic impact of a bioterrorist attack: Are prevention and postattack intervention programs justifiable? Emerg Infect Dis 3: 83–94.
47. Daszak P (2009) A call for "smart surveillance": A lesson learned from H1N1. EcoHealth 6: 1–2.

15

Evaluation of a gp63–PCR Based Assay as a Molecular Diagnosis Tool in Canine Leishmaniasis in Tunisia

Souheila Guerbouj[1,2], Fattouma Djilani[2], Jihene Bettaieb[3], Bronwen Lambson[4¤a], Mohamed Fethi Diouani[2¤b], Afif Ben Salah[3], Riadh Ben Ismail[2¤c], Ikram Guizani[1,2]*

1 Laboratory of Molecular Epidemiology and Experimental Pathology, Pasteur Institute of Tunis, Université de Tunis el Manar, Tunis, Tunisia, 2 Laboratory of Epidemiology and Ecology of Parasitic Diseases, Pasteur Institute of Tunis, Tunis, Tunisia, 3 Laboratory of Medical Epidemiology, Pasteur Institute of Tunis, Tunis, Tunisia, 4 Molteno Institute for Parasitology, Department of Pathology, University of Cambridge, Cambridge, United Kingdom

Abstract

A gp63PCR method was evaluated for the detection and characterization of *Leishmania (Leishmania)* (*L.*) parasites in canine lymph node aspirates. This tool was tested and compared to other PCRs based on the amplification of 18S ribosomal genes, a *L. infantum* specific repetitive sequence and kinetoplastic DNA minicircles, and to classical parasitological (smear examination and/or culture) or serological (IFAT) techniques on a sample of 40 dogs, originating from different *L. infantum* endemic regions in Tunisia. Sensitivity and specificity of all the PCR assays were evaluated on parasitologically confirmed dogs within this sample (N = 18) and control dogs (N = 45) originating from non–endemic countries in northern Europe and Australia. The gp63 PCR had 83.5% sensitivity and 100% specificity, a performance comparable to the kinetoplast PCR assay and better than the other assays. These assays had comparable results when the gels were southern transferred and hybridized with a radioactive probe. As different infection rates were found according to the technique, concordance of the results was estimated by (κ) test. Best concordance values were between the gp63PCR and parasitological methods (74.6%, 95% confidence intervals CI: 58.8–95.4%) or serology IFAT technique (47.4%, 95% CI: 23.5–71.3%). However, taken together Gp63 and Rib assays covered most of the samples found positive making of them a good alternative for determination of infection rates. Potential of the gp63PCR-RFLP assay for analysis of parasite genetic diversity within samples was also evaluated using 5 restriction enzymes. RFLP analysis confirmed assignment of the parasites infecting the dogs to *L. infantum* species and illustrated occurrence of multiple variants in the different endemic foci. Gp63 PCR assay thus constitutes a useful tool in molecular diagnosis of *L. infantum* infections in dogs in Tunisia.

Editor: Jason Mulvenna, Queensland Institute of Medical Research, Australia

Funding: This work received financial support from the EU-DGXII STD3 (CT930253) and INCO-DC (CT970256) programs and from the Ministry of Higher Education and Research in Tunisia (LR00SP04 & LR11IPT04). The funders had no role in study design, data collection and analysis, decision to publish, or preparation of the manuscript.

Competing Interests: The authors have declared that no competing interests exist.

* Email: ikram.guizani@pasteur.rns.tn

¤a Current address: Centre for HIV and STI, National Institute for Communicable Diseases of the National Health Laboratory Service, Johannesburg, South Africa
¤b Current address: Laboratory of Veterinary Epidemiology and Microbiology, Pasteur Institute of Tunis, Tunis, Tunisia
¤c Current address: World Health Organization – Eastern Mediterranean Regional Office (WHO – EMRO), Cairo, Egypt

Introduction

Visceral leishmaniasis due to *Leishmania infantum* is endemic in Mediterranean basin countries, Middle East, Latin America and Asia. Canines are the major reservoir of the infection [1]. Infected dogs present either a range of clinical manifestations of a viscero-cutaneous form or an asymptomatic status. These latter are considered as carriers since they are for sand flies as infectious as the symptomatic ones [2,3]. Canine leishmaniasis (CanL) is a major veterinary and public health problem not only in old endemic foci but also in non endemic areas where outbreaks are occasionally reported, such as in the United States and Canada [4] and in northern Europe [5]. For epidemiological purposes, there is a need for a precise estimation of the number of infected dogs to evaluate the real extent of infection and better elaborate control programs. Several diagnostic techniques are available for detection of canine infection or diagnosis of the disease. These can be achieved either by demonstrating the parasites microscopically in stained smears [6] or after *in vitro* cultivation [7]. Indirect methods use mainly serological means, like the enzyme-linked immunosorbant assay (ELISA) [8,9], the indirect immunofluorescence assay (IFAT) [10,11] and the direct agglutination test (DAT) [12,13]. However, these diagnostic methods present limitations essentially due to their sensitivity and specificity: parasitological techniques are characteristically insensitive and serological tests are limited by their inability to distinguish between past and present infections and the possibility of cross-reactions with other infectious agents [8,14,15]. With the advent of DNA-based methods and the polymerase chain reaction particularly, more sensitive and rapid detection of parasites has become possible. Although several groups have tested PCR assays in different types of biological samples (fresh, frozen, formalin-fixed or paraffin-embedded biopsies) for the detection of *Leishmania* [9,16,17,18], their values in diagnosis of canine leishmaniasis were partially evaluated.

Here we evaluate a gp63PCR-based technique [19] for molecular diagnosis of *Leishmania* infection in dogs collected from *L. infantum* stable transmission areas in Tunisia, comparing it to classical parasitological and serological techniques and to other molecular assays based on PCR amplification of 18S ribosomal genes, an *L. infantum* specific repetitive sequence and kinetoplast DNA minicircles.

Materials and Methods

Ethics statement

All canine sampling was conducted during routine veterinary care in primary practices. Sampling of Tunisian dogs was conducted during a previous survey study within leishmaniasis endemic regions in Tunisia [20], where (with the exception of 7 dogs that were received at the clinic of the veterinary school for diagnosis) stray dogs were collected during campaigns performed jointly by the Ministries of health and of the Interior, integrating analysis of *Leishmania* prevalence to anti-rabies control programs (stray dog culling). At the time of the study as the veterinarians of our institute took care of these dogs under humane conditions, we did not request ethical consent from the recently installed ethics committee at our institution, to take and use samples of stray dogs that were caught for elimination, or dog samples taken to confirm diagnosis of clinically patent dogs. We used in this last case, remains of the aspirate taken for culture to extract DNAs. Nevertheless, collection of dogs was performed in compliance with the directive 86/609/EEC of the European parliament and the council on the protection of animals used for scientific purposes, in agreement with the guidelines of International Guiding Principles for Biomedical Research Involving Animals.

The second group is composed of 45 control dogs living in regions free from leishmaniasis in northern Europe and Australia (Table S2). Extracted DNAs from samples of these dogs were kindly provided by Dr. David Sargan (University of Cambridge, UK). Sampling of these control dogs was in a range of clinical tests. In all cases the owners gave informed consent that any excess of samples taken during clinical testing could be used in research so long as that excess formed a minority of the sample. This was in accordance with UK Home Office Guidelines. Dogs were not anesthetized. The samples represent, in the case of the Cardigan Welsh Corgis and the Irish setter, DNA from excess blood (<1 ml) after a DNA based test for the rcd3 and rcd1 PRA mutations, respectively. The blood (2–5 ml) was collected as clinical samples into EDTA tubes without anesthesia. This was done by veterinary surgeons in primary practices. In the case of the Irish wolfhound, surplus blood (<1 ml) from clinical collection (usually 2 ml) was taken by a veterinary surgeon for blood ammonia and other tests as part of work up in surveillance for portosystemic shunt. Collections took place at a number of referral clinics. In the cases of the Cocker spaniel and Labrador retriever these were excess (< 1 ml) from cases where EDTA blood, usually 2–5 ml, was collected for routine hematological work up in the clinics of the Queen's Veterinary Hospital, University of Cambridge.

Dogs and samples

Two groups of dogs were studied. The first group corresponded to a total of 40 dogs, from endemic areas of leishmaniasis in Tunisia (Table S1). Lymph node aspirates (~100 µl) were taken by veterinary surgeons in primary practices and stored at −80°C before DNA extraction. Dogs were not anesthetized and sampling did not make any suffering. This dog group has been previously characterized in our laboratory, using parasitological (Giemsa stained smear examination and in vitro culture), serological (IFAT)

and molecular (PCR) tests (Table S1). Only seven dogs (J1– J7) from this group have acute leishmaniasis that presented with clinical and biological features of the disease to the clinic of Sidi Thabet Veterinary school (Tunisia). The remaining 33 dogs did not have patent leishmaniasis; some of them were however oligosymptomatic. The 18 dogs that were positive either by smear examination or culture inoculation (parasitologically confirmed dogs) constituted the positive control group.

The second group is composed of 45 control dogs living in regions free from leishmaniasis in northern Europe and Australia (Table S2). Extracted DNAs from samples of these dogs were kindly provided by Dr. David Sargan (University of Cambridge, UK). Details about the samples are provided in the ethics statement section.

DNA extraction

Frozen lymph node aspirates were suspended in a lysis solution (50 mM NaCl, 10 mM EDTA, 50 mM Tris–HCl pH 7.4) and incubated overnight at 55°C with 100 µg/ml Proteinase K and 0.05% SDS. Total DNA was phenol/chloroform purified and ethanol precipitated as previously described [21].

PCR amplification

Different PCR tests were applied to dog DNA samples. The first PCR targets the coding region of gp63 genes of *Leishmania*, using specific primers SG1 and SG2 as previously described [19]. The second PCR amplifies a central region of a ribosomal gene encoding for the 18S subunit (RIB PCR) present in all *Leishmania* parasites [22]. The third PCR used in this study targets a repetitive genomic sequence found in *L. infantum* species (INF PCR, Genebank Accession No. L42486.1) [23]. KIN PCR used primers KINF and KINR to amplify minicircles of the kinetoplastic DNA of *Leishmania* [24]. Table 1 summarizes the primers sequences used for the different PCRs and the amplified fragments sizes expected. Reaction and cycling conditions are also presented on Table 1.

Another PCR used in this study amplifies a dog gene (acidic ribosomal phosphoprotein fragment, PO) in order to assess for possible sample degradation prior to analysis or inhibition of amplification. PO primers (Table 1), designed from human, rat and mouse PO gene sequences, cross-react with dog DNA and allow amplification of a 470 bp fragment [25]. Products from the different PCRs were analyzed by agarose gel electrophoresis.

In all PCR reactions, multiple negative controls (no DNA) were included in order to monitor for possible contamination. Furthermore, to avoid contamination of samples during carryover and processing, separated laboratory spaces were used for PCR reaction preparation and for analysis of amplified products (gel preparation and migration). Filter-filled tips were also used to set up the PCR reactions. All results were confirmed by hybridization to specific radio-labeled probes.

Probes and hybridization

All PCR gels were transferred onto Hybond N+ membranes according to the Southern method [21] and hybridized to specific probes at 65°C. RIB, INF and KIN PCRs unique fragments (650 bp, 100 bp and 800 bp, respectively) amplified from a positive control corresponding to an *L. infantum* DNA (MHOM/TN/96/Drep15), were gel-extracted, purified using the Qiaquick gel extraction kit (Qiagen, Paris, France) and used as probes. Whereas, a 2 kb fragment corresponding to the coding region of the *L. infantum* gp63 gene was used for gp63PCRs, as previously described [19]. Probes were labeled with $\alpha^{32}P$ dCTP using the random primer labeling kit (Amersham–HVD, Athens,

Table 1. PCR primers sequences, reaction and cycling conditions used.

PCR code	Target	Forward primer Sequence (5' – 3')	Reverse primer sequence (5' – 3')	Amplified fragment size (bp)	Annealing temperature (°C)	Agarose gel percentage	Reaction conditions (25 µl final volume)	Cycling conditions
Gp63	Gp63 gene family	SG1: GTCTCCACCGAG GACCTCACCGA	SG2: TGATGTAGCC GCCCTCCTCGAAG	1300	65	1,2%	22,5 pmol each primer; 0,2 mM dNTPs; 1 mM MgCl$_2$; 0,5 units Taq DNA polymerase (PerkinElmer, France); 50 ng template DNA; 5% DMSO	94°C: 5 min; 35 cycles of 94°C: 30 sec; annealing: 30 sec; 72°C: 1 min; 72°C: 10 min
RIB	18S ribosomal gene	RIBF: GGTTCCTTTCC TGATTTACG	RIBR: GGCCGGTAA AGGCCGAATAG	650	60	1,6%	22,5 pmol each primer; 0,2 mM dNTPs; 1 mM MgCl$_2$; 0,5 units Taq DNA polymerase (PerkinElmer, France); 50 ng template DNA	94°C: 5 min; 35 cycles of 94°C: 30 sec; annealing: 30 sec; 72°C: 1 min; 72°C: 10 min
INF	Repetitive genomic sequence	INFF: ACGAGGTCAGC TCCACTCC	INFR: CTGCAACG CCTGTGTCTAC	100	59	2%	22,5 pmol each primer; 0,2 mM dNTPs; 1 mM MgCl$_2$; 0,5 units Taq DNA polymerase (PerkinElmer, France); 50 ng template DNA	94°C: 5 min; 35 cycles of 94°C: 30 sec; annealing: 30 sec; 72°C: 1 min; 72°C: 10 min
KIN	Minicircles of the kinetoplastic DNA	KINF: GGGGTTGGTGTAAA ATAGGGCGG	KINR: CCAGTTT CCCGCCCGGAG	800	67	1,5%	22,5 pmol each primer; 0,2 mM dNTPs; 1 mM MgCl$_2$; 0,5 units Taq DNA polymerase (PerkinElmer, France); 50 ng template DNA	94°C: 5 min; 35 cycles of 94°C: 30 sec; annealing: 30 sec; 72°C: 1 min; 72°C: 10 min
PO	Acidic ribosomal phosphoprotein	POF: TCATTGTGGGA GCAGACA	POR: GGAGAAG GGGGAGATGTT	470	51	1,5%	20 pmol each primer; 0,2 mM dNTPs; 1,5 mM MgCl$_2$; 1,25 units Taq DNA polymerase (PerkinElmer, France); 20 ng template DNA	94°C: 5 min; 35 cycles of 94°C: 30 sec; annealing: 30 sec; 72°C: 1 min; 72°C: 10 min

Greece) and used to hybridize blots of all the gels. After high stringency washes, labeled hybrid DNA was visualized on X–ray sensitive auto-radiographic films.

Gp63 PCR-RFLP and cluster analysis

Amplified gp63 fragments were digested with *BsiE*I, *Msc*I, *Hinc*II, *BsmB*I and *Sal*I restriction enzymes (Amersham–HVD, Athens, Greece) as previously described [19]. PCR-RFLP profiles were analyzed after overnight electrophoresis in 3% agarose gels and subsequently hybridized to the ^{32}P-labelled gp63 probe. Restriction bands obtained with all the restriction enzymes were scored 1 or 0 for presence or absence of bands, respectively. Genetic distances according to the Nei-modified method were calculated from RFLP data. This data served to construct a dendrogram according to the Kitch method [26], using the PHYLIP package (version 3.69). The Kitch program constructs a tree by successive (agglomerative) clustering, using an average-linkage method of clustering, similar to that used in the UPGMA method. However, this method was chosen as it assumes a molecular clock, allowing the total length of branches from the root to any species to be the same. In addition, this program has options that allow after the tree is constructed to remove and re-add each group, and to try alternative topologies, thus improving the result [26].

Concordance test

The concordance between results of the parasitological, serological or molecular tests was estimated by determining the kappa coefficient (95% CI) using the kappa (k) test of concordance [27]. The Kappa coefficient is interpreted in accordance with Landis and Koch [28] as almost perfect (1.00–0.81), substantial (0.80–0.61), moderate (0.60–0.41), fair (0.40–0.21) and slight (0.20–0.0). The statistical analysis was carried out using the SPSS software package (Version 13.0).

Results

Assessment of DNA quality by PO PCR

The PO primers expected to amplify a 470 bp fragment of a mitochondrial phosphoprotein gene present in mammals [25] were used to evaluate occurrence of inhibition during amplification in dog samples DNAs. All the 40 Tunisian dogs'DNAs generated the expected fragment size of 470 bp (Table 2 and Table S1). Among the control group (N = 45), 3 DNAs were negative (Table 2 and Table S2), indicating PCR inhibition or DNA degradation.

Leishmania DNA PCR amplification from dog samples

The different PCR tests applied to the 85 dog DNA samples of the study showed that 26, 24, 20 and 17 dogs, all from the Tunisian group, were positive using RIB, INF, KIN and gp63 PCRs, respectively (Table 2) with fragments at the expected 650 bp, 100 bp, 800 bp and 1300 bp size, respectively. All control dogs, originating from non–endemic regions for leishmaniasis, did not present any amplification with the different PCR tests (Table 2).

In order to verify the specificity of the PCR products obtained and to assess the possibility of false negative results, all electrophoresis gels were Southern transferred onto a Nylon membrane and amplified products were hybridized to corresponding ^{32}P labeled probes. Results obtained after Ethidium bromide (EtBr) staining and UV observation (before hybridization) and after probe hybridization were compared (Table 2 and Table S1). All bands observed on the gels were confirmed by the probe

Table 2. Results of parasitology, serology and PCR investigations on Tunisian and control dogs.

	Parasitology	Serology	PO PCR[a]	RIB PCR[b] EtBr	RIB PCR[b] 32P	INF PCR[b] EtBr	INF PCR[b] 32P	KIN PCR[b] EtBr	KIN PCR[b] 32P	gp63 PCR[b] EtBr	gp63 PCR[b] 32P
Tunisian dogs (N = 40) Positive results	18/40	26/40	40/40	26/40	35/40	24/40	39/40	20/40	33/40	17/40	17/40
Sensitivity[c] (%)				55.6 (10/18)	83.5 (15/18)	83.5 (15/18)	100 (18/18)	61.1 (11/18)	83.5 (15/18)	83.5 (15/18)	83.5 (15/18)
Infection rate[d] (%)	45.0 (18/40)	65.0 (26/40)			87.5 (35/40)		97.5 (39/40)		82.5 (33/40)		42.5 (17/40)
Control dogs (N = 45) Positive results			42/45	0/45	3/45	0/45	5/45	0/45	0/45	0/45	1/45
Specificity[e] (%)				100	93.3 (42/45)	100	88.9 (40/45)	100	100	100	97.8 (44/45)

[a]PO PCR targets a mammalian mitochondrial phosphoprotein gene.
[b]RIB, INF, KIN and gp63 PCRs target a central region of 18S ribosomal gene, a repetitive genomic sequence, minicircles of the kinetoplastic DNA and gp63 family coding sequences, respectively in *Leishmania*.
[c]Sensitivity of the different PCR assays corresponds to the proportion of positive dogs among the 18 parasitologically confirmed ones.
[d]Infection rates are the proportion of positive dogs among the total dog number.
[e]specificity of the different PCR assays corresponds to the number of negative dogs among the control dog group.
Abbreviations: EtBr, Ethidium bromide staining and reading under UV light; ^{32}P, autoradiographic reading after hybridization with a ^{32}P labeled probe.

hybridizations. This step also increased the number of positive Tunisian dogs to 35, 39 and 33 with RIB, INF and KIN PCRs, respectively while the number of gp63 PCR positive dogs did not change after hybridization (Table 2).

Sensitivity and Specificity of PCR tests

Sensitivity of the different PCR tests was measured as the proportion of positive dogs among the positive control group of 18 parasitologically confirmed dogs (Table 2). RIB, INF, KIN and gp63 PCRs had a sensitivity of 55.6% (10/18), 83.5% (15/18), 61.1% (11/18) and 83.5% (15/18), respectively. After ^{32}P labeled probe hybridization, sensitivity changed to 83.5% (15/18), 100% and 83.5% (15/18) for RIB, INF, and KIN PCRs, respectively but it remained the same for gp63PCR (Table 2).

Specificity of the PCR tests was estimated as the proportion of the negative control dogs (originating from non–endemic regions for leishmaniasis) that were negative in the assays. 100% of specificity was achieved by all PCR tests after analysis of EtBr stained gels, while 93.3% (42/45), 88.9% (40/45) and 97.8% (44/45) were found for RIB, INF and gp63 PCRs, respectively, after autoradiography analysis (Table 2 and Table S2). This decrease was due to the presence of positive signals after hybridization in the case of several dogs (9/45) (Table S2). No change was observed for KIN PCR, after hybridization (Table 2).

Comparative evaluation of parasitological, serological and molecular tools for diagnosis of canine leishmaniasis

Infection rate within our sample was estimated using the parasitological, serological and molecular techniques. Parasitological tests using direct examination of amastigotes within biopsies (stained smears) and *in vitro* isolation in culture media of promastigotes indicated a 45% (18/40) infection rate (Table 2). Using IFAT, the infection rate was 65% (26/40) (Table 2). With the PCR assays, considering the dogs were infected when positive signals were observed before or after hybridization, the infection rates reached 87.5% (35/40), 97.5% (39/40) and 82.5% (33/40) for RIB, INF and KIN PCRs, respectively while with the gp63PCR it was 42.5% (17/40) (Table 2). Given the differences in measures of infection rates, concordance of the results was investigated computing the proportion of identical results found by different tools and comparing them in a pair wise way (Table 3). The best concordance kappa (κ) values were found between the gp63PCR test and parasitological (74.6%, 95% confidence interval (CI): 0.588, 0.954) or serological IFAT (47.4%, 95%CI: 0.235, 0.713) methods (Table 3), with a substantial and moderate agreement between these tools, respectively. Concordance between the RIB, INF and KIN PCRs and parasitological or serological methods showed negative or close to zero (−0.304 to 0.041) kappa values, indicating a disagreement (Table 3). In addition, when the PCR tools were pair-wise compared, fair concordance kappa values were found between KIN and RIB (22%, 95%CI: −0.158, 0.598) and between KIN and INF (21.6%, 95%CI: −0.143, 0.575) PCRs (Table 3).

Species identification and analysis of intra-specific parasite polymorphism by gp63 PCR-RFLP

The gp63PCR products obtained for 15 parasitological positive dogs and representative strains of *L. infantum*, *L. donovani*, *L. archibaldi*, *L. major*, *L. tropica* and *L. aethiopica* species were purified from the gels, digested with *BsiE*I, *Sal*I, *Msc*I, *BsmB*I and *Hinc*II restriction enzymes and analyzed for restriction length polymorphisms by electrophoresis and southern blot analysis using a ^{32}P labeled gp63 probe, as previously described [19]. Restriction

Table 3. Pair wise concordance values calculated using the kappa coefficient for parasitology, serology and PCR investigations.

| | Parasitology | | Serology (IFAT) | | PCRs | | | | | | | |
| | | | | | RIB | | INF | | KIN | |
	Kappa	95% CI*	Kappa	95% CI*	Kappa	95% CI*	Kappa	95% CI*	Kappa	95% CI*
Serology (IFAT)	0.515	0.274, 0.756								
PCRs										
RIB	−0.070	−0.264, 0.124	−0.226	−0.387, −0.065						
INF	0.041	−0.039, 0.121	−0.049	−0.141, 0.043	−0.043	−0.116, 0.029				
KIN	0.014	−0.205, 0.233	−0.304	−0.473, −0.135	0.220	−0.158, 0.598	0.216	−0.143, 0.575		
gp63	0.746	0.588, 0.954	0.474	0.235, 0.713	0.011	−0.169, 0.191	0.037	−0.035, 0.109	0.089	−0.117, 0.295

*CI, Confidence interval.
RIB, INF, KIN and gp63 PCRs target a central region of 18S ribosomal gene, a repetitive genomic sequence, minicercles of the kinetoplastic DNA and gp63 family coding sequences, respectively in *Leishmania*.

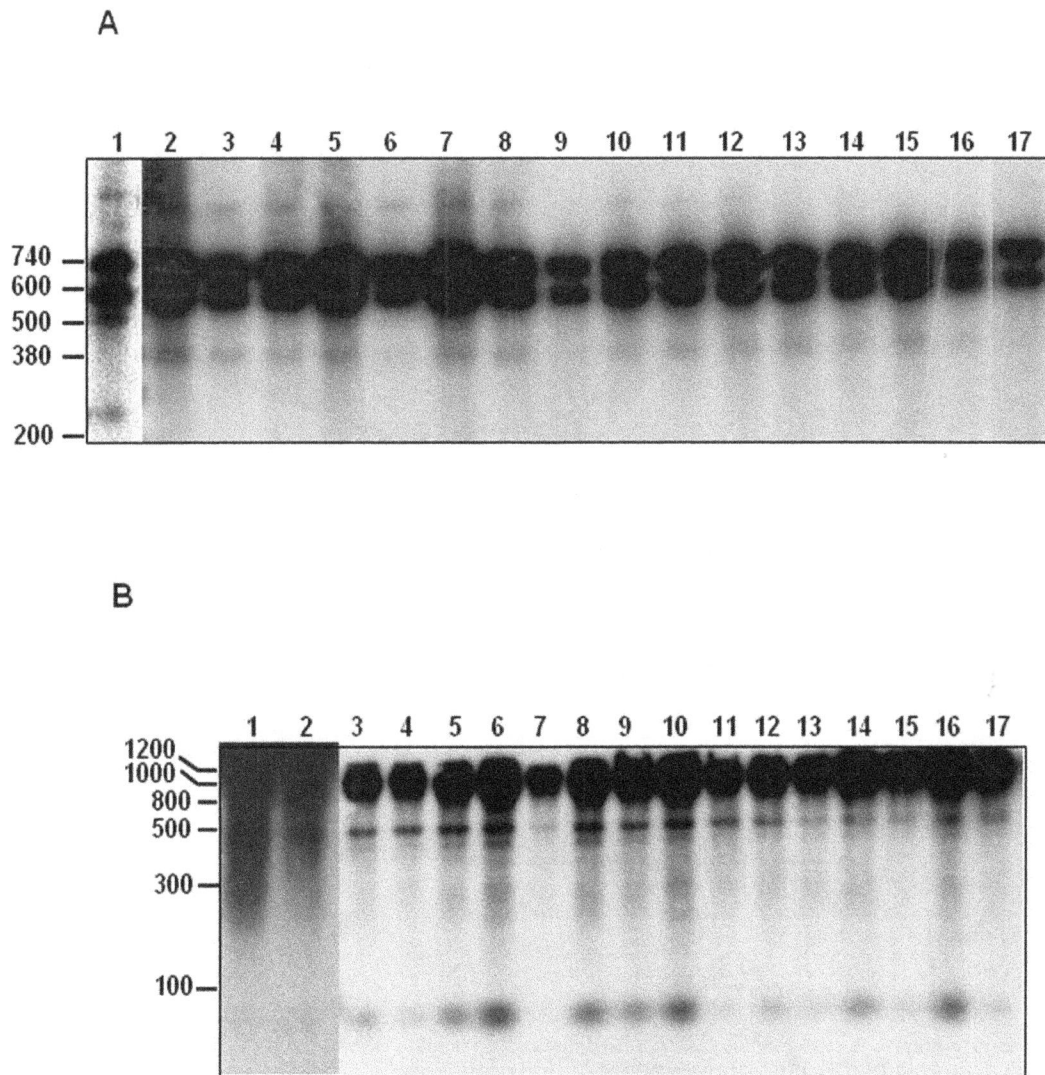

Figure 1. Gp63PCR-RFLP patterns of *Leishmania* **parasites obtained from dog biopsies.** A: digestion with *Msc*I restriction enzyme; B: digestion with *Sal*I restriction enzyme. 1: *L. donovani*, 2: *L. infantum*, 3: LN112, 4: LN129, 5: LN26, 6: LN11, 7: LN80, 8: LN2, 9: LN39, 10: LN77, 11: LN102, 12: LN110, 13: J1, 14: J3, 15: J5, 16: J6, 17: J7. All sizes are indicated in bp.

profiles were polymorphic but species- specific fragments like the presence of an *L. infantum* specific 380 bp *Msc*I fragment and the absence of a 500 bp and a 220 bp *L. donovani* specific *Msc*I fragments [19], allowed identification of the dog *Leishmania* parasites as members of the *L. donovani* complex, more precisely belonging to the *L. infantum* species (Figure 1). In order to better illustrate diversity and phenetic relationships of the amastigotes infecting the studied dogs, the restriction profiles were used to calculate Nei-modified distances and the generated data matrix was then used to construct a dendrogram (Kitch-Margoliash, Phylip package). All dog parasites clustered together with the *L. infantum* reference strain, distinctly from *L. donovani* and *L. archibaldi* representative strains (Figure 2). Whereas, strains representing other Old World species, *L. major*, *L. tropica* and *L. aethiopica* were individualized on separate branches (Figure 2). However, within the dogs' clade, small clusters were observed that were not correlated to epidemiological features like geographical origin, sex or age of dogs. This however highlights occurrence of multiple parasite variants (variability index = 0.47 (7/15))

characterized by gp63 genes coding for surface antigens having variable, either exposed or buried residues. Three of these variants were shared by 11 parasites (Figure 2). Of relevance to molecular tracking of parasites, different variants were observed in the same transmission area while a same variant was observed in different endemic regions. Moreover, the study here brings information on 2 parasites (LN36 and LN100) that could not be isolated and maintained by *in vitro* culture (Table S1), which illustrates an additional value of the gp63 PCR based assays for molecular diagnosis of canine leishmaniasis.

Discussion

Variable clinical and biological manifestations characterize *Leishmania* canine infection and leishmaniasis. Its diagnosis still constitutes a major epidemiological problem. Within Tunisian endemic foci, for instance, 50% to 90% of infected dogs are asymptomatic [29,30], which further show the necessity to use sensitive diagnostic techniques. In spite of their limits, parasito-

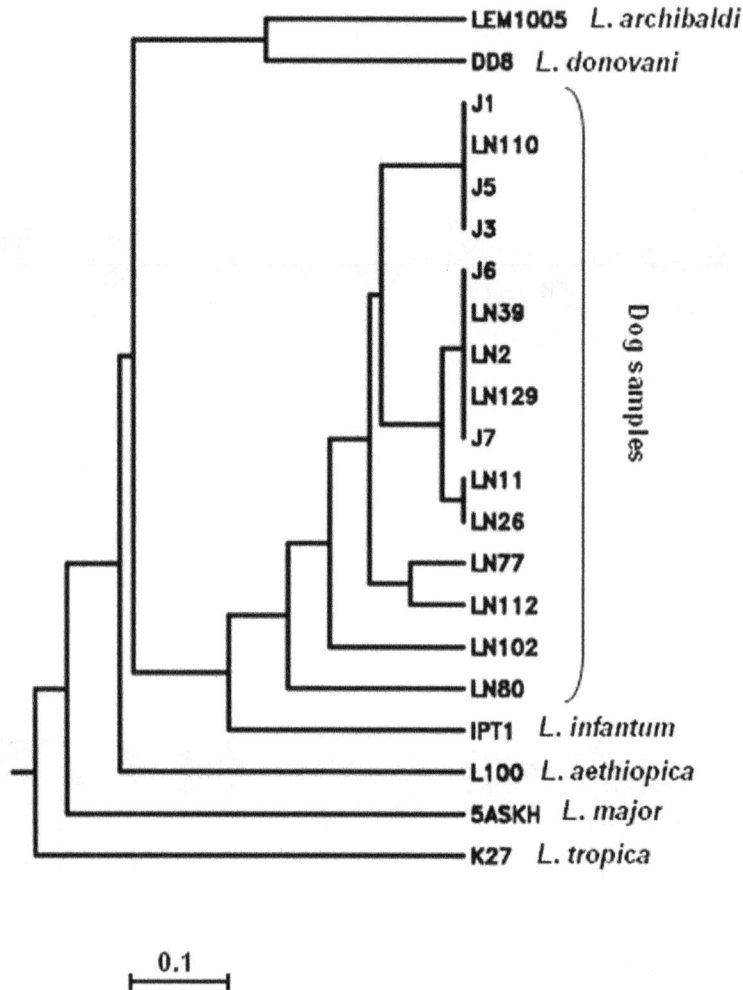

Figure 2. Kitch dendrogram constructed using Nei-modified distances calculated from gp63PCR-RFLP results obtained with lymph node biopsies of dogs from Tunisia. Branches corresponding to Old World representative *Leishmania* strains are indicated.

logical and serological techniques are still the most common methods used to diagnose canine leishmaniasis and are considered as gold standards [31,32]. With the advent of molecular tools like PCR, a more sensitive and rapid detection of parasites has become possible. The potential of a gp63 amplification–based tool in molecular diagnosis of canine leishmaniasis was here evaluated. Sensitivity and specificity of this gp63PCR were estimated and compared to parasitological (direct examination and *in vitro* culture), and serological (IFAT) techniques, as well as to other PCR assays. DNAs purified from lymph node (LN) biopsies, taken from 40 Tunisian dogs were PCR amplified in 5 assays targeting, the intra-genic regions of gp63 genes (gp63 PCR), a central region of 18S encoding ribosomal gene (RIB PCR), an *L. infantum* specific repetitive sequence (INF PCR), minicircles of kinetoplast DNA (KIN PCR) and a mammalian phosphorotein gene (PO PCR). This latter PCR was used to verify the absence of inhibitors within the DNA preparations. All PCR products were hybridized to their respective ^{32}P labeled probe, which allowed (i) to validate specificity of the obtained signal and (ii) to check for absence of false negative results. An 83.5% sensitivity was calculated for the gp63PCR tool while in controlled laboratory conditions using purified DNA the test could detect 0.01 pg of DNA, which correspond to 0.1 promastigote [19]. This could be explained by

differences at the level of amplification efficacy, in relation with parasite burden, presence of host material (including inhibitors) or reaction conditions. Sensitivity of PCR tests was shown to vary outstandingly when applied either on cultured parasites or on peripheral blood samples of infected dogs [18,33]. Specificity of gp63PCR was estimated on a group of control dogs, constituted by non-infected dogs originating from countries where leishmaniasis is not endemic. Consequently, 100% of specificity was found after EtBr reading. This percentage decreased to a value of 97.8% after hybridization with a ^{32}P labeled gp63 probe. Using the same dog sample, 100% of specificity was achieved with EtBr reading for PCRs amplifying genomic sequences (RIB and INF PCRs) while a decrease of specificity (93% for RIB PCR and 89% for INF PCR) was noticed with ^{32}P reading. Previous studies that used the INF PCR showed a specificity of 97% when this tool was applied to detect *Leishmania* DNA from patients presenting with visceral leishmaniasis [23]. Here, no certified explanation for the positive (and very faint) signals observed could be provided, travel history of the dogs could be a reason; non–specific amplification or cross-reactivity with other microbes could be other reasons. Nevertheless, it is important to notice that only a few studies have used hybridization with ^{32}P labeled probes consecutively after EtBr detection of PCR signals.

Parasitological, serological and molecular techniques, in addition to gp63PCR tool, are methods that showed different rates of infection when tested on our study sample. In other studies that amplified the conserved region of *Leishmania* kDNA minicircles, a prevalence of 67% was found in Spain [16], 24.7% is detected in dogs from an urban area in Brazil [34] while 51.88% was found in western China [35] and 29% in Greece [36]. PCRs using ribosomal genes detected 79.8% of dog infection in southern France [37] and 11.5% in the West Bank, Palestine [38]. However, 58.1% was found in Greece with INF PCR targeting a specific fragment of a repetitive sequence of *L. infantum* DNA [36]. Disparity of the measured rates of infection could be explained by (i) epidemiological differences, (ii) biases introduced when selecting negative dogs or (iii) by efficiency in amplification of different size fragments. Consequently, measure of concordance between results of different tools would allow a better evaluation. Thus, κ concordance values between the different tools showed a substantial and moderate agreement between gp63PCR and parasitological methods (74.6%) and serology IFAT technique (47.4%), respectively, which was higher than that achieved with the other PCR tools. This underscores need for using several methods to diagnose canine infection. Previous studies have in fact shown that a canine infection could be under-estimated when only one technique is used [31,32]. However, if we consider the appropriate situations where these different techniques could be used, several comments could be advanced. Indeed, although its weak sensitivity, parasitological diagnosis remains a method of choice in individual cases like veterinary consultation, where dogs having patent disease are specifically recruited and for which this kind of examination is sensitive [39]. *In vitro* culture, in these cases, constitutes a limitation, since up to several weeks could be necessary before a result could be advanced. Besides, it is a laborious diagnostic technique mostly performed in research laboratories. It is precisely in these cases that PCR tools are the most useful, since they allow the detection of *Leishmania* DNA with a high sensitivity and specificity, thus providing a rapid diagnosis [32]. Concerning serological methods, these are based on the presence of IgG antibodies within dogs' sera. However, a positive result may indicate an exposure to the parasite but not necessarily an active infection [2,3]. Moreover, these techniques are not able to reveal the real prevalence, nor the transmission intensity of the infection, since it is difficult to differentiate between an active and a non-active state of the infection [3,7,32]. Another challenge in comparative evaluation of tools is the selection of negative control dogs in countries endemic for leishmaniasis. Thus, using simultaneously several diagnostic methods, including PCR, seems to be necessary for canine leishmaniasis diagnosis. In this context, use of gp63PCR (EtBr reading) associated with another PCR tool like RIB PCR, which was most discordant, will allow maximizing possibilities to find positive responses. Gp63

PCR in addition to RIB PCR could constitute a good diagnostic procedure in canine leishmaniasis that would complement parasitological and IFAT methods or constitute alternatives to detect infection. Moreover, a gp63 PCR positive signal was found in the case of 2 dogs, from which *Leishmania* parasites could not be isolated in culture. This further emphasized the interesting potential of this gp63PCR as a molecular tool, able of detecting and studying parasites, bypassing *in vitro* culture steps. On the other hand, the gp63 assay did not detect parasites of cases that were positive by the classical techniques. Presence of specific inhibitors to this assay or parasites having polymorphic priming sites may be causes affecting PCR efficiency. PO primers amplified all the Tunisian dog samples inferring that other causes than PCR inhibition may explain this sensitivity default.

Intra-specific polymorphism of parasites within infected dogs' lymph nodes was evaluated by RFLP analysis of the amplified gp63PCR fragments by several restriction enzymes [19] followed by phenetic analysis using Nei-modified distances. The dendrogram confirmed the identity of the studied dog parasites as belonging to the *L. donovani* complex and more precisely to the *L. infantum* species. Polymorphic PCR-RFLP profiles highlighted their genetic variability constituting in some cases small groups that clustered together on the dendrogram. However this variability did not correlate with epidemiological features like geographical origin, sex or age of dogs. Gp63 PCR-RFLP highlighted geographical structuring of *L. infantum* and *L. donovani* parasites and importance of host selection pressures were hypothesized [19]. Thus, it appears important to develop further studies comparing parasites having diverse host origins. Nevertheless, this gp63PCR constitutes an innovative approach that allows study of *L. infantum* variability within the reservoir to assess occurrence of parasite variants in a concomitant way to their detection.

Supporting Information

Table S1 Panel of dogs collected from leishmaniasis endemic regions in Tunisia and results of parasitology, serology and PCR investigations.

Table S2 Panel of control dogs collected from non-endemic countries for leishmaniasis and PCR results.

Author Contributions

Conceived and designed the experiments: SG BL IG RBI. Performed the experiments: SG FD. Analyzed the data: SG JB IG FD RBI. Contributed reagents/materials/analysis tools: SG IG FD JB BL MFD ABS RBI. Wrote the paper: SG IG.

References

1. jeux P (2001) The increase in risk factors for leishmaniasis worldwide. Trans R Soc Trop Med Hyg 95: 239–243.
2. ina R, Amela C, Nieto J, San Andres M, Gonzalez F, et al. (1994) Infectivity of dogs naturally infected with *Leishmania infantum* to colonized *Phlebotomus perniciosus*. Trans Roy Soc Trop Med Hyg 88: 491–493.
3. halsky EM, Rocha MF, Da Rocha Lima AC, França-Silva JC, Pires MQ, et al. (2007) Infectivity of seropositive dogs, showing different clinical forms of leishmaniasis, to *Lutzomyia longipalpis* phlebotomine sand flies. Vet Parasitol 147: 67–76.
4. Schantz PM, Steurer FJ, Duprey ZH, Kurpel KP, Barr SC, et al. (2005) Autochthonous visceral leishmaniasis in dogs in North America. J Am Vet Med Assoc 226: 1316–1322.
5. Gramiccia M, Gradoni L (2007) The leishmaniases of Southern Europe. In: Takken W, Knols W, Bart GJ, editors.Emerging pests and vector-borne diseases

in Europe. Ecology and control of vector-borne diseases, vol. 1. Wageningen Academic Publishers, Wageningen. pp. 75–95.
6. Giudice, Passantino A (2011) Detection of eishmania mastigotes in peripheral blood from four dogs. Acta Vet Hung 59: 205–213.
7. Gramiccia M (2011) Recent advances in leishmaniasis in pet animals: Epidemiology, diagnostics and anti-vectorial prophylaxis. Vet Parasitol 181: 23–30.
8. Porrozzi R, Santos da Costa MV, Teva A, Falqueto A, Ferreira AL, et al. (2007) Comparative evaluation of enzyme-linked immunosorbent assays based on crude and recombinant leishmanial antigens for serodiagnosis of symptomatic and asymptomatic *Leishmania infantum* visceral infections in dogs. Clin Vaccine Immunol 14: 544–548.
9. Gomes Y, Paiva M, Cavalcanti M, Lira RA, Abath FG, et al. (2008) Diagnosis of canine visceral leishmaniasis: biotechnological advances. Vet J 175: 45–52.

10. Ferroglio E, Centaro E, Mignone W, Trisciuoglio A (2007) Evaluation of an ELISA rapid device for the serological diagnosis of *Leishmania infantum* infection in dog as compared with immunofluorescence assay and Western blot. Vet Parasitol 144: 162–166.

11. Maia C, Campino L (2008) Methods for diagnosis of canine leishmaniasis and immune response to infection. Vet Parasitol 158: 274–287.

12. Oskam L, Slappendel RJ, Beijer EG, Kroon NC, van Ingen CW, et al (1996) Dog–DAT: a direct agglutination test using stabilized, freeze–dried antigen for the serodiagnosis of canine visceral leishmaniasis. FEMS Immunol Med Microbiol 16: 235–239.

13. Ferreira Ede C, de Lana M, Carneiro M, Reis AB, Paes DV, et al. (2007) Comparison of serological assays for the diagnosis of canine visceral leishmaniasis in animals presenting different clinical manifestations. Vet Parasitol 146: 235–241.

14. Alvar J, Cañavate C, Molina R, Moreno J, Nieto J (2004) Canine leishmaniasis. Adv Parasitol 57: 1–88.

15. Srividya G, Kulshrestha A, Singh R, Salotra P (2012) Diagnosis of visceral leishmaniasis: developments over the last decade. Parasitol Res 110: 1065–1078.

16. Solano-Gallego L, Morell P, Arboix M, Alberola J, Ferrer L (2001) Prevalence of *Leishmania infantum* infection in dogs living in an area of canine leishmaniasis endemicity using PCR on several tissues and serology. J Clin Microbiol 39: 560–563.

17. Schönian G, Nasereddin A, Dinse N, Schweynoch C, Schallig HD, et al. (2003) PCR diagnosis and characterization of *Leishmania* in local and imported clinical samples. Diagn Microbiol Infect Dis 47: 349–358.

18. Solcà Mda S, Guedes CE, Nascimento EG, Oliveira GG, dos Santos WL, et al. (2012) Qualitative and quantitative polymerase chain reaction (PCR) for detection of *Leishmania* in spleen samples from naturally infected dogs. Vet Parasitol 184: 133–140.

19. Guerbouj S, Victoir K, Guizani I, Seridi N, Nuwayri-Salti N, et al. (2001) Gp63 gene polymorphism and population structure of *Leishmania donovani* complex: influence of the host selection pressure? Parasitology 122: 25–35.

20. Boelaert M, Aoun K, Liinev J, Goetghebeur E, Van der Stuyft P (1999) The potential of latent class analysis in diagnostic test validation for canine *Leishmania infantum* infection. Epidemiol Infect 123: 499–506.

21. Guizani I, Van Eys GJJM, Ben Ismail R, Dellagi K (1994) Use of recombinant DNA probes for species identification of Old World *Leishmania* isolates. Am J Trop Med Hyg 50: 632–640.

22. Van Eys GJJM, Schoone GJ, Kroon NCM, Ebeling SB (1992) Sequence analysis of small subunit ribosomal RNA genes and its use for detection and identification of *Leishmania* parasites. Mol Biochem Parasitol 51: 133–142.

23. Piarroux R, Azaiez R, Lossi AM, Reynier P, Muscatelli F, et al. (1993) Isolation and characterization of a repetitive DNA sequence from *Leishmania infantum*: development of a visceral leishmaniasis polymerase chain reaction. Am J Trop Med Hyg 49: 364–369.

24. Smyth AJ, Ghosh A, Hassan MQ, Basu D, De Bruijn MHL, et al. (1992) Rapid and sensitive detection of *Leishmania* kinetoplast DNA from spleen and blood samples of kala-azar patients. Parasitology 105: 183–192.

25. Ashford DA, Bozza M, Freire M, Miranda JC, Sherlock I, et al. (1995) Comparison of the polymerase chain reaction and serology for the detection of canine visceral leishmaniasis. Am J Trop Med Hyg 53: 251–255.

26. Felsenstein J (1984) Distance methods for inferring phylogenies: a justification. Evolution 38: 16–24.

27. Sim JJ, Wright CC (2005) The Kappa Statistic in Reliability Studies: Use, Interpretation, and Sample Size Requirements. Phys Therapy 85: 257–268.

28. Landis JR, Koch GG (1977) The measurement of observer agreement for categorical data. Biometrics 33: 159–174.

29. Chargui N, aouas N, orcii M, ahmar S, uesmi M, et al (2009) Use of PCR, IFAT and in vitro culture in the detection of Leishmania infantum infection in ogs nd evaluation of the prevalence of anine leishmaniasis n a low endemic area in unisia. Parasite 16: 65–69.

30. Diouani MF, en Alaya Bouafif N, ettaib J, ouzir H, edidi S, et al. (2008) Dogs. infantum infection from an endemic region of the north of unisia: a prospective study. Arch Inst Pasteur Tunis 85: 55–61.

31. Miró G, Cardoso L, Pennisi MG, Oliva G, Baneth G (2008) Canine leishmaniosis – new concepts and insights on an expanding zoonosis: part two. Trends Parasit 24: 371–377.

32. Solano-Gallego L, Miró G, Koutinas A, Cardoso L, Pennisi MG, et al. (2011) LeishVet guidelines for the practical management of canine leishmaniosis. Parasites & Vectors 4: 86–101.

33. Lachaud L, Marchergui-Hammami S, Chabbert E, Dereure J, Dedet JP, et al. (2002) Comparison of six PCR methods using peripheral blood for detection of canine visceral leishmaniasis. J Clin Microbiol 40: 210–215.

34. Coura-Vital W, Marques MJ, Veloso VM, Roatt BM, Aguiar-Soares RD, et al. (2011) Prevalence and factors associated with *Leishmania infantum* infection of dogs from an urban area of Brazil as identified by molecular methods. PLoS Negl Trop Dis 5: e1291.

35. Wang JY, Ha Y, Gao CH, ang, Yang YT, et al. (2011) The prevalence of canine *eishmania nfantum* infection in western China detected by PCR and serological tests. Parasites & Vectors. 4: 69–76.

36. Andreadou, Liandris E, Kasampalidis IN, Taka S, Antoniou M, et al. (2012) Evaluation of the performance of selected in-house and commercially available PCR and real-time PCR assays for the detection of *Leishmania* DNA in canine clinical samples. Exp Parasitol 131: 419–424.

37. Lachaud L, habbert E, ubessay P, ereure J, amothe J, t al. (2002) Value of two PCR methods for the diagnosis of canine visceral leishmaniasis and the detection of asymptomatic carriers. Parasitology 125: 197–207.

38. Hamarsheh, Nasereddin A, Damaj S, Sawalha S, Al-Jawabreh H, et al. (2012) Serological and molecular survey of *Leishmania* parasites in apparently healthy dogs in the West Bank, Palestine. Parasites & Vectors 5: 183–190.

39. Oliva G, Scalone A, Foglia Manzillo V, Gramiccia M, Pagano A, et al. (2006) Incidence and time course of *eishmania nfantum* infections examined by parasitological, serologic, and nested–PCR techniques in a cohort of naive dogs exposed to three consecutive transmission seasons. J Clin Microbiol 44: 1318–1322.

16

Treatment of an Intramammary Bacterial Infection with 25-Hydroxyvitamin D$_3$

John D. Lippolis[1]*, Timothy A. Reinhardt[1], Randy A. Sacco[1], Brian J. Nonnecke[1], Corwin D. Nelson[2]

1 Ruminant Diseases and Immunology Research Unit, National Animal Disease Center, Agricultural Research Service (ARS), United States Department of Agriculture (USDA), Ames, Iowa, United States of America, **2** Department of Biochemistry, University of Wisconsin-Madison, Madison, Wisconsin, United States of America

Abstract

Deficiency of serum levels of 25-hydroxyvitamin D$_3$ has been correlated with increased risk of infectious diseases such as tuberculosis and influenza. A plausible reason for this association is that expression of genes encoding important antimicrobial proteins depends on concentrations of 1,25-dihydroxyvitamin D$_3$ produced by activated immune cells at sites of infection, and that synthesis of 1,25-dihydroxyvitamin D$_3$ is dependent on the availability of 25-hydroxyvitamin D$_3$. Thus, increasing the availability of 25(OH)D$_3$ for immune cell synthesis of 1,25-dihydroxyvitamin D$_3$ at sites of infection has been hypothesized to aid in clearance of the infection. This report details the treatment of an acute intramammary infection with infusion of 25-hydroxyvitamin D$_3$ to the site of infection. Ten lactating cows were infected with in one quarter of their mammary glands. Half of the animals were treated intramammary with 25-hydroxyvitamin D$_3$. The 25-hydroxyvitamin D$_3$ treated animal showed significantly lower bacterial counts in milk and showed reduced symptomatic affects of the mastitis. It is significant that treatment with 25-hydroxyvitamin D$_3$ reduced the severity of an acute bacterial infection. This finding suggested a significant non-antibiotic complimentary role for 25-hydroxyvitamin D$_3$ in the treatment of infections in compartments naturally low in 25-hydroxyvitamin D$_3$ such as the mammary gland and by extension, possibly upper respiratory tract infections.

Editor: Jürgen Schauber, Ludwig-Maximilian-University, Germany

Funding: United States Department of Agriculture (USDA) was the sole funder for this research. USDA determines the research priorities of all research that it funds. Publication of research is subject to review of USDA officials. Specific study design, data collection, data analysis, and preparation of the manuscript is under the control of the individual researchers.

Competing Interests: A patent application has been filed for the use of 25(OH)vitamin D in the treatment of mastitis.

* E-mail: john.lippolis@ars.usda.gov

Introduction

The relationship between vitamin D status and the ability of that animal's immune system to effectively prevent disease is a topic of much research in both human and veterinary medicine [1–5]. Vitamin D, following its conversion to its active form 1, 25-dihydroxyvitamin D$_3$ (1,25(OH)$_2$D$_3$), the active form of vitamin D, is a primary regulator of calcium and skeletal homeostasis [1]. However, additional functions in the immune system became evident in the early 1980s when it was found that 1,25(OH)$_2$D$_3$ was produced by monocytes in diseased tissue, the vitamin D receptor was identified in immune tissues and some immune functions were shown to be influenced by 1,25(OH)$_2$D$_3$ [6–11]. More that 80 years prior to the demonstration of the role of vitamin D in immune function, cod liver oil or exposure to sun, both sources of vitamin D, were used to treat tuberculosis (Reviewed in: [2,12]. Then in 1986, Rook and co-workers showed that 1,25(OH)2D3 induced anti-tuberculosis activity in cultured monocytes [13]. Additionally, 1,25(OH)$_2$D$_3$ has been found to affect monocyte chemotaxis [14] and act as an adjuvant in the production of bacterial-specific antibodies [15]. In 2006, a seminal paper was published by Liu *et. al.* [16] in which they demonstrated that toll-like receptor (TLR) activation of monocytes induced 25-hydroxyvitamin D-1α-hydroxylase (1α -hydroxylase). 1-hydroxylase converts 25-hydroxyvitamin D$_3$ (25(OH)D$_3$) to the active 1,25(OH)$_2$D$_3$. 1,25(OH)$_2$D$_3$ induced

the antimicrobial peptide cathelicidin and inhibited the growth of *Mycobacterium tuberculosis*. Furthermore, they showed that cathelicidin induction was compromised when using serum from donors with low 25(OH)D$_3$. This suggested that maintaining vitamin D status above that needed for normal calcium homeostasis was required for optimal immune responses via this newly highlighted intracrine pathway.

Associations between serum 25(OH)D$_3$ concentrations and optimal immune function is now a subject of significant scrutiny. Levels of serum 25(OH)D$_3$, sufficient for full functionality of the immune system are thought to be higher than levels needed for proper skeletal formation [17,18]. Using samples collected as part of the National Health and Nutrition Examination Survey, researcher determined the levels of 25(OH)D$_3$ in various populations [19]. Their data indicated that in humans only 20–25% of the population has 25(OH)D$_3$ levels considered immunologically sufficient (>30 ng/ml) [17,19]. There is an inverse correlation between serum 25(OH)D$_3$ levels and the risk for upper respiratory tract infections [20], tuberculosis [21], and multiple sclerosis [22]. Dietary supplementation of vitamin D has been shown to decrease the risk of relapse in multiple sclerosis patients [23] and decreases the risk of influenza A infections [24]. Together this information indicates an important role of vitamin D in the clearance of infections and containment of inflammation by the body's immune cells.

Mastitis in dairy cattle allows for unique studies of immune cells and the role of vitamin D in modulating the immune system's response to pathogens. First, it is known that intramammary infections activate bovine macrophages found in the milk through the TLR pathways resulting in the upregulation of the expression of the 1α-hydroxylase gene. The expression of 1α-hydroxylase is responsible for the conversion of $25(OH)D_3$ to active hormone $1,25(OH)_2D_3$ [4]. The production of $1,25(OH)_2D_3$ leads to changes in gene expression in macrophages isolated from milk of an infected gland [3]. Therefore, the intracrine pathway described in humans [16] is active in the bovine mammary gland macrophages during a bacterial infection, but fails to induce the induction of cathelicidin [4]. A second important aspect of studying the role of vitamin D in mammary gland infections, is that milk is deficient in $25(OH)D_3$. The levels of $25(OH)D_3$ in milk are only 0.3–0.6 ng/ml [25], thus immune cells are devoid of a source of $25(OH)D_3$ after they enter the infected mammary gland. The hypothesis tested in these experiments was that infusion of $25(OH)D_3$ into the mammary gland of a dairy cow infected with *Streptococcus uberis* would reduce the severity of the infection.

Materials and Methods

Animals

Ten mid-lactation primiparous Holstein cows at the USDA National Animal Disease Center were used for this study. The National Animal Disease Center animal care and use committee approved all animal-related procedures used in this study (Protocol ARS-4001). Prior to the study, all cows were healthy and bacteria were not detected in their milk prior to the study. Cows were feed a standard ration, which included between 30,000 and 40,000 IU of vitamin D per day. Cows were milked two times a day.

Infection and Treatment

Mammary gland infection was induced by infusion of approximately 500 cfu of *Streptococcus uberis* strain 0140 (*S. uberis*; a gift from Dr. Max Paape, USDA, Beltsville, MD) suspended in 10 mL of FBS into one quarter of all ten cows. Infected animals were randomly divided into two treatment groups: the first group received 100 ug of $25(OH)D_3$ in 10 ml of FBS in the infected quarter at the completion of each milking, starting at the time of infection and continuing throughout the experiment. The second group received 10 ml of FBS only in the infected quarter at the completion of each milking. Antibiotics were not used during the study.

Collection of milk, blood and temperature data

Milk samples were aseptically collected from infected quarters at each milking (twice daily) throughout the study. Milk was used for determination of bacterial counts, somatic cell counts, determination of bovine serum albumin (BSA) levels, and $25(OH)D_3$ levels. Milk was serially diluted in sterile phosphate-buffered saline and spread on blood agar plates, then incubated for 24 h at 37°C. Following incubation, plates were examined for bacterial growth and colonies enumerated.

Milk somatic cell counts were determined by sampling milk, adding a preservative, and counting at a Dairy Herd Information Association (DHIA) (Dubuque, IA) approved facility. Bovine serum albumin levels in the milk were measured using a commercial ELISA quantitation kit (Bethyl Laboratories, Montgomery, TX). The kit was used according to manufacturer's protocol and protein concentrations determined using the included standards.

Blood samples (10 ml) were taken by venipuncture of the jugular vein once a day. Serum was obtained by centrifugation. The levels of $25(OH)D_3$ in the serum were determined by a radioimmunoassay [26].

Rectal temperatures were obtained twice a day, at the time of milking.

Statistical analysis

Data were analyzed as a completely randomized design (JMP version 7 SAS Institute Inc., Cary, NC). Cow served as the experimental unit in the analysis of all data. Effects of treatments on variables (i.e. bacterial counts, rectal temperatures, somatic cell counts, serum albumin, feed intake, milk production) were analyzed with repeated-measures ANOVA. Bacterial and somatic cell counts were log10 transformed prior to analysis. The model included the fixed effects of treatment, time, and treatment x time interaction. Post hoc tests were applied when treatment, time, or treatment x time effects were detected. The values presented for all variables are the means and standard errors of the mean.

Results

All ten animals were successfully infected with *S. uberis*. Establishment of infection was indicated by at least one time point having a bacterial count of greater than 1000 cfu/ml (data not shown). Figure 1 shows the mean bacterial counts of the $25(OH)D_3$ treated group and the control group. There was a significant effect ($P<0.05$) of the $25(OH)D_3$ treatment (figure 1). In addition, there were significant reductions ($P<0.05$) in milk bacterial counts at the fourth, sixth, and ninth milkings in the $25(OH)D_3$ treatment group compared to the control group.

Additional indicators of a mammary gland infection were monitored, including rectal temperatures, somatic cell counts, and BSA in the milk. Rectal temperatures showed a $25(OH)D_3$ treatment effect with a $P = 0.065$ and are plotted in figure 2. There was a continuation of the trend that the $25(OH)D_3$ treated group had a better clinical outcome, in that somatic cell counts were lower in the $25(OH)D_3$ treated group (figure 3). Acute bacterial infections are known to increase mammary vascular permeability, an indicator of this change is increased BSA levels in milk [27]. Milk from the morning milking was tested by ELISA for BSA (figure 4). Day 3 levels of BSA were higher in the control animals compared to the $25(OH)D_3$ treated animals ($P = 0.07$).

Mastitis causes reduction of both feed intake and milk productions, and the level of reduction correlates with the severity of the infection. The pre-infected feed intake and milk production was calculated as the average of the values from the four days prior to the infection. There was a trend for the $25(OH)D_3$ treated animals to have higher average feed intake (figure 5). There was a significant ($P <0.05$) time x treatment effect, as the $25(OH)D_3$ treated animals milk production decline due to the infection occurred later in the infection compared to control cows (figure 6).

Table 1 shows the blood serum levels of $25(OH)D_3$ in the control animals compared to the $25(OH)D_3$ treated animals. This data demonstrates that the dose of 100 ug $25(OH)D_3$ twice daily did not affect ($P>0.10$) blood serum $25(OH)D_3$ levels.

Discussion

In a recent review it was stated that "Data from several models of infection have so far not supported a role of vitamin D in affecting the course of disease" [28]. These authors' conclusions are based on 1) the lack of in vivo evidence for an effect of vitamin D status on the course of disease and 2) the findings that 1,

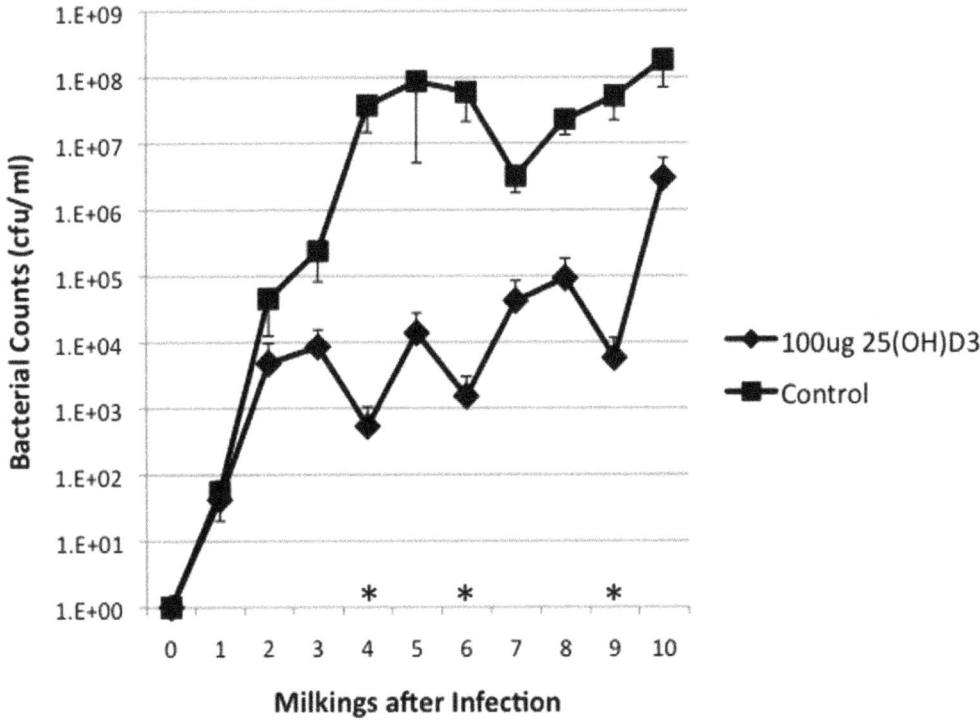

Figure 1. Bacterial Counts in Control and 25(OH)D₃ Treated Animals. Ten dairy cattle were infused with approximately 500 cfu of *S. uberis* in one quarter of their mammary gland. Five cows were immediately treated with 100 ug of 25(OH)D₃ in FBS and the remain five cows were treated with FBS alone. Cows were subsequently treated after each milking (twice daily) with 25(OH)D₃ or FBS for 10 milkings (5 days). Milk sample were isolated from each cow and serially diluted and plated on blood agar plates. Average bacterial counts were determined for 25(OH)D₃ treated (υ) and control animals(v). Time points with statistically significant differences are indicated with (*).

$25(OH)_2D_3$ inhibits T helper cell functions that are important in many infections and which we have characterized in vitro using a cow model [29]. The data presented in this study demonstrate that in vivo administration of $25(OH)D_3$, used as a treatment, reduces the severity of an intramammary infection. The effectiveness of $25(OH)D_3$ may be due to many factors, including a predominant

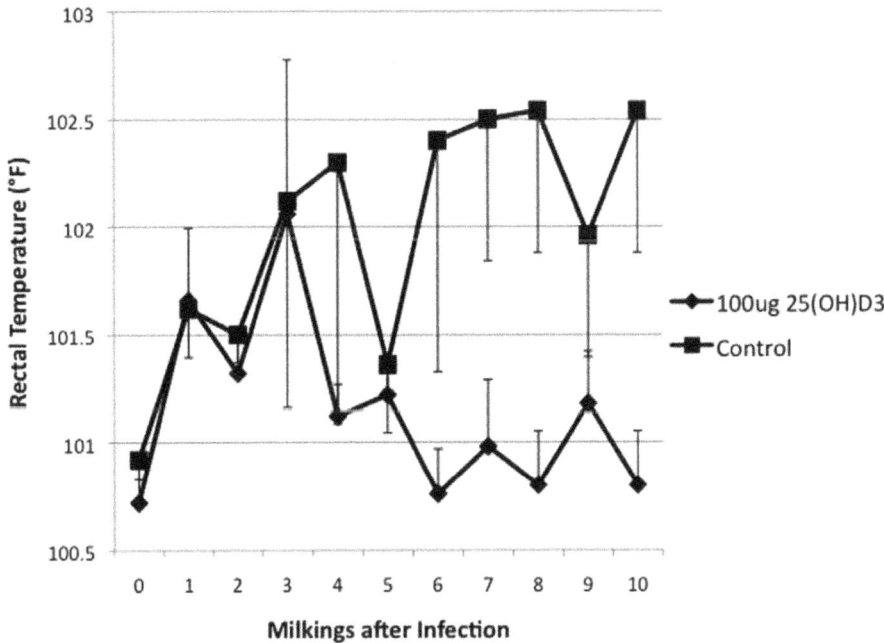

Figure 2. Rectal Temperature in Control and 25(OH)D₃ Treated Animals. Rectal temperature were taken twice daily, at each milking, and the average was determined for 25(OH)D₃ treated (υ) and control animals(v).

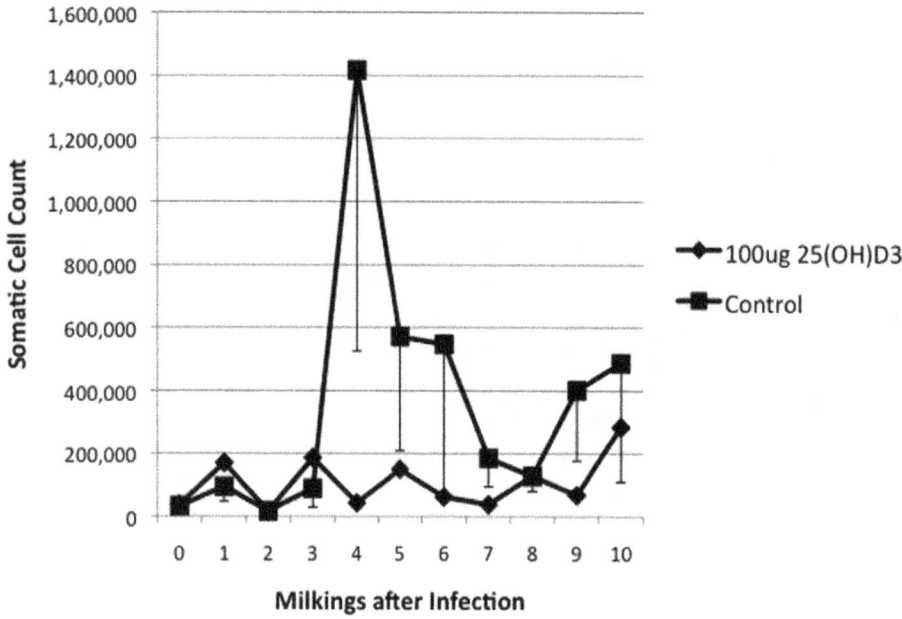

Figure 3. Somatic Cell Counts in Control and 25(OH)D₃ Treated Animals. Milk samples for somatic cells counts (SCC) were taken at each milking and sent to a DHIA facility for counting. The average SCC were determined for 25(OH)D₃ treated (υ) and control animals(v).

role of the innate immune response in mastitis and that the milk normally has low 25(OH)D₃ levels. Monocytes/macrophages play a critical role in the immune response to mastitis [30] and intracrine produced 1,25(OH)2D3 effects many aspects of the innate immune system [31] and specifically macrophages antimicrobial mechanisms [2,5]. Our ability to demonstrate in

vivo efficacy of 25(OH)D₃ on a bacterial infection (figure 1) may be due to the fact that the milk compartment of the mammary gland is relatively devoid of 25(OH)D₃, even though systemic vitamin D status is excellent (table 1). Concentrations of 25(OH)D₃ in milk are only 0.3–0.6 ng/ml compared to 35 ng/ml in serum considered necessary for full immune function [17,18,25]. It may

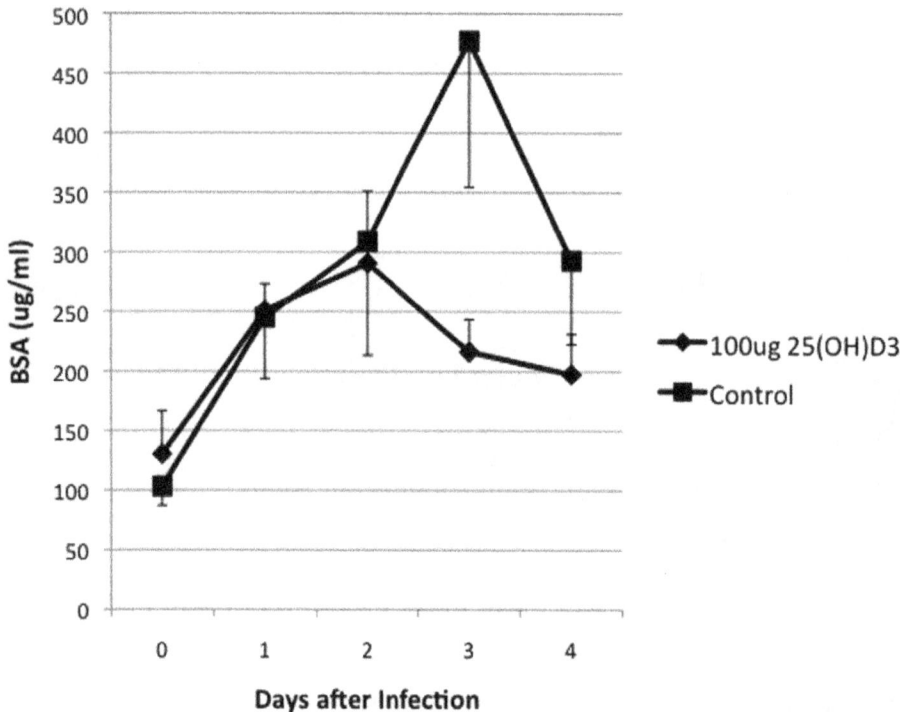

Figure 4. Bovine Serum Albumin in Milk of Control and 25(OH)D₃ Treated Animals. Milk samples were tested for BSA levels at each time point and the average was determined for 25(OH)D₃ treated (υ) and control animals(v).

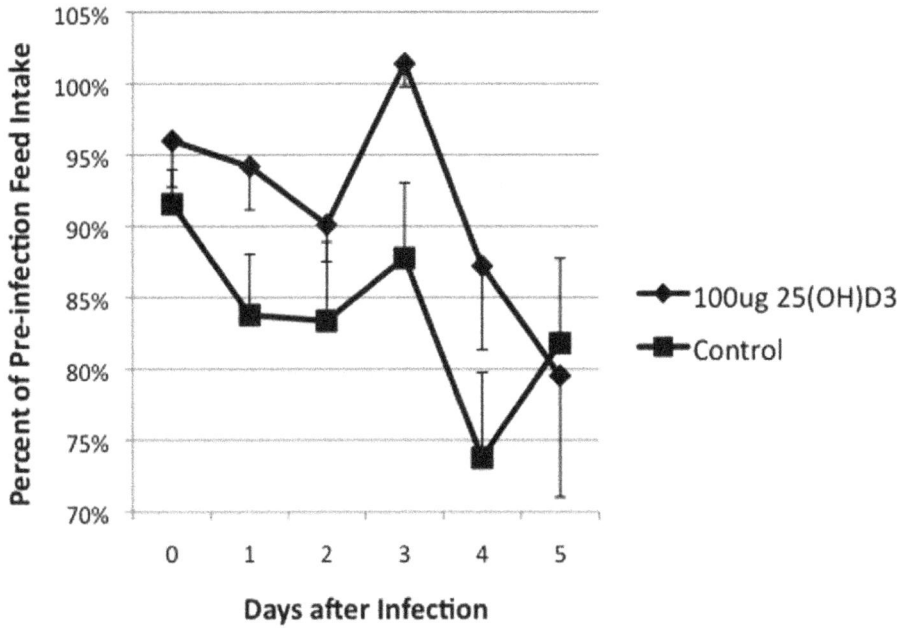

Figure 5. Feed Intake in Control and 25(OH)D₃ Treated Animals. Daily feed intake was determined for each cow. Data are expressed as a percentage of the pre-infections (the average of the 4 days feed intake prior to infection). Each the average was determined for 25(OH)D₃ treated (υ) and control animals(ν).

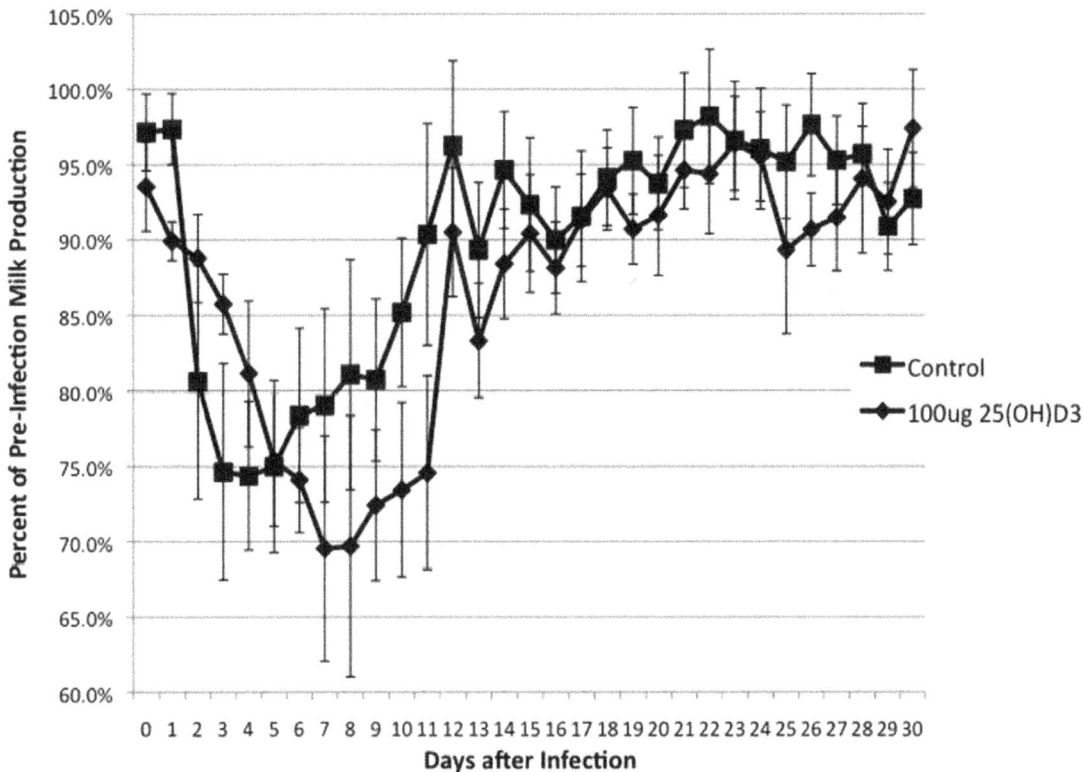

Figure 6. Milk Production in Control and 25(OH)D₃ Treated Animals. Daily milk production was determined for each cow. Data are expressed as a percentage of the pre-infections (the average of the 4 days milk production prior to infection). Each the average was determined for 25(OH)D₃ treated (υ) and control animals(ν). Repeated measures analysis showed a significant treatment x time effect.

Table 1. Serum levels of 25(OH)D$_3$ in the cows treated with 100 ug 25(OH)D$_3$ infused into the mammary gland and cows untreated.

	No treatment (ng/ml)	25(OH)D3 (ng/ml)
Day 0	50.9±3.0	47.7±4.8
Day 4	52.6±7.5	54.3±7.5
Day 10	60.0±8.3	59.7±9.8

Numbers represent the mean±standard error of the mean.

be that treatment with 25(OH)D$_3$ in individuals with sufficient circulating 25(OH)D$_3$, will only be effective for infections in anatomical locations with low concentrations of 25(OH)D$_3$, such as the mammary gland, and possilby the lung, and upper respiratory tract. It is thus important to note that the data presented here did not directly address the broader issue of "systemic vitamin D status" on the course of disease. However, these data clearly demonstrate that increasing 25(OH)D$_3$ concentrations in a tissue with low 25(OH)D$_3$ concentrations can positively influence the early course of the disease.

In this study, the treatment of an intramammary infection with 25(OH)D$_3$ reduced bacterial counts (figure 1), decreased the severity of the disease (figures 2, 3, 4, 5), and delayed loss of milk production (figure 6). Based on human studies [16] these results would depend on the ability of activated monocytes/macrophages to produce 1,25(OH)$_2$D$_3$ from 25(OH)D$_3$ and to induce antibacterial peptides such as cathelicidin. Bovine monocytes/macrophages produces 1,25(OH)$_2$D$_3$ from 25(OH)D$_3$ both in vitro [4] and in vivo [3] following bacterial activation. Unlike human monocytes, bovine moncytes stimulated with 1,25(OH)$_2$D$_3$ does not lead to the induction of antibacterial cathelicidins in the cattle [4]. To date, only a few genes in bovine have been identified as responsive to 1,25(OH)$_2$D$_3$, namely, nitric oxide synthetase , the chemokine RANTES, vitamin D receptor, S100 calcium binding protein A12 (S100A12), and 24-hydroxylase [3,4,29]. Presumably other immune mediators are involved in the vitamin D immune pathway and experiments to determine them are ongoing. We do not know whether the lower bacterial counts in the 25(OH)D$_3$ treated animal are the result of enhanced nitric oxide killing, specific leukocyte recruitment, and/or production of a yet unidentified antibacterial peptide.

Administration of 25(OH)D$_3$ is known to affect the innate immune system [2,17,31]. In the case of humans 1,25(OH)$_2$D$_3$ treatment can cause increased expression of cathelicidins or defensins [32], and in the case of cattle 1,25(OH)$_2$D$_3$ treatment can cause increased expression in nitric oxide and RANTES [4]. Since the first significant affect of 25(OH)D$_3$ treatment was seen at 48 hours (fourth milking) of infection, it is likely that the affect of 1,25(OH)$_2$D$_3$ treatment is on the innate immune system. However, we have recently shown that the bovine adaptive immune system is also sensitive to 25(OH)D$_3$ treatment [29]. In those experiments, cattle were immunized with an antigen several weeks prior to the experiment. We showed that antigen-stimulated PBMC from those immunized cattle, when treated with antigen and 25(OH)D$_3$ suppressed IFN-γ and IL-17F in T cells. The role of T cells in bovine mastitis is not well defined, however, reinfection of animals treated and not treated with 25(OH)D$_3$ would begin to assess the role of the affect of vitamin D on the adaptive immune system during an infection.

At the end of this experiment all animals were treated with antibiotics to eliminate the *S. uberis* infections indicating that 25(OH)D$_3$ treatment alone was not an effective in eliminating the infection. However, the reduction in the number of bacteria and severity of disease shown in this study suggests that 25(OH)D$_3$ may be effective in combination with antibiotics. This combined-treatment approach may allow for reductions in antibiotic use and diminish concerns about antibiotic residues in the dairy products and development of antibiotic resistance in food animals. Although not evaluated in the present study a combined antibiotic and vitamin D therapy may provide an effective treatment strategy for chronic infections that are not effectively treated by antibiotics alone.

In conclusion we demonstrated for the first time a positive in vivo effect of intramammary administration of 25(OH)D$_3$ on the course of a bacterial infection in the mammary gland. This finding suggested a significant non-antibiotic complimentary role for 25(OH)D$_3$ in the treatment of infections in compartments naturally low in 25(OH)D$_3$ such as the mammary gland and by extension, a potentially useful treatment of lung/respiratory tract infections via aerosol administration. These experiments were designed to focus on the early innate immune response to experimental intramammary infection and do not address to affect of 25(OH)D$_3$ on adaptive immunity to bacterial infections. Further studies will be needed to address these important questions.

Acknowledgments

We thank Duane Zimmerman, Randy Atchison, and Derrel Hoy (USDA National Animal Disease Center, Ames, IA) for their technical assistance.

Author Contributions

Conceived and designed the experiments: JDL TAR. Performed the experiments: JDL. Analyzed the data: JDL TAR RAS CDN. Contributed reagents/materials/analysis tools: JDL TAR BJN. Wrote the paper: JDL TAR RAS BJN CDN.

References

1. Adams JS, Hewison M (2008) Unexpected actions of vitamin D: new perspectives on the regulation of innate and adaptive immunity. Nat Clin Pract Endocrinol Metab 4: 80–90. doi:10.1038/ncpendmet0716.

2. Liu PT, Modlin RL (2008) Human macrophage host defense against Mycobacterium tuberculosis. Current Opinion in Immunology 20: 371–376. doi:10.1016/j.coi.2008.05.014.

3. Nelson CD, Reinhardt TA, Beitz DC, Lippolis JD (2010) In vivo activation of the intracrine vitamin d pathway in innate immune cells and mammary tissue during a bacterial infection. PLoS ONE 5: e15469. doi:10.1371/journal.pone.0015469.

4. Nelson CD, Reinhardt TA, Thacker TC, Beitz DC, Lippolis JD (2010) Modulation of the bovine innate immune response by production of 1alpha,25-dihydroxyvitamin D(3) in bovine monocytes. J Dairy Sci 93: 1041–1049. doi:10.3168/jds.2009-2663.

5. Adams JS, Ren S, Liu PT, Chun RF, Lagishetty V, et al. (2009) Vitamin d-directed rheostatic regulation of monocyte antibacterial responses. J Immunol 182: 4289–4295. doi:10.4049/jimmunol.0803736.

6. Barbour GL, Coburn JW, Slatopolsky E, Norman AW, Horst RL (1981) Hypercalcemia in an anephric patient with sarcoidosis: evidence for extrarenal generation of 1,25-dihydroxyvitamin D. N. Engl. J. Med. 305: 440–443. doi:10.1056/NEJM198108203050807.

7. Adams JS, Sharma OP, Gacad MA, Singer FR (1983) Metabolism of 25-hydroxyvitamin D3 by cultured pulmonary alveolar macrophages in sarcoidosis. J Clin Invest 72: 1856–1860. doi:10.1172/JCI111147.

8. Reinhardt TA, Horst RL, Littledike ET, Beitz DC (1982) 1,25-Dihydroxyvitamin D3 receptor in bovine thymus gland. Biochemical and Biophysical Research Communications 106: 1012–1018.

9. Lemire JM, Adams JS, Sakai R, Jordan SC (1984) 1 alpha,25-dihydroxyvitamin D3 suppresses proliferation and immunoglobulin production by normal human peripheral blood mononuclear cells. J Clin Invest 74: 657–661. doi:10.1172/JCI111465.

10. Provvedini DM, Tsoukas CD, Deftos LJ, Manolagas SC (1983) 1,25-dihydroxyvitamin D3 receptors in human leukocytes. Science 221: 1181–1183.

11. Bhalla AK, Amento EP, Clemens TL, Holick MF, Krane SM (1983) Specific high-affinity receptors for 1,25-dihydroxyvitamin D3 in human peripheral blood mononuclear cells: presence in monocytes and induction in T lymphocytes following activation. J Clin Endocrinol Metab 57: 1308–1310.

12. Chocano-Bedoya P, Ronnenberg AG (2009) Vitamin D and tuberculosis. Nutrition Reviews 67: 289–293. doi:10.1111/j.1753-4887.2009.00195.x.

13. Rook GA, Steele J, Fraher L, Barker S, Karmali R, et al. (1986) Vitamin D3, gamma interferon, and control of proliferation of Mycobacterium tuberculosis by human monocytes. Immunology 57: 159–163.

14. Girasole G, Wang JM, Pedrazzoni M, Pioli G, Balotta C, et al. (1990) Augmentation of monocyte chemotaxis by 1 alpha,25-dihydroxyvitamin D3. Stimulation of defective migration of AIDS patients. J Immunol 145: 2459–2464.

15. Reinhardt TA, Stabel JR, Goff JP (1999) 1,25-dihydroxyvitamin D3 enhances milk antibody titers to Escherichia coli J5 vaccine. J Dairy Sci 82: 1904–1909.

16. Liu PT, Stenger S, Li H, Wenzel L, Tan BH, et al. (2006) Toll-like receptor triggering of a vitamin D-mediated human antimicrobial response. Science 311: 1770–1773. doi:10.1126/science.1123933.

17. Adams JS, Hewison M (2010) Update in vitamin D. J Clin Endocrinol Metab 95: 471–478. doi:10.1210/jc.2009-1773.

18. Hollis BW (2005) Circulating 25-hydroxyvitamin D levels indicative of vitamin D sufficiency: implications for establishing a new effective dietary intake recommendation for vitamin D. J Nutr 135: 317–322.

19. Ginde AA, Liu MC, Camargo CA (2009) Demographic differences and trends of vitamin D insufficiency in the US population, 1988-2004. Arch. Intern. Med. 169: 626–632. doi:10.1001/archinternmed.2008.604.

20. Ginde AA, Mansbach JM, Camargo CA (2009) Vitamin D, respiratory infections, and asthma. Curr Allergy Asthma Rep 9: 81–87.

21. Nnoaham KE, Clarke A (2008) Low serum vitamin D levels and tuberculosis: a systematic review and meta-analysis. Int J Epidemiol 37: 113–119. doi:10.1093/ije/dym247.

22. Munger KL, Levin LI, Hollis BW, Howard NS, Ascherio A (2006) Serum 25-hydroxyvitamin D levels and risk of multiple sclerosis. JAMA 296: 2832–2838. doi:10.1001/jama.296.23.2832.

23. Burton JM, Kimball S, Vieth R, Bar-Or A, Dosch H-M, et al. (2010) A phase I/II dose-escalation trial of vitamin D3 and calcium in multiple sclerosis. Neurology 74: 1852–1859. doi:10.1212/WNL.0b013e3181e1cec2.

24. Urashima M, Segawa T, Okazaki M, Kurihara M, Wada Y, et al. (2010) Randomized trial of vitamin D supplementation to prevent seasonal influenza A in schoolchildren. Am J Clin Nutr 91: 1255–1260. doi:10.3945/ajcn.2009.29094.

25. Hollis BW, Roos BA, Draper HH, Lambert PW (1981) Vitamin D and its metabolites in human and bovine milk. J Nutr 111: 1240–1248.

26. Hollis BW, Kamerud JQ, Selvaag SR, Lorenz JD, Napoli JL (1993) Determination of vitamin D status by radioimmunoassay with an 125I-labeled tracer. Clin Chem 39: 529–533.

27. Bannerman DD, Paape MJ, Goff JP, Kimura K, Lippolis JD, et al. (2004) Innate immune response to intramammary infection with Serratia marcescens and Streptococcus uberis. Vet. Res. 35: 681–700. doi:10.1051/vetres:2004040.

28. Bruce D, Ooi JH, Yu S, Cantorna MT (2010) Vitamin D and host resistance to infection? Putting the cart in front of the horse. Exp Biol Med (Maywood) 235: 921–927. doi:10.1258/ebm.2010.010061.

29. Nelson CD, Nonnecke BJ, Reinhardt TA, Waters WR, Beitz DC, et al. (2011) Regulation of mycobacterium-specific mononuclear cell responses by 25-hydroxyvitamin d(3). PLoS ONE 6: e21674. doi:10.1371/journal.pone.0021674.

30. Sordillo LM, Shafer-Weaver K, DeRosa D (1997) Immunobiology of the mammary gland. J Dairy Sci 80: 1851–1865. doi:10.3168/jds.S0022-0302(97)76121-6.

31. Hewison M (2010) Vitamin D and the intracrinology of innate immunity. Molecular and cellular endocrinology 321: 103–111. doi:10.1016/j.mce.2010.02.013.

32. Adams JS, Liu PT, Chun R, Modlin RL, Hewison M (2007) Vitamin D in defense of the human immune response. Annals of the New York Academy of Sciences 1117: 94–105. doi:10.1196/annals.1402.036.

17

Meloxicam and Buprenorphine Treatment after Ovarian Transplantation Does Not Affect Estrous Cyclicity and Follicular Integrity in Aged CBA/J Mice

Anna H. Le, Luis A. Bonachea, Shelley L. Cargill*

Department of Biological Sciences, San José State University, San José, California, United States of America

Abstract

Angiogenesis, the formation of new blood vessels, is important for the survival of ovarian transplants and the restoration of ovarian functions. Without angiogenesis, transplanted ovarian tissue becomes more susceptible to tissue damage and necrosis. Administration of analgesics for pain management has been shown to decrease angiogenesis, which can influence transplant success especially in aged animals. Aging and the effects of hypoxia after transplantation decrease reproductive viability of the ovarian transplant; therefore, it is important to understand the additional effects of analgesics on aged animal models. The present study investigated the effects of two analgesics, buprenorphine, an opiate, and meloxicam, a non-steroidal anti-inflammatory drug (NSAID), on the reproductive indicators related to estrous cyclicity and follicular integrity after ovarian transplantation of young ovaries into aged CBA/J mice. These aged females did not show any different reproductive responses when treated with either buprenorphine or meloxicam. No significant differences were observed in estrous cycle length, the onset of estrous cycling, the regularity of estrous cycles, and the proportion of viable follicles and total number of follicles per ovarian sample across treatment groups.

Editor: Shree Ram Singh, National Cancer Institute, United States of America

Funding: This work was supported by: California State University Research Funds to SC; Junior Faculty Career Development Grant to SC; John and Betty Davison Fellowship to AL. The funders had no role in study design, data collection and analysis, decision to publish, or preparation of the manuscript.

Competing Interests: The authors have declared that no competing interests exist.

* Email: shelley.cargill@sjsu.edu

Introduction

Angiogenesis, the development of new blood vessels, is important during normal tissue development and healing. Angiogenesis, therefore, is an important determinant in the outcomes of organ transplantation as tissues require a continuous supply of nutrients, oxygen, and hormones as well as a route for removal of wastes in order to maintain viability. Angiogenic processes in normal tissue, as opposed to tumors, decrease into adulthood but occur regularly in the adult female reproductive system [1], [2]. In female rodents, angiogenesis is particularly important for the estrous cycle, which regulates varying levels of estrogen and progesterone for ovarian functions [3], [4], [5].

While the use of analgesics is advised in survival surgeries to minimize pain and discomfort in research animals, analgesics can reduce angiogenesis [6], [7], [8], [9], [10]. Although not all of the interactions of analgesics and angiogenesis have been elucidated, the putative anti-angiogenic effects of the two classes of analgesics, opiates and NSAIDs, have been investigated in some *in vivo* and *in vitro* studies [6], [7], [8], [9], [10].

In a previous aging study, the transplantation of ovaries from young CBA mice into aged, late-reproductive female mice significantly increased the remaining life expectancy of the recipients [11]. In that experiment, nearly all transplantations performed were successful, as was indicated by the restoration of estrous cyclicity. Further experiments were performed, with all procedural details kept consistent except for the additional use of post-surgery buprenorphine [12]. However, unpublished data from the same experiment suggested several unsuccessful transplants, as indicated by the lack of estrous cyclicity after surgery. It is possible that the post-surgical administration of analgesics negatively influenced transplantation success by decreasing angiogenesis and thereby decreasing the blood supply to the transplant [6], [7], [8], [9], [10].

Aging has long been acknowledged in its role in decreased female fertility [13], [14]. Angiogenesis becomes deficient with age [15] and may negatively influence reproductive function. Aged 40–48 week old female ICR mice showed a higher frequency of oocytes with DNA fragmentation, implying increased apoptotic cells compared with young 7–8 week old mice and 20–24 week old mice [13]. Estrous cycles become extended in aged mice, often leading to the cessation of cycling [14]. In addition to the effects of aging, ischemic injury due to transplantation may cause decreased viability of ovarian transplants [16], [17]. It has been demonstrated that ovarian size and the number of follicles were dramatically decreased after orthotopic grafting in mice [16]. Although mice have also demonstrated the restoration of reproductive cycling after transplantation, distinguishable estrous cycles were not always clear [17]. The use of aged models that are subject to treatment with analgesics for ovarian transplantation may have compounding effects on reproductive function. This highlights the importance of evaluating analgesic effects in aged transplant recipients to understand its impact in future transplantation studies in aged animals.

The effects of two analgesics, buprenorphine and meloxicam, on ovarian transplant success in aged females were evaluated and compared using follicular analysis, ovarian size, and estrous cyclicity post-surgery as indicators of transplant viability. A decrease in the viability of the transplant would indicate decreased angiogenesis [4], [5]. As the two different classes of analgesics have different mechanisms of action, the two analgesics may have different effects on angiogenesis and transplant viability [18], [19], [20].

Materials and Methods

Ethics Statement

This study was carried out in strict accordance with the recommendations in the Guide for the Care and Use of Laboratory Animals of the National Institutes of Health. All experimental procedures were approved by the Institutional Animal Care and Use Committee at San Jose State University (Protocol #959). Surgery was performed under sodium pentobarbital anesthesia, and all efforts were made to minimize suffering.

Mice

Adult CBA/J strain female mice (Jackson Laboratory, Sacramento, CA) were housed under controlled conditions of temperature ($21 \pm 2°C$), humidity (minimum 50%) and lighting (12L:12D, lights on at 0700 hours) in accordance to the University Animal Care guidelines with approval by the San José State University Institutional Animal Care and Use Committee. Animals received feed (Purina Mouse Chow 5008: 23.5% protein, 6.5% fat; Purina Mills. St Louis, MO) and water (deionized) *ad libitum*. Through power analysis, we determined that a sample size of nine focal animals per treatment group would be needed to detect a one-tailed mean difference between groups in the range of 1.5–2 standard deviations from the control animals for a single response. A sample size of 10 animals per group was chosen to account for the roughly 5% transplant failure rate and 5% seizure loss rate observed in previous studies (pers. obs.). For every experimental animal, a donor female was used to supply transplant ovaries, giving a total of 60 female mice anticipated for use in this study. As a note for other researchers, while CBA/J mice are known to be prone to seizures [21], we did not anticipate the high percentage of animals that died of seizures before the end of the study (n = 4, roughly 13%). Prior to surgery, three females died due to seizures and were excluded from the study. As a result, 27 recipient and 27 donor females were used in the transplantation procedures. Recipient and donor females were group housed with 5 animals per $26 \times 17 \times 13$-cm cage until surgery. After surgery, each recipient female was housed individually in a $26 \times 17 \times 13$-cm cage for the duration of the experiment. Male mice were housed in cages adjacent to female mice to promote estrous cycling in females [22].

Surgical Procedures and Vaginal Cytology

Bilateral ovariectomies of and ovarian transplantations to recipients at 11 months of age were carried out as previously described [23] with the following exception: the ovarian bursa was closed with one suture of 7-0 Ethilon nylon filament (Ethicon, San Angelo, TX) instead of the 6-0 suture [23]. The transplanted ovaries were from 2-month old females of the same strain [23]. Reproductive data in the form of vaginal cytology were collected via vaginal lavage daily at 0730 hours for one month when the recipient females were 5 months old (pre-surgery), for 14 days immediately prior to ovarian transplantation surgery, and daily starting three days after ovarian transplantation surgery for approximately 75 days (73–76 days) until the end of the experiment. All vaginal cytology data were assessed as wet mounts without staining. Donor mice were housed in close proximity to males for 1–3 weeks prior to use and were at an age considered to be reproductively competent [11] [12]. Donor mice estrous cyclicity was confirmed after surgery, as all ovarian transplant recipients cycled within 10 days after receiving the transplant. At recipient female ovariectomy, complete removal of all recipient ovarian tissue was visually confirmed under stereomicroscopy. At sacrifice, the presence of only transplanted ovarian tissue was visually confirmed under stereomicroscopy, and upon removal for analysis, no residual ovarian fragments from the ovariectomized recipient ovary were observed.

Analgesic Administration

For administration of drug treatments after surgeries, meloxicam, buprenorphine, and 0.9% saline (no analgesics) were randomly assigned to nine females each. Two saline-treated females died during the course of the experiment. One female died during the transplantation process due to anesthesia complications. CBA/J mice are susceptible to seizures, which may have been the cause of an approximately 1 month post-surgery premature death for the second female [21]. Both of these females from the saline control group were excluded from the study, for a new n of seven. After the unplanned losses in the saline group, the final sample size of n = 7 for the saline group would have allowed us to detect a difference as small as 1.9 SD from the mean of the saline group. The meloxicam treatment group received IP meloxicam (Boehringer Ingelheim, St. Joseph, MO) doses of 5 mg/kg of body weight, the buprenorphine treatment group received IP buprenorphine (Reckitt Benckiser Healthcare, Hull, England) doses of 0.05 mg/kg of body weight, and the saline-control group received IP 0.9% saline (Vedco, Inc., St. Joseph, MO) with the same volumes given with analgesic treatments. The analgesic doses administered were in accordance of veterinary recommendations and previous studies [12], [24], [25], [26]. These treatments were administered every 12 hours for 48 hours post-surgery, with the first dose of treatment administered at the end of surgery prior to recovery from anesthesia.

Fixation and Preservation of Ovaries

All female mice were randomly reassigned a new identification number for subsequent follicular analysis and sacrificed by cervical dislocation. Immediately after sacrifice, one ovary from each female was placed into optimal cutting temperature (OCT) medium (Sakura Finetek, Torrance, CA) and frozen over isopentane (Fisher Scientific, Fair Lawn, NJ) and dry ice (Praxair Distribution Inc., San Jose, CA). The fixed and frozen ovaries were transported overnight by FedEx to IHC World (Ellicott City, MD) to be sectioned using a cryostat. Serial consecutive sections of 6 μm thickness were placed onto glass microscope slides (TruBond, Woodstock, MD) and shipped to San Jose, CA. Upon receipt of the shipment, slides were immediately stored in $-80°C$ until staining with hematoxylin and eosin. Nine consecutive sections per ovary were used for follicular analysis. Analyses made from these nine tissue sections are referred to as a single ovarian sample.

Histological Staining and Assessment

After removal of slides from $-80°C$ storage, slides were warmed to room temperature, fixed in ice cold acetone (Fisher Scientific,

Santa Clara, CA) and rinsed twice in phosphate buffered saline (PBS). The primary stain, Mayer's hematoxylin (Thermo Fisher Lab Vision, Fremont, CA), was applied for five seconds, then rinsed under running tap water for 30 seconds. Slides were counterstained with 0.5% eosin Y in 95% ethanol (Allied Chemical & Dye Corp, New York, NY) for two minutes and rinsed with distilled water by dipping the slide ten times. Slides were dehydrated using 95% ethanol followed by 100% ethanol (Fisher Scientific, Pittsburgh, PA), cleared using xylene (Fisher Scientific, Fair Lawn, NJ) and a coverslip was applied using SecureMount^{TM} mounting medium (Fisher Scientific, Kalamazoo, MI).

Hematoxylin and eosin stained slides were utilized for determination of follicle numbers and the mean cross sectional area from each ovarian sample. Follicular data were collected from images captured on a Leica ICC550HD camera (JH Technologies, Fremont, CA) that had been fitted on a Leica DM500 microscope (JH Technologies, Fremont, CA) at a total magnification of 100X. Cross sectional area per ovarian sample was measured in ImageJ software (National Institutes of Health, Bethesda, MD).

Both viable and atretic follicles were counted from serial sections of each ovarian sample and viable follicles were analyzed as a proportion of the total number of follicles counted. To avoid duplication of follicle numbers, only the follicles with nuclei present in the section were counted. If a follicle did not have a nucleus present on any of the sections, the relative position of the follicle was noted to ensure the follicle was counted only once. Follicular classifications were determined based on previously described classifications [1], [27]. Representative follicle types in this study are depicted in Figure 1.

Statistical Analyses

All vaginal smear data and follicular analyses were recorded and analyzed blind with respect to treatment. Prior to vaginal cytology analyses and follicular analyses, all animals were randomly reassigned a new identification number, which was not disclosed to the person observing the slides or performing estrous stage classification.

Estrous cycle length was determined by counting the number of days from proestrus to the next proestrus [15], [28], [29]. The 75 days of post ovarian transplantation vaginal smears were divided into three blocks of 25 days: Block 1 (days 1–25 after surgeries), Block 2 (days 26–50 after surgeries), and Block 3 (days 51–75 after surgeries). The mean estrous cycle length across treatment groups was analyzed for all 75 days and for each block. In addition, the onset of estrous cycle was determined by the number of days after surgery to the first proestrus. Finally, the estrous cycles from each animal were classified into three categories: regular (4–5 days in length with either 1–2 days of estrus or 2–3 days of diestrus), extended (3–4 consecutive days of estrus or 4–5 consecutive days of diestrus), and abnormal (more than 4 consecutive days of estrus or more than 6 consecutive days of diestrus) [28].

Estrous cycle lengths (days) for all 75-days post-surgery and the onset of estrous cycle (days) across treatment groups were compared using Kruskal-Wallis ANOVA as the data failed the Shapiro-Wilk Test for normality. The estrous cycle lengths (days) for the three blocks were rank transformed and analyzed using MANOVA as the data were not normally distributed as determined by the Shapiro-Wilk Test. Whether or not individuals from each treatment group cycled until the end of the study was compared using a Chi-square Test of Independence. The differences in the number of regular, extended, and abnormal cycles between treatments were rank transformed and compared using MANOVA as the data failed the Shapiro-Wilk Test for normality. Classifications of estrous cycles were also compared using the Chi-square Test of Independence for differences in the percentage of females between treatments that exhibited abnormal cycles *versus* those that did not. A separate Chi-square Test of Independence was used to test the differences in the percentage of females between treatments that did and did not exhibit extended cycles. Percentage of viable follicles and the total number of follicles counted per ovarian sample were compared using MANOVA. The cross sectional area per ovarian sample of each treatment group was compared using Kruskal-Wallis ANOVA as the data failed the Levene's Test for Homogeneity of Variances.

Results

Estrous Cyclicity

Estrous cycle length was not significantly different across groups (Kruskal-Wallis ANOVA: $\chi^2 = 0.92$, df = 2, $p = 0.63$; Figure 2A). The median estrous cycle length for the saline-control was 7.7 days ($n = 6$, $Q_1 = 7.3$, $Q_3 = 8.1$), for the buprenorphine-treated was 6.9 days ($n = 8$, $Q_1 = 6.2$, $Q_3 = 9.1$), and for the meloxicam-treated was 7.2 days ($n = 8$, $Q_1 = 6.1$, $Q_3 = 8.3$). One female from each treatment group was excluded from analysis due to abnormal cycle lengths (>3 standard deviations from the sample mean).

The cycle lengths during Block 1 (days 1–25 after surgeries), Block 2 (days 26–50), and Block 3 (days 51–75) were not

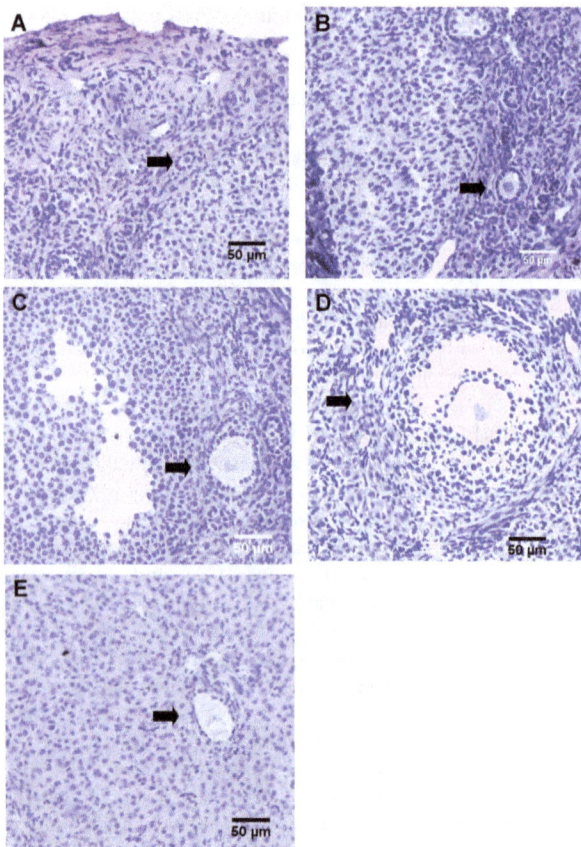

Figure 1. Representative follicle types, H&E stain, 100X total magnification. (A) primordial follicle, (B) primary follicle, (C) secondary follicle, (D) antral follicle, (F) atretic follicle. Corresponding follicles are marked by arrows.

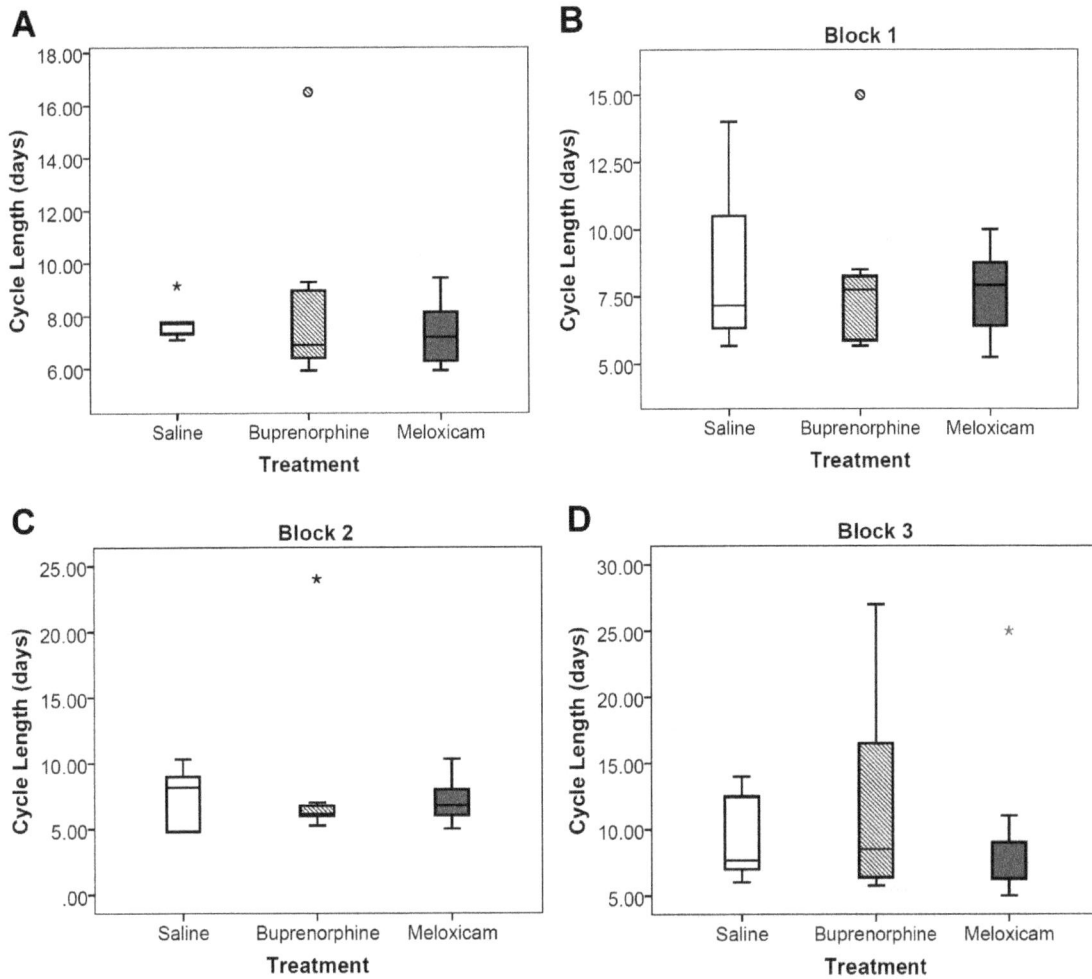

Figure 2. Boxplots of the estrous cycle length in days taken from daily vaginal cytology for each time block after surgery. (A) all 75 days (Kruskal-Wallis ANOVA: $\chi^2 = 0.92$, df = 2, $p = 0.63$). (B) block 1, days 1–25 after surgery. (C) block 2 days 26–50 after surgery. (D) block 3, days 51–75 after surgery. $N = 22$, saline ($n = 6$), buprenorphine ($n = 8$), meloxicam ($n = 8$). (Rank transformed, MANOVA: F(6,34) = 0.27, $p = 0.95$). The horizontal line in each box interior represents the median, the upper and lower whiskers show the maximum and minimum values, the upper hinge represents the 75th percentile, the lower hinge represents the 25th percentile, "o" represents an outside value, and asterisk (*) represents a far outside value.

significantly different across treatment groups in any of the three time blocks (Rank transformed, MANOVA: F(6,34) = 0.27, $p - 0.95$; Figure 2B, 2C, 2D). The median cycle length during Block 1 was 7.2 days for the saline-control ($n = 6$, $Q_1 = 6.2$, $Q_3 = 11.4$), 7.8 days for the buprenorphine-treated ($n = 8$, $Q_1 = 5.8$, $Q_3 = 8.4$), and 7.9 days for the meloxicam-treated ($n = 8$, $Q_1 = 6.4$. $Q_3 = 8.9$). During Block 2, the median cycle length was 8.2 days for saline ($Q_1 = 4.8$, $Q_3 = 9.3$), 6.1 days for buprenorphine ($Q_1 = 6.0$, $Q_3 = 6.9$), and 6.0 days for meloxicam ($Q_1 = 5.9$, $Q_3 = 8.0$). During Block 3, the median cycle length was 7.7 days for saline ($Q_1 = 6.8$, $Q_3 = 12.9$), 8.5 days for buprenorphine ($Q_1 = 6.2$, $Q_3 = 18.8$), and 6.3 days for meloxicam ($Q_1 = 6.3$, $Q_3 = 10.0$). One female from each treatment group was excluded from analysis due to no cycling in at least one of the blocks.

There was no significant difference in the time until the onset of estrous cycling between groups (Kruskal-Wallis ANOVA: $\chi^2 = 3.64$, df = 2, $p = 0.16$). Median number of days to the onset of cycling was 9.0 days for the saline-control ($n = 7$, $Q_1 = 7.00$, $Q_3 = 12.00$), 6.0 days for the buprenorphine-treated ($n = 9$, $Q_1 = 5.00$, $Q_3 = 9.00$), and 7.0 days for the meloxicam-treated ($n = 9$, $Q_1 = 5.50$, $Q_3 = 7.50$). The onset of cycling was seen as

early as 5 days post-surgery and the mean onset of estrous cycling across all treatment groups was 10 days ($SD = 10.52$) post-surgery. All females across all treatment groups exhibited estrous cyclicity after ovarian transplantation indicating successful transplantation for all recipient females.

Estrous cycle analysis showed no significant relationship between treatment and duration of cycling (whether or not a female cycled until the end of the study, Day 75) (Chi-square Test of Independence. $\chi^2 - 3.87$, df – 2, $p - 0.15$). Two females from the buprenorphine-treated group exhibited early cessation of cycling (approximately 20 days before sacrifice), while the other seven buprenorphine-treated females (77.8%) cycled until the end of the study. All females (100%) from the saline-control and meloxicam-treated groups cycled until the end of the study.

There was no significant difference across treatments in the number of regular, extended, or abnormal cycles exhibited in the 75 days post-surgery (Rank transformed, MANOVA: F(6,40) = 0.60, $p = 0.73$; Figure 3). The saline group ($n = 7$) exhibited a median of 4 regular cycles ($Q_1 = 3.0$, $Q_3 = 6.0$), 1 extended cycle ($Q_1 = 0.0$, $Q_3 = 3.0$), and 2 abnormal cycles ($Q_1 = 1.0$, $Q_3 = 3.0$). The buprenorphine group ($n = 9$) exhibited

A

B

C

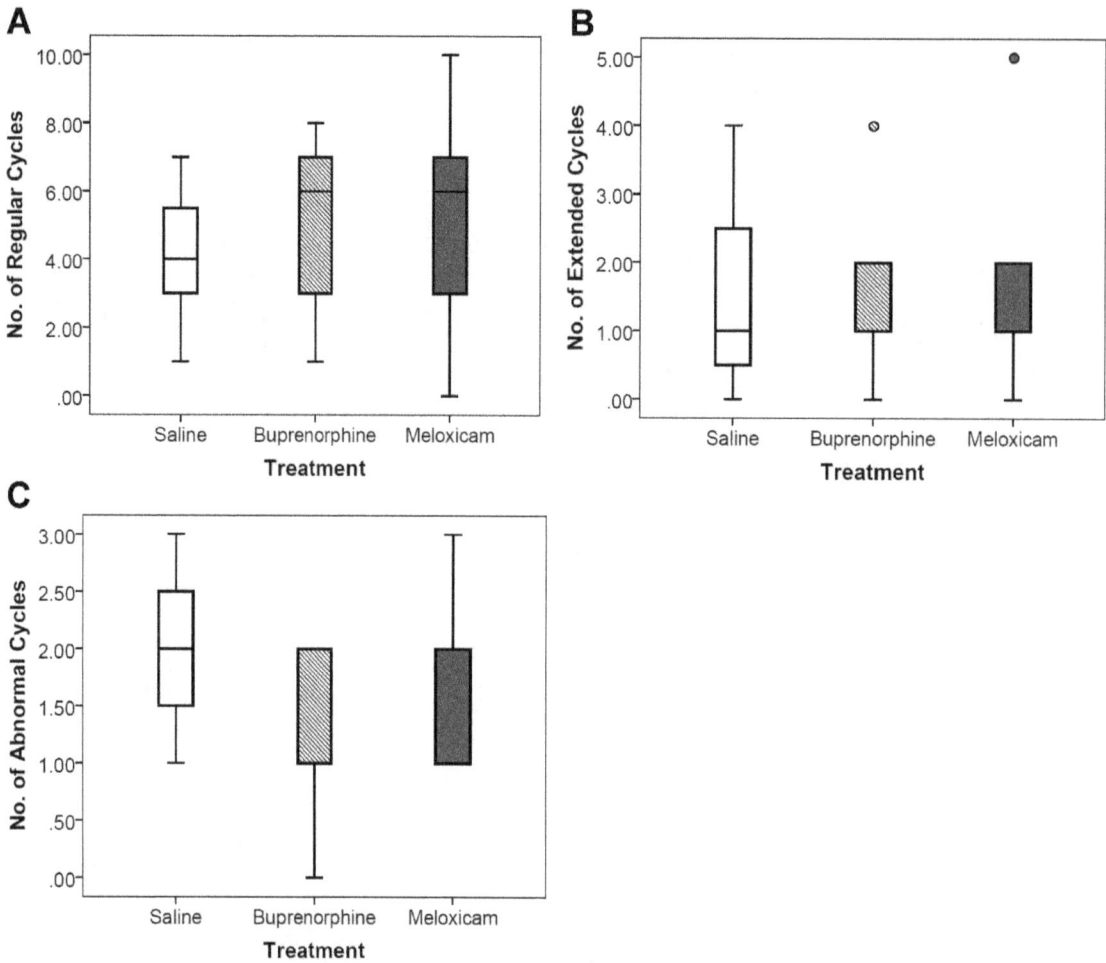

Figure 3. Boxplots of the estrous cycle classifications for each treatment. (A) regular, defined by 4–5 days in length. (B) extended, defined by 3–4 consecutive days of estrus or 4–5 consecutive days of diestrus. (C) abnormal, defined by having >4 days consecutive days of estrus or >6 consecutive days of diestrus. $N = 25$, saline ($n = 7$), buprenorphine ($n = 9$), meloxicam ($n = 9$). (Rank transformed, MANOVA: $F(6,40) = 0.60$, $p = 0.73$). The horizontal line in each box interior represents the median, the upper and lower whiskers show the maximum and minimum values, the upper hinge represents the 75th percentile, the lower hinge represents the 25th percentile, "o" represents an outside value, and asterisk (*) represents a far outside value.

a median of 6 regular cycles ($Q_1 = 3.0$, $Q_3 = 7.0$), 1 extended cycle ($Q_1 = 1.0$, $Q_3 = 2.0$), and 2 abnormal cycles ($Q_1 = 0.5$, $Q_3 = 2.0$). The meloxicam group ($n = 9$) exhibited a median of 6 regular cycles ($Q_1 = 3.0$, $Q_3 = 6.0$), 1 extended cycle ($Q_1 = 0.5$, $Q_3 = 2.0$), and 2 abnormal cycles ($Q_1 = 1.0$, $Q_3 = 2.5$).

All females in the saline-control ($n = 7$) group and the meloxicam-treated group ($n = 9$) exhibited abnormal estrous cycles (more than 4 consecutive days of estrus or more than 6 consecutive days of diestrus) compared with seven females (77.8%) in the buprenorphine-treated ($n = 9$) group. The percentages of each treatment exhibiting abnormal estrous cycles as opposed to not

Table 1. Percentage of females from each treatment exhibiting the three categories of estrous cycles: regular, extended, and abnormal.

Treatment	n	Females with Regular Cycles (%)	Females with Extended Cycles (%)	Females with Abnormal Cycles (%)
Saline	7	100	71.4	100
Buprenorphine	9	100	77.8	77.8
Meloxicam	9	88.9	77.8	100

Regular cycles defined by cycle lengths of 4–5 days, extended cycles defined by 3–4 days of consecutive estrus or 4–5 days of diestrus, and abnormal cycles defined by >4 days or consecutive estrus or >5 days of diestrus, (Chi-square Test of Independence, Regular $\chi^2 = 1.85$ and $p = 0.40$, Extended $\chi^2 = 0.11$ and $p = 0.95$, Abnormal $\chi^2 = 3.87$ and $p = 0.15$).

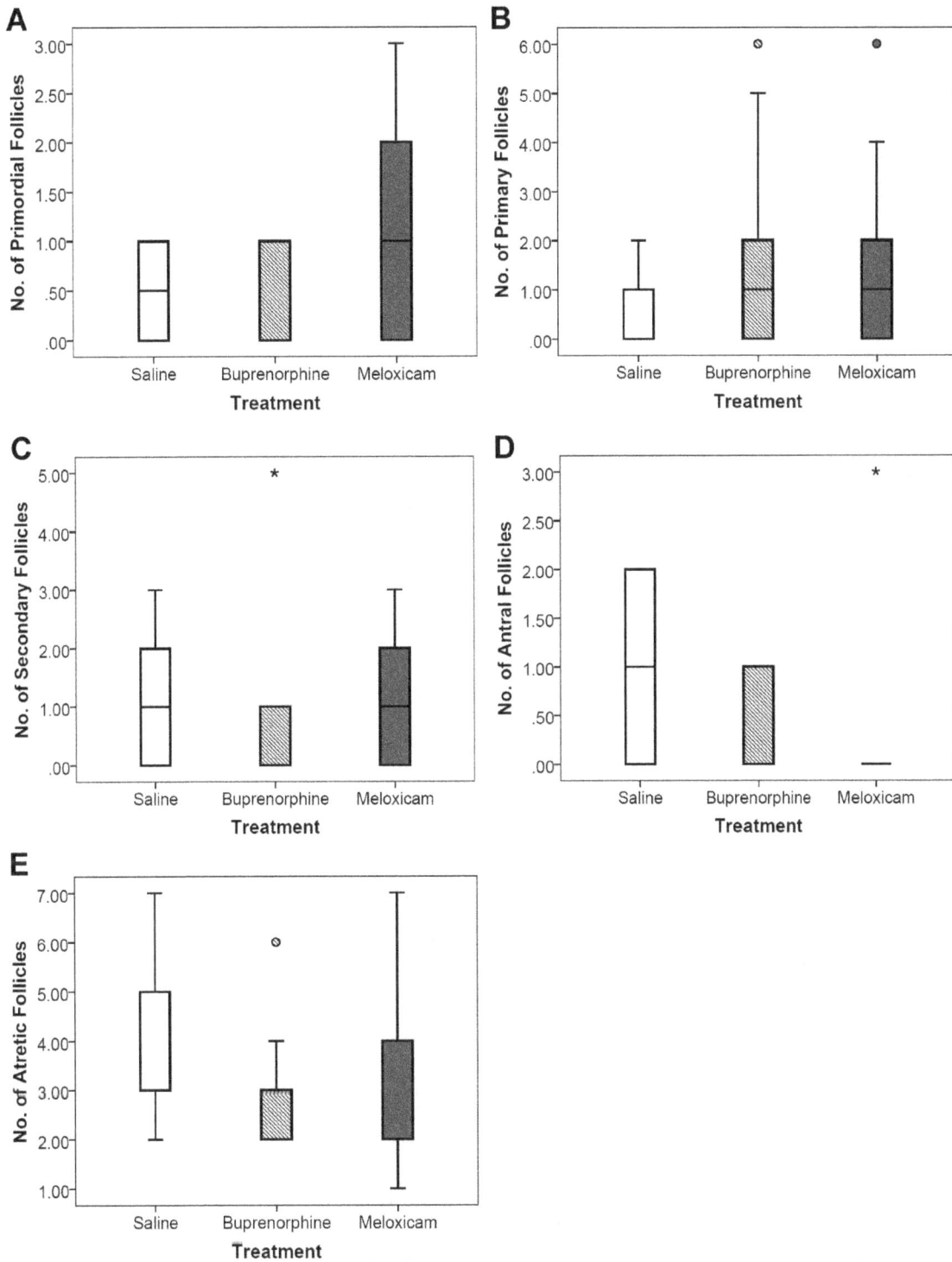

Figure 4. Boxplots of the number of each follicle type per ovarian sample (each ovarian sample consists of nine tissue sections). $N = 24$, saline ($n = 6$), buprenorphine ($n = 9$), meloxicam ($n = 9$). (Rank transformed, MANOVA: $F(10,34) = 0.45$, $p = 0.91$). (A) primordial follicles. (B) primary follicles. (C) secondary follicles. (D) early antral follicles. (E) antral follicles. (F) atretic follicles. The horizontal line in each box interior represents the median, the upper and lower whiskers show the maximum and minimum values, the upper hinge represents the 75th percentile, the lower hinge represents the 25th percentile, "o" represents an outside value, and asterisk (*) represents a far outside value.

exhibiting abnormal cycles were not significantly different (Chi-square Test of Independence: $\chi^2 = 3.87$, df = 2, $p = 0.15$, Table 1). Five saline-control, seven buprenorphine-treated, and seven meloxicam-treated females exhibited extended estrous cycles (3–4 consecutive days of estrus or 4–5 consecutive days of diestrus). The proportions of each treatment group exhibiting extended estrous cycles was also not significant (Chi-square Test of Independence: $\chi^2 = 0.11$, df = 2, $p = 0.95$, Table 1). All saline-

Table 2. The proportion of viable follicles and the total number of follicles per ovarian sample for each treatment.

Treatment	n	Proportion of Viable Follicles per ovarian sample	Total No. of Follicles per ovarian sample
Saline	6	0.48±0.18	7.3±2.07
Buprenorphine	9	0.44±0.26	6.9±5.09
Meloxicam	9	0.51±0.24	7.6±4.33

Data are shown as mean ± SD. Each ovarian sample consists of nine tissue sections. The total number of follicles per ovarian sample includes counts from viable and atretic follicles. (MANOVA, $F_{(4,40)} = 0.10$, $p = 0.98$).

control and buprenorphine-treated females and eight meloxicam-treated females exhibited at least one regular estrous cycle (Chi-square Test of Independence: $\chi^2 = 1.85$, df = 2, $p = 0.40$, Table 1).

Histological Analysis

One female from the saline-control group was excluded from all histological analyses, as tissue sections from this female were lacking ovarian tissue. The number of each follicle type across treatment groups was not significantly different (Rank transformed, MANOVA: $F_{(10,34)} = 0.45$, $p = 0.91$; Figure 4). Treatment did not have any significant effect on the proportion of viable follicles and the number of total follicles observed per ovarian sample (MANOVA: $F_{(4,40)} = 0.10$, $p = 0.98$; Table 2). The mean proportion of viable follicles was approximately 47.8% for the saline-control group, 43.7% for the buprenorphine-treated group, and 50.9% for the meloxicam-treated group. The mean total number of follicles (including viable and atretic follicles) counted from each ovarian sample was 7.3 for the saline-control, 6.9 for the buprenorphine-treated, and 7.6 for the meloxicam-treated groups.

No significant differences were observed in the cross-sectional area of the ovary across treatments (Kruskal-Wallis ANOVA: $\chi^2 = 0.76$, df = 2, $p = 0.69$). The median cross sectional area of the saline-control group was 1.33 mm^2 ($n = 6$, $Q_1 = 0.91$, $Q_3 = 1.62$), of the buprenorphine-treated group was 1.64 mm^2 ($n = 9$, $Q_1 = 0.91$, $Q_3 = 2.00$), and of the meloxicam-treated group was 1.40 mm^2 ($n = 9$, $Q_1 = 1.30$, $Q_3 = 1.69$).

Discussion

Indicators of ovarian transplant success, estrous cyclicity, and viability of follicles revealed no significant differences between treatment groups. Previous studies have found that both opiates and NSAIDs negatively affect angiogenesis with some conflicting results regarding increased or decreased angiogenesis with opiate treatments [6], [8], [9], [30], [31]. Most of these studies have employed high doses of analgesics for prolonged periods, which do not represent the veterinary recommended doses utilized in the current study [6], [8], [9], [27], [28]. The results from this study indicate that recommended doses for a moderate time period do not negatively affect the transplanted ovary in aged females beyond what is expected by the surgical process itself.

Neovascularization of an ovarian heterotopic autotransplant could be observed as soon as three days after transplantation in mice and two days in rats [32], [33], [34]. Restoration of ovarian cycling has been reported to occur as soon as 10–14 days after transplantation of whole ovary transplants and ovarian grafts [16], [17], [35]. However, after transplantation of whole ovaries in this study, as opposed to transplantation of ovarian grafts in previous studies, the onset of estrous cycle occurred as early as five days post-surgery with a mean of 10 days for all females.

Animal models of ovarian transplantations are especially sensitive to the effects of aging. In the present study, ovaries from 2-month old females were transplanted into 11-month old females. The CBA/J mice used in the current study have a lifespan of 647 days [36] with a decline in fecundity at approximately 11 months of age [37]. Total follicle numbers in young 6–8 week old C3H/HeNCrlBR and B6129SF1/J ovaries that had been grafted into 6–8 week old B6C3F1/J and B6129SF1/J recipients was lower than intact ovary total follicle numbers and have been estimated to be about 100 follicles per ovary [16] due to the hypoxia experienced with ovarian transplantation [5]. Also of importance is that gonadotropin levels decrease with age, reducing gonadotropic input to the ovaries [38], [39]. In middle-aged rodents, a significant decrease was seen in the levels of LH during an LH surge as well as a delayed occurrence of the LH surge compared with young rodents [39]. GnRH levels may not change with age, but the LH response to GnRH decreases with age [38]. These age-associated factors could lead to decreased follicular development and thus to decreased follicular counts in the aged recipients of this study. These factors may have contributed to the early cessation of cycling seen in two of the buprenorphine-treated animals. It is also possible that those two animals experienced decreased vascularization of the transplanted ovary but it is unclear whether this can be attributed to the analgesic buprenorphine.

The effects of analgesics on ovarian transplant success in aged females require further investigation. This study suggests that at the recommended veterinary doses [12], [24], [25], [26], the two analgesics studied do not decrease angiogenesis to the extent that there are alterations in estrous cycle length or the proportion of viable follicles and the total number of follicles per ovary. This would imply that the veterinary recommended doses of analgesic do not induce additional damage after ovarian transplantation nor significantly affect the function of the transplanted ovary. Thus, the recommended dosages for buprenorphine and meloxicam may be beneficial to decrease surgical pain in mice without negatively affecting ovarian transplant survival as assessed by estrous cycle length and follicle count.

Acknowledgments

We thank Michael Sneary and Rachael French for sharing their scientific expertise and Gary B. Anderson for his insightful review of the manuscript.

Author Contributions

Conceived and designed the experiments: SC AL. Performed the experiments: AL SC. Analyzed the data: AL LB. Contributed reagents/materials/analysis tools: AL SC LB. Contributed to the writing of the manuscript: AL SC LB.

References

1. Bassett DL (1943) The changes in the vascular pattern of the ovary of the albino rat during the estrous cycle. Am J Anat 73(2): 251–291.

2. Shweiki D, Itin A, Neufeld G, Gitay-Goren H, Keshet E (1993) Patterns of expression of vascular endothelial growth factor (VEGF) and VEGF receptors in mice suggest a role in hormonally regulated angiogenesis. J Clin Invest 91(5): 2235–2243.

3. Fevold HL, Hisaw FL, Leonard SL (1931) The gonad stimulating and the luteinizing hormones of the anterior lobe of the hypophesis. Am J Physiol 97(2): 291–301.

4. Israely T, Dafni H, Granot D, Nevo N, Tsafriri A, et al. (2003) Vascular remodeling and angiogenesis in ectopic ovarian transplants: a crucial role of pericytes and vascular smooth muscle cells in maintenance of ovarian grafts. Biol Reprod 68(6): 2055–2064.

5. Kim SS, Yang HW, Kang HG, Lee HH, Lee HC, et al. (2004) Quantitative assessment of ischemic tissue damage in ovarian cortical tissue with or without antioxidant (ascorbic acid) treatment. Fertil Steril 82(3): 679–685.

6. Hsiao PN, Chang MC, Cheng WF, Chen CA, Lin HW, et al. (2009) Morphine induces apoptosis of human endothelial cells through nitric oxide and reactive oxygen species pathways. Toxicol 256(1): 83–91.

7. Jones MK, Wang H, Peskar BM, Levin E, Itani RM, et al. (1999) Inhibition of angiogenesis by nonsteroidal anti-inflammatory drugs: insight into mechanisms and implications for cancer growth and ulcer healing. Nat Med 5(12): 1418–1423.

8. Lam CF, Chang PJ, Huang YS, Sung YH, Huang CC, et al. (2008) Prolonged use of high-dose morphine impairs angiogenesis and mobilization of endothelial progenitor cells in mice. Anesth Analg 107(2): 686–692.

9. Liu HC, Anday JK, House SD, Chang SL (2004) Dual effects of morphine on permeability and apoptosis of vascular endothelial cells: morphine potentiates lipopolysaccharide-induced permeability and apoptosis of vascular endothelial cells. J Neuroimmunol 146(1): 13–21.

10. Zúñiga J, Fuenzalida M, Guerrero G, Illanes J, Dabancens A, et al. (2003) Effects of steroidal and non steroidal drugs on the neovascularization response induced by tumoral TA3 supernatant on CAM from chick embryo. Biol Res 36(2): 233–240.

11. Cargill SL, Carey JR, Müller HG, Anderson G (2003) Age of ovary determines remaining life expectancy in old ovariectomized mice. Aging Cell 2(3): 185–190.

12. Mason JB, Cargill SL, Anderson GB, Carey JR (2009) Transplantation of young ovaries to old mice increased life span in transplant recipients J Gerontol A Biol Sci Med Sci 64(12): 1207–1211.

13. Fujing Y, Ozaki K, Yamamasu S, Ito F, Matsuoka I, et al. (1996) DNA fragmentation of oocytes in aged mice. Mol Hum Reprod 11(7): 1480–1483.

14. Nelson JF, Felicio LS, Randall PK, Sims C, Finch CE (1982) A longitudinal study of estrous cyclicity in aging C57BL/6J mice: I. Cycle frequency, length and vaginal cytology. Biol Reprod 27(2): 327–339.

15. Rivard A, Fabre JE, Silver M, Chen D, Murohara T, et al. (1999) Age-dependent impairment of angiogenesis. Circulation 99(1): 111–120.

16. Liu L, Wood GA, Morikawa L, Ayearst R, Fleming C, et al. (2008) Restoration of fertility by orthotopic transplantation of frozen adult mouse ovaries. Hum Reprod 23(1): 122–128.

17. Gunasena KT, Villines PM, Critser ES, Critser JK (1997) Live births after autologous transplant of cryopreserved mouse ovaries. Hum Reprod 12(1): 101–106.

18. Kamei J, Saitoh A, Suzuki T, Misawa M, Nagase H, et al. (1995) Buprenorphine exerts its antinociceptive activity via μ1-opioid receptors. Life Sci 56(15): PL285–PL290.

19. Tarnawski AS, Jones MK (2003) Inhibition of angiogenesis by NSAIDs: molecular mechanisms and clinical implications. J Mol Med 81: 627–636.

20. Vane JR, Botting RM (1996) Mechanism of action of anti-inflammatory drugs. Scand J Rheumatol 25: 9–21.

21. Fuller JL, Sjursen Jr FH (1967) Audiogenic seizures in eleven mouse strains. J Hered 58(3): 135–140.

22. Whitten WK (1956) Modification of the oestrous cycle of the mouse by external stimuli associated with the male. J Endocrinol 13(4): 399–404.

23. Cargill SL, Medrano JF, Anderson GB (1999) Infertility in a line of mice with the high growth mutation is due to luteal insufficiency resulting from disruption at the hypothalamic-pituitary axis. Biol Reprod 61: 283–287.

24. Flecknell P (2009) Laboratory Animal Anesthesia. Burlington: Academic Press. 300 p.

25. Plumb DC (2002) Veterinary Drug Handbook. White Bear Lake: Iowa State Press. 1208 p.

26. Wright-Williams SL, Courade JP, Richardson CA, Roughan JA, Flecknell PA (2007) Effects of vasectomy surgery and meloxicam treatment of faecal corticosterone levels and behaviour in two strains of laboratory mouse. Pain 130: 108–118.

27. Myers M, Britt KL, Wreford NGM, Ebling FJP, Kerr JB (2004) Methods for quantifying follicular numbers within the mouse ovary. Reprod 127(5): 569–580.

28. Goldman JM, Murr AS, Cooper RL (2007) The rodent estrous cycle: characterization of vaginal cytology and its utility in toxicological studies. Birth Defects Res B Dev Reprod Toxicol 80(2): 84–97.

29. Lohff JC, Christian PJ, Marion SL, Arrandale A, Hoyer PB (2005) Characterization of cyclicity and hormonal profile with impending ovarian failure in a novel chemical-induced mouse model of perimenopause. Comp Med 55(6): 523–527.

30. Dai X, Song H, Cui S, Wang T, Liu Q, et al. (2010) The stimulative effects of endogenous opioids on endothelial cell proliferation, migration, and angiogenesis in vitro. Eur J Pharmacol 628: 42–50.

31. Gupta K, Kshirsagar S, Chang L, Schwartz RS, Law PY, et al. (2002) Morphine stimulates angiogenesis by activating proangiogenic and survival-promoting signaling and promotes breast tumor growth. Cancer Res 62: 4491–4498.

32. Dissen GA, Lara HE, Fahrenbach WH, Costa ME, Ojeda SR (1994) Immature rat ovaries become revascularized rapidly after autotransplantation and show a gonadotropin-dependent increase in angiogenic factor gene expression. Endocrinol 134(3): 1146–1154.

33. Nugent D, Newton H, Gallivan L, Gosden RG (1998) Protective effect of vitamin E on ischaemia-reperfusion injury in ovarian grafts. J Reprod Fertil 114(2): 341–346.

34. Wang Y, Chang Q, Sun J, Dang L, Ma W, et al. (2012) Effects of HMG on revascularization and follicular survival in heterotopic autotransplants of mouse ovarian tissue. Reprod Biomed Online 24(6): 646–653.

35. Harris M, Eakin RM (1949) Survival of transplanted ovaries in rats. J Exp Zool 112(1): 131–163.

36. Yuan R, Tsaih SW, Petkova SB, Evsikova CM, Xing S, et al. (2009) Aging in inbred strains of mice: study design and interim report on median lifespans and circulating IGF1 levels. Aging Cell 8: 277–287.

37. Gosden RG (1975) Ovarian support of pregnancy in ageing inbred mice. J Reprod Fert 42: 423–430.

38. Arias P, Carbone S, Szwarcfarb B, Feleder C, Rodríguez M, et al. (1996) Effects of aging on N-methyl-D-aspartate (NMDA)-induced GnRH and LH release in female rats. Brain Res 740(1): 234–238.

39. Cooper RL, Conn PM, Walker RF (1980) Characterization of the LH surge in middle-aged female rats. Biol Reprod 23(3): 611–615.

18

Radiographic Risk Factors for Contralateral Rupture in Dogs with Unilateral Cranial Cruciate Ligament Rupture

Connie Chuang, Megan A. Ramaker, Sirjaut Kaur, Rebecca A. Csomos, Kevin T. Kroner, Jason A. Bleedorn, Susan L. Schaefer, Peter Muir*

Comparative Orthopaedic Research Laboratory, and the Department of Surgical Sciences, School of Veterinary Medicine, University of Wisconsin-Madison, Madison, Wisconsin, United States of America

Abstract

Background: Complete cranial cruciate ligament rupture (CR) is a common cause of pelvic limb lameness in dogs. Dogs with unilateral CR often develop contralateral CR over time. Although radiographic signs of contralateral stifle joint osteoarthritis (OA) influence risk of subsequent contralateral CR, this risk has not been studied in detail.

Methodology/Principal Findings: We conducted a retrospective longitudinal cohort study of client-owned dogs with unilateral CR to determine how severity of radiographic stifle synovial effusion and osteophytosis influence risk of contralateral CR over time. Detailed survival analysis was performed for a cohort of 85 dogs after case filtering of an initial sample population of 513 dogs. This population was stratified based on radiographic severity of synovial effusion (graded on a scale of 0, 1, and 2) and severity of osteophytosis (graded on a scale of 0, 1, 2, and 3) of both index and contralateral stifle joints using a reproducible scoring method. Severity of osteophytosis in the index and contralateral stifles was significantly correlated. Rupture of the contralateral cranial cruciate ligament was significantly influenced by radiographic OA in both the index and contralateral stifles at diagnosis. Odds ratio for development of contralateral CR in dogs with severe contralateral radiographic stifle effusion was 13.4 at one year after diagnosis and 11.4 at two years. Odds ratio for development of contralateral CR in dogs with severe contralateral osteophytosis was 9.9 at one year after diagnosis. These odds ratios were associated with decreased time to contralateral CR. Breed, age, body weight, gender, and tibial plateau angle did not significantly influence time to contralateral CR.

Conclusion: Subsequent contralateral CR is significantly influenced by severity of radiographic stifle effusion and osteophytosis in the contralateral stifle, suggesting that synovitis and arthritic joint degeneration are significant factors in the disease mechanism underlying the arthropathy.

Editor: Cheryl London, The Ohio State University, United States of America

Funding: Connie Chuang was supported by the Merial Summer Scholars Program, University of Wisconsin-Madison, School of Veterinary Medicine. The project described was also supported by the Clinical and Translational Science Award (CTSA) program, through the NIH National Center for Advancing Translational Sciences (NCATS), grant UL1TR000427. The funders had no role in study design, data collection and analysis, decision to publish, or preparation of the manuscript. The content is solely the responsibility of the authors and does not necessarily represent the official views of the NIH.

Competing Interests: The authors have declared that no competing interests exist.

* Email: muirp@vetmed.wisc.edu

Introduction

Complete cranial cruciate ligament rupture (CR) is an important cause of stifle instability and associated pelvic limb lameness in dogs in which fiber damage to the caudal cruciate ligament is also common [1,2]. Each year, at least one billion dollars are spent in the United States on treatment of CR and associated meniscal tearing [3]. While CR can result from trauma, a large majority of dogs develop CR during normal activity in association with pre-existing degeneration of the stifle joint and the cruciate ligament complex [4,5]. Among dogs presented with unilateral CR, a large proportion of patients will develop contralateral CR within 12 to 24 months of initial diagnosis [6,7]. In previous work, analysis of this risk has been reported as an incidence after surgery (percentage of patients within the cohort). This risk is in the range of 22–54% at 6 to 17 months of diagnosis [6,8–11]. More recently survival analysis has been used to evaluate risk factors for development of contralateral CR [7,12].

Many studies have investigated the disease mechanism and examined clinically relevant markers of disease or risk factors for development of CR. A current hypothesis relevant to the CR disease mechanism is that stifle joint inflammation precedes development of stifle instability from CR. Development of synovitis is an early event in the incipient phase of the condition that precedes development of clinically detectable joint instability, based on arthoscopic examination of the stifle [2]. Development of stifle synovitis also increases the risk of subsequent contralateral CR in dogs [13].

Moderate to severe osteoarthritis (OA) is usually detectable radiographically in the affected index stifle at the time of diagnosis of unilateral CR [14,15]. Radiographic signs of OA are often present in clinically stable contralateral stifle joints at the time of diagnosis [2,12,14,15], but underestimate severity of synovitis [2].

Clinical Trial Flow Diagram

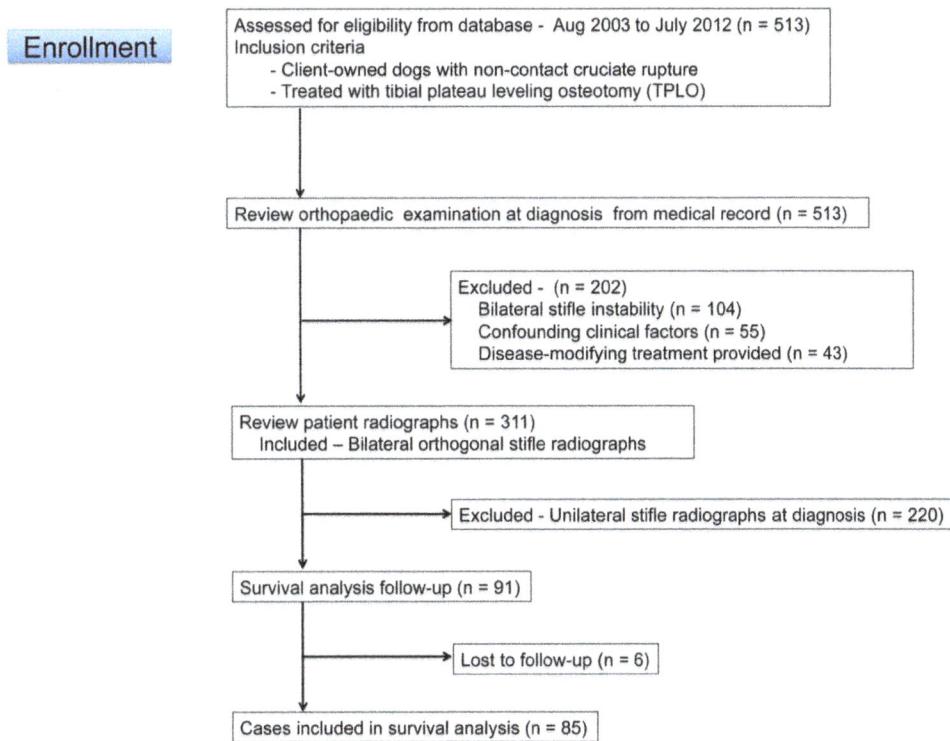

Figure 1. Flow diagram for case inclusion and exclusion. Of the 513 cases identified from the initial medical records search, 85 dogs were ultimately included in the survival analysis.

It has been recognized for some time that radiographic signs of contralateral stifle joint degeneration in dogs with unilateral CR influence risk of contralateral CR [6,9]. However, these analyses were limited to determining that global scoring of radiographic change, including synovial effusion and osteophytosis, influenced risk of contralateral CR.

In a previous experiment, survival analysis of time to contralateral CR in a large group of dogs presented with unilateral CR was conducted using cases from three referral centers to examine the pattern of contralateral CR in the affected population studying a variety of surgical stabilizing treatments [7]. The median time to contralateral CR for the entire affected population was 947 days [7]. However, survival analysis in this previous study did not consider radiographic change or type of surgical treatment at the time of diagnosis in the statistical model. Past research suggests that both synovial effusion and osteophytosis assessed radiographically would significantly influence time to contralateral CR. More recently, the presence of radiographic synovial effusion and osteophytosis in the contralateral stifle at diagnosis of unilateral CR has been shown to be a significant risk factor for development of contralateral cruciate rupture over time [12], supporting the concept that radiographic abnormalities at the time of initial diagnosis are predictive of clinical outcome. Functional outcome after treatment of CR with a stabilizing surgical procedure is procedure-dependent. Consequently, surgical procedure could also influence time to contralateral CR. Functional outcome at 12 months after treatment with tibial plateau leveling osteotomy (TPLO) is superior to treatment with a lateral fabellar suture [16,17], and meta-analysis of surgical treatments suggests that evidence most strongly supports the ability of TPLO to return dogs to normal function [18].

The present study aimed to evaluate severity of radiographic change in the unstable index and stable contralateral stifle joints at the time of diagnosis of unilateral CR and examine synovial effusion and osteophytosis as risk factors for contralateral CR. We hypothesized that risk of contralateral CR would be significantly influenced by the severity of synovial effusion and osteophytosis in both stifles at the time of initial diagnosis of unilateral CR. Confirmation that radiography is an important predictive marker for risk of subsequent contralateral CR could be relevant to clinical management of affected dogs. We designed this study to provide baseline date for ongoing longitudinal studies of disease-modifying treatment for the underlying arthropathy.

Materials and Methods

Dogs

Medical records of dogs that were admitted to the Small Animal Orthopaedic Surgery Service at the University of Wisconsin-Madison UW Veterinary Care Hospital for unilateral (TPLO) treatment of CR between Aug 2003 and July 2012 were reviewed. Because functional outcome after treatment of CR with a stabilizing surgical procedure is procedure-dependent and meta-analysis of surgical treatments suggests that evidence most strongly supports the ability of TPLO to return dogs to normal function [16–18], the study was limited to TPLO-treated dogs to minimize any variation in time to contralateral CR associated with different surgical treatments. The initial medical record search identified 513 dogs that were treated with TPLO. To be included in the study, dogs had to meet the following criteria: Diagnosis of unilateral CR with radiographs of both stifles made at the time of diagnosis. Dogs were excluded for the following reasons: Diagnosis of bilateral CR, unilateral stifle radiographs at the time of diagnosis, the presence of confounding clinical factors that could affect patient mobility and a normal convalescence after surgery, and lack of clinical follow-up. Medical records from 428 dogs were excluded after filtering (**Fig. 1**). Records from 85 dogs were then reviewed in detail as described below.

Medical Records Review and Diagnosis of Cranial Cruciate Ligament Rupture

Diagnosis of CR was defined by the detection of stifle instability clinically. CR was confirmed by physical examination and detection of cranial tibial translation using the cranial drawer and cranial tibial thrust tests [19], as well as assessment of periarticular fibrosis and joint thickening. Age, gender, breed, and body weight for the study cohort were obtained from the medical record.

Radiography

Synovial effusion and osteophytosis were used to evaluate the severity of stifle OA. These criteria were selected based on high reproducibility [15,20]. The most important early radiographic sign of stifle OA is development of synovial effusion and associated compression of the infrapatellar fat pad [14]. Orthogonal cranio-caudal and medio-lateral radiographic views of the index stifle that was treated with TPLO were reviewed. Radiographic views of the contralateral stifle were similarly reviewed. Synovial effusion was graded subjectively on a scale from 0–2 (0 - normal, 1 - mild, 2 - severe) (**Fig. 2**). Both cranial and caudal stifle joint spaces were examined in this assessment. Cranially, the extent of effusion and the shape of the infrapatellar fat pad were considered. Caudal bulging of the joint capsule was also evaluated during grading. Osteophytosis was graded subjectively on a scale from 0–3 (0 - normal, 1 - mild, 2 - moderate, 3 - severe) based on the severity of osteophytosis at the margins of the stifle joint (**Fig. 3**). Grading was based on previously described numerical rating scales [15]. Radiographic scoring was performed by a single observer (CC), after training was provided by an experienced clinician (PM). In addition, the tibial plateau angle (TPA) was calculated from the lateral radiographic views of the index and contralateral tibias with the stifle and tarsus held in ninety degrees of flexion. For lateral radiographs which did not include the entire tibia, a longitudinal reference axis as long as possible was used [21].

Clinical Follow-Up

Clinical follow-up was done by medical record review, telephone conversation with the owner of the dog or the primary veterinarian, or orthopaedic examination at the UW Veterinary Care Hospital. The presence of contralateral CR was confirmed by detection of stifle instability by a veterinarian. During telephone follow-up with owners, the presence or absence of contralateral pelvic limb lameness and any relevant clinical findings made by their primary veterinarian were determined. Dogs that had experienced contralateral CR were coded as a complete case and time from initial diagnosis to contralateral CR was calculated in days. If an individual dog had not experienced contralateral CR at time of follow-up, the case was coded as censored and the time from initial diagnosis to clinical follow-up was calculated in days. If the dog did not return to the UW Veterinary Hospital after surgery or the owner was lost to follow-up, then the case was excluded from the analysis.

Statistical Analysis

Data were reported as mean ± standard deviation or median (range) as appropriate. The Student's t test for paired data was used to compare TPA in index and contralateral stifles. The Spearman Rank test was used to determine whether severity of synovial effusion and osteophytosis in index and contralateral stifles were correlated and whether clinical parameters were correlated with radiographic change. Precision of radiographic scoring for synovial effusion and arthritis degeneration of the stifle was determined. One observer (RAC) evaluated a series of orthogonal stifle radiographs from 15 dogs that represented the range of severity for synovial effusion and osteophytosis three times in a blinded fashion to determine intra-observer repeatability of the scoring system using the intraclass correlation coefficient (ICC) statistic. The series of radiographs from 15 dogs were also graded by two other observers (CC, KTK) in a blinded fashion. Collectively, these observations were used to determine inter-observer reproducibility of the scoring system using the ICC. ICC ≤0.3 were considered weak, coefficients >0.3 and <0.75 were considered moderate, and ≥0.75 were considered strong.

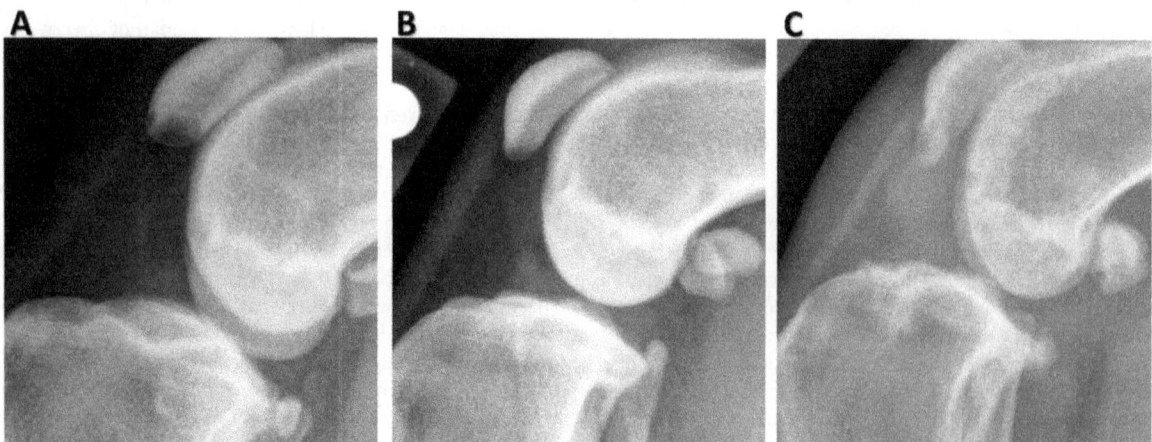

Figure 2. Severity scoring of stifle radiographs for synovial effusion. (A–C) Severity of synovial effusion was graded as 0 = normal (A), 1 = mild (B), or 2 = severe (C), using the medial-lateral radiographic view. Severity scoring was based on the magnitude of the soft tissue density within the stifle joint and the dimensions of the intra-patellar fat pad density in the cranial part of the joint. Grading was based on a previously published scale [15].

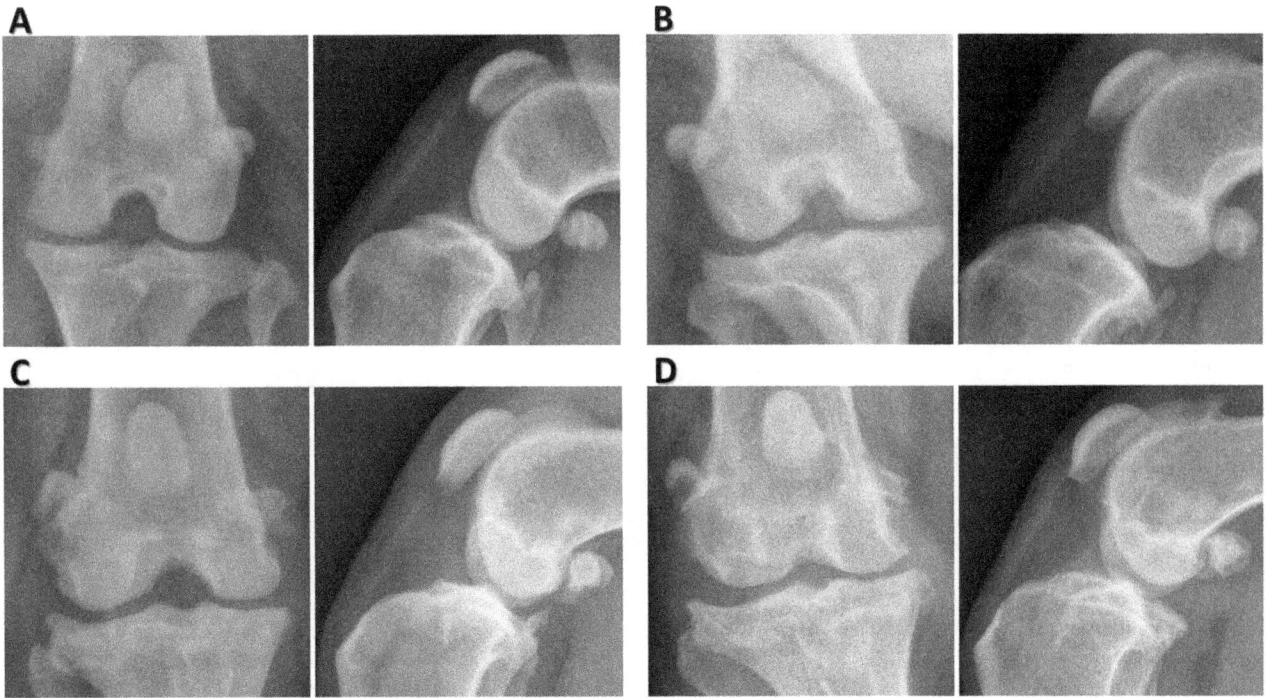

Figure 3. Severity scoring of stifle radiographs for osteophytosis. (A–D) Severity of osteophytosis was graded as 0 = normal (A), 1 = mild (B), 2 = moderate (C) or 3 = severe (D) respectively after evaluation of orthogonal views of the stifle. Severity scoring was based on the magnitude and severity of osteophyte formation around the joint margins, including the proximal and distal poles of the patella, the lateral and medial aspects of the trochlear ridges of the distal femur, and the lateral, medial, cranial, and caudal aspects of the proximal tibia, and the fabellae. Grading was based on a previously published scale [15].

Data from clinical follow-up of the cohort was used for survival analysis. Contingency tables for radiographic grading of severity of synovial effusion and osteophytosis in both the index and contralateral stifle were made for development of contralateral CR at one year and at two years after diagnosis and treatment of the index stifle with TPLO. The effect of severity of synovial effusion and osteophytosis of the index and contralateral stifle joints on development of contralateral cruciate rupture was examined using a Monte-Carlo simulation Chi-square test [22]. For tables with a significant disease association, Chi-square or Fisher exact testing, as appropriate, was used to determine which grades of synovial effusion or osteophytosis had significant effects on time to contralateral CR. Odds ratios and 95% confidence limits were also calculated for each grade.

Logistic regression and Cox's Proportional Hazards models were also used to determine which clinical factors might influence risk of contralateral CR. Initially, putative risk factors were analyzed in a univariate model. Factors considered in the univariate model included age, gender, body weight, dog breed, TPA, and severity of synovial effusion and osteophytosis in the index and contralateral stifles. Univariate parameters with $p < 0.2$ were then considered further in a multivariate model. Survival curves stratified by radiographic scoring of synovial effusion and osteophytosis severity were also compared using the Logrank (Mantel-Cox) test. All results were considered significant at $p \leq 0.05$.

Results

Study Cohort

The initial medical records search identified 513 dogs treated with TPLO. Case filtering excluded 428 dogs. Dogs with bilateral stifle instability at diagnosis were excluded (n = 104). Dogs with confounding factors that could affect patient mobility, normal weight bearing, or a normal outcome from TPLO surgery were excluded (n = 55, **Table 1**). Furthermore, dogs given medical treatments after surgery that could be disease-modifying were also excluded (n = 43). These treatments included bilateral arthroscopy with associated joint lavage, leflunomide treatment and doxycycline treatment. Radiographs for the remaining 311 dogs were then reviewed. Of these 311 dogs, 220 were excluded because bilateral orthogonal radiographic views at diagnosis were lacking, and 6 dogs were lost to follow-up. After the filtering process, data from 85 dogs were available for survival analysis (**Fig. 1**).

The age of the study population was 5.3±2.7 years old and ranged from <1 to 11 years. Body weight was 40.5±15.1 kg and ranged from 12.4 to 83 kg. Included in the study were 2 males, 38 castrated males, 1 female, and 44 ovariohysterectomized females. A range of breeds was represented, with 67 pure breeds and 18 mixed breed dogs. The most common breeds were Labrador Retriever (n = 21), Golden Retriever (n = 11), Newfoundland (n = 6), and German Shepherd (n = 5). Other breeds included Bernese Mountain Dog, Chesapeake Bay Retriever, Great Dane, Rottweiler, Boxer, Mastiff, Shar Pei, Bulldog, Brittany Spaniel, Siberian Husky, Standard Poodle, and Wirehaired Pointing Griffon (listed from high to low frequency; each with <5 dogs, total n = 24). Labrador Retriever crosses were the most common type of mixed breed dog (n = 5). Among these 85 dogs, 45 dogs

Table 1. Confounding factors for case exclusion.

Confounding factor	Number of Dogs
Previous stifle surgery	30
TPLO treatment for a stable partial cruciate rupture	9
TPLO implant removal after surgery	8
Implant-associated infection	2
Polyarthritis	1
Premature physeal closure in the distal femur	1
Femoral osteochondritis dissecans	1
Femoral osteoproliferation	1
Pelvic limb amputation	1
Popliteal tendon avulsion	1
Failed tibial plateau leveling osteotomy	1
Femoral head ostectomy	1

Note: 55 dogs in total were excluded during case filtering because of confounding clinical factors. More than one confounding factor was found in some dogs.

had left CR and 40 dogs had right CR at diagnosis. No dog had a history of traumatic injury.

Radiography

In the index stifle, Grade 2 synovial effusion was found in 76 of 85 dogs (89%). Grade 2 effusion in the contralateral stifle was found in 22 of 85 dogs (26%). In the index stifle, Grade 3 osteophytosis was found in 34 of 85 dogs (40%). Grade 3 osteophytosis was found in 6 of 85 dogs (7%) in the contralateral stifle. In the index stifle, median severity of synovial effusion and osteophytosis was 2 (0,2) and 3 (0,3) respectively. In the contralateral stifle, median severity of synovial effusion and osteophytosis was 1 (0,2) and 1 (0,3) respectively. Severity of synovial effusion and osteophytosis was increased in the index stifle, when compared with the contralateral stifle ($p<0.001$). Severity of osteophytosis ($S_R = 0.39$, $p<0.0005$), but not synovial effusion ($S_R = 0.17$, $p = 0.13$) in the index and contralateral stifles were significantly correlated (**Fig. 4**). Body weight was not significantly correlated with either synovial effusion or osteophytosis in either the index or contralateral stifle. TPA in the index and contralateral stifles was 28 ± 3 and 27 ± 3 degrees respectively. There was no significance in TPA between index and contralateral stifles. TPA ranged from 21 to 35 in the index stifle and 19 to 34 in the contralateral stifle.

Intra-observer reproducibility for scoring of synovial effusion and osteophytosis on orthogonal stifle radiographs was 0.87 (95% confidence interval −0.73–0.95) and 0.82 (95% confidence interval −0.64–0.93) respectively. Inter-observer reproducibility for scoring of synovial effusion and osteophytosis was 0.83 (95% confidence interval −0.64–0.93) and 0.84 (95% confidence interval −0.67–0.94) respectively.

Survival Analysis

Overall, 28 of 85 dogs (33%) developed contralateral CR within the study period. At the end of the study period of 2,516 days, 67% of dogs had not developed a contralateral CR. In the lower quartile of the cohort, time to contralateral CR was 498 days. Development of contralateral CR was significantly influenced by radiographic change in both stifles.

At one year (365 days) after diagnosis, development of contralateral CR was significantly influenced by severity of

radiographic effusion in the contralateral stifle ($p = 0.0001$), but not the index stifle (**Tables 2–3**). A similar result was found at two years (730 days) after diagnosis (**Tables 2–3**). The odds ratio for development of contralateral CR in dogs with Grade 2 stifle effusion in the contralateral stifle was 13.4 by one year and 11.4 at two years after diagnosis. Similarly, at one year after diagnosis, development of contralateral CR was significantly influenced by severity of radiographic osteophytosis in the contralateral stifle ($p < 0.05$), but not the index stifle (**Tables 4–5**). At two years after diagnosis, this effect was no longer significant ($p = 0.11$). The odds ratio for development of contralateral CR in dogs with Grade 3 osteophytosis in the contralateral stifle was 9.9 by one year after diagnosis.

When data were analyzed using a univariate logistic regression model, development of contralateral CR at one year after diagnosis was significantly influenced by severity of radiographic effusion (odds ratio [unit change] = 4.7, $p<0.005$) and osteophytosis (odds ratio [unit change] = 2.1, $p = 0.01$) in the contralateral stifle. The effects of breed, age, body weight, gender, TPA, index effusion, and index osteophytosis ($p = 0.08$) were not significant. In the final multivariate model, development of contralateral CR was significantly influenced by radiographic effusion in the contralateral stifle (odds ratio [unit change] = 5.0), radiographic osteophytosis in the index stifle (odds ratio [unit change] = 2.0), and radiographic osteophytosis in the contralateral stifle (odds ratio [unit change] = 0.9) ($p<0.001$). Similar results were obtained when development of contralateral CR at two years after diagnosis was analyzed. In the two-year univariate model, risk of contralateral CR after diagnosis was significantly influenced by severity of radiographic osteophytosis in the index stifle (odds ratio [unit change] = 6.28, $p<0.005$) and severity of radiographic effusion in the contralateral stifle (odds ratio [unit change] = 2.07, $p<0.05$). The effects of breed, age, body weight, gender, TPA, index effusion, and contralateral osteophytosis ($p = 0.06$) were not significant. In the final multivariate model, development of contralateral CR was significantly influenced by radiographic effusion in the contralateral stifle (odds ratio [unit change] −2.60), radiographic osteophytosis in the index stifle (odds ratio [unit change] −2.78), and radiographic osteophytosis in the contralateral stifle (odds ratio [unit change] −0.74) ($p<0.005$).

Data were also analyzed using the Cox's Proportional Hazards model. In the univariate model, development of contralateral CR

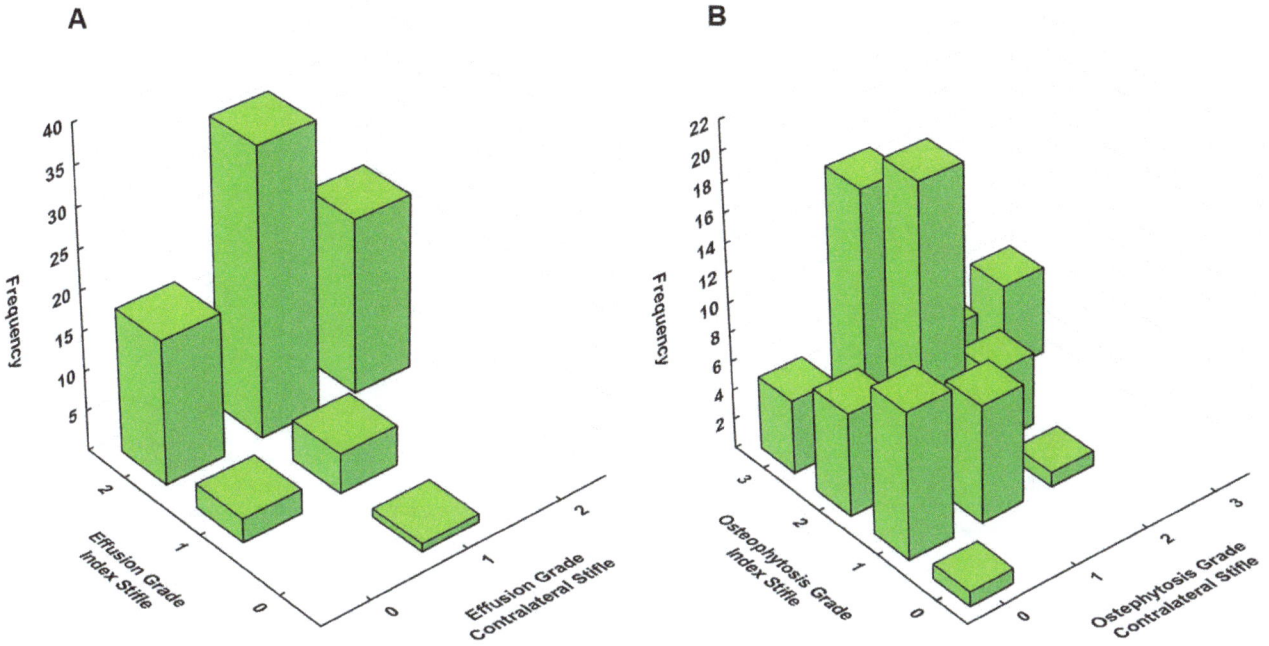

Figure 4. Relationship of osteoarthritic changes in the index and contralateral stifles. (**A**) Bivariate histogram of radiographic synovial effusion grade in index and contralateral stifles. (**B**) Bivariate histogram of osteophytosis grade in index and contralateral stifles. Severity of osteophytosis ($S_R = 0.39$, $p < 0.0005$), but not synovial effusion ($S_R = 0.17$, $p = 0.13$) in the index and contralateral stifles were correlated.

after diagnosis was significantly influenced by severity of radiographic effusion (hazard ratio [unit change] = 2.4, $p < 0.005$) in the contralateral stifle and osteophytosis (hazard ratio [unit change] = 1.64, $p = 0.05$) in the index stifle. The effects of breed, age, body weight, gender, TPA, index effusion, and contralateral OA ($p = 0.08$) were not significant. In the final multivariate model, development of contralateral CR was significantly influenced by radiographic effusion in the contralateral stifle (hazard ratio [unit change] = 2.8, $p < 0.005$), radiographic osteophytosis in the index stifle (hazard ratio [unit change] = 2.0), but not radiographic osteophytosis in the contralateral stifle (hazard ratio [unit change] = 0.78, $p = 0.37$).

When survival curves stratified by radiographic grading of severity of synovial effusion and osteophytosis were compared using the Logrank (Mantel-Cox) test, it was found that time to contralateral CR was not significantly influenced by severity of radiographic effusion or osteophytosis in the index stifle (**Fig. 5**). However, time to contralateral CR was significantly decreased in dogs with Grade 2 radiographic effusion of the contralateral stifle at diagnosis, when compared with the grades of 0 or 1 ($p < 0.001$) (**Fig. 6A**). Time to contralateral CR was also significantly decreased in dogs with Grade 3 osteophytosis of the contralateral stifle at diagnosis when compared with the grades of 0 or 2 ($p < 0.05$) (**Fig. 6B**).

Table 2. Relationship of radiographic synovial effusion in the index stifle to contralateral cranial cruciate ligament rupture at one and two years after surgery.

One year after surgery					
Effusion Grade	**Ruptured**	**Not ruptured**	**Odds ratio**	**95% CI**	**Significance**
0	0	1	1.25	0.05–31.98	$p = 0.89$
1	2	6	1.33	0.24–7.28	$p = 0.74$
2	15	59	0.89	0.17–4.73	$p = 0.89$
Two years after surgery					
0	0	1	0.61	0.02–15.72	$p = 0.77$
1	2	5	0.74	0.13–4.16	$p = 0.73$
2	20	36	1.67	0.31–9.04	$p = 0.55$

Note: At one year after surgery, n = 83 dogs; 2 dogs were censored at <365 days. Overall, radiographic synovial effusion in the index stifle was not significantly associated with risk of rupture at 1 year ($p = 1.0$). At two years after surgery, n = 64 dogs; 21 dogs were censored at <730 days. Overall, radiographic synovial effusion in the index stifle was not significantly associated with risk of rupture at 2 years ($p = 1.0$).

Table 3. Relationship of radiographic synovial effusion in the contralateral stifle to contralateral cranial cruciate ligament rupture at one and two years after surgery.

One year after surgery					
Effusion Grade	Ruptured	Not ruptured	Odds ratio	95% CI	Significance
0	1	19	0.15	0.02–1.25	$p = 0.08$
1	4	37	0.24	0.07–0.82	$p = 0.02$
2	12	10	13.44	3.88–46.51	$p = 0.0001$
Two years after surgery					
0	4	11	0.63	0.17–2.26	$p = 0.47$
1	6	27	0.21	0.07–0.65	$p = 0.007$
2	12	4	11.40	3.02–46.05	$p = 0.0003$

Note: At one year after surgery, n = 83 dogs; 2 dogs were censored at <365 days. Overall, radiographic synovial effusion in the contralateral stifle was significantly associated with risk of rupture at 1 year ($p = 0.0001$). At two years after surgery, n = 64 dogs; 21 dogs were censored at <730 days. Overall, radiographic synovial effusion in the contralateral stifle was significantly associated with risk of rupture at 2 years ($p = 0.0001$).

Discussion

Collectively, past observations suggest that the CR condition is a progressive, acquired degenerative condition in the dog. However, the disease mechanism remains poorly understood. Stifle synovitis develops in the initial phase of the condition and is often associated with some degree of fiber rupture in the cruciate ligament complex and an increased risk of subsequent contralateral CR [2,12,13]. Since radiography is routinely used for stifle joint evaluation in veterinary practice, the present study aimed to evaluate radiographic features for association with development of contralateral CR. We found that both effusion and osteophytosis of both stifles influenced the pattern of contralateral CR. Effusion of the contralateral stifle, in particular, was a highly significant risk factor for disease progression and development of contralateral CR, with an odds ratio of 13.4 for development of a contralateral CR by 1 year after diagnosis. We also found that radiographic

scoring had excellent reproducibility, suggesting that it could successfully be used clinically.

It has been recognized for at least 25 years that dogs affected with unilateral CR often go on to develop contralateral CR. In a recent study, 11% of dogs were diagnosed with bilateral CR at diagnosis [11]. Risk of contralateral CR ranges from 22–54% at 6 to 17 months of diagnosis [6,8–11]. The signalment of the cohort in the present study was typical for the condition and 33% of dogs developed contralateral rupture within the study period. Since this proportion was less than 50%, we were not able to define median time to contralateral CR. However, survival time for the lower quartile of the cohort was 498 days.

Past epidemiological studies have suggested that increasing age [23], neutering of male and female dogs [24], and breed [23] influence risk of CR. In addition, breeds at high risk of CR include the Newfoundland, Rottweiler, Labrador Retriever, Boxer, and Bulldog [23]. The CR trait has been shown to have moderate to high heritability in the Newfoundland and Boxer [25,26]. In

Table 4. Relationship of radiographic osteophytosis in the index stifle to contralateral cranial cruciate ligament rupture at one and two years after surgery.

One year after surgery					
Osteophytosis Grade	Ruptured	Not ruptured	Odds ratio	95% CI	Significance
0	0	1	1.25	0.05–31.98	$p = 0.89$
1	2	17	0.38	0.08–1.86	$p = 0.23$
2	6	25	0.89	0.29–2.72	$p = 0.84$
3	9	23	2.10	0.72–6.18	$p = 0.18$
Two years after surgery					
0	0	1	0.61	0.02–15.72	$p = 0.77$
1	3	14	0.32	0.08–1.25	$p = 0.10$
2	7	16	0.76	0.25–2.26	$p = 0.62$
3	12	11	3.38	1.14–10.00	$p = 0.03$

Note: At one year after surgery, n = 83 dogs; 2 dogs were censored at <365 days. Overall, radiographic osteophytosis in the index stifle was not significantly associated with risk of rupture at 1 year ($p = 0.49$). At two years after surgery, n = 64 dogs; 21 dogs were censored at <730 days. Overall, radiographic osteophytosis in the index stifle was not significantly associated with risk of rupture at 2 years ($p = 0.09$).

Table 5. Relationship of radiographic osteophytosis in the contralateral stifle to contralateral cranial cruciate ligament rupture at one and two years after surgery.

One year after surgery					
Osteophytosis Grade	Ruptured	Not ruptured	Odds ratio	95% CI	Significance
0	1	21	0.13	0.02–1.08	$p = 0.06$
1	10	34	1.34	0.46–3.96	$p = 0.59$
2	2	9	0.84	0.16–4.33	$p = 0.84$
3	4	2	9.85	1.63–59.51	$p = 0.01$
Two years after surgery					
0	3	14	0.32	0.08–1.25	$p = 0.10$
1	13	22	1.31	0.46–3.73	$p = 0.61$
2	2	5	0.74	1.13–4.16	$p = 0.73$
3	4	1	9.11	0.95–87.34	$p = 0.06$

Note: At one year after surgery, n = 83 dogs; 2 dogs were censored at <365 days. Overall, radiographic osteophytosis in the contralateral stifle was significantly associated with risk of rupture at 1 year ($p = 0.03$). At two years after surgery, n = 64 dogs; 21 dogs were censored at <730 days. Overall, radiographic osteophytosis in the contralateral stifle was not significantly associated with risk of rupture at 2 years ($p = 0.11$).

addition, proximal tibial conformation, including TPA, has also been considered an important risk factor for CR [27,28]. In the present study, effects of breed, age, body weight, gender, and TPA did not significantly influence time to contralateral CR, in contrast to radiographic OA in the index and contralateral stifles, particularly the contralateral stifle. There is no evidence of homotypic variation in TPA in dogs [29] and very high TPA values were not present in our cohort in either the index or contralateral stifles. Whilst various epidemiological factors may be important for disease initiation, our results suggest that breed, age, body weight, gender, and TPA are not important factors affecting disease progression over time. These findings are similar to other recently published work [12]. Indirectly, this may suggest that risk factors for disease initiation and disease progression are different. The present study is not able to advance understanding of risk factors for disease initiation. Therefore, the relationship between initiation of fiber fraying in the cruciate ligament complex and development of contralateral stifle synovial effusion and osteoarthritis remains to be determined.

OA is usually detectable radiographically in CR-affected stifles at time of diagnosis [2,14,15]. We found Grade 2 effusion was present in a large majority of index stifles, with 40% of index stifles also affected with Grade 3 osteophytosis. Radiographic signs of contralateral stifle OA in dogs with unilateral CR influence risk of contralateral CR, based on global assessment of synovial effusion, osteophytosis, and subchondral sclerosis [6,9]. However, past analyses have been limited to determining that global scoring of radiographic change, including synovial effusion and osteophytosis, influenced risk of contralateral CR. At diagnosis, we found that Grade 2 effusion was present in the contralateral stifle in 26% of dogs, with Grade 3 osteophytosis being identified in 7% of dogs. Severity of OA was increased in the index stifle. We also found that severity of stifle osteophytosis in the index and contralateral stifles was significantly correlated, suggesting that the disease mechanism influences OA progression in both stifles. Severity of radiographic synovial effusion and osteophytosis was not significantly correlated with body weight, suggesting body weight does not confound interpretation of radiographic change.

In a previous study, we used survival analysis of time to contralateral CR in a large group of dogs presented with unilateral

CR to examine the pattern of contralateral CR [7]. The median time to contralateral CR for the entire affected population was 947 days [7]. However, we did not consider radiographic change at the time of diagnosis in the statistical model. Furthermore, various types of surgical treatment were provided that could have influenced overall mobility after surgery [16–18]; in the present study all dogs were treated with TPLO. In the current study, we found that both severity of radiographic synovial effusion and osteophytosis in the contralateral stifle were significant factors for contralateral rupture associated with a high odds ratio for contralateral CR, particularly at one year after diagnosis. Although a similar trend was identified at 2 years after diagnosis, analysis at this time point had some limitations because not all censored cases had two or more years of follow-up. Kaplan-Meir survival curves for severe Grade 2 radiographic synovial effusion and Grade 3 osteophytosis in the contralateral stifle had significantly reduced time to contralateral CR, when compared with dogs with less severe radiographic grades. Differences between Grade 3 and Grade 1 osteophytosis curves were not significantly different, likely because of low statistical power.

Results were not significant for radiographic synovial effusion in the index stifle, because Grade 2 effusion is typically present once ligament rupture is sufficient to induce joint instability. Survival analysis using logistic regression and the Cox's Proportional Hazard model yielded similar results, although these analyses also suggested that severity of osteophytosis in the index stifle is a significant risk factor for contralateral CR.

It has been hypothesized that stifle synovitis may be an important factor contributing to development of the CR condition. It is known that synovitis is present in clinically stable stifles and that histologic synovitis increases the risk of subsequent contralateral CR [2,13]. Results from the present study, particularly radiographic assessment of synovial effusion in the contralateral stifle, suggest that stifle synovitis is a significant factor in the mechanism that promotes progressive rupture of cruciate ligament fibers over time. This finding is not surprising, since experimental induction of stifle synovitis leads to a significant reduction in cranial cruciate ligament tensile properties [30], likely because the cruciate ligament complex is supplied by fluid flow from both the ligament vascular supply as well as stifle synovial fluid [31]. These

A. Index Effusion

B. Index Osteophytosis

A. Contralateral Effusion

B. Contralateral Osteophytosis

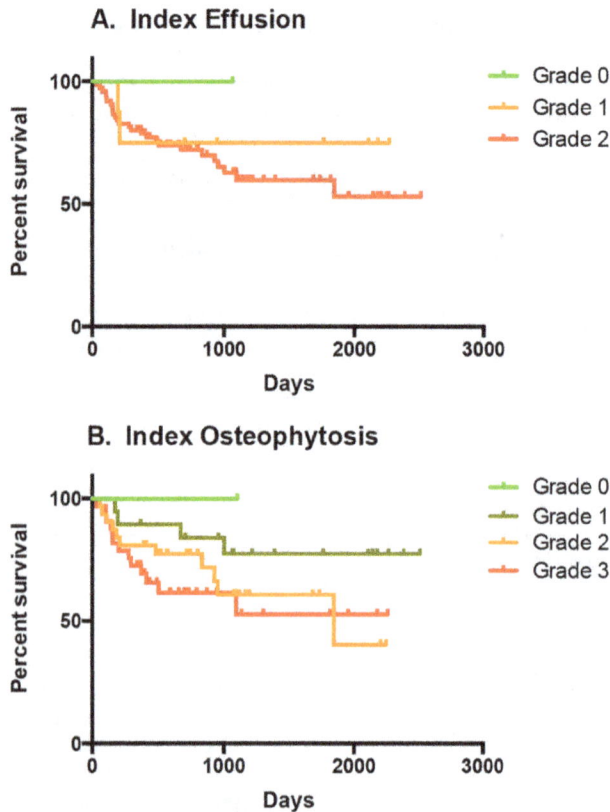

Figure 5. Time to contralateral cranial cruciate ligament rupture stratified by severity of synovial effusion and osteoarthritis in the index stifle. Kaplan-Meier plots for a population of 85 client-owned dogs. Time to contralateral cranial cruciate ligament rupture was not significantly influenced by severity of synovial effusion (**A**) or osteophytosis (**B**) in the index stifle.

Figure 6. Time to contralateral cranial cruciate ligament rupture stratified by severity of synovial effusion or osteoarthritis in the contralateral stifle. Kaplan-Meier plots for a population of 85 client-owned dogs. (**A**) Time to contralateral cranial cruciate ligament rupture was significantly decreased in dogs with Grade 2 radiographic synovial effusion of the contralateral stifle at diagnosis, when compared with the grades of 0 or 1 ($p<0.001$). (**B**) Time to contralateral cranial cruciate ligament rupture was significantly decreased in dogs with Grade 3 osteophytosis of the contralateral stifle at diagnosis, when compared with the grade 0 and grade 2 ($p<0.05$).

findings suggest that the immune mechanisms that lead to stifle synovitis [4,32] should be a focus for future work. Stifle synovitis likely represents a target for disease-modifying therapy aimed at blocking disease progression.

There were several limitations to this study. Our survival analysis was based on a group of 85 dogs treated with TPLO collected from a large cohort of client-owned dogs. However, many dogs were excluded in the initial case filtering, particularly because bilateral stifle radiographs at the time of diagnosis were lacking. This retrospective study reviewed case material over a nine-year period. During this period, it was not standard of care in small animal orthopaedic specialty practice to obtain bilateral stifle radiographs at the time of diagnosis. Consequently, a large number of cases were screened in order to yield an appropriate cohort of dogs for survival analysis. Although significant, results of some statistical analyses were associated with a relatively large confidence interval. Our conclusions may have been strengthened by analysis of longitudinal data from a larger number of dogs. Radiographic scoring was performed subjectively but yielded similar results to other work, in which synovial effusion or osteophytosis was graded as present or absent [12]. Our results strongly support the concept that bilateral radiographic views should be made routinely to fully assess both stifles for OA when dogs are suspected to have unilateral CR [12]. Furthermore, because of the retrospective nature of the study, there was some variation in the follow-up assessment that could have affected case

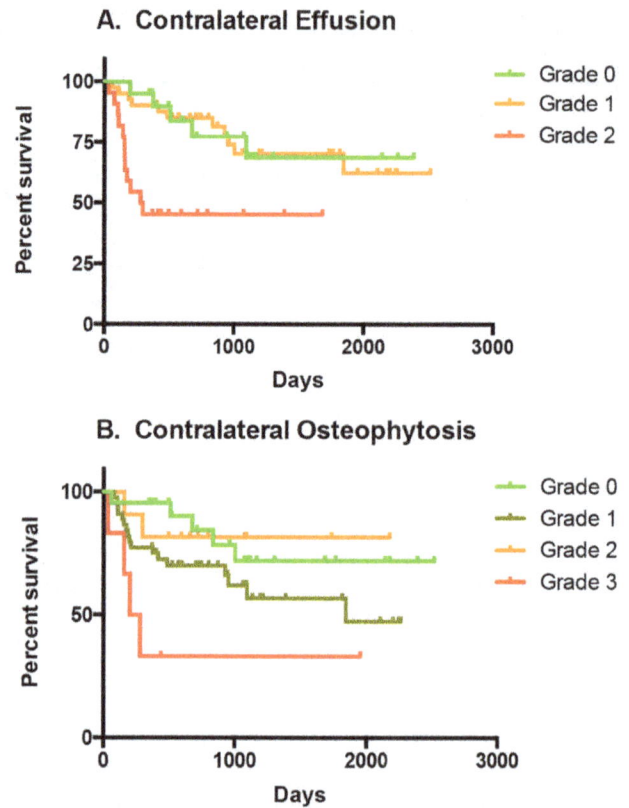

coding. In particular, it is possible that owners may have failed to identify lameness associated with development of contralateral rupture.

In conclusion, subsequent contralateral CR is common in client-owned dogs. Radiographic synovial effusion and osteophytosis in the contralateral stifle of dogs with unilateral CR are significant, clinically relevant markers for risk of contralateral CR. Severe synovial effusion or osteophytosis in the contralateral stifle results in an approximately ten-fold increase in risk of contralateral CR. Our results suggest that stifle radiography provides a predictive marker for risk of contralateral CR that could be used to inform clinical treatment of affected dogs. Since stifle synovitis is a target for disease-modifying therapy, stifle radiography could also be a valuable tool for longitudinal studies of disease-modify treatment for the CR arthropathy. In future work, analysis of stifle magnetic resonance imaging would appear warranted, since synovitis, associated synovial thickening, and joint effusion can be more directly examined [33,34].

Acknowledgments

The authors gratefully acknowledge the help of Victoria Rajamanickam for advice regarding statistical analysis of data.

Author Contributions

Conceived and designed the experiments: PM. Performed the experiments: CC MAR SK RC KTK JAB SLS PM. Analyzed the data: CC MAR PM. Wrote the paper: CC PM.

References

1. Sumner JP, Markel MD, Muir P (2010) Caudal cruciate ligament damage in dogs with cranial cruciate ligament rupture. Vet Surg 39: 936–941.
2. Bleedorn JA, Greuel EN, Manley PA, Schaefer SL, Markel MD, et al (2011) Synovitis in dogs with stable stifle joints and incipient cranial cruciate ligament rupture: A cross-sectional study. Vet Surg 40: 531–543.
3. Wilke VL, Robinson DA, Evans RB, Rothschild MF, Conzemius MG (2005) Estimate of the annual economic impact of treatment of cranial cruciate ligament injury in dogs in the United States. J Am Vet Med Assoc 227: 1604–1607.
4. Doom M, de Bruin T, de Rooster H, van Bree H, Cox E (2008) Immunopathological mechanisms in dogs with rupture of the cranial cruciate ligament. Vet Immunol Immunopathol 125: 143–161.
5. Comerford EJ, Smith K, Hayashi K (2011) Update on the aetiopathogenesis of canine cranial cruciate ligament disease. Vet Comp Orthop Traumatol 24, 91–98.
6. Doverspike M, Vasseur PB, Harb MF, Walls CM (1993) Contralateral cranial cruciate ligament rupture: incidence in 114 dogs. J Am Anim Hosp Assoc 29: 167–170.
7. Muir P, Schwartz Z, Malek S, Kreines A, Cabrera SY, et al. (2011) Contralateral cruciate survival in dogs with unilateral non-contact cranial cruciate ligament rupture. PLoS One 6: e25331.
8. Moore KW, Read RA (1995) Cranial cruciate ligament rupture in the dog – a retrospective study comparing surgical techniques. Aust Vet J 72: 281–285.
9. de Bruin T, de Rooster H, Bosmans T, Duchateau L. van Bree H, et al. (2007) Radiographic assessment of the progression of osteoarthrosis in the contralateral stifle joint of dogs with a ruptured cranial cruciate ligament. Vet Rec 161: 745–750.
10. Cabrera SY, Owen TJ, Mueller MG, Kass PH (2008) Comparison of tibial plateau angles in dogs with unilateral versus bilateral cranial cruciate ligament rupture: 150 cases (2000–2006). J Am Vet Med Assoc 232: 889–892.
11. Buote N, Fusco J, Radasch R (2009) Age, tibial plateau angle, sex, and weight as risk factors for contralateral rupture of the cranial cruciate ligament in Labradors. Vet Surg 38: 481–489.
12. Fuller MC, Hayashi K, Bruecker KA, Holsworth IG, Sutton JS, et al. (2014) Evaluation of the radiographic infrapatellar fat pad sign of the contralateral stifle joint as a risk factor for subsequent contralateral cranial cruciate ligament rupture in dogs with unilateral rupture: 96 cases (2006–2007). J Am Vet Med Assoc 244: 328–338.
13. Erne JB, Goring RL, Kennedy FA, Schoenborn WC (2009) Prevalence of lymphoplasmacytic synovitis in dogs with naturally occurring cranial cruciate ligament rupture. J Am Vet Med Assoc 235: 386–390.
14. Bennett D, Tennant B, Lewis DG, Baughan J, May C, et al. (1988) A reappraisal of anterior cruciate ligament disease in the dog. J Small Anim Pract 29: 275–297.
15. Innes JF, Costello M, Barr FJ, Rudorf H, Barr ARS (2004) Radiographic progression of osteoarthritis of the canine stifle joint: a prospective study. Vet Radiol Ultrasound 45: 143–148.
16. Gordon-Evans WJ, Griffon DJ, Bubb C, Knap KM, Sullivan M, et al. (2013) Comparison of lateral fabellar suture and tibial plateau leveling osteotomy techniques for treatment of dogs with cranial cruciate ligament disease. J Am Vet Med Assoc 243: 675–680.
17. Nelson SA, Krotscheck U, Rawlinson J, Todhunter RJ, Zhang Z, et al. (2013) Long-term functional outcome of tibial plateau leveling osteotomy versus extracapsular repair in a heterogenous population of dogs. Vet Surg 42: 38–50.
18. Bergh MS, Sullivan C, Ferrell CL, Troy J, Budsberg SC (2014) Systematic review of surgical treatments for cranial cruciate ligament disease in dogs. J Am Anim Hosp Assoc 50: epub.
19. Might KR, Bachelez A, Martinez SA, Gay JM (2013) Evaluation of the drawer test and the tibial compression test for differentiating between cranial and caudal stifle subluxation associated with cruciate ligament instability. Vet Surg 42: 392–397.
20. Cooper C, Cushnaghan J, Kirwan JR, Dieppe PA, Rogers J, et al. (1992) Radiographic assessment of the knee joint in osteoarthritis. Ann Rheum Dis 51: 80–82.
21. Abel SB, Hammer DL, Shott S (2003) Use of the proximal portion of the tibia for measurement of the tibial plateau angle in dogs. Am J Vet Res 64: 1117–1123.
22. Sham PC, Curtis D (1995) Monte Carlo tests for associations between disease and alleles at highly polymorphic loci. Ann Hum Genet 59: 97–105.
23. Witsberger TH, Villamil JA, Schultz LG, Hahn AW, Cook JL (2008) Prevalence of and risk factors for hip dysplasia and cranial cruciate ligament deficiency in dogs. J Am Vet Med Assoc 232: 1818–1824.
24. Whitehair JG, Vasseur PB, Willits NH (1993) Epidemiology of cranial cruciate ligament rupture in dogs. J Am Vet Med Assoc 203: 1016–1019.
25. Wilke VL, Conzemius MG, Kinghorn BP, Macrossan PE, Cai W, et al. (2006) Inheritance of rupture of the cranial cruciate ligament in Newfoundlands. J Am Vet Med Assoc 228: 61–64.
26. Nielen ALJ, Janss LLG, Knol BW (2001) Heritability estimations for diseases, coat color, body weight, and height in a birth cohort of Boxers. Am J Vet Res 62: 1198–1206.
27. Inauen R, Koch D, Bass M, Haessig M (2009) Tibial tuberosity conformation as a risk factor for cranial cruciate ligament rupture in the dog. Vet Comp Orthop Traumatol 22: 16–20.
28. Mostafa AA, Griffon DJ, Thomas MW, Constable PD (2009) Morphometric characteristics of the pelvic limbs of Labrador retrievers with and without cranial cruciate ligament deficiency. Am J Vet Res 70: 498–507.
29. Sabanci SS, Ocal MK (2014) Lateral and medial tibial plateau angles in normal dogs. Vet Comp Orthop Traumat 27: 135–140.
30. Goldberg VM, Burstein A, Dawson M (1982) The influence of an experimental immune synovitis on the failure mode and strength of the rabbit anterior cruciate ligament. J Bone Joint Surg 64A: 900–906.
31. Kobayashi S, Baba H, Uchida K, Negoro K, Sato M, et al. (2006) Microvascular system of the anterior cruciate ligament in dogs. J Orthop Res 24: 1509–1520.
32. Muir P, Kelly JL, Marvel SJ, Heinrich DA, Schaefer SL, et al. (2011) Lymphocyte populations in joint tissues from dogs with inflammatory stifle arthritis and degenerative cranial cruciate ligament rupture. Vet Surg 40, 753–761.
33. Krasnokutsky S, Belitskaya-Lévy I, Bencardino J, Samuels J, Attuer M, et al. (2011) Quantitative magnetic resonance imaging evidence of synovial proliferation is associated with radiographic severity of knee osteoarthritis. Arthritis Rheum 63: 2983–2991.
34. Hill CL, Gale DG, Chaisson CE, Skinner K, Kazis L, et al (2001) Knee effusions, popliteal cysts, and synovial thickening: association with knee pain in osteoarthritis. J Rheumatol 28: 1330–1337.

19

Computer-Assisted Radiographic Calculation of Spinal Curvature in Brachycephalic "Screw-Tailed" Dog Breeds with Congenital Thoracic Vertebral Malformations: Reliability and Clinical Evaluation

Julien Guevar, Jacques Penderis, Kiterie Faller, Carmen Yeamans, Catherine Stalin, Rodrigo Gutierrez-Quintana*

School of Veterinary Medicine, College of Medical, Veterinary and Life Sciences, University of Glasgow, Glasgow, United Kingdom

Abstract

The objectives of this study were: To investigate computer-assisted digital radiographic measurement of Cobb angles in dogs with congenital thoracic vertebral malformations, to determine its intra- and inter-observer reliability and its association with the presence of neurological deficits. Medical records were reviewed (2009–2013) to identify brachycephalic screw-tailed dog breeds with radiographic studies of the thoracic vertebral column and with at least one vertebral malformation present. Twenty-eight dogs were included in the study. The end vertebrae were defined as the cranial end plate of the vertebra cranial to the malformed vertebra and the caudal end plate of the vertebra caudal to the malformed vertebra. Three observers performed the measurements twice. Intraclass correlation coefficients were used to calculate the intra- and inter-observer reliabilities. The intraclass correlation coefficient was excellent for all intra- and inter-observer measurements using this method. There was a significant difference in the kyphotic Cobb angle between dogs with and without associated neurological deficits. The majority of dogs with neurological deficits had a kyphotic Cobb angle higher than 35°. No significant difference in the scoliotic Cobb angle was observed. We concluded that the computer assisted digital radiographic measurement of the Cobb angle for kyphosis and scoliosis is a valid, reproducible and reliable method to quantify the degree of spinal curvature in brachycephalic screw-tailed dog breeds with congenital thoracic vertebral malformations.

Editor: Claire Wade, University of Sydney, Australia

Funding: The authors have no support or funding to report.

Competing Interests: The authors have declared that no competing interests exist.

* Email: Rodrigo.GutierrezQuintana@Glasgow.ac.uk

Introduction

Congenital vertebral malformations causing secondary kyphosis (dorsal curvature of the vertebral column) and scoliosis (lateral curvature of the vertebral column) are relatively common in dogs, especially in the brachycephalic "screw-tailed" breeds such as the English bulldog, French bulldog, Boston terrier and Pug [1–3]. Patients with congenital vertebral malformations are often asymptomatic with malformations representing incidental findings identified during unrelated radiographic studies. Clinical signs observed in the affected population are usually those of a progressive myelopathy secondary to vertebral canal stenosis, but also to vertebral instability related to the degree of spinal curvature [1,2,4,5]. The prevalence of clinically affected brachycephalic screw-tailed dogs with congenital vertebral malformations is unknown, but could represent an important "spontaneous" model of spinal deformity.

An important factor evaluated in human patients with congenital vertebral malformations causing kyphosis and scoliosis

is the degree of spinal curvature. The angular magnitude of a spinal deformity is usually quantified using the Cobb angle [6]. This method is used to guide decisions regarding progression, physiotherapy, orthotic options and surgical interventions [7–9]. Various techniques have been used to determine the Cobb angle in humans, including manual, digital computer-assisted (semi-automatic), automatic and even smartphone procedures [9–13].

To the authors' knowledge there are just three previous studies that attempted to quantify the degree of spinal curvature in dogs, and none of them used a computer-assisted method [2,4,5]. In the setting of congenital vertebral malformations in dogs, validating a reliable method is an essential first step towards assessment of disease severity, progression, prognostic significance and it may be used to guide treatment. As a first step in understanding the effect of vertebral malformations in dogs, assessing the reliability of a computer-assisted Cobb angle measurement is therefore important.

The aims of the present study were to investigate the use of Cobb angle measurements in dogs with congenital thoracic vertebral malformations in order to objectively quantify the degree of spinal curvature (kyphosis and scoliosis) using a open-access, computer assisted, digital radiographic measurement system and also to determine if the degree of spinal curvature was associated with the presence of neurological deficits in dogs with thoracic vertebral malformations. We hypothesized that the method would be reproducible and reliable and that neurological deficits would be more likely in dogs with more severe kyphosis.

Materials and Methods

Ethics statement

This study was considered as sub-threshold for specific ethical approval by the convenor of the school of veterinary medicine ethics committee, as the work involved only analysis of data routinely recorded from normal and necessary clinical procedures.

Cases

The medical records of the University of Glasgow Small Animal Hospital were retrospectively reviewed from September 2009 to April 2013 to identify French bulldogs, English bulldogs, Boston terriers and Pugs with or without neurological deficits that had lateral and ventro-dorsal digital radiographs of the thoracic spine with at least a single vertebral congenital malformation present. The breed, age and sex were recorded. If there were any neurological deficits associated with the vertebral malformation identified, then the neurological grade at presentation was recorded, using the standard grading system (Table 1) [14]. Patients were then divided into two groups, one where the vertebral malformation was associated with neurological deficits (Group 1) and one without associated neurological deficits (Group 2). The cases used in the present study were also included in a previous study on classification of congenital vertebral malformations [15]. All dogs in group1 had magnetic resonance imaging which confirmed the compressive myelopathy to be secondary to the vertebral malformation on sagittal and transverse T2 weighted images.

Radiographic assessment

Radiographs of the thoracic spine (lateral and ventro-dorsal views) were performed using a digital radiography system (Siemens, Camberley, United Kingdom). They were then evaluated by three observers using an open-source PACS Workstation DICOM viewer (Osirix Imaging Software, v 3.9.2, Pixmeo, Geneva, Switzerland) that measured the Cobb angle automatically. Observers included two board certified veterinary neurologists (RG, JP) and a veterinary neurology resident (JG) that were blinded to the dog groups. Radiographs were reviewed on the same monitor of a laptop computer (Mac Book Pro, Apple,

Cupertino, California, USA) on two occasions and several weeks apart.

The degree of spinal curvature was assessed on the ventro-dorsal view for scoliosis and on the lateral view for kyphosis of the vertebral malformation leading to spinal curvature. Two reference lines, including a line parallel to the cranial vertebral end plate of the first vertebra cranial to the malformed vertebra and a line parallel to the caudal vertebral end plate of the first caudal vertebra, were traced and the Cobb angle was automatically calculated by the software (Figure 1). If multiple malformations were present, each was evaluated individually unless they were adjacent, in which case the most significant vertebral malformation was selected.

Statistics

The intraclass correlation coefficient (ICC) two-way mixed model on absolute agreement was used to analyse the measurement reliability and it was calculated for both intra- and inter-observer reliability [16]. The value can range from zero to one, with a higher value indicating better reliability. ICC less than 0.40 was considered as poor; 0.40 to 0.59 as fair; 0.60 to 0.74 as good, and 0.75 to 1.00 as excellent [17]. Descriptive statistics were reported as mean, median, range and standard deviation (SD). The Mann-Whitney test was used to compare both groups as the data was not normally distributed. Statistical significance was set for $P<0.05$. When statistics were calculated to compare the two groups, only one set of values from one observer was used (as the ICC values were excellent). When multiple vertebral malformations were present the one with the highest kyphotic and or scoliotic angle was used for the comparison between groups. Data was analyzed using statistical software (Minitab 16.0, Minitab Inc, Coventry, UK and SPSS 21, IBM Corp, Chicago, IL, USA).

Results

Data on the groups and the neurological status are summarized in Table 1 and Table 2. Twenty-one dogs had a single congenital vertebral malformation causing some degree of kyphosis and/or scoliosis, five had two malformations and two had three malformations.

The mean Cobb angle of all measured radiographs for kyphosis was 24.02° (n: 222; median: 16.94°; range: 0.02°–87°), and 5.69° for scoliosis (n: 222; median: 3.02°; range: 0°–49.72°). The mean Cobb angle for kyphosis of group 1 (dogs with associated neurological deficits) was 45.67° (n: 72; median: 49.35°, range: 7.7°–87°) and 16.89° for group 2 (dogs without associated neurological deficits) (n: 96; median: 14.62°; range: 1.50°–47.90°). The mean Cobb angle for scoliosis of group 1 was 9.35° (n: 72; median: 4.10°; range 0°–49.72°) and 3.82° (n: 96; median: 2.39°; range: 0°–17.6°) for group 2.

Table 1. Clinical 0 to 5 grading scale for thoracolumbar spinal cord lesions [14] and incidence in the two groups.

Grade	Clinical signs	Group1	Group2
0	Normal		16/16 (100%)
1	Spinal pain	0/12 (0%)	
2	Ambulatory paraparesis	9/12 (75%)	
3	Non-ambulatory paraparesis	2/12 (17%)	
4	Paraplegia with intact deep pain perception	1/12 (8%)	
5	Paraplegia with absent deep pain perception	0/12 (0%)	

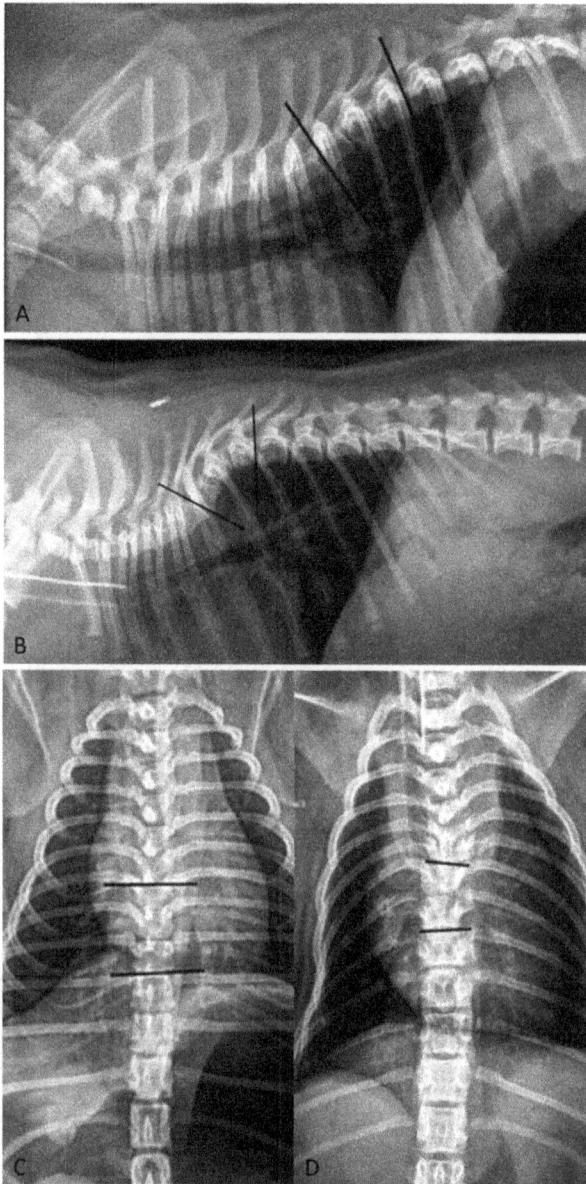

Figure 1. Cobb angles measurements. Lateral and ventro-dorsal radiographs of a neurologically normal Pug with a congenital vertebral malformation at the eighth thoracic vertebra (T8) identified as an incidental finding (A,C) and a clinically affected Pug with a related congenital vertebral malformation at the seventh thoracic vertebra (T7) (B,D). The placement of the reference lines for the calculation of the kyphotic (lateral radiograph) and scoliotic (ventro-dorsal radiograph) angles is shown. The lines pass over the cranial vertebral end plate of T7 and over the caudal vertebral end plate of the ninth thoracic vertebra (T9) in the normal pug (A,C); and similarly over the vertebral end plates of the sixth thoracic vertebra (T6) and T8 in the affected pug (B,D).

There was a statistically significant difference between the kyphotic angles of the two groups ($P<0.001$), but there was no statistically significant difference between its scoliotic angles ($P = 0.55$) (Figure 2). A kyphotic angle $>35°$ had a positive predictive value of 75% for related neurological deficits (negative predictive value of 100%), with a sensitivity and specificity of 100% and 84% respectively.

The intra-and the inter-observer ICC were both excellent when assessing the Cobb angle to quantify spinal curvature on digital radiographs; when the confidence interval was set at 95% (CI 95%), it remained excellent. Table 3 outlines the intra- and inter-observer correlation coefficients for the Cobb angles and their CI 95%.

Discussion

To the authors' knowledge, this is the first study assessing the reliability of a computer-assisted digital radiographic measurement method to calculate the Cobb angle in veterinary medicine, despite the method being one of the most commonly used in human medicine for assessment of kyphosis and scoliosis [18,19]. We confirmed the hypothesis that the evaluation of the Cobb angle on digital radiographs is a feasible and reliable method to quantify the degree of spinal curvature in dogs. Three previous veterinary studies investigated spinal curvature in dogs: one studied a manual technique to measure the degree of kyphosis and its relationship with neurological deficit, and the other two mentioned the use of the Cobb angle manual technique to assess the deformity prior to surgery in dogs without assessing its reliability [2,4,5].

As digital imaging techniques are available in most veterinary practices and hospitals, we aimed to evaluate the feasibility and the reproducibility of Cobb angle measurements in patients with abnormal spinal curvatures, such as kyphosis and scoliosis, via a computer assisted, commercially available plug-in for digital radiography. We confirmed that this method was easy to use and that its reproducibility was excellent, with ICC values over 0.9. When assessing the confidence interval set at 95%, we could conclude that it remained excellent. Assessing this method on digitalized radiography offered the advantage of evaluating a technique which is accessible for general practitioners, and where image size and contrast could be modulated to better define the vertebral end plates, without influencing the results.

Cobb angle measurements have been reported to have a high variability due to incorrect definition of the end vertebra, as well as defective angle measurement [20]. The rationale for the use of a software plug-in that automatically calculates the Cobb angle and for the use of pre-selected and constant end-vertebrae was to reduce these sources of error [20,21]. It is clear however that inaccuracy in angle measurement exists and was inherent to the method itself as measurement of a three-dimensional structure was attempted in a two-dimensional radiographic plane. This was in part explained by the difficulty in drawing a line through a vertebral end plate, which was not evident as a straight line on the radiographs, as well as the difficulty in defining some of the vertebral endplates when vertebrae were superimposed, in particular on ventro-dorsal view radiographs.

The mean scoliotic angles for the two groups were lower than $10°$, which should therefore not be classified as scoliosis *per se* [22]. This, in part, explains why scoliosis was identified in many dogs in our population, without it being related to the presence of neurological deficits.

Kyphosis was the main spinal deformity observed in association with clinical signs, as previously reported [1,2,5]. In the affected group of 12 dogs, in two dogs the neurological deficits could be ascribed to extrusion of an intervertebral disc adjacent to the congenital vertebral malformation or due to empyema secondary to discospondylitis adjacent to the congenital vertebral malformation. Early degeneration of intervertebral discs adjacent to malformed vertebrae has recently been highlighted in dogs, and may have been the predisposing factor in that patient [23]. If those

Table 2. Incidence, breed, sex and age (n = 28).

Variables	Group1	Group2	Total population
Population	12 (43%)	16 (57%)	28 (100%)
Breed	Pug: 9 (75%)	Pug: 2 (12.5%)	Pug: 11 (39%)
	EB: 2 (17%)	EB: 9 (56%)	EB: 11 (39%)
	BT: 0	BT: 3 (19%)	BT: 3 (10.5%)
	FB: 1 (8%)	FB: 2 (12.5%)	FB: 3 (10.5%)
Sex	Female: 6 (50%)	Female: 2 (12.5%)	Female: 8 (28%)
	Male: 6 (50%)	Male: 14 (87.5%)	Male: 20 (72%)
Age	Mean: 2.4 y	Mean: 2.6 y	Mean: 2.5 y
	Range: 4 m-7.5 y	Range: 7 m-14 y	Range: 4 m-14 y
	SD: 2.4 y	SD: 3.2 y	SD: 2.86 y

EB: English bulldog, FB: French bulldog, BT: Boston terrier, m: months, y: years and SD: Standard deviation.

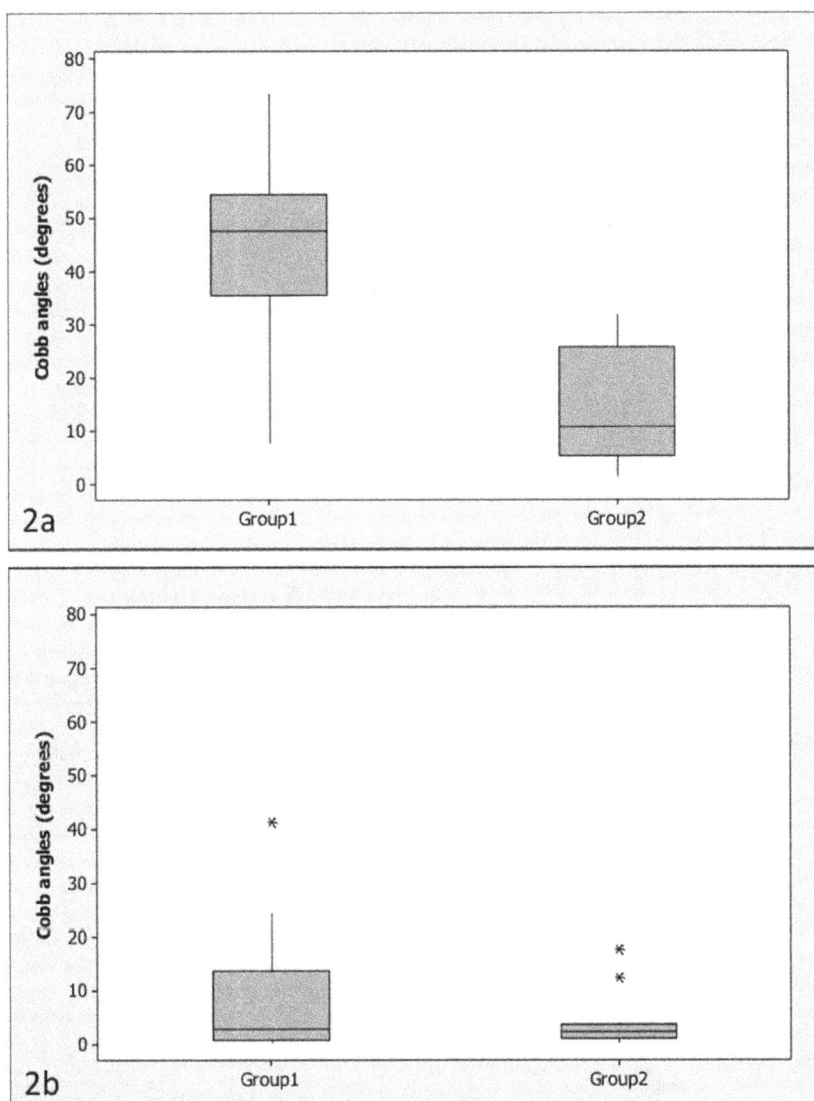

Figure 2. Boxplots of the two groups. Boxplots of the kyphotic Cobb angles for group1 (dogs with associated neurological deficits) and group 2 (dogs without associated neurological deficits) (2a) ($P < 0.001$) and boxplots of the scoliotic angles of groups 1 and 2 (2b) ($P = 0.55$). The Mann-Whitney test was used to compare both groups. The bottom and top lines of the box represent the first and third quartiles, the band inside the box represents the median and the asterisks outside the box and whisker plot represent outliers.

Table 3. Intraclass correlation coefficient (ICC) and 95% coefficient intervals for digital measurement of the Cobb angles (n = 222).

		Data	ICC	CI 95%
		Intraobserver1	0.996	0.992–0.998
		Intraobserver2	0.989	0.980–0.995
	Kyphosis	Intraobserver3	0.984	0.969–0.992
		Interobserver1,2,3	0.982	0.967–0.990
		Interobserver,2,3	0.972	0.950–0.985
Cobb angles				
		Intraobserver1	0.99	0.980–0.995
		Intraobserver2	0.958	0.915–0.979
	Scoliosis	Intraobserver3	0.936	0.876–0.967
		Interobserver1,2,3	0.957	0.926–0.976
		Interobserver1,2,3	0.964	0.936–0.981

CI: Coefficient Interval; 1,2,3: refer to the 3 observers. ICC: intra class correlation coefficients.

two cases are excluded from our affected population, then a cut-off appears around a kyphotic angle of 35°. This finding would suggest that, if indeed kyphotic angles are of progressive nature, [1,24] healthy young dogs with a kyphotic angle below, but close to, 35° may benefit from monitoring for the subsequent appearance of neurological deficits. Serial Cobb angle measurements in these patients would also allow objective determination of progression of vertebral angulation. There is currently no supportive data to suggest any advantages for preventive stabilization with spinal surgery in dogs without neurological deficits; although early intervention may be warranted to prevent them.

Although this study has limitations in its retrospective nature and its small sample size, it advances evidence for the computer-assisted digital radiographic measurement of the Cobb angle as a reliable, reproducible and easy to use method to quantify the degree of spinal curvature in dogs. Further prospective studies, most likely multicenter with larger populations, would be valuable to assess the exact correlation between the degree of spinal curvature and the neurological status in pre-defined dog breeds; as determined by the Cobb angle measurement.

Conclusions

The goal of this study was to assess the use of the Cobb angle method in dogs with spinal curvature and to determine the interobserver and intraobserver reliability of the technique. We concluded that the use of digital imaging and software allowed accurate and reproducible measurement of the Cobb angle in a canine group with congenital vertebral malformations. We also identified in our groups, that a Cobb angle value greater than 35° indicated a high probability of related neurological deficits.

Acknowledgments

The authors thank Michael P. Grevitt from the Centre for Spinal Studies and Surgery at Nottingham University Hospitals Trust for his review and comments of the present paper.

Author Contributions

Conceived and designed the experiments: RGQ JG JP. Performed the experiments: RGQ JG JP. Analyzed the data: RGQ JG KF. Contributed reagents/materials/analysis tools: CS CY. Contributed to the writing of the manuscript: JG JP KF CY CS RGQ.

References

1. Westworth DR, Sturges BK (2010) Congenital spinal malformations in small animals. Vet Clin North Am Small Anim Pract 40: 951–981.
2. Moissonier P, Gossot P, Scotti S (2011) Thoracic kyphosis associated with hemivertebra. Vet Surg 40: 1029–1032.
3. Done SH, Drew RA, Robins G, Robins GM, Lane JG (1975) Hemivertebra in the dog: clinical and pathological observations. Vet Record 96: 313–317
4. Aikawa T, Shibata M, Asano M, Hara Y, Tagawa M, et al. (2014) A Comparison of Thoracolumbar Intervertebral Disc Extrusion in French Bulldogs and Dachshunds and Association With Congenital Vertebral Anomalies. Vet Surg 43: 301–307.
5. Aikawa T, Kanazono S, Yoshigae Y, Sharp NJ, Muñana KR (2007) Vertebral Stabilization Using Positively Threaded Profile Pins and Polymethylmethacry-late, with or Without Laminectomy, for Spinal Canal Stenosis and Vertebral Instability Caused by Congenital Thoracic Vertebral Anomalies. Vet Surg 36: 432–441.
6. Cobb J (1948) Outline for the study of scoliosis. Am Acad Orthop Surg Instr Course Lect; 5: 261–275.
7. Nasca RJ, Stelling FH, Steel HH (1975) Progression of congenital scoliosis due to hemivertebrae and hemivertebrae with bars. J Bone Joint Surg Am 57: 456–466.
8. McMaster M, Singh H (1999) Natural history of congenital kyphosis and kyphoscoliosis: A study of one hundred and twelve patients. J Bone Joint Surg Am 81: 1367–1383.
9. Langensiepen S, Semler O, Sobottke R, Fricke O, Franklin J, et al. (2013) Measuring procedures to determine the Cobb angle in idiopathic scoliosis: a systematic review. Eur Spine J 22: 2360–2371.
10. Srinivasalu S, Modi H, Smehta S, Suh SW, Chen T (2008) Measurement of scoliosis and kyphosis radiographs. Intraobserver and interobserver variation. Asian Spine J 2: 90–93.
11. Tanure MC, Pinheiro AP, Oliveira AS (2010) Reliability assessment of Cobb angle measurements using manual and digital methods. Spine J 10: 769–774.
12. Zhang J, Lou E, Hill D, Raso JV, Wang Y, et al. (2010) Computer-aided assessment of scoliosis on posteroanterior radiographs. Med Biol Eng Comput 48: 185–195.
13. Qiao J, Liu Z, Xu L, Wu T, Zheng X, et al. (2012) Reliability analysis of a smartphone-aided measurement method for Cobb angle scoliosis. J Spinal Disord Tech 25: E88–E92.

14. Sharp N, Wheeler S (2005) Thoracolumbar disc disease. In: Sharp N, Wheeler S, Editors.Small animal spinal disorders: Diagnosis and surgery. Philadelphia, Elsevier Mosby. pp. 121–159

15. Gutierrez-Quintana R, Guevar J, Stalin C, Faller K, Yeamans C, et al. (2014) A proposed radiographic classification of congenital thoracic vertebral malformations in brachycephalic "screw-tailed" dog breeds. Vet Radiol Ultrasound In Press.

16. Shrout P, Fleiss J (1979) Intraclass correlations: Uses in assessing rater reliability. Psychol Bull 86, 420–428.

17. Fleiss JL (1986) Reliability of Measurement. In: Fleiss JL, editor.The Design and Analysis of Clinical Experiments. Toronto, Wiley. pp1–32

18. Harrison DE, Harrison DD, Cailliet R, Janik TJ, Holland B (2001) Radiographic analysis of lumbar lordosis: centroid, cobb, TRALL, and Harrison posterior tangent methods. Spine 26: E235–E242.

19. Morissy RT, Goldsmith GS, Hall EC, Kehl D, Cowie GH (1990) Measurement of the Cobb Angle on radiographs of patients who have scoliosis. J Bone Joint Surg Am 72: 320–327.

20. Gstoetner M, Sekyra K, Wallochnik N, Winter P, Wachter R, et al. (2007) Inter- and intraobserver reliability assessment of the Cobb angle: manual versus digital measurement tools. Eur Spine J 16: 1587–1592.

21. Shea KG, Stevens PM, Nelson M, Smith JT, Masters KS, et al. (1998) A comparison of manual versus computer-assisted radiographic measurement. Intraobserver measurement variability for Cobb angles. Spine 23: 551–555.

22. Angevine PD, Deutsch H (2008) Idiopathic scoliosis. Neurosurgery 63: A86–A93.

23. Faller K, Penderis J, Stalin C, Guevar J, Yeamans C, et al. (2014) The effect of kyphoscoliosis on intervertebral disc degeneration in dogs. Vet J 200: 449–451.

24. Philips MF, Dormans J, Drummond D, Schut L, Sutton LN (1997) Progressive Congenital Kyphosis: Report of Five Cases and Review of the Literature. Pediatr Neurosurg 26: 130–143.

20

Clinical Risk Factors Associated with Anti-Epileptic Drug Responsiveness in Canine Epilepsy

Rowena M. A. Packer[1], Nadia K. Shihab[¶1,2], Bruno B. J. Torres[¶3], Holger A. Volk[1]*

1 Department of Clinical Science and Services, Royal Veterinary College, Hatfield, Hertfordshire, United Kingdom, 2 Department of Neurology/Neurosurgery, Southern Counties Veterinary Specialists, Ringwood, Hampshire, United Kingdom, 3 Department of Veterinary Medicine and Surgery, Federal University of Minas Gerais, Belo Horizonte, Minas Gerais, Brazil

Abstract

The nature and occurrence of remission, and conversely, pharmacoresistance following epilepsy treatment is still not fully understood in human or veterinary medicine. As such, predicting which patients will have good or poor treatment outcomes is imprecise, impeding patient management. In the present study, we use a naturally occurring animal model of pharmacoresistant epilepsy to investigate clinical risk factors associated with treatment outcome. Dogs with idiopathic epilepsy, for which no underlying cause was identified, were treated at a canine epilepsy clinic and monitored following discharge from a small animal referral hospital. Clinical data was gained via standardised owner questionnaires and longitudinal follow up data was gained via telephone interview with the dogs' owners. At follow up, 14% of treated dogs were in seizure-free remission. Dogs that did not achieve remission were more likely to be male, and to have previously experienced cluster seizures. Seizure frequency or the total number of seizures prior to treatment were not significant predictors of pharmacoresistance, demonstrating that seizure density, that is, the temporal pattern of seizure activity, is a more influential predictor of pharmacoresistance. These results are in line with clinical studies of human epilepsy, and experimental rodent models of epilepsy, that patients experiencing episodes of high seizure density (cluster seizures), not just a high seizure frequency pre-treatment, are at an increased risk of drug-refractoriness. These data provide further evidence that the dog could be a useful naturally occurring epilepsy model in the study of pharmacoresistant epilepsy.

Editor: Giuseppe Biagini, University of Modena and Reggio Emilia, Italy

Funding: The authors have no funding or support to report.

Competing Interests: Nadia K. Shihab is employed by Southern Counties Veterinary Specialists. There are no patents, products in development or marketed products to declare.

* Email: hvolk@rvc.ac.uk

¶ NKS and BBJT are joint second authors on this work.

Introduction

Epilepsy is the most common chronic neurological condition in humans and dogs, with estimated prevalences of 0.4–1% [1] and 0.6%, respectively [2]. In human medicine, the best improvement in Quality of Life (QoL) for epilepsy patients is achieved when treatment leads to remission (seizure freedom) [3–5]. Indeed, in one study, no significant change in QoL was found after treatment for subjects that did *not* achieve seizure freedom [4]. In addition to anti-epileptic drug (AED) therapy, surgical interventions are utilised to achieve seizure freedom in medically intractable cases [6]. The dog has been considered as a naturally occurring model of human epilepsy [7,8]. There are considerable parallels in the diagnosis of human and canine epilepsy, with similarly high levels of workup, for example and the use of advanced diagnostic imaging and in limited cases, the use of electroencephalography (EEG) [9]. However, in veterinary medicine, most epilepsy trials have primarily focused on reducing seizure frequency, rather than achieving seizure freedom. Indeed, an ≥50% reduction in seizure frequency has been the definition of AED efficacy in the majority of canine epilepsy studies (e.g. [10–17]). This may not be a

satisfactory outcome for the carers (the owners), with nearly one third considering only complete seizure freedom as an acceptable outcome [18]. More than two thirds of dogs with epilepsy will continue to have seizures long-term [19–22] and around 20–30% will remain poorly controlled (<50% reduction of seizure frequency) despite adequate treatment with phenobarbitone (PB) and/or potassium bromide (KBr) [23–25]. Consequently, there is a need to identify those dogs that are likely to have poor outcomes so that owners have realistic, evidence-based expectations of their dog's treatment. This has been an area of focus in human epilepsy, with analyses identifying risk factors for pharmacoresistance and poor outcome (e.g. [26–28]). In contrast, it has been recognised that more epidemiologic studies are needed to further document the nature and occurrence of remission of epilepsy in dogs [29], and identify risk factors associated with positive and negative outcomes. For those dogs that are unresponsive to AEDs, 'alternative' non-pharmacological treatment options need to be developed to improve their quantity and quality of life, for example, dietary and surgical interventions [30].

Remission with or without medication has been observed in canine epilepsy cases, demonstrating that epilepsy in dogs is not *necessarily* a lifelong condition. Remission rates vary between studies, for example in a study of Danish Labrador Retrievers, 24% of dogs were classed as being in remission; with only 1 (6%) of these receiving antiepileptic treatment (drug-induced remission) [21]. In a further Danish study of 63 dogs with epilepsy, the remission rate (both spontaneous remission and remission with treatment) was 15% [22]. In these studies, remission was classified as being seizure free for two years or three years seizure free, respectively. In a Swiss study of Labrador Retrievers, 30% of dogs treated with phenobarbitone became seizure-free, with an average follow-up period of 4.8 years [19]. In a study of the efficacy of phenobarbital compared with KBr as a first line treatment, complete seizure freedom was achieved in 85% and 52%, respectively, of treated dogs [31]. This study only lasted for six months however, and it is possible that the percentage of dogs experiencing seizure freedom would be lower given a longer follow-up period. In addition, higher % treatment success rates may reflect studying animals in first opinion practice environment, where seizure phenotypes are likely to be less severe than animals seen at referral practices.

Several factors related to the natural history of the disease and clinical factors have been implicated in both the experimental and clinical literature as influencing the likelihood of successful treatment with AEDs (either remission or <50% reduction in seizure frequency). For example, recent rodent studies found that early treatment [32] had a positive influence on the likelihood of remission being achieved in certain types of epilepsy. Indeed, in human epilepsy it was thought that patients should be treated with AEDs immediately after a seizure to increase the likelihood of achieving remission. However, evidence that remission rates in countries with and without ready access to AEDs are similar [33] implies that AEDs may act to suppress seizures, but have no influence on achieving remission. In addition, there is increasing evidence from both canine, rodent and human studies, that other aspects of disease e.g. different markers of severity *can* influence drug responsiveness and treatment outcome [19,29,34–36]. This includes a high seizure frequency before treatment, and the presence of cluster seizures and/or status epilepticus. Much of the canine epilepsy literature in this area is derived from single breed studies, thus the aim of this retrospective study was to investigate factors associated with remission in a large population of dogs with epilepsy treated at a multi-breed canine specific epilepsy clinic.

Materials and Methods

Data from dogs treated at a multi-breed canine specific epilepsy clinic at the Royal Veterinary College Small Animal Referral Hospital (RVC SARH) between 2005–2011 was retrospectively collected from RVC's electronic patient records. Clinical data was originally gained via standardised owner questionnaires for epilepsy patients at their first appointment, and longitudinal follow up data was gained via telephone interview with the dogs' owners. All dogs received a uniform diagnostic protocol (including complete blood cell count; serum biochemical profile and dynamic bile acid testing; MRI of the brain, 1.5-Tesla Gyroscan NT, Philips Medical Systems) and a neurological examination to rule out an underlying cause of the seizure activity. Only dogs which were reported in the records to be diagnosed with idiopathic epilepsy, for which a cause was not identified (no remarkable findings on interictal neurological examination, haematology, biochemistry, brain magnetic resonance imaging and cerebrospinal fluid examination), were included in the study. A genetic or hereditary basis cannot be confirmed for every case included in the study, and it is possible that the cause could have been identified

with continuous EEG recording. Only dogs receiving AEDs were included in the study.

Seizures were classified according to the former guidelines of the International League Against Epilepsy, modified for veterinary patients (Berendt and Gram, 1999; Licht et al., 2002). Epilepsy was defined of at least two unprovoked seizures >24 h apart. Cluster seizures were defined as an episode where more than one seizure occurred within a 24 h period, with full recovery of consciousness between seizures. Status epilepticus was defined as seizure activity lasting longer than 10 min without gaining consciousness. Seizure activity lasting less than 10 min without gaining consciousness was classed as a single seizure episode. A consistent history was collected with the help of a questionnaire developed for a previous study [10]. The data collected included: signalment, age presented to the hospital (days), age of dog at the time of the first seizure (days), time until diagnosis (days), duration of the disorder before treatment (days), number of seizures prior to any treatment with an AED, seizure frequency per month before medication, type of seizures experienced, and experience of cluster seizures (yes/no) and status epilepticus (yes/no). Medication administered was recorded, specifically whether phenobarbitone (PB), potassium bromide (KBr) or other 3rd line drugs were prescribed, and response to these drugs recorded as responsive or unresponsive. Follow up time was recorded in days. Treatment success was recorded as:

(i)   Seizure-free remission (with or without medication) (1/0)

(ii) ≥50% reduction in seizure frequency (1/0)

Non-responsiveness to an AED was classified as a less than 50% reduction in seizure frequency, despite being within the reference range for the prescribed AED(s) and titrated to the maximum tolerated effective dose. As these data were derived from a clinical population, decision-making leading to the maximum dose of any AED was made by both the clinician and the owner, taking into account adverse effects of the drug and its efficacy. Serum levels of phenobarbitone and/or potassium bromide were checked by the attending clinician, and recorded from the clinical records where available, to ensure the dog was within the reference range for these AEDs and receiving adequate therapy, and to test the effect of this variable.

Ethics statement

This study was approved by the Royal Veterinary College's Ethics and Welfare Committee. The owners of the dogs gave permission for their animals to be used in this study.

Statistical analysis

Differences between outcome variables were tested with a Fisher's exact test for categorical variables with expected values < 10, and the Pearson's chi squared test for expected values >10. The Mann Whitney U-test was used for continuous variables. Generalised linear mixed models for binary outcomes were then used to identify risk factors in a multivariate analysis for successful treatment outcomes, using the lmer function in R from the lme4 package. Treatment outcomes (i) seizure free remission with or without medication (1/0) and (ii) ≥50% reduction in seizure frequency (1/0) were used as the response variables in models. Follow-up time and serum AED values were tested in the models to verify that they did not have an effect on treatment success. Breed was included as a random effect, with all cross breeds coded plainly as 'cross breed' due to the unknown parentage of many of these dogs. This random effect took into account the genetic non-independence of multiple members of the same breed in the study

Table 1. Association between clinical variables and being in seizure-free remission in canine epilepsy patients.

		Remission		Statistics	
		No (%)	Yes (%)	Fishers exact (2 sided)	P
Sex	Male	75.1	53.6	5.56	0.024
	Female	24.9	46.4		
Neuter status	Neutered	53.2	75.0	4.53	0.038
	Entire	46.8	25.0		
Seizure severity	Status epilepticus	20.0	0.0	0.25	0.802
	No Status epilepticus	80.0	100.0		
	Cluster seizures	62.8	17.9	19.63	<0.001
	No Cluster seizures	37.2	82.1		
		Median (25th–75th percentile)	Median (25th–75th percentile)	Mann Whitney U	P
Age presented to hospital (days)		1080 (720–1800)	1440 (1080–2085)	1933	0.61
Time until diagnosis (days)		180 (62.3–378.8)	90 (15–225)	1204	0.79
Age at onset seizures (days)		720 (441–1286)	1170 (720–1725)	2971	0.026
Duration of disorder before treatment (days)		90 (30–180)	60 (26–120)	578	0.31
Number of seizures before start of treatment		5 (3–8.5)	4 (3–5.3)	1286	0.09
Seizure frequency per month before medication		3 (1–6)	2 (1.25–3.75)	1582	0.39

population, and possible demographic and environmental factors. Predictors including age, sex and neuter status were tested in all models. Multicollinearity was checked for in all models, identified from inflated standard errors in the models, and thus avoided. Model fit was assessed using the deviance and Akaike's information criterion. Data is presented as median with 25th and 75th percentiles and all tests were used two-sided with $P<0.05$ being considered statistically significant.

Results

Population demographics

122 dogs were lost to follow and 344 dogs were included in the analysis, of which 89.5% were pure bred and 10.5% were cross-breeds. The five most common breeds were the Labrador Retriever (14.8%), cross breed (10.5%), Border Collie (9.9%), German Shepherd Dog (8.7%) and the Staffordshire Bull Terrier (5.5%). The majority of dogs were male (70.3%), with 57% of all dogs neutered. The median age (in days) at presentation to the small animal referral hospital was 1260 days (720–2008) (approximately 3.5 years).

Clinical data

The median age at onset of seizures was 780 days (360–1447.5). The median time until diagnosis was 150 days (38–360), with the median duration of the disorder before treatment 67.5 days (30–180). The median number of seizures before the start of treatment was 4.5 (3–7.25) with a median seizure frequency (per month) before medication of 3 (1–5). The median follow up time was 656 days (330–960).

A minority of dogs had experienced status epilepticus (13.1%), whereas nearly half of dogs had experienced cluster seizures (48%). There was a significant association between the presence of status epilepticus and cluster seizures ($X^2 = 8.05$, $P = 0.004$), with 9.8% of dogs experiencing both status epilepticus and cluster seizures. There was no difference between male and female dogs experiencing cluster seizures (48.9% vs. 45.8%; $X^2 = 0.26$, $P = 0.61$); however, more male dogs experienced status epilepticus than female dogs (15.5% vs. 5.2%; $X^2 = 4.12$, $P = 0.041$). At the univariate level (Table 1) dogs without cluster seizures were significantly more likely to go into remission, but there was no difference in dogs with or without status epilepticus.

The most common seizure type was complex-focal seizures with secondary tonic-clonic generalisation (35.7%), followed by generalised tonic-clonic (32.6%), complex-focal (14.1%), and simple-focal seizures with secondary tonic-clonic generalisation (13.7%). The rarest seizure type was simple-focal seizures with only 11 cases (3.8%).

Of the 113 dogs for which PB concentrations were available, they were well within the reference range (29.1±1.60 µg/ml, reference range from our laboratory of 15–45 µg/ml). KBr concentrations were available for 53 dogs and were 1.61±0.11 mg/ml, again well within the reference range from our laboratory of 0.5–1.9 mg/ml.

The majority of dogs were receiving PB at follow up (67.2%), with a further 38.4% of cases receiving KBr, and 27% of all cases receiving PB and KBr in combination. A minority of cases (10.2%) were prescribed a third line AED (e.g. gabapentin, pregabalin, levetiracetam and zonisamide). In addition, 5.4% of cases received

Table 2. Association between clinical variables and ≥50% reduction in seizure frequency in canine epilepsy patients.

		≥50% reduction		Statistics	
		No (%)	Yes (%)	Fishers exact (2 sided)	P
Sex	Male	78.5	64.5	5.54	0.025
	Female	21.5	35.5		
Neuter status	Neutered	50.0	63.2	3.62	0.040
	Entire	50.0	36.8		
Seizure severity	Status epilepticus	21.1	10.2	4.35	0.052
	No Status epilepticus	78.9	89.8		
	Cluster seizures	71.7	33.5	34.01	<0.001
	No Cluster seizures	28.3	66.5		
		Median (25th–75th percentile)	Median (25th–75th percentile)	Mann Whitney U	P
Age presented to hospital (days)		990 (720–1514.8)	1424.5 (840–2094.5)	5795	0.011
Time until diagnosis (days)		183 (72.5–360)	150 (34–360)	4225.5	0.216
Age at onset seizures (days)		720 (360–1125)	968 (447.8–1699)	9893	0.007
Duration of disorder before treatment (days)		37.5 (22.5–142.5)	90 (30–180)	833.5	0.064
Number of seizures before start of treatment		5 (3.3–8.8)	4.5 (3–7.8)	2762	0.276
Seizure frequency per month before medication		3 (1–5)	2 (1–5)	5022.5	0.569

emergency rectal diazepam treatment and 8.1% received pulsed intermittent treatment with levetiracetam.

Risk factors for remission

Fourteen per cent of dogs were in remission on PB treatment. When ≥50% reduction in seizure frequency is used as the outcome measure, success rates are markedly higher with 64.5% of dogs achieving this level of seizure reduction. At the univariate level, several factors were associated with an increased likelihood of achieving remission (Table 1), namely: being female, neutered, no previous experience of cluster seizures and an older age at onset of seizures. The same four factors were also associated with an increased likelihood of achieving an ≥50% reduction in seizure frequency, with the addition of an older age at presentation to hospital (Table 2).

When tested in a multivariate mixed model (Table 3), two categorical variables were significantly associated with the likelihood of remission being achieved; sex and cluster seizures, with female dogs over two times more likely to achieve remission, and dogs with no previous experience of cluster seizures over six times more likely to achieve remission. No effects of neuter status or previous episodes of status epilepticus were found in any model, and were not found to improve model fit (determined by Akaike Information Criterion [AIC] and % correct classification), and as such they were not included in the final model. There were no significant effects of time until diagnosis, duration of time before treatment, the number of seizures before treatment or the seizure frequency per month before medication. No effects of follow up time or serum AED values were found. There were no significant effects of seizure type on the likelihood of remission (p = 0.208);

Table 3. Risk factors for remission in canine epilepsy cases.

Predictor	Odds Ratio (95% CI OR)	SE (coef)	Z	P
Sex				
Female	2.39 (1.01–5.64)	0.44	2.00	0.047
Male	Ref			
Cluster Seizures				
No	6.08 (2.35–15.70)	0.49	3.75	<0.001
Yes	ref			

Table 4. Risk factors for an ≥50% reduction in seizure frequency in canine epilepsy cases.

Predictor	Odds Ratio (95% CI OR)	SE (coef)	Z	P
Sex				
Female	2.15 (1.12–4.15)	0.33	2.32	0.021
Male	ref			
Cluster Seizures				
No	4.66 (2.58–8.39)	0.30	5.14	<0.001
Yes	ref			
Age at onset of seizures (days)	1.00 (1.00–1.01)	0.00	2.51	0.013

however the seizure types with the lowest remission rates were simple-focal (0% remission) and complex-focal seizure with secondary tonic-clonic generalisation (14.1% remission).

When an ≥50% reduction in seizure frequency is used as the outcome measure (Table 2 and 4), the same two factors were found to significantly predict the likelihood of achieving remission in a multivariate model (Table 4), with the addition of age at onset of seizures. As age at onset of seizures increases, the likelihood of achieving an ≥50% reduction in seizure frequency increases.

Breeds

Dogs of fifteen different breeds achieved seizure freedom, and dogs of fifty-two breeds achieved an ≥50% reduction in seizure frequency. There was no statistically significant effect of breed on the likelihood of dogs going into remission or having an ≥50% reduction in seizure frequency when tested at the univariate level. Of the breeds with over 10 dogs for which data was available (the Labrador Retriever, Cross Breed, German Shepherd, Border Collie and Staffordshire Bull Terrier), the breed least likely to go into remission or have an ≥50% reduction in seizure frequency was the Border Collie (0% and 40% respectively), followed by the German Shepherd (11% and 35%) and Staffordshire Bull Terrier (0% and 57%). Fishers exact tests revealed only significant effects of being a Border Collie or German Shepherd on the likelihood of entering remission or experiencing an ≥50% reduction in seizure frequency (Table 5). When these breeds were included in multivariate analyses as binary variables, no significant effects were found.

Discussion

The results of this retrospective study provide evidence that the presence of cluster seizures and thus seizure *density* (the temporal pattern of seizure activity) is a more influential risk factor on the likelihood of achieving remission in canine epilepsy than seizure

frequency or the total number of seizures prior to treatment. Nearly half (48%) of dogs in the study population had experienced cluster seizures, of which only 17.9% achieved remission and 33.5% achieved an ≥50% reduction in seizure frequency. This result has previously been found in human epilepsy [37]. The number of epileptic dogs that experience cluster seizures varies between studies, with recent reports between 38% and 64% [20,38]. The breed least likely to achieve remission in this study was the Border Collie, a breed previously demonstrated to have a higher level of cluster seizures than other breeds (84.6% affected) [20], with similar levels reported in other studies (e.g. 94%; [29]). A remission rate of 14.2% was observed in this study, similar to a previous Danish study of canine epilepsy (15%) [22]. These were both mixed study populations; however, in studies of Labrador Retrievers in isolation, higher levels of remission have been observed (24–40%) [19,21]. When >50% reduction in seizure frequency is used as the outcome measure, success rates are markedly higher at 64.5%.

Seizure *density* as well as frequency has been demonstrated to influence the likelihood of remission in humans, with individuals who experience an episode of status epilepticus [39–41], or cluster seizures [37] less likely to go into remission. These results were also seen in a recent study of predictors of pharmacoresistance in rats, where the average seizure frequency per day of 13 rats nonresponsive to medication was 4.31/day, indicating some rats having cluster seizures [36]. This frequency was significantly higher than 20 drug-responsive rats (mean 0.54/day). It is further notable, that of the 13 rats that were unresponsive to medication, a subgroup of six rats (18%) experienced high levels of cluster seizures, with an average of 8.94 seizures per day [36]. Intact male and female dogs have a higher likelihood of having cluster seizures [42] which may have a negative impact on their prognosis. Evidence from canine epilepsy is not clear however, with 89% (8/9) of Border Collies in remission having a history of cluster seizures, status epilepticus, or both [29]. A severe epilepsy

Table 5. Top five breeds most likely to lack drug response.

Breed	% remission	p	% ≥50% reduction	P
Border Collie	0	0.02	40	0.01
German Shepherd	11	0.51	35	0.01
Staffordshire Bull Terrier	0	0.18	57	0.37
Cross Breed	19	0.30	61	0.38
Labrador Retriever	23	0.14	76	0.07

phenotype is often seen in this breed, thus data from a larger population with a diversity of breeds represented would be valuable to gain an insight into this relationship in a wider population with a variety of disease phenotypes.

No evidence was found to support the results of a recent rodent study that found early treatment [32] influenced the likelihood of remission being achieved. There are divergent opinions within the veterinary profession regarding time to treatment after diagnosis of epilepsy, a topic also debated in human medicine [43]. One school of thought advises treatment of seizures as soon as a dog is diagnosed as having recurrent seizures (i.e. after the second seizure episode). However, the impact of AED side effects on QoL may be considerable, with this being the top reason cited by owners for a decreased QoL in their dogs (28% of 25 owners questioned) [44]. As such, the second school of thought considers that there should be a balance between the benefits gained from using AEDs with the potential adverse effects they cause. The results of this study indicated no effect of time to treatment; however, there is mixed evidence regarding its effects on treatment outcome. In clinical studies of epilepsy in dogs, decreased time to treatment has not been observed as a positive influence upon treatment outcome, indeed, one study demonstrated that Labrador Retrievers that were in remission received medication a longer period of time after their first seizure than those dogs which continued to seizure [19]. It should be acknowledged that this result may be biased by animals with a more severe seizure phenotype receiving treatment earlier, due to owner and/or veterinarian concerns. It is currently not veterinary practice to initiate treatment after the first seizure. Early initation of treatment has also proven unsuccessful in several human studies [45–47]. Time to treatment is additionally likely to be influenced by disease severity, for example it was shorter in dogs with episodes of status epilepticus [48], thus being confounding factors in statistical analyses.

A large number of seizures before treatment has been identified as a poor prognostic factor in several previous human studies of epilepsy [34,41,49], with patients experiencing a greater number of seizures prior to initiation of treatment more likely to have refractory epilepsy. In rats, it was recently demonstrated that seizure frequency in the early phase of epilepsy is a strong predictor of refractoriness [36]. This has also been seen in dogs, with refractory dogs having a significantly higher number of seizures prior to presentation and beginning of treatment in Labradors [19] and an initially higher seizure frequency in Border Collies [29]. It has been discussed whether this initial high seizure frequency and subsequent refractoriness may be an effect of kindling (Reynolds, 1995). However, as time to treatment has not been found to be a strong predictor of refractoriness in dogs and humans, initial high seizure frequency has been considered more likely to be the result, rather than the cause of the pathophysi-ological changes that are later manifested as refractory epilepsy [34,50]. Indeed, in this study and another previous study of canine epilepsy, the number of seizures before treatment was not significantly different between dogs positive vs. negative treatment outcomes [48]. In addition, no effect was found of seizure type upon the likelihood of remission; however, the most common seizure type in dogs that did not achieve remission (39.6%) was complex-focal seizures, also seen in human epilepsy [51,52], adding evidence to the belief that focal seizures are more challenging to treat.

Males were found to be less likely to achieve remission than female dogs. Historically, male dogs are thought to seizure more than female dogs [53], and recent epidemiological studies of idiopathic epilepsy have confirmed a male overrepresentation for this disorder [2,38]. With regard to the impact of sex upon

treatment outcome, little existing data is available. One study noted that female dogs with epilepsy lived longer with the disorder than male dogs, with a median age at death two years greater (8 vs. 6 years, respectively) [22]; however, this outcome measure may be influenced by owner euthanasia decisions, so can only be a proxy of treatment success. In previous studies, male dogs were found to be more highly affected by cluster seizures than female dogs [42]. This result was not found in the current study, and indeed sex and the presence of cluster seizures were found to be independently significant risk factors, thus further investigation is warranted into the effect of sex on treatment outcome.

Age at onset of disease was found to significantly influence the likelihood of achieving an $\geq 50\%$ reduction in seizure frequency, with dogs experiencing their first seizure at an older age more likely to achieve this level of reduction. This has previously been demonstrated in Border Collies, with the mean age at onset significantly higher in dogs with remission compared to those with active epilepsy [29], and in Labradors, with dogs classed as having excellent or good results (defined as those that were seizure-free, or had an improvement in their seizure frequency, strength and/or duration) having a significantly higher age at onset than uncontrolled dogs [19]. Early age at seizure onset has been previously identified in children to be a predictor of pharmacore-sistance [54]. In contrast, in a study of canine juvenile epilepsy (where the first seizure occurs before the age of one year), age at onset had no influence on survival outcome [20].

There are recognised limitations to studying epilepsy in a veterinary referral population [20] due to a bias towards a more severe seizure phenotype, and thus may not be representative of the whole canine epilepsy population. As such, further studies of epilepsy in the first opinion practice population may be warranted, although the level of diagnostic work up may be lower owing to availability of equipment and specialist expertise, and thus confidence in diagnosis may be variable. A further limitation of this study is the varied follow up time of cases. In previous studies, remission was strictly classified as dogs that were seizure free for two or three years [21,22]. In human epilepsy, seizures may re-occur after a period of months of seizure freedom, without alterations to treatment [55]. As such, some of the dogs classified as seizure free in this study may have later experienced seizures. This may be due to a variety of factors including drug tolerance, deterioration of the epilepsy phenotype, acquired drug resistance and poor owner compliance [55]. The median follow up time, however, was 656 days and thus is in line with the follow-up standards of comparable epilepsy studies in the veterinary environment. There are limitations to which variables could be controlled for in this study, introduced by data being collected in a clinical environment with naturally occurring disease in client owned animals. Due to the expense of medication it is possible that clients may decline third line AEDs that may affect the response rate, which may mean the figures here are an underestimate of how many dogs could biologically achieve remission. In addition, EEG is not routinely used in the Canine Epilepsy Clinic data were sourced from, or in veterinary medicine in general at present, and thus there is no confirmation that the 'seizure' episodes reported by owners was indeed seizure activity. A further limitation of this study is that serum AED levels were not available for all dogs; however, clinicians contributing to this dataset routinely checked AED serum levels were within the reference ranges and thus, this is naturally standardised across the sample. Furthermore, not all serum levels were conducted at the same laboratory and therefore could not be analysed in the same dataset. No statistical association between AED levels and treatment outcome were found; however, future studies could include this variable to check this result was not due to the lower power of this sub-sample.

Conclusions

In conclusion, the present provides evidence that it is not merely the absolute *number* of seizures prior to treatment that predicts refractoriness, but their temporal pattern, with those patients experiencing cluster seizures (more than one seizure within a 24 h period) more likely to be pharmacoresistant. Whether this result is an effect of cluster seizures promoting epileptogenesis and causing brain damage that results in seizures resistant to medication, or is actually a reflection of a more aggressive disease phenotype that is harder to treat is unknown, and warrants further investigation. The present study further demonstrates similarities between this naturally occurring model of epilepsy and both experimental rodent models [36], and human clinical studies [37]. The similarity between clinical environments, high level of diagnostic work up, and shared living environments between humans and dogs further strengthens the use of this readily available animal model.

Acknowledgments

The paper was internally approved for submission (Manuscript ID number CSD_00726).

Author Contributions

Conceived and designed the experiments: NKS BBJT HAV. Performed the experiments: NKS BBJT. Analyzed the data: RMAP. Contributed reagents/materials/analysis tools: RMAP. Contributed to the writing of the manuscript: HAV RMAP.

References

1. Sander JW, Shorvon SD (1996) Epidemiology of the epilepsies. Journal of Neurology, Neurosurgery, and Psychiatry 61: 433–443.
2. Kearsley-Fleet L, O'Neill DG, Volk HA, Church DB, Brodbelt DC (2013) Prevalence and risk factors for canine epilepsy of unknown origin in the UK. Veterinary Record 172.
3. Poochikian-Sarkissian S, Sidani S, Wennberg R, Devins G (2008) Seizure Freedom Reduces Illness Intrusiveness and Improves Quality of Life in Epilepsy. The Canadian Journal of Neurological Sciences 35: 280–286.
4. Birbeck Gretchen L, Hays Ron D, Cui X, Vickrey Barbara G (2002) Seizure Reduction and Quality of Life Improvements in People with Epilepsy. Epilepsia 43: 535–538.
5. Kwan P, Arzimanoglou A, Berg AT, Brodie MJ, Allen Hauser W, et al. (2010) Definition of drug resistant epilepsy: consensus proposal by the ad hoc task force of the ILAE Commission on Therapeutic Strategies. Epilepsia 51: 1069–1077.
6. Ramey WL, Martirosyan NL, Lieu CM, Hasham HA, Lemole Jr GM, et al. (2013) Current management and surgical outcomes of medically intractable epilepsy. Clinical Neurology and Neurosurgery 115: 2411–2418.
7. Löscher W, Schwartz-Porsche D, Frey HH, Schmidt D (1985) Evaluation of epileptic dogs as an animal model of human epilepsy. Arzneimittelforschung 35(1): 82–7.
8. Potschka H, Fischer A, von Rüden E-L, Hülsmeyer V, Baumgärtner W (2013) Canine epilepsy as a translational model? Epilepsia 54: 571–579.
9. Berendt M, Høgenhaven H, Flagstad A, Dam M (1999) Electroencephalography in dogs with epilepsy: similarities between human and canine findings. Acta Neurologica Scandinavica 99: 276–283.
10. Volk HA, Matiasek LA, Luján Feliu-Pascual A, Platt SR, Chandler KE (2008) The efficacy and tolerability of levetiracetam in pharmacoresistant epileptic dogs. The Veterinary Journal 176: 310–319.
11. Platt SR, Adams V, Garosi LS, Abramson CJ, Penderis J, et al. (2006) Treatment with gabapentin of 11 dogs with refractory idiopathic epilepsy. Veterinary Record 159: 881–884.
12. Dewey CW, Cerda-Gonzalez S, Levine JM, Badgley BL, Ducoté JM, et al. (2009) Pregabalin as an adjunct to phenobarbital, potassium bromide, or a combination of phenobarbital and potassium bromide for treatment of dogs with suspected idiopathic epilepsy. Journal of the American Veterinary Medical Association 235: 1442–1449.
13. Dewey CW, Guiliano R, Boothe DM, Berg JM, Kortz GD, et al. (2004) Zonisamide therapy for refractory idiopathic epilepsy in dogs. Journal of the American Animal Hospital Association 40.
14. von Klopmann T, Rambeck B, Tipold A (2007) Prospective study of zonisamide therapy for refractory idiopathic epilepsy in dogs. Journal of Small Animal Practice 48: 134–138.
15. Andrew SE (2008) Immune-mediated canine and feline keratitis. Veterinary Clinics of North America-Small Animal Practice 38: 269-+.
16. Muñana KR, Nettifee-Osborne JA, Bergman RL, Jr., Mealey KL (2012a) Association between ABCB1 genotype and seizure outcome in collies with epilepsy. Journal of Veterinary Internal Medicine 26: 1358–1364.
17. Muñana KR, Thomas WB, Inzana KD, Nettifee-Osborne JA, McLucas KJ, et al. (2012b) Evaluation of levetiracetam as adjunctive treatment for refractory canine epilepsy: a randomized, placebo-controlled, crossover trial. Journal of Veterinary Internal Medicine 26: 341–348.
18. Wessmann A, Volk H, Parkin T, Ortega M, Anderson TJ (2012) Living with canine idiopathic epilepsy: a questionnaire-based evaluation of quality of life. Proceedings of the 24th Symposium ESVN-ECVN. J Vet Intern Med 26: 823–852.
19. Heynold Y, Faissler D, Steffen F, Jaggy A (1997) Clinical, epidemiological and treatment results of idiopathic epilepsy in 54 labrador retrievers: a long-term study. Journal of Small Animal Practice 38: 7–14.
20. Arrol L, Penderis J, Garosi L, Cripps P, Gutierrez-Quintana R, et al. (2012) Aetiology and long-term outcome of juvenile epilepsy in 136 dogs. Veterinary Record 170: 335.
21. Berendt M, Gredal H, Pedersen LG, Alban L, Alving J (2002) A Cross-Sectional Study of Epilepsy in Danish Labrador Retrievers: Prevalence and Selected Risk Factors. Journal of Veterinary Internal Medicine 16: 262–268.
22. Berendt M, Gredal H, Ersbøll AK, Alving J (2007) Premature Death, Risk Factors, and Life Patterns in Dogs with Epilepsy. Journal of Veterinary Internal Medicine 21: 754–759.
23. Trepanier L, Schwark W, Van Schoick A, Carrillo J (1998) Therapeutic serum drug concentrations in epileptic dogs treated with potassium bromide alone or in combination with other anticonvulsants: 122 cases (1992–1996). J Am Vet Med Assoc 213: 1449–1453.
24. Schwartz-Porsche D, Löscher W, Frey H (1985) Therapeutic efficacy of phenobarbital and primidone in canine epilepsy: a comparison. J Vet Pharmacol Ther 8: 113–119.
25. Podell M, Fenner W (1993) Bromide therapy in refractory canine idiopathic epilepsy. Journal of Veterinary Internal Medicine 7: 318–327.
26. Cockerell O, Johnson A, Sander J (1994) Remission of epilepsy: results from the National General Practice Study of Epilepsy. Lancet 346: 140–144.
27. Bonnett LJ, Tudur Smith C, Smith D, Williamson PR, Chadwick D, et al. (2014) Time to 12-month remission and treatment failure for generalised and unclassified epilepsy. Journal of Neurology, Neurosurgery & Psychiatry 85: 603–610.
28. MacDonald BK, Johnson AL, Goodridge DM, Cockerell OC, Sander JWAS, et al. (2000) Factors predicting prognosis of epilepsy after presentation with seizures. Annals of Neurology 48: 833–841.
29. Hülsmeyer V, Zimmermann R, Brauer C, Sauter-Louis C, Fischer A (2010) Epilepsy in Border Collies: Clinical Manifestation, Outcome, and Mode of Inheritance. Journal of Veterinary Internal Medicine 24: 171–178.
30. Martlé V, Van Ham L, Raedt R, Vonck K, Boon P, et al. (2014) Non-pharmacological treatment options for refractory epilepsy: An overview of human treatment modalities and their potential utility in dogs. The Veterinary Journal 199: 332–339.
31. Boothe DM, Dewey C, Carpenter DM (2012) Comparison of phenobarbital with bromide as a first-choice antiepileptic drug for treatment of epilepsy in dogs. J Am Vet Med Assoc 240: 1073–1083.
32. Blumenfeld H, Klein JP, Schridde U, Vestal M, Rice T, et al. (2008) Early treatment suppresses the development of spike-wave epilepsy in a rat model. Epilepsia 49: 400–409.
33. Placencia M, Sander JWAS, Shorvon SD, Roman M, Alarcon F, et al. (1993) Antiepileptic drug treatment in a community health care setting in northern Ecuador: a prospective 12-month assessment. Epilepsy Research 14: 237–244.
34. Kwan P, Brodie MJ (2000) Early Identification of Refractory Epilepsy. New England Journal of Medicine 342: 314–319.
35. Weissl J, Hulsmeyer V, Brauer C, Tipold A, Koskinen LL, et al. (2012) Disease progression and treatment response of idiopathic epilepsy in Australian Shepherd dogs. Journal of Veterinary Internal Medicine 26: 116–125.
36. Löscher W, Brandt C (2010) High seizure frequency prior to antiepileptic treatment is a predictor of pharmacoresistant epilepsy in a rat model of temporal lobe epilepsy. Epilepsia 51: 89–97.
37. Sillanpää M, Schmidt D (2008) Seizure clustering during drug treatment affects seizure outcome and mortality of childhood-onset epilepsy. Brain 131: 938–944.
38. Short AD, Dunne A, Lohi H, Boulton S, Carter SD, et al. (2011) Characteristics of epileptic episodes in UK dog breeds: an epidemiological approach. Veterinary Record 169: 48.
39. Hauser WA (1990) Status epilepticus: epidemiologic considerations. Neurology 40: 9–13.

40. Callaghan BC, Anand K, Hesdorffer D, Hauser WA, French JA (2007) Likelihood of seizure remission in an adult population with refractory epilepsy. Annals of Neurology 62: 382–389.

41. Sillanpää M (1993) Remission of Seizures and Predictors of Intractability in Long-Term Follow-Up. Epilepsia 34: 930–936.

42. Monteiro R, Adams V, Keys D, Platt SR (2012) Canine idiopathic epilepsy: prevalence, risk factors and outcome associated with cluster seizures and status epilepticus. Journal of Small Animal Practice 53: 526–533.

43. Marson AG (2008) When to start antiepileptic drug treatment and with what evidence? Epilepsia 49: 3–6.

44. Chang Y, Mellor DJ, Anderson TJ (2006) Idiopathic epilepsy in dogs: owners' perspectives on management with phenobarbitone and/or potassium bromide. Journal of Small Animal Practice 47: 574–581.

45. Musicco M, Beghi E, Solari A, Viani F (1997) Treatment of first tonic-clonic seizure does not improve the prognosis of epilepsy. Neurology 49: 991–998.

46. Camfield C, Camfield P, Gordon K, Dooley J (1996) Does the number of seizures before treatment influence ease of control or remission of childhood epilepsy? Not if the number is 10 or less. Neurology 46: 41–44.

47. Avanzini G, Depaulis A, Tassinari A, de Curtis M (2013) Do seizures and epileptic activity worsen epilepsy and deteriorate cognitive function? Epilepsia 54: 14–21.

48. Saito M, Muñana K, Sharp N, Olby N (2001) Risk factors for development of status epilepticus in dogs with idiopathic epilepsy and effects of status epilepticus on outcome and survival time: 32 cases (1990–1996). J Am Vet Med Assoc 219: 618–623.

49. Collaborative Group for the Study of Epilepsy (1992) Prognosis of Epilepsy in Newly Referred Patients: A Multicenter Prospective Study of the Effects of Monotherapy on the Long-Term Course of Epilepsy. Epilepsia 33: 45–51.

50. Berg AT, Shinnar S (1997) Do Seizures Beget Seizures? An Assessment of the Clinical Evidence in Humans. Journal of Clinical Neurophysiology Secondary Epileptogenesis 14: 102–110.

51. Regesta G, Tanganelli P (1999) Clinical aspects and biological bases of drug-resistant epilepsies. Epilepsy Research 34: 109–122.

52. Reynolds EH, Elwes RDC, Shorvon SD (1983) Why Does Epilepsy Become Intractable - Prevention of Chronic Epilepsy. Lancet 2: 952–954.

53. Bielfelt SW, Redman HC, McClellan RO (1971) Sire- and sex-related differences in rates of epileptiform seizures in a purebred beagle dog colony. American Journal of Veterinary Research 32: 2039–2048.

54. Cockerell OC, Johnson AL, Sander JW, Shorvon SD (1997) Prognosis of epilepsy: a review and further analysis of the first nine years of the British National General Practice Study of Epilepsy, a prospective population-based study. Epilepsia 38: 31–46.

55. Löscher W, Schmidt D (2006) Experimental and Clinical Evidence for Loss of Effect (Tolerance) during Prolonged Treatment with Antiepileptic Drugs. Epilepsia 47: 1253–1284.

21

Bacterial Diversity Dynamics Associated with Different Diets and Different Primer Pairs in the Rumen of Kankrej Cattle

Dipti W. Pitta[1]*, Nidhi Parmar[2], Amrut K. Patel[2], Nagaraju Indugu[1], Sanjay Kumar[1], Karsanbhai B. Prajapathi[3], Anand B. Patel[2], Bhaskar Reddy[2], Chaitanya Joshi[2]

1 Center for Animal Health and Productivity, School of Veterinary Medicine, University of Pennsylvania, Philadelphia, Pennsylvania, United States of America, 2 Ome Research Facility, Department of Animal Biotechnology, Anand Agricultural University, Anand, Gujarat, India, 3 Livestock Production and Management Department, College of Veterinary Science and Animal Husbandry, Sardar Krushi Nagar Dantiwada Agricultural University, Sardar Krushi Nagar, Gujarat, India

Abstract

The ruminal microbiome in herbivores plays a dominant role in the digestion of lignocellulose and has potential to improve animal productivity. Kankrej cattle, a popular native breed of the Indian subcontinent, were used to investigate the effect of different dietary treatments on the bacterial diversity in ruminal fractions using different primer pairs. Two groups of four cows were assigned to two primary diets of either dry or green forages. Each group was fed one of three dietary treatments for six weeks each. Dietary treatments were; K1 (50% dry/green roughage: 50% concentrate), K2 (75% dry/green roughage: 25% concentrate) and K3 (100% dry/green roughage). Rumen samples were collected using stomach tube at the end of each dietary period and separated into solid and liquid fractions. The DNA was extracted and amplified for V1–V3, V4–V5 and V6–V8 hypervariable regions using P1, P2 and P3 primer pairs, sequenced on a 454 Roche platform and analyzed using QIIME. Community compositions and the abundance of most bacterial lineages were driven by interactions between primer pair, dietary treatment and fraction. The most abundant bacterial phyla identified were *Bacteroidetes* and *Firmicutes* however, the abundance of these phyla varied between different primer pairs; in each primer pair the abundance was dependent on the dietary treatment and fraction. The abundance of *Bacteroidetes* in cattle receiving K1 treatment indicate their diverse functional capabilities in the digestion of both carbohydrate and protein while the predominance of *Firmicutes* in the K2 and K3 treatments signifies their metabolic role in fibre digestion. It is apparent that both liquid and solid fractions had distinct bacterial community patterns (P<0.001) congruent to changes in the dietary treatments. It can be concluded that the P1 primer pair flanking the V1–V3 hyper-variable region provided greater species richness and diversity of bacterial populations in the rumen of Kankrej cattle.

Editor: Kostas Bourtzis, International Atomic Energy Agency, Austria

Funding: Funding was received from the Indian Council of Agricultural Research. The funders had no role in study design, data collection and analysis, decision to publish, or preparation of the manuscript.

Competing Interests: The authors have declared that no competing interests exist.

* Email: dpitta@vet.upenn.edu

Introduction

The bovine populations of the Indian subcontinent represent a diverse genetic resource formed through various natural selective pressures such as varying supplies of nutrients, climatic conditions, and within species competition. Further, local environment and economic traits continues this selection process which leads to shaping entirely new species [1,2].

Based on phenotypic characterization, the National Bureau of Animal Genetic Resources reported 30 cattle breeds in India. Over millions of years ruminants and rumen microbiota have co-evolved and thus the rumen contains a complex and diverse bionetwork of bacteria, fungi and protozoa that facilitate fibre digestion. Unlike developed countries, domestic ruminants in developing and under-developed countries are often fed an abundance of fibre and little protein supplement (concentrate mix). When ruminants are fed fibre-rich rations the microbial ecology is altered. Since bacteria play an important role in all facets of rumen fermentation it is important to understand the rumen microbial ecology in domesticated ruminants that are maintained on local forages.

The breed Kankrej originated from Zebu cattle, native to the North Western part of India and is known for its dual (milk and draught) purpose and resilience to tropical weather conditions [3]. Kankrej cattle are native to the state of Gujarat and are held in high prestige there, being known to thrive on locally available forages with an average milk production of 6–10 L per day with 5% fat (unpublished data). As the composition of the rumen microbiome is primarily driven by diet [4] and the fact that Kankrej can utilize locally available feed resources efficiently for milk production, we were interested to determine diet-induced shifts in the rumen microbiome of Kankrej cattle.

In the recent past, next generation sequencing technology offered the most cost-effective platform to characterize community microbial populations at much greater resolution. Recently, we explored diversity in the metabolically active bacterial communities of water buffalo recovered by different primer pairs and investigated diet-induced shifts in the bacterial community compositions when water buffaloes were fed different proportions of forage and concentrate [5]. In this study, we used 454 Roche sequencing technology to investigate dynamics in the rumen microbiome of Kankrej cattle fed different roughages sources (dry and green) supplemented with a commercially available concentrate mixture.

Materials and Methods

All animal management and research procedures were conducted under animal use protocols approved by the University Animal Ethics Committee (Permit number: AAU/GVC/CPCSEA-IAEC/108/2013), Anand Agricultural University (AAU), Anand, Gujarat, India.

Experimental design and rumen sampling

Eight 5–6 year old healthy (approx. 450 kg) non-pregnant and non-lactating multiparous Kankrej cows were maintained before the start of the experiment on locally available roughages at the Livestock Research Station, Anand Agricultural University (AAU), Gujarat. Two groups of four cows were assigned to two primary diets of either dry or green roughages. Within each diet, dietary treatments were designed to have an increasing proportion of dry and green roughage and a decreasing proportion of the concentrate mix. The dietary treatments (dry/green roughage: concentrate) were K1 (50:50); K2 (75:25) and K3 (100:0). The experimental animals received the K1 diet for six weeks followed by K2 for six weeks and then K3 for the subsequent six weeks. On the last day of each experimental feeding period, rumen samples were collected three hours post feeding using gastric lavage. Each rumen sample was further separated into solid and liquid fractions by squeezing through a four-layered muslin cloth and pH of the liquid fraction was measured immediately. Samples were placed on ice, transported to the laboratory and then stored at −80°C prior to analyses.

DNA extraction

The archived rumen samples were thawed and processed separately. Solid samples were processed with PBS buffer for an hour to improve the yields of fibre adherent bacteria attached to the solid semi digested plant particles. Both solid and liquid rumen samples were then extracted for DNA using QIAamp DNA Stool Mini Kit (Qiagen, Valencia, CA). The genomic DNA was quantified and quality checked using Nanodrop (ND1000; Thermo Fisher Scientific, Wilmington, DE, USA) spectrophotometry as well as on 0.8% agarose gel electrophoresis.

Amplification and sequencing

The choice of primers is one of the most critical steps for accurate rDNA amplicon analysis. However, there is little information available on the impact of targeting different hypervariable regions of rDNA genes to explore bacterial diversity, particularly in the rumen system. Choosing a sub-optimal or more precise primer pairs can lead to either under-representation or over-representation of particular species or even the entire phylum, and consequently leads to questionable biological conclusions [6–8]. Therefore, in the current study, we sought to cover the entire 16S rDNA gene using three different primer pairs

and to identify the most suitable primer pair(s) that can provide a better coverage of bacterial diversity, including the rare species, in complex environments such as the rumen microbiome. The extracted DNA from both liquid and fibre rumen samples was amplified using three sets of primers (Table 1; P1: V1–V3; P2: V4–V5; P3: V6–V8) in a PCR reaction containing 5X amplification mix (5.0 µL); emPCR additive (2.0 µL); 100% DMSO (1.5 µL); 10 pM forward primer (1.0 µL); 10 pM reverse primer (1.0 µL); nuclease free water (12.5 µL); emPCR enzyme mix (1.0 µL) and 30 ng of template (1 µL). All PCR reactions were run on a thermal cycler with an initial denaturation at 95°C for 3 min followed by 35 cycles with each cycle containing denaturation at 95°C for 30 sec; annealing at 60°C for 1 min and extension at 72°C for 1 min and then a concluding step of extension at 72°C for 7 min. The amplified PCR products were size selected (+/− 50 bp) using the gel cutting method, eluted using Qiaquick gel extraction kit (Qiagen, Valencia, CA) and quantified using Qubit DNA HS assay (Life Technologies, Grand Island, NY). The amplicons from the three primer pairs generated for each sample were pooled in equimolar concentration. The pyrosequencing of amplicons was performed at the OME Research Facility (Anand, Gujarat, India) using a 454 Roche Platform (GS FLX Titanium; Roche 454 Life Sciences, Branford, CT).

Data analysis

The 16S pyrosequence reads were analyzed using the QIIME pipeline [9], followed by statistical analysis in R [10]. Reads were discarded if they did not match the expected sample-specific barcode and 16S primer sequences, shorter than 200 bp or longer than 1000 bp, or contained a homopolymer sequence in excess of 6 bp. Operational taxonomic units (OTUs) were formed at 97% similarity using UCLUST [11]. Representative sequences from each OTU were aligned to 16S reference sequences with PyNAST [12] and used to infer a phylogenetic tree with FastTree [13]. Taxonomic assignments within the GreenGenes taxonomy [12/10 release, [14] were generated using the RDP Classifier version 2.2 [15]. Alpha diversity of samples was calculated between samples of different forages, dietary treatments, rumen fractions and primer pairs at different rarefaction depths (i.e. 200, 5000 and 7000) using available preferences such as the chao1 estimator for species richness, and the Shannon diversity index, which estimates total diversity taking into account both species richness and evenness for each rarefaction depth. A non-parametric permutational multivariate ANOVA test [16], implemented in the vegan package for R [17,18], was used to test the effects of primer pairs, dietary treatments and fraction on overall community composition, as measured by weighted UniFrac distance [19]. To test for differences in taxon abundance, a generalized non-linear model was constructed with the nlme package for R [20].

Results

Details of dietary composition

The nutrient and chemical composition of the two main forages along with the dietary levels (treatments) and the mean ruminal pH values in the respective dietary treatments are presented in Table 2. The dietary treatments differed in their total protein and crude fibre concentrations. DK1 and GK1 treatments contained higher protein concentrations, while DK3 and GK3 treatments had higher crude fibre concentrations. The ruminal pH for dietary treatments containing 50% concentrate (DK1 and GK1) had different pH values while K2 and K3 treatments in both dry and green roughage diets had similar pH values.

Table 1. PCR primer pair targeting different hyper variable regions of 16S rDNA.

Primer Pair Name	Primer pair	Sequence (5'-3')	Region targeted	Amplicon length (bp)	Reference
P1	8F	AGA GTT TGA TCC TGG CTC AG	V1, V2 & V3	527	[73,74]
	534R	ATT ACC GCG GCT GCT GGC			
P2	517F	GCC AGC AGC CGC GGT AA	V4 & V5	410	[49]
	926R	CCG TCA ATT YYT TTR AGT TT			[49]
P3	917F	GAA TTG ACG GGG RCC C	V6, V7 & V8	452	[49,75]
	1386R	GCG GTG TGT GCA AGG AGC			

Bacterial community comparisons

A total of 748,700 reads from 144 different bacterial communities were analyzed in this study. Alignments and phylogenetic assignments of 16S pyrotags was performed at 97% similarity which resulted in the identification of 21 phyla and 453 genera in the bacterial domain (Table S1, S2, S3, S4). Distinct differences in species richness and diversity were evident by primer pair (Fig. 1a, b, and c). The effect of different dietary regimes is relatively small when compared to the effect of primer pairs on the distribution patterns of different bacterial species in the rumen (Fig. S1, S2 and S3).

Comparisons between bacterial communities were based on the UniFrac distances calculated by primer pair, dietary treatment and fraction and visualized using principle coordinate analysis (Fig. 2). Clustering of communities was influenced by the interactions between primer pair, treatment, and fraction (P<0.001; Fig. 2; Table 3). The effect of primer pair on the community composition was significant (P<0.001; Fig. 2). Bacterial community composition was influenced by dietary treatment (P<0.001) (Fig. 2; Table 3), both within and between primer pairs. It is apparent that both liquid and solid fractions had distinct community compositions (P<0.001; Fig. 2). However, there was no effect of forage (dry or green) on community composition (results not shown).

Phylogenetic characterization of bacterial lineages

Across all communities the most predominant phyla were *Bacteroidetes* and *Firmicutes* comprising up to 90% (Fig. 3a, b). We found that as the animals transitioned from K1 to K3 diets, lineages from *Bacteroidetes* reduced and that of *Firmicutes* increased in both fractions across all primer pairs (Fig. 4 a, b). Other phyla that contributed to greater than 1% abundance were *Fibrobacteres*, *Proteobacteria*, *Tenericutes*, *Lentisphaerae* and *Verrucomicrobia*. The lineages from the *Bacteroidetes* phylum were mostly assigned to the *Prevotellaceae* family. About 11 genera (including unclassified genera) were identified from the *Bacteroidetes* lineages that contributed to more than 0.2% abundance in a majority of communities (Fig. 5a, b). However, *Prevotella* was the most dominant genus across all communities. The lineages from *Firmicutes* were dominated by *Ruminococcaceae*, *Lachnospiraceae*, and *Veillonellaceae* members represented by a substantial number of genera (Fig. 5a, b).

Shifts in the bacterial phylotypes

Effects of interaction. Shifts in the abundance of bacterial populations were apparent from phylum through genus (Fig. 3a, b; 4a, b; 5a, b; Table S1, S2, S3, S4). The abundance of individual bacterial populations was highly influenced by interactions

between primer pair, dietary treatments and fractions (P×T×F; P×T; P×F and T×F; Table 3 and 4).

Among the bacterial phyla, *Bacteriodetes*, *Fibrobacteres*, *and Tenericutes were* greatly influenced (P<0.001) by P×T×F; P×T; P×F and T×F interactions (Table 3; Tables S1, S2). Among the *Bacteroidetes* representatives, *Prevotellaceae* (*Prevotella*, YRC22) and *Sphingobacteriaceae* (*Sphingobacterium*) were influenced by nearly all interactions. Similarly the clans of *Firmicutes* such as *Clostridia* (*Clostridium*, *Cristensella*, *Dehalobacterium*), *Lachnospiraceae* (*Butyrivibrio*, *Syntrophococcus*, *Psuedobutyrivibrio*), *Ruminococcaceae* (*Oscillospira*, *Ruminococcus*) and *Veillonellaceae* (*Schwartzia*, *Selenomonas*, *Succiniclasticum*) changed due to interactions. Genus *Fibrobacter* of the phylum *Fibrobacteres* and the *Desulfovibrio* and *Succinivibrio* lineages of *Proteobacteria* were also significantly influenced by the interactions among primer, fraction and treatment (Table 4; Tables S3, S4).

Distinction between community profiles of the fibre and liquid fraction

Although the same bacterial lineages were commonly present in fibre and liquid fractions, their percent abundance varied (P<0.001) between the two fractions (Fig. 3a, b; Fig. 5a, b).

In the liquid fraction, among communities associated with primer pair 1, the predominant phylum was *Bacteroidetes* (up to > 70%). The proportion of *Bacteroidetes* was altered with changes in dietary treatments with K1 showing higher abundance of *Bacteroidetes* while the abundance was reduced from K1 to K3 (P<0.001). Green roughage fed animals had a slightly higher abundance of *Bacteroidetes* than dry roughage fed animals. Although the contribution from *Firmicutes* was substantial, there was little differentiation between the K1, K2 and K3 treatments. A higher abundance of *Proteobacteria* and *Fibrobacter* was noticed in the K2 treatment (P<0.001).

Across bacterial communities recovered from primer pair 2 in the liquid fraction, the dominant phylum was dependent on the dietary treatment. The K1 treatment had a significant (P<0.001) abundance of *Bacteroidetes* (60–80%) which reduced to 3.0% in the K2 and K3 treatments. In contrast, *Firmicutes* was 20% in the K1 treatments which significantly (P<0.001) increased to 60% abundance in the K3 treatment. The abundance of *Proteobacteria* and *Fibrobacter* was also substantial in the K2 and K3 treatments compared to the K1 treatment.

Primer pair 3 derived bacterial communities showed a similar pattern to that of primer pair 2 in the liquid fraction. However, the abundance of *Firmicutes* was much higher (about 90%) in the K2 and K3 treatments. Also the recovery of *Proteobacteria* and *Fibrobacteres* was lower with primer pair 3 as compared to other primer pairs.

Table 2. Nutrient and chemical composition (%) of experimental dietary treatments and the mean ruminal pH.

Nutrient (%)	Dry	Green	Concentrate	Nutrient composition in the dietary treatments					
				DKI	DK2	DK3	GK1	GK2	GK3
Moisture	6.31	82.26	5.74	ND	ND	ND	ND	ND	ND
Crude protein	5.32	7.75	20.21	12.77	9.04	5.32	13.98	10.86	7.75
Crude fat	1.44	0.94	1.87	1.66	1.55	1.44	1.40	1.17	0.94
Crude fibre	31.00	32.85	12.57	21.79	26.39	31.00	22.71	27.78	32.85
Acid insoluble ash	2.53	3.36	3.84	3.19	2.86	2.55	3.6	3.48	3.36
Ruminal pH				7.29±0.06c	7.09±0.06b	7.08±0.05b	6.88±0.05a	6.97±0.07ab	6.99±0.08ab

DK1: 50% dry forage: 50% concentrate; DK2: 75% dry forage: 25% concentrate and DK3: 100% dry forage; GK1: 50% green forage: 50% concentrate; GK2: 75% green forage: 25% concentrate; GK3: 100% green forage; ND: Not detected;
a, b, c: means in a row having different superscript are statistically different (P<0.05).
±: standard error of means (n=4).

In the solid fraction, P1 associated bacterial communities showed lower abundance values for *Bacteroidetes* and higher values for *Firmicutes* compared to the liquid fraction. Across P2 communities, K1 treatment had a comparable profile to that of K1 in P1 associated communities. However, K3 treatments were dominated by *Firmicutes* (up to 75%). In K2 treatments, the contribution from *Firmicutes* was up to 55% while *Proteobacteria*, *Fibrobacteres* and *Actinobacteria* together contributed up to 45%. The abundance of *Bacteroidetes* in K2 and K3 regimen was minimal (1–3%). In P3 associated communities, the abundance of *Bacteroidetes* and *Firmicutes* was 60:20 in the K1 diets. However, on K2 and K3 dietary treatments, *Firmicutes* alone comprised more than 95% abundance.

Comparison of bacterial fingerprints at the lowest level of lineage

We chose to present the abundance (>0.2%) of bacterial lineages at the OTU level for each of the samples in both fractions (Fig. 5a and b). For ease of interpretation, fingerprints were presented by primer pair, dietary treatments and fractions. The effect of interactions between primer pair, treatment, and fraction on the abundance of bacterial genera is presented (Table 4).

In the liquid fraction, about 55 lineages were identified with 11 lineages from *Bacteroidetes* and 20 lineages from *Firmicutes* across all samples. In P1 associated communities, genus *Prevotella* was well represented along with several other *Bacteroidetes* lineages. The majority (about 19 out of 20) of lineages from *Firmicutes* except for *Clostridiaceae* (02d06) were recovered by P1. However, *Ruminobacter*, *Desulfovibrio* and *Succinovibrionaceae members* were not recovered; representatives from *Verrucomicrobia*, and *Elusimicrobia* were weakly represented across P1 associated communities. In P2 associated profiles, K1 had contrasting profiles compared to K2 and K3. Notably, except for the weak presence of *Prevotella*, all other lineages of *Bacteroidetes* were not detected in K2 and K3 treatments. On the contrary, diversity in *Firmicutes* was high with more representative OTUs present in all P2 associated communities; however, their abundance was much higher in K2 and K3 treatment profiles. Also, the abundance of *Fibrobacteres* was much more evident in K2 followed by K3 communities. The P3 associated communities showed different profiles compared to P1 and P2 primer pairs. Among the *Bacteroidetes* lineages, lineages from *Prevotellaceae* were only detected in K1 communities. The abundance of *Prevotella* was much higher in K1 compared to K2 and K3. The representatives from *Christensenellaceae*, *Ruminococcaceae*, *Clostridiales* and *Vellionellaceae* were abundant on K2 and K3 treatments among P3 communities. The OTUs from *Planctomycete* and *Tenericutes* were not recovered by primer pair 3.

In the solid fraction, 49% lineages were identified from *Firmicutes* and 22% from *Bacteroidetes*. In P1 associated communities, all the lineages from *Bacteroidetes* and *Firmicutes* were well represented in K1, K2 and K3 dietary treatments except *Firmicutes* 02d06. However, members of *Proteobacteria* (*Desulfovibrio*, *Luteimonas*) and *Verrucomicrobia* (RFP12) were either weakly recovered or not detected in K1, K2 and K3 treatments. In P2 associated patterns, lineages from *Bacteroidetes* were more abundant in K1 compared to K2 and K3, where most of the lineages were not detected. Among *Firmicutes*, *Clostridium* followed by *Lachnospiraceae*, *Succiniclasticum* and *Butyrivibrio* were more abundant in K2 and K3 whereas *Ruminococcaceae* was abundant in K1 treatment. Primer pair 2 showed higher abundance of *Fibrobacter* in K2 and K3 compared to P1 and P3. The OTUs from *Verrucomicrobia* RFP12 and *Tenericutes*

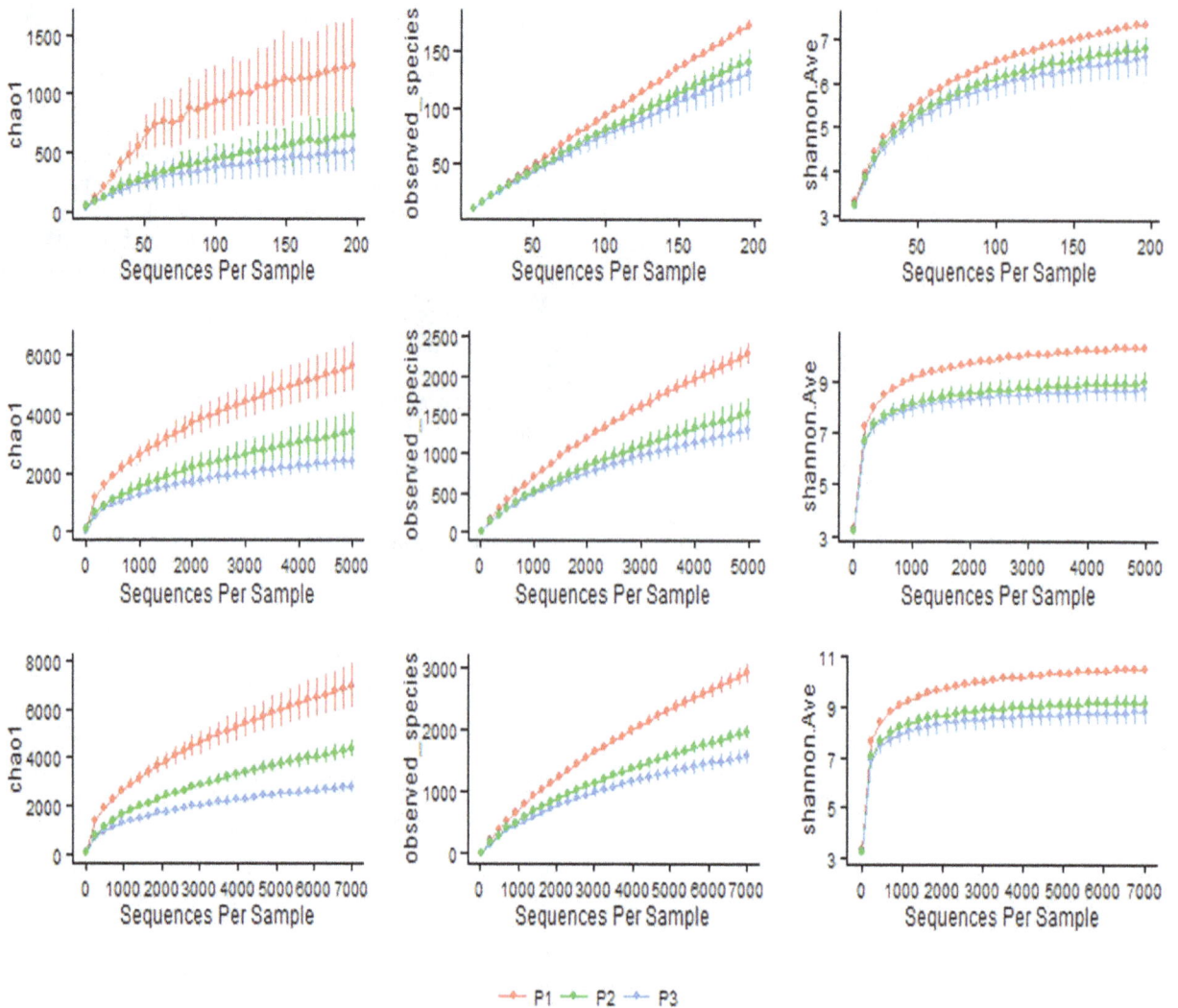

Figure 1. Rarefaction plots for three different primer pairs. Sequence depths a) 200, b) 5000 and c) 7000 displaying species richness (Chao 1 and Observed species) and phylogenetic relationship (Shannon index); (P1: targeting V1–V3 region; P2: targeting V4–V5 region and P3: targeting V6–V8 region).

RF39 were not detected in K2 and K3 with P2 whereas TM7 F16 was identified in all the treatments.

In P3 associated microbial profiles, results for *Bacteroidetes* lineage were similar to that of P2 in K1 diet whereas in K2 and K3 more *Bacteroidetes* lineages were recovered by P3 compared to P2. The abundance of *Christensenellaceae*, *Clostridiales*, *Clostridium*, *Ruminococcus*, *Succiniclasticum* and *Veillonellaceae* were much higher in K2 and K3, whereas *Bulleidia* and *Firmicutes* RFN20 were not detected in these diets. The members of *Proteobacteria* (*Ruminobacter* and *Succinivibrionaceae*) were not detected in K2 and K3 compared to K1. The OTUs from *Anareoplasmataceae*, *Firmicutes* RF39, and *Verrucomicrobia* LD1-PB3 were not recovered by primer pair 3.

Discussion

The concept of the "microbiome" (microbes, their genes and interactions with the host/habitat) is currently being evaluated in many aspects of biological science, and studies over the past decade have been dramatically advanced by Next Generation Sequencing (NGS) technology [21,22]. For example, character-

ization of the rumen microbiome and its associated repertoire of glycoside hydroxylase (GH) enzymes in steers using NGS revealed that the microbiome composition, including GH content, is driven primarily by diet [23].

Our study intends to characterize the rumen microbiome of Kankrej cattle, an indigenous bovine breed of the Indian subcontinent which is commonly reared to serve multiple needs such as milk, meat and draft purposes. The aim of this study is to understand the rumen microbiome of this indigenous breed and also elucidate the dynamics in the rumen microbial communities mediated by a difference in primer pairs, fractions and dietary treatments in the rumen contents using 16S rDNA pyrotag sequencing technology.

Bacterial populations within the rumen microbiome have been categorized into three major groups based on their location designated as adherent bacteria (bound to feed particles), planktonic bacteria (free-living in the liquid) and the epimural community (associated with rumen epithelium) [24,25]. Previously, either whole rumen contents or the squeezed rumen fluid was used for bacterial diversity analysis; however, differentiating

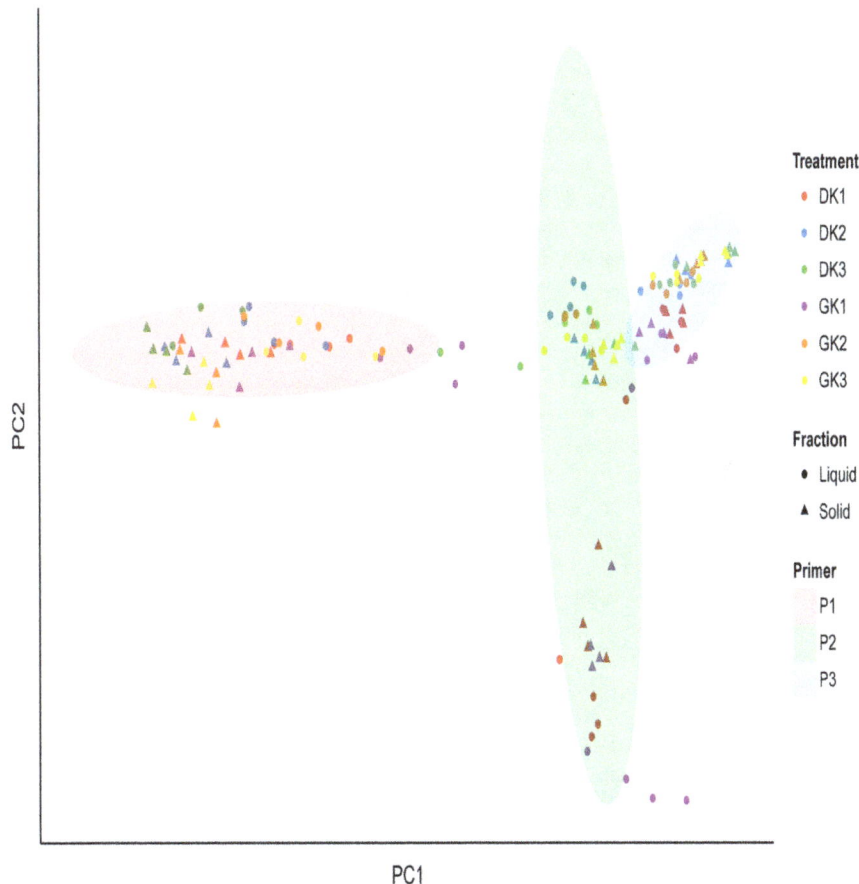

Figure 2. Principal coordinate analysis based on weighted Unifrac distances. Primer pair (P1: targeting V1–V3 region; P2: targeting V4–V5 region and P3: targeting V6–V8 region); treatment: (DK1: 50% dry forage: 50% concentrate; DK2: 75% dry forage: 25% concentrate and DK3: 100% dry forage; GK1: 50% green forage: 50% concentrate; GK2: 75% green forage: 25% concentrate; GK3: 100% green forage) and fraction: solid (S) and liquid (L).

microbial communities by rumen fraction has recently become more common due to the efficiency and lower cost of NGS technology [5,23–29]. Similar to our findings distinct microbial communities associated with each of the rumen fractions have been observed across several reports [5,29,30]. Further, we found a contrasting difference in the phylogenetic composition of each fraction at the phylum level with a higher abundance of *Bacteroidetes* in the liquid fraction similar to findings of [5] and a higher abundance of *Firmicutes* in the solid fraction analogous to the reports of [21,31]. *Firmicutes* lineages are known to utilize readily available fermentable carbohydrates [31] and also participate in the initial colonization of the peripheral side chains of cellulosic matrix [23] thus showing their metabolic role in carbohydrate digestion. In contrast, *Bacteroidetes* lineages are reported to have diverse metabolic capabilities including the degradation of protein and polysaccharides [31,32].

A majority of studies rely on 16S rRNA gene to understand the phylogenetic composition of bacterial communities utilizing either cultivation [33,34] or cultivation independent DNA derived next generation sequencing technology [5,35–37]. However, amplification of 16S rDNA gene fragments can be biased owing to differences in primer pairs used to target different hyper-variable regions of the 16S rDNA gene [5,38–41]. In addition, differences in sampling procedure used to harvest rumen contents (gastric tube vs. cannulated animal) and sample type (whole rumen

contents vs. separate rumen fractions) can have a huge impact on microbial diversity [42–44]. Considering the above factors that account for variation, and for the fact that we have identified a strong influence of primer pair on the recovery of bacterial populations in the rumen of water buffalo [5], we investigated the influence of different primer pairs on the rumen microbiome of Kankrej cattle.

Congruent to our earlier report [5], we found that bacterial diversity was contingent upon the choice of primer pairs. However, we have identified that the effect of interactions between primer pair, dietary treatment and fraction had a strong influence on the community composition as well as upon the abundance of individual bacterial lineages. In agreement with previous studies [5,23,29], *Bacteroidetes* and *Firmicutes* were found to comprise about 90% of the bacterial populations regardless of the difference in dietary treatment, primer and fraction. Within each primer pair, the effect of dietary treatments was more pronounced on the abundance of either *Bacteroidetes* or *Firmicutes* in P2 and P3 associated communities while both phyla were co-dominant in P1 associated communities. Our previous report [5] showed a greater recovery of *Bacteroidetes* with the P2 primer pair in contrast to this study. Differences in the recovery of *Bacteroidetes* between Pitta et al [5] and the current study is largely explained by the amplification of cDNA from metabolically active bacteria in our previous work compared to total bacterial DNA (live and dead) in

Table 3. Effect of dietary treatment, fraction and primer and their interactions on relative abundance of rumen bacterial phyla.

Bacterial Phyla	Individual effect			Interactions			
	P	T	F	PxT	PxF	TxF	PxTxF
Bacteroidetes	***	***	***	***	***	***	***
Firmicutes	***	***	***	***	***	**	NS
Fibrobacteres	***	***	***	***	***	***	***
Proteobacteria	***	***	***	***	NS	*	NS
Tenericutes	***	***	***	***	***	***	***
Lentisphaerae	***	***	***	***	**	***	***
Cyanobacteria	***	***	***	***	***	***	***
TM7	***	NS	**	*	***	NS	NS
Spirochaetes	***	***	***	NS	***	**	NS
Verrucomicrobia	***	***	***	***	***	***	**
Actinobacteria	*	**	**	-	NS	-	NS
WPS.2	***	***	NS	***	-	NS	NS
Synergistetes	NS	***	NS	NS	NS	NS	NS
Elusimicrobia	***	***	***	*	***	**	-
Chloroflexi	*	-	*	**	NS	NS	NS
SR1	***	*	*	***	*	NS	*
Armatimonadetes	***	***	**	NS	-	NS	**
LD1	***	NS	**	***	**	NS	NS
X.Thermi	NS	***	*	NS	NS	**	NS
Planctomycetes	***	***	NS	***	-	**	***

P: primer; T: treatment; F: fraction; NS: Non-significant;

***: P<0.001;

**: P<0.01;

*: P<0.05.

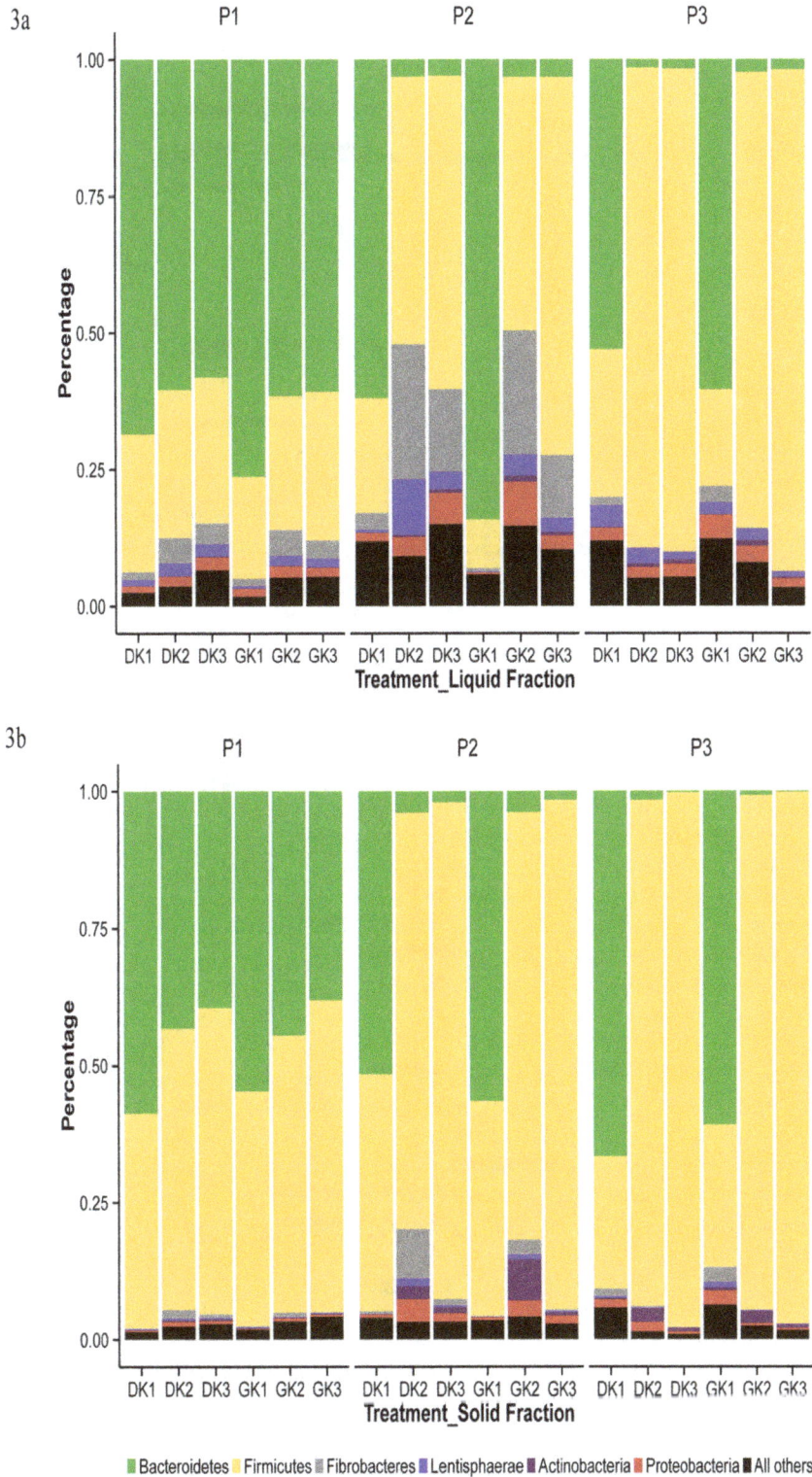

Figure 3. Phylogenetic composition by primer pairs and dietary treatments. Rumen fraction a) liquid; b) solid; Primer pair (P1: targeting V1–V3 region; P2: targeting V4–V5 region and P3 targeting V6–V8 region), treatment: (DK1: 50% dry forage: 50% concentrate; DK2: 75% dry forage: 25% concentrate and DK3: 100% dry forage; GK1: 50% green forage: 50% concentrate; GK2: 75% green forage: 25% concentrate; GK3: 100% green forage) and fraction: solid (S) and liquid (L).

the present study. In addition, differences in the host animal (water buffalo vs Kankrej cattle) could also be a confounding factor in bacterial diversity determination. Previous reports [5,45–47] have

also demonstrated that the bacterial diversity is host specific. Future work should aim to investigate bacterial diversity based upon both DNA-derived and cDNA-derived 16S rDNA amplicons

4a

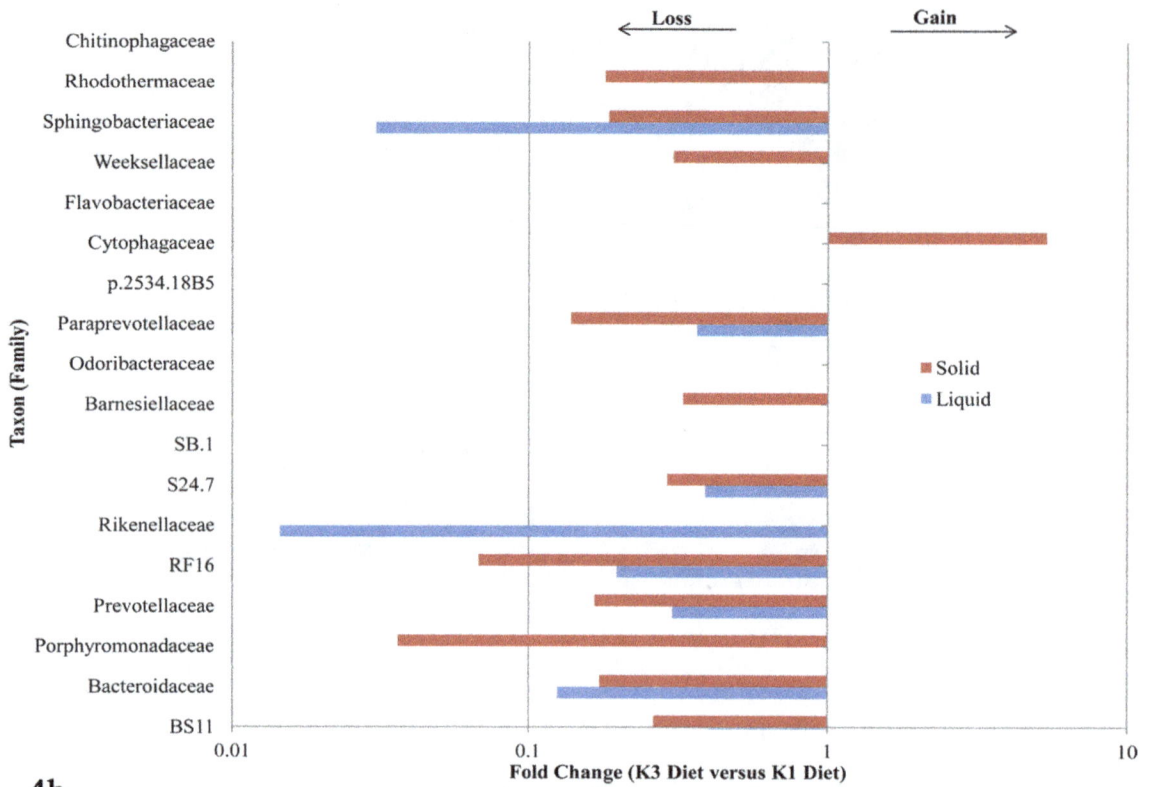

4b

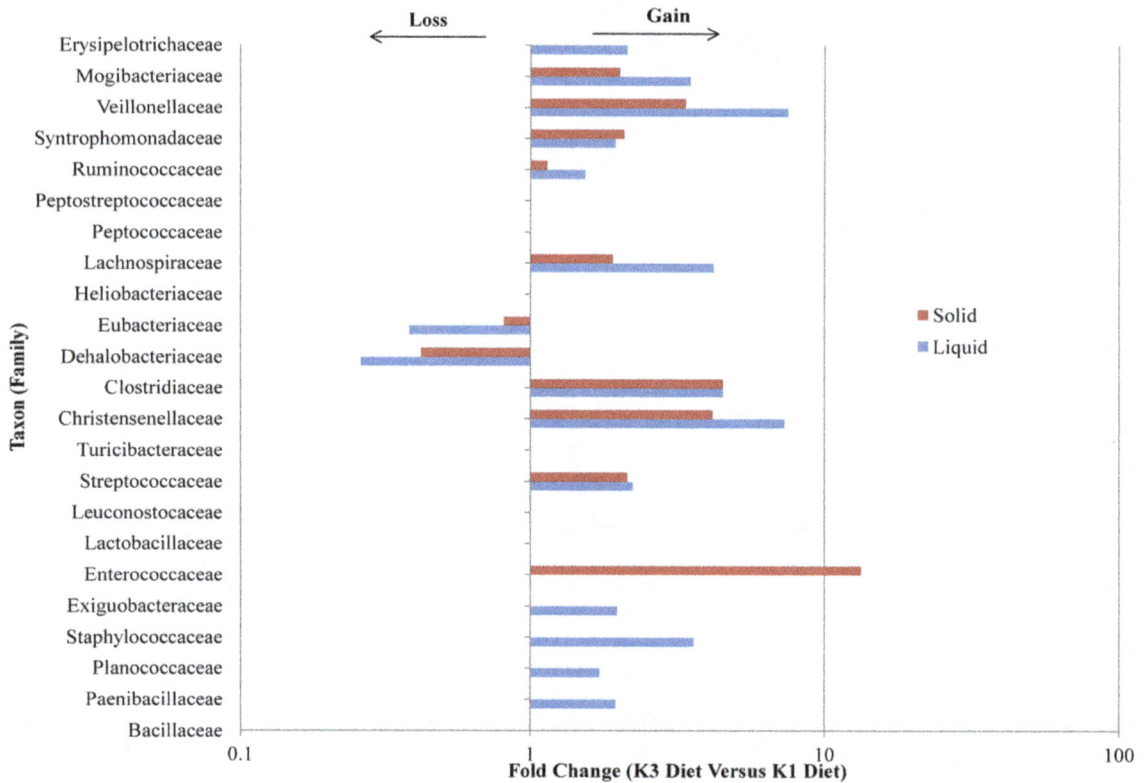

Figure 4. Fold changes in STabundant bacterial lineages at family level. Bacterial lineages a) loss of lineages in *Bacteroidetes*; b) gain in lineages in *Firmicutes*, across both fractions and primers, as the animals transitioned from K1 (50% dry/green forage: 50% concentrate) to K3 (100% dry/green forage).

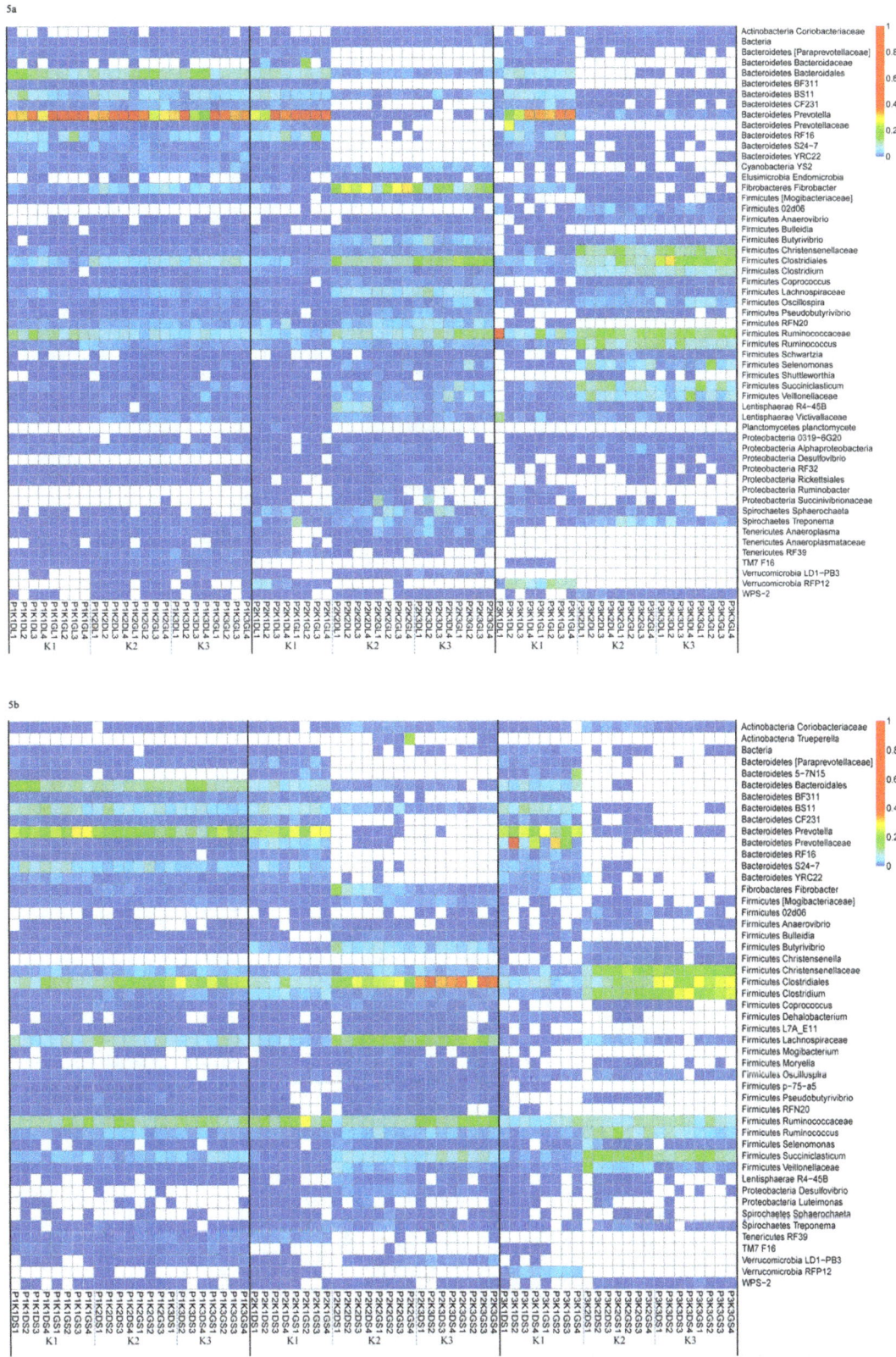

Figure 5. Thermal double dendrogram of the most abundant bacterial operational taxonomic units (OTUs). Rumen fraction a) liquid; b) solid; Primer pair (P1: targeting V1–V3 region; P2: targeting V4–V5 region and P3: targeting V6–V8 region), treatment: (DK1: 50% dry forage: 50% concentrate; DK2: 75% dry forage: 25% concentrate and DK3: 100% dry forage; GK1: 50% green forage: 50% concentrate; GK2: 75% green forage: 25% concentrate; GK3: 100% green forage).

Table 4. Effect of dietary treatment, fraction and primer and their interactions on relative abundance of rumen bacterial taxa at the genus level.

Bacterial taxa	Individual effect			Interactions			
	P	T	F	PxT	PxF	TxF	PxTxF
Bacteroidetes; BS11	***	***	***	***	NS	***	NS
Bacteroidetes; Bacteroidaceae; BF311	***	***	***	***	NS	NS	NS
Bacteroidetes; Porphyromonadaceae; Parabacteroides	*	**	NS	***	NS	NS	NS
Bacteroidetes; Prevotellaceae; Prevotella	***	***	***	***	***	***	-
Bacteroidetes; RF16	*	***	***	-	***	***	NS
Bacteroidetes; S24.7	***	***	***	NS	***	***	NS
Bacteroidetes; Paraprevotellaceae; CF231	***	***	***	***	**	NS	NS
Bacteroidetes; Paraprevotellaceae; YRC22	***	***	***	**	-	***	-
Bacteroidetes; Sphingobacteriaceae; Sphingobacterium	*	***	*	***	*	***	**
Bacteroidetes; Rhodothermaceae; Rubricoccus	*	*	**	NS	*	*	NS
Fibrobacteres; Fibrobacteraceae; Fibrobacter	***	***	***	***	***	***	***
Firmicutes; Christensenellaceae; Christensenella	***	***	***	***	***	***	***
Firmicutes; Clostridiaceae; 02d06	***	***	***	***	***	NS	NS
Firmicutes; Clostridiaceae; Clostridium	***	***	***	***	***	***	***
Firmicutes; Dehalobacteriaceae; Dehalobacterium	***	***	***	***	*	*	***
Firmicutes; Lachnospiraceae; Butyrivibrio	***	***	**	***	*	-	NS
Firmicutes; Lachnospiraceae; Clostridium	**	-	-	**	NS	NS	*
Firmicutes; Lachnospiraceae; Coprococcus	***	***	NS	***	*	-	NS
Firmicutes; Lachnospiraceae; Moryella	***	***	***	*	***	NS	NS
Firmicutes; Lachnospiraceae; Pseudobutyrivibrio	***	***	***	**	***	***	NS
Firmicutes; Lachnospiraceae; Syntrophococcus	***	-	**	*	***	**	*
Firmicutes; Ruminococcaceae; Oscillospira	***	***	***	**	***	***	NS
Firmicutes; Ruminococcaceae; Ruminococcus	***	***	NS	***	*	*	NS
Firmicutes; Veillonellaceae; Anaerovibrio	***	***	*	***	***	***	NS
Firmicutes; Veillonellaceae; Mitsuokella	**	**	**	***	*	*	**
Firmicutes; Veillonellaceae; Schwartzia	***	***	***	***	***	***	***
Firmicutes; Veillonellaceae; Selenomonas	***	***	***	***	***	***	-
Firmicutes; Veillonellaceae; Succiniclasticum	***	***	***	***	NS	***	-
Lentisphaerae; R4.45B	***	***	***	***	***	***	***
Proteobacteria; Caulobacteraceae; Mycoplana	***	***	**	***	***	***	***
Proteobacteria; Desulfovibrionaceae; Desulfovibrio	***	***	***	***	***	***	***
Proteobacteria; Succinivibrionaceae; Ruminobacter	***	***	*	***	*	*	NS
Proteobacteria; Succinivibrionaceae; Succinivibrio	***	***	***	***	***	***	***

Table 4. Cont.

Bacterial taxa	Individual effect			Interactions			
	P	T	F	PxT	PxF	TxF	PxTxF
Tenericutes; Anaeroplasmataceae; Anaeroplasma	***	***	***	**	***	***	**
Verrucomicrobia; RFP12	***	***	***	***	***	***	***

P: primer; T: treatment; F: fraction; NS: Non-significant;
***: P<0.001;
**: P<0.01;
*: P<0.05.

from a single species of ruminants to study the influence of primer pair on total and metabolically active bacterial diversity.

Notably, primer pair P2 was able to retrieve lineages of *Proteobacteria, Fibrobacteres, Tenericutes* and *Spirochaetes* much more efficiently at the expense of *Bacteroidetes* particularly in the liquid portion than the other two primer pairs possibly due to an interaction effect of dietary treatment, fraction and primer pair. From these results it is apparent that the detection and/or recovery of certain phyla are primer dependent. This primer effect has been reported in other microbial ecosystems. The effect of seven different primer pairs, targeting different hypervariable regions of DNA derived from activated sludge [38] and marine samples [6] demonstrated that combining V3 and V4 regions yielded better diversity patterns. It was also reported that V3–V4 and V4–V5 hyper variable regions were recommended for optimal bacterial profiling based on *in silico* analysis [38,48–50]. Across different ecosystems including the rumen microbiome, the use of primer pairs that flank V3–V4 hypervariable regions resulted in the recovery of a majority of bacterial populations [5,41,49–53] which partially concurs with this study. However, Claesson et al. [48] revealed significant amplification bias with the experimental sequencing of the V3–V4 region compared to the other regions, accentuating the necessity for more experimental validation of primer pairs. Based on our results, P1 primer pair, targeting V1–V3 hyper-variable region, was found to offer the more informative fingerprinting profiles with the rumen fractions (solid and liquid) as well as with the dietary treatments compared to P2 and P3 primer pairs. Yu and Morrison [54] also suggested amplification of V1 and V3 region for gut microbiome studies with short amplicon size, and thus corroborate well with our study.

Diet has a direct influence on the composition of the rumen microbiome [4,34] and studies have elucidated diet-induced shifts in the microbiome using different molecular techniques [5,26,29,52,53,55,56]. In our study, animals had access to either dry or green roughage in increasing proportion while the proportion of concentrate declined as the animals moved from K1 to K3 diets. As the ratio between the concentrate and roughage changed, a corresponding change was noticed in the phylogenetic composition of rumen bacterial populations in Kankrej cattle. Moreover, difference in phylogenetic composition was also noticed due to different primer pairs.

Similar to previous findings [5,55], we have noted a higher abundance of *Bacteroidetes* with increasing proportion of concentrate in the dietary treatment with P1 primer in both solid and liquid fractions compared to P2 and P3. Coverage of *Prevotella* and other *Bacteroidetes* lineages was greater with P1 primer pair covering the V1–V3 region. The abundance of lineages of *Firmicutes* (*Coprococcus, Lactonifactor, Sporobacter*) and *Fibrobacteres* (*Fibrobacter*) was also well represented with P1 and P2 primer pairs compared to P3 whereas TM7 was not recovered with P2. Although the percent abundance was different due to the dietary effects in both solid and liquid fractions, the P1 primer pair offered more information on different bacterial phyla and covered more diverse bacterial lineages. The coverage of observed number of sequences, diversity and species richness with V1–V3 based primer (P1) was higher and in agreement with the results of [27,57]. The present data also relates with our transition cow study which showed better coverage of bacterial lineages using V1–V2 region based primer [58]. Results from metagenomic studies (unpublished data) are also in agreement which showed more than 80% abundance of *Bacteroidetes* and *Firmicutes* in the rumen microbiome followed by *Proteobacteria*. It was reported that the main functional role of *Bacteroidetes* is polysaccharide degradation [32]. However, lineages of *Bacteroidetes* are plastic as they continue to evolve and adapt to dietary substrates that become available in the host. Therefore, *Bacteroidetes* complement host metabolism and develop the repertoire of enzymes that can target polysaccharides such as cellulose, pectin and xylan [32], oligosaccharides [59], and also host derived carbohydrates such as mucin and chondroitin sulfates containing N-glycans [60]. Comparative analysis of *Bacteroidetes* genomes revealed that these lineages contain numerous carbohydrate enzymes that can degrade different substrates originated from plant, algae and fungi due to the presence of Polysaccharide Utilizing Loci that help ligate and uptake of carbohydrate substrate and TonB receptors that transport these complexes into the cytoplasm [32]. In addition, certain lineages of *Bacteroidetes* such as *P. ruminocola* [61] and *P. albensis* [62] found in the rumen are inclined towards utilizing the dipeptides due to the presence of dipeptidyl peptidases. The abundance of *Prevotellaceae* and *Porphyromonadaceae* among the *Bacteroidetes* on concentrate diets as observed in this study is congruent with previous reports [5,55,63,64]. It could be inferred that our findings corroborate with Thomas et al [32] on the diverse nature of *Bacteroidetes* and its participation in the degradation of protein and polysaccharides, both of which are available in the K1 dietary treatments.

Firmicutes are primarily comprised of Gram positive, low G+C content bacteria [65] and include a majority of the fibre-adherent rumen bacterial populations [23] and also in animals fed high forage diets [55]. In our study, *Firmicutes* constituted the majority of bacterial populations particularly in the solid fraction on K2 and K3 dietary treatments which were rich in crude fibre content. Among the *Firmicutes* group, families such as *Lachnospiraceae*, *Ruminococcaceae*, *Veillonellaceae* and unclassified *Clostridiales* were abundant in our study similar to previous findings [44,57,66]. Several reports emphasize the role of *Firmicutes*, in particular members of *Clostridiales*, *Ruminococcaceae* and *Lachnospiraceae* in fibre digestion [67–72] and therefore their abundance on K2 and K3 diets in the rumen of Kankrej cattle was expected.

While the abundance of *Bacteroidetes* and *Firmicutes*, including their possible metabolic capacities were evident, the shifts noted in other minor groups such as *Proteobacteria, Fibrobacteres, Verrucomicrobia, Spirochaetes* and unclassified bacteria that were detected in the present study remain obscure. However, their abundance was driven by interactions between primer pairs, dietary treatment and fractions. This study illustrates that the rumen microbiome of Kankrej cattle is sensitive to changes in the diet and that distinct microbial communities were identified in each of the rumen fractions. The recovery of rumen bacterial populations was dependent on primer choice, however, community and individual bacterial populations within a primer pair were driven by an interaction effect. Further, a period of six weeks was found to be adequate to identify differences in the bacterial communities due to a change in the diet. Prolonged feeding of these experimental diets could have led to the identification of a core microbial consortium that is specific for either concentrate or fibre rich diets. It is evident that the rumen microbiome of Kankrej cattle is sensitive to external stimuli and therefore further investigations can lead to novel insights to the microbial ecology as well as biotechnology research in biofuel production.

Supporting Information

Figure S1 Rarefaction plots for two different forages. Sequence depths a) 200, b) 5000 and c) 7000 displaying species richness (Chao 1 and Observed species) and phylogenetic relationship (Shannon index); (D: dry and G: green).

Figure S2 Rarefaction plots for six different dietary treatments. Sequence depths a) 200, b) 5000 and c) 7000 displaying species richness (Chao 1 and Observed species) and phylogenetic relationship (Shannon index); (DK1: 50% dry forage: 50% concentrate; DK2: 75% dry forage: 25% concentrate and DK3: 100% dry forage; GK1: 50% green forage: 50% concentrate; GK2: 75% green forage: 25% concentrate; GK3: 100% green forage).

Figure S3 Rarefaction plots for two different fractions. Sequence depths a) 200, b) 5000 and c) 7000 displaying species richness (Chao 1 and Observed species) and phylogenetic relationship (Shannon index); (S: solid and L: liquid).

Table S1 Mean values of bacterial phyla in the liquid fraction presented for each dietary treatment retrieved by each primer pair in the rumen of Kankrej cattle. Primer pair (P1: targeting V1–V3 region; P2: targeting V4–V5 region and P3: targeting V6–V8 region), treatment: (DK1: 50% dry forage: 50% concentrate; DK2: 75% dry forage: 25% concentrate and DK3: 100% dry forage; GK1: 50% green forage: 50% concentrate; GK2: 75% green forage: 25% concentrate; GK3: 100% green forage).

Table S2 Mean values of bacterial phyla in the solid fraction presented for each dietary treatment retrieved by each primer pair in the rumen of Kankrej cattle. Primer pair (P1: targeting V1–V3 region; P2: targeting V4–V5 region and P3: targeting V6–V8 region), treatment: (DK1: 50% dry forage: 50% concentrate; DK2: 75% dry forage: 25% concentrate and DK3: 100% dry forage; GK1: 50% green forage: 50% concentrate; GK2: 75% green forage: 25% concentrate; GK3: 100% green forage).

Table S3 Mean values of bacterial genus in the liquid fraction presented for each dietary treatment retrieved by each primer pair in the rumen of Kankrej cattle. Primer pair (P1: targeting V1–V3 region; P2: targeting V4–V5 region and P3: targeting V6–V8 region), treatment: (DK1: 50% dry forage: 50% concentrate; DK2: 75% dry forage: 25% concentrate and DK3: 100% dry forage; GK1: 50% green forage: 50% concentrate; GK2: 75% green forage: 25% concentrate; GK3: 100% green forage).

Table S4 Mean values of bacterial phyla in the solid fraction presented for each dietary treatment retrieved by each primer pair in the rumen of Kankrej cattle. Primer pair (P1: targeting V1–V3 region; P2: targeting V4–V5 region and P3: targeting V6–V8 region), treatment: (DK1: 50% dry forage: 50% concentrate; DK2: 75% dry forage: 25% concentrate and DK3: 100% dry forage; GK1: 50% green forage: 50% concentrate; GK2: 75% green forage: 25% concentrate; GK3: 100% green forage).

Author Contributions

Conceived and designed the experiments: CJ KBP. Performed the experiments: CJ NP ABP AKP BR KBP. Analyzed the data: DP SK NI. Contributed reagents/materials/analysis tools: DP SK NI CJ NP ABP AKP BR. Contributed to the writing of the manuscript: DP SK NI CJ NP ABP AKP BR.

References

1. Kale D, Rank D, Joshi C, Yadav B, Koringa P, et al. (2010) Genetic diversity among Indian Gir, Deoni and Kankrej cattle breeds based on microsatellite markers. Indian Journal of Biotechnology 9: 126–130.

2. Mona U, Farah NF (2012) Genetic diversity study of indigenous cattle (Gir and Kankrej) population of Rajasthan using microsatellite markers. African Journal of Biotechnology 11: 16313–16319.

3. Mukesh M, Sodhi M, Kataria R, Mishra B (2009) Use of microsatellite multilocus genotypic data for individual assignment assay in six native cattle breeds from north-western region of India. Livestock Science 121: 72–77.

4. Edwards JE, McEwan NR, Travis AJ, Wallace RJ (2004) 16S rDNA library-based analysis of ruminal bacterial diversity. Antonie Van Leeuwenhoek 86: 263–281.

5. Pitta D, Kumar S, Veiccharelli B, Parmar N, Reddy B, et al. (2014) Bacterial diversity associated with feeding dry forage at different dietary concentrations in the rumen contents of Mehsana buffalo (*Bubalus bubalis*) using 16S pyrotags. Anaerobe 25: 31–41.

6. Klindworth A, Pruesse E, Schweer T, Peplies J, Quast C, et al. (2012) Evaluation of general 16S ribosomal RNA gene PCR primers for classical and next-generation sequencing-based diversity studies. Nucleic acids research: 1–11.

7. Baker G, Cowan DA (2004) 16 S rDNA primers and the unbiased assessment of thermophile diversity. Biochemical Society of Transactions 32: 218–221.

8. Sipos R, Székely AJ, Palatinszky M, Révész S, Márialigeti K, et al. (2007) Effect of primer mismatch, annealing temperature and PCR cycle number on 16S rRNA gene-targetting bacterial community analysis. FEMS Microbiology Ecology 60: 341–350.

9. Caporaso JG, Kuczynski J, Stombaugh J, Bittinger K, Bushman FD, et al. (2010) QIIME allows analysis of high-throughput community sequencing data. Nature Methods 7: 335–336.

10. Team RC (2013) R: a language and environment for statistical computing. Version 3.0. 1, R Foundation for Statistical Computing, Vienna.

11. Edgar RC (2010) Search and clustering orders of magnitude faster than BLAST. Bioinformatics 26: 2460–2461.

12. Caporaso JG, Bittinger K, Bushman FD, DeSantis TZ, Andersen GL, et al. (2010) PyNAST: a flexible tool for aligning sequences to a template alignment. Bioinformatics 26: 266–267.

13. Price MN, Dehal PS, Arkin AP (2010) FastTree 2–approximately maximum-likelihood trees for large alignments. PloS One 5: e9490.

14. McDonald D, Price MN, Goodrich J, Nawrocki EP, DeSantis TZ, et al. (2011) An improved Greengenes taxonomy with explicit ranks for ecological and evolutionary analyses of bacteria and archaea. The ISME Journal 6: 610–618.

15. Wang Q, Garrity GM, Tiedje JM, Cole JR (2007) Naive Bayesian classifier for rapid assignment of rRNA sequences into the new bacterial taxonomy. Applied and Environmental Microbiology 73: 5261–5267.

16. Anderson MJ (2001) A new method for non-parametric multivariate analysis of variance. Austral Ecology 26: 32–46.

17. Bates D, Maechler M Bolker (2013) lme4: Linear mixed-effects models using S4 classes. R package version 0999999–2.

18. Oksanen J, Blanchet F, Kindt R, Legendre P, O'Hara R, et al. vegan: Community Ecology Package. 2013. R package version 2.0–7.

19. Lozupone C, Knight R (2005) UniFrac: a new phylogenetic method for comparing microbial communities. Applied and Environmental Microbiology 71: 8228–8235.

20. Pinheiro J, Bates D, Saikat D, Sarkar D team RC (2013) nlme: Linear and Nonlinear Mixed Effects Models. R package version 3.1–113.

21. Chaucheyras-Durand F, Ossa F (2014) Review: The rumen microbiome: Composition, abundance, diversity, and new investigative tools. The Professional Animal Scientist 30: 1–12.

22. Morgavi D, Kelly W, Janssen P, Attwood G (2013) Rumen microbial (meta) genomics and its application to ruminant production. Animal 7: 184 201.

23. Brulc JM, Antonopoulos DA, Miller MEB, Wilson MK, Yannarell AC, et al. (2009) Gene-centric metagenomics of the fiber-adherent bovine rumen microbiome reveals forage specific glycoside hydrolases. Proceedings of the National Academy of Sciences 106: 1948–1953.

24. McAllister T, Bae H, Jones G, Cheng K (1994) Microbial attachment and feed digestion in the rumen. Journal of Animal Science 72: 3004–3018.

25. Wallace R, Cheng K-J, Dinsdale D, Ørskov E (1979) An independent microbial flora of the epithelium and its role in the ecomicrobiology of the rumen. Nature 279: 424–426.

26. Kong Y, Teather R, Forster R (2010) Composition, spatial distribution, and diversity of the bacterial communities in the rumen of cows fed different forages. FEMS Microbiology Ecology 74: 612–622.

27. Petri R, Schwaiger T, Penner G, Beauchemin K, Forster R, et al. (2013) Changes in the rumen epimural bacterial diversity of beef cattle as affected by diet and induced ruminal acidosis. Applied and Environmental Microbiology 79: 3744–3755.

28. Pinloche E, McEwan N, Marden J-P, Bayourthe C, Auclair E, et al. (2013) The effects of a probiotic yeast on the bacterial diversity and population structure in the rumen of cattle. PloS One 8: e67824.

29. Pitta DW, Pinchak WE, Dowd SE, Osterstock J, Gontcharova V, et al. (2010) Rumen bacterial diversity dynamics associated with changing from bermuda-grass hay to grazed winter wheat diets. Microbial Ecology 59: 511–522.

30. Larue R, Yu Z, Parisi VA, Egan AR, Morrison M (2005) Novel microbial diversity adherent to plant biomass in the herbivore gastrointestinal tract, as revealed by ribosomal intergenic spacer analysis and rrs gene sequencing. Environmental Microbiology 7: 530–543.

31. Huo W, Zhu W, Mao S (2014) Impact of subacute ruminal acidosis on the diversity of liquid and solid-associated bacteria in the rumen of goats. World Journal of Microbiology and Biotechnology 30: 669–680.

32. Thomas F, Hehemann J-H, Rebuffet E, Czjzek M, Michel G (2011) Environmental and gut bacteroidetes: the food connection. Frontiers in Microbiology 2.

33. Hungate R (1969) Chapter IV A Roll Tube Method for Cultivation of Strict Anaerobes. Methods in Microbiology 3: 117–132.

34. Hungate RE (1966) The rumen and its microbes. New York: Academic Press.

35. Amend AS, Seifert KA, Bruns TD (2010) Quantifying microbial communities with 454 pyrosequencing: does read abundance count? Molecular Ecology 19: 5555–5565.

36. Engelbrektson A, Kunin V, Wrighton KC, Zvenigorodsky N, Chen F, et al. (2010) Experimental factors affecting PCR-based estimates of microbial species richness and evenness. The ISME Journal 4: 642–647.

37. Jumpponen A (2007) Soil fungal communities underneath willow canopies on a primary successional glacier forefront: rDNA sequence results can be affected by primer selection and chimeric data. Microbial Ecology 53: 233–246.

38. Cai L, Ye L, Tong AHY, Lok S, Zhang T (2013) Biased diversity metrics revealed by bacterial 16S pyrotags derived from different primer sets. PloS One 8: e53649.

39. Polz MF, Cavanaugh CM (1998) Bias in template-to-product ratios in multitemplate PCR. Applied and Environmental Microbiology 64: 3724–3730.

40. Větrovský T, Baldrian P (2013) The variability of the 16S rRNA gene in bacterial genomes and its consequences for bacterial community analyses. PLoS One 8: e57923.

41. Yu Z, Morrison M (2004) Improved extraction of PCR-quality community DNA from digesta and fecal samples. Biotechniques 36: 808–813.

42. Cardona S, Eck A, Cassellas M, Gallart M, Alastrue C, et al. (2012) Storage conditions of intestinal microbiota matter in metagenomic analysis. BMC Microbiology 12: 158.

43. Kim M, Morrison M, Yu Z (2011) Evaluation of different partial 16S rRNA gene sequence regions for phylogenetic analysis of microbiomes. Journal of Microbiological Methods 84: 81–87.

44. Kim M, Morrison M, Yu Z (2011) Status of the phylogenetic diversity census of ruminal microbiomes. FEMS Microbiology Ecology 76: 49–63.

45. Gruninger RJ, Sensen CW, McAllister TA, Forster RJ (2014) Diversity of Rumen Bacteria in Canadian Cervids. PloS One 9: e89682.

46. Hernandez-Sanabria E, Goonewardene LA, Wang Z, Zhou M, Moore SS (2013) Influence of sire breed on the interplay among rumen microbial populations inhabiting the rumen liquid of the progeny in beef cattle. PloS One 8: e58461.

47. Li ZP, Liu HL, Li GY, Bao K, Wang KY, et al. (2013) Molecular diversity of rumen bacterial communities from tannin-rich and fiber-rich forage fed domestic Sika deer (Cervus nippon) in China. BMC Microbiology 13: 151.

48. Claesson MJ, Wang Q, O'Sullivan O, Greene-Diniz R, Cole JR, et al. (2010) Comparison of two next-generation sequencing technologies for resolving highly complex microbiota composition using tandem variable 16S rRNA gene regions. Nucleic acids research: 38: e200.

49. Nossa CW, Oberdorf WE, Yang L, Aas JA, Paster BJ, et al. (2010) Design of 16S rRNA gene primers for 454 pyrosequencing of the human foregut microbiome. World Journal of Gastroenterology 16: 4135.

50. Wang Y, Qian P-Y (2009) Conservative fragments in bacterial 16S rRNA genes and primer design for 16S ribosomal DNA amplicons in metagenomic studies. PloS One 4: e7401.

51. Claesson MJ, O'Sullivan O, Wang Q, Nikkilä J, Marchesi JR, et al. (2009) Comparative analysis of pyrosequencing and a phylogenetic microarray for exploring microbial community structures in the human distal intestine. PloS One 4: e6669.

52. Dethlefsen L, Huse S, Sogin ML, Relman DA (2008) The pervasive effects of an antibiotic on the human gut microbiota, as revealed by deep 16S rRNA sequencing. PLoS Biology 6: e280.

53. Tajima K, Aminov R, Nagamine T, Matsui H, Nakamura M, et al. (2001) Diet-dependent shifts in the bacterial population of the rumen revealed with real-time PCR. Applied and Environmental Microbiology 67: 2766–2774.

54. Yu Z, Morrison M (2004) Comparisons of different hypervariable regions of rrs genes for use in fingerprinting of microbial communities by PCR-denaturing gradient gel electrophoresis. Applied and Environmental Microbiology 70: 4800–4806.

55. Fernando SC, Purvis H, Najar F, Sukharnikov L, Krehbiel C, et al. (2010) Rumen microbial population dynamics during adaptation to a high-grain diet. Applied and Environmental Microbiology 76: 7482–7490.

56. Khafipour E, Li S, Plaizier JC, Krause DO (2009) Rumen microbiome composition determined using two nutritional models of subacute ruminal acidosis. Applied and Environmental Microbiology 75: 7115–7124.

57. Fouts DE, Szpakowski S, Purushe J, Torralba M, Waterman RC, et al. (2012) Next generation sequencing to define prokaryotic and fungal diversity in the bovine rumen. PloS One 7: e48289.

58. Pitta D, Kumar S, Vecchiarelli B, Shirley D, Bittinger K, et al. (2014) Temporal dynamics in the ruminal microbiome of dairy cows during the transition period. Journal of Animal Science 92: 4014–4022.

59. Leser TD, Amenuvor JZ, Jensen TK, Lindecrona RH, Boye M, et al. (2002) Culture-independent analysis of gut bacteria: the pig gastrointestinal tract microbiota revisited. Applied and Environmental Microbiology 68: 673–690.

60. Wallace RJ (1996) Ruminal microbial metabolism of peptides and amino acids. The Journal of Nutrition 126: 1326S–1334S.

61. Salyers A, Vercellotti J, West S, Wilkins T (1977) Fermentation of mucin and plant polysaccharides by strains of Bacteroides from the human colon. Applied and Environmental Microbiology 33: 319–322.

62. Walker JA, Kilroy GE, Xing J, Shewale J, Sinha SK, et al. (2003) Human DNA quantitation using *Alu* element-based polymerase chain reaction. Analytical biochemistry 315: 122–128.

63. Callaway T, Dowd S, Edrington T, Anderson R, Krueger N, et al. (2010) Evaluation of bacterial diversity in the rumen and feces of cattle fed different levels of dried distillers grains plus solubles using bacterial tag-encoded FLX amplicon pyrosequencing. Journal of Animal Science 88: 3977–3983.

64. Kittelmann S, Seedorf H, Walters WA, Clemente JC, Knight R, et al. (2013) Simultaneous amplicon sequencing to explore co-occurrence patterns of bacterial, archaeal and eukaryotic microorganisms in rumen microbial communities. PloS One 8: e47879.

65. Holt JG, Krieg NR, Sneath PH, Staley JT, Williams ST (1994) Bergey's manual of determinative bacteriology. Baltimore: Williams and Wilkins 75: 121.

66. de Menezes AB, Lewis E, O'Donovan M, O'Neill BF, Clipson N, et al. (2011) Microbiome analysis of dairy cows fed pasture or total mixed ration diets. FEMS Microbiology Ecology 78: 256–265.

67. Koike S, Kobayashi Y (2001) Development and use of competitive PCR assays for the rumen cellulolytic bacteria: *Fibrobacter succinogenes*, *Ruminococcus albus* and *Ruminococcus flavefaciens*. FEMS Microbiology Letters 204: 361–366.

68. Michalet-Doreau B, Fernandez I, Fonty G (2002) A comparison of enzymatic and molecular approaches to characterize the cellulolytic microbial ecosystems of the rumen and the cecum. Journal of Animal Science 80: 790–796.

69. Michalet-Doreau B, Fernandez I, Peyron C, Millet L, Fonty G (2001) Fibrolytic activities and cellulolytic bacterial community structure in the solid and liquid phases of rumen contents. Reproduction Nutrition Development 41: 187.

70. Saro C, Ranilla MJ, Carro M (2012) Postprandial changes of fiber-degrading microbes in the rumen of sheep fed diets varying in type of forage as monitored by real-time PCR and automated ribosomal intergenic spacer analysis. Journal of Animal Science 90: 4487–4494.

71. Koike S, Yoshitani S, Kobayashi Y, Tanaka K (2003) Phylogenetic analysis of fiber-associated rumen bacterial community and PCR detection of uncultured bacteria. FEMS Microbiology Letters 229: 23–30.

72. Mosoni P, Chaucheyras-Durand F, Béra-Maillet C, Forano E (2007) Quantification by real-time PCR of cellulolytic bacteria in the rumen of sheep after supplementation of a forage diet with readily fermentable carbohydrates: effect of a yeast additive. Journal of Applied Microbiology 103: 2676–2685.

73. Edwards U, Rogall T, Blöcker H, Emde M, Böttger EC (1989) Isolation and direct complete nucleotide determination of entire genes. Characterization of a gene coding for 16S ribosomal RNA. Nucleic Acids Research 17: 7843–7853.

74. Muyzer G, De Waal EC, Uitterlinden AG (1993) Profiling of complex microbial populations by denaturing gradient gel electrophoresis analysis of polymerase chain reaction-amplified genes coding for 16S rRNA. Applied and Environmental Microbiology 59: 695–700.

75. Skillman LC, Evans PN, Naylor GE, Morvan B, Jarvis GN, et al. (2004) 16S ribosomal DNA-directed PCR primers for ruminal methanogens and identification of methanogens colonising young lambs. Anaerobe 10: 277–285.

22

Large Outbreak Caused by Methicillin Resistant *Staphylococcus pseudintermedius* ST71 in a Finnish Veterinary Teaching Hospital – From Outbreak Control to Outbreak Prevention

Thomas Grönthal[1]*, **Arshnee Moodley**[2], **Suvi Nykäsenoja**[3], **Jouni Junnila**[4], **Luca Guardabassi**[2], **Katariina Thomson**[5], **Merja Rantala**[1]

1 Central Laboratory, Department of Equine and Small Animal Medicine, University of Helsinki, Helsinki, Finland, **2** Department of Veterinary Disease Biology, Faculty of Health and Medical Sciences, University of Copenhagen, Copenhagen, Denmark, **3** Food and Feed Microbiology Research Unit, Finnish Food Safety Authority Evira, Helsinki, Finland, **4** 4Pharma Ltd., Espoo, Finland, **5** Veterinary Teaching Hospital, University of Helsinki, Helsinki, Finland

Abstract

Introduction: The purpose of this study was to describe a nosocomial outbreak caused by methicillin resistant *Staphylococcus pseudintermedius* (MRSP) ST71 SCC*mec* II-III in dogs and cats at the Veterinary Teaching Hospital of the University of Helsinki in November 2010 – January 2012, and to determine the risk factors for acquiring MRSP. In addition, measures to control the outbreak and current policy for MRSP prevention are presented.

Methods: Data of patients were collected from the hospital patient record software. MRSP surveillance data were acquired from the laboratory information system. Risk factors for MRSP acquisition were analyzed from 55 cases and 213 controls using multivariable logistic regression in a case-control study design. Forty-seven MRSP isolates were analyzed by pulsed field gel electrophoresis and three were further analyzed with multi-locus sequence and SCC*mec* typing.

Results: Sixty-three MRSP cases were identified, including 27 infections. MRSPs from the cases shared a specific multi-drug resistant antibiogram and PFGE-pattern indicated clonal spread. Four risk factors were identified; skin lesion (OR = 6.2; CI$_{95\%}$ 2.3–17.0, $P = 0.0003$), antimicrobial treatment (OR = 3.8, CI$_{95\%}$ 1.0–13.9, $P = 0.0442$), cumulative number of days in the intensive care unit (OR = 1.3, CI$_{95\%}$ 1.1–1.6, $P = 0.0007$) or in the surgery ward (OR = 1.1, CI$_{95\%}$ 1.0–1.3, $P = 0.0401$). Tracing and screening of contact patients, enhanced hand hygiene, cohorting and barrier nursing, as well as cleaning and disinfection were used to control the outbreak. To avoid future outbreaks and spread of MRSP a search-and-isolate policy was implemented. Currently nearly all new MRSP findings are detected in screening targeted to risk patients on admission.

Conclusion: Multidrug resistant MRSP is capable of causing a large outbreak difficult to control. Skin lesions, antimicrobial treatment and prolonged hospital stay increase the probability of acquiring MRSP. Rigorous control measures were needed to control the outbreak. We recommend the implementation of a search-and-isolate policy to reduce the burden of MRSP.

Editor: Paul J. Planet, Columbia University, United States of America

Funding: TG was funded by Finnish Foundation of Veterinary Research; http://www.sels.fi/index_eng.htm, grant number 3-291-29. 4Pharma Ltd., provided support in the form of a salary for author JJ. The funders had no role in the study design, data collection and analysis, decision to publish, or preparation of the manuscript.

Competing Interests: JJ is an employee of 4Pharma Ltd. There are no patents, products in development or marketed products to declare.

* Email: thomas.gronthal@helsinki.fi

Introduction

Methicillin-resistant *Staphylococcus pseudintermedius* (MRSP) has emerged as a major animal pathogen in veterinary medicine [1], similar to methicillin resistant *Staphylococcus aureus* (MRSA) in human medicine [2]. MRSP can cause a wide variety of infections that are difficult to treat due to multi-drug resistance [1]. Transmission is mainly due to global spread of epidemic clones such as ST71, the predominant clone in Europe, and ST68, the predominant clone in North America [3]. Among others, hospitalization and antimicrobial treatment have been recognized as risk factors for MRSP colonization or infection [4–7]. Indistinguishable or closely related MRSP isolates from patients, environmental sites and staff members at veterinary clinics have been reported [8,9] suggestive of veterinary care associated spread of MRSP. However, to our best knowledge, no nosocomial outbreak reports of MRSP have yet been published. In addition, little information exists about infection control and preventive measures in practical situations.

The Veterinary Teaching Hospital of the University of Helsinki experienced a nosocomial MRSP outbreak between November 2010 and January 2012 with 63 confirmed cases among canine and feline patients. Prior to this MRSP was a very rare finding among patients of the Veterinary Teaching Hospital (Figure 1). The goal of this study was to (i) identify and characterize the strain causing the outbreak, (ii) to describe the outbreak and determine risk factors for acquiring MRSP, (iii) to describe the control measures implemented to contain the outbreak and (iv) to present our current policy for prevention of further outbreaks and the spread of MRSP. The hypothesis was that in addition to previously recognized risk factors, many variables related to patient condition, duration of surgical procedures, as well as the length of antimicrobial therapy increases the risk for MRSP acquisition during an outbreak.

Materials and methods

The hospital setting

The Veterinary Teaching Hospital of the University of Helsinki is a national primary care and referral animal hospital in Finland. The hospital provides 24/7 emergency and intensive care services for animals primarily in the Greater Helsinki area. The Small Animal Hospital of the unit has approximately 18 000 visits annually, with nearly 2000 surgical procedures. Approximately 80% of patients are dogs, 17% cats and the rest are other species. Bacteriological specimens from the hospital are investigated by the Clinical Microbiology Laboratory of the Faculty of Veterinary Medicine. The laboratory receives specimens from all over Finland. Apart from investigation of clinical specimens the

laboratory is responsible for resistance surveillance of small animal pathogens in the hospital and in Finland.

Epidemiological investigation and definitions

The study population consisted of dogs and cats that had been hospitalized for 1 day or more at the Small Animal Hospital during the outbreak period (November 2010 – January 2012) and thus were potentially exposed to nosocomial MRSP. Cases were either colonized (MRSP cultured only from mucous membranes) or infected (MRSP cultured from an infection site) with MRSP displaying the following antibiogram; resistance to oxacillin (and thus all beta-lactams), erythromycin, clindamycin, sulfamethoxazole-trimethoprim, gentamicin, tetracycline and enrofloxacin and susceptibility to fusidic acid and amikacin. To exclude community acquired MRSPs, only infections detected in the outbreak period either after surgical procedures performed at the hospital or other infections which appeared after prolonged or several treatment periods in the hospital were included. Colonized patients were enrolled if the MRSP was detected after at least 1 day of hospitalization and the animal had been treated in the same wards as MRSP positive patients. Controls were patients from the same population as cases but were negative in MRSP screening. Patients with a positive MRSP specimen on first admission, and non-hospitalized (polyclinic) patients were excluded from the study.

The investigation extended over a total of 26 months comprising the outbreak period (November 2010 – January 2012) and the follow-up period (February 2012 – November 2012). Treatment histories of the patients were gathered from the hospital patient registry software (Provet YES 1.1, Finnish Net Solutions Oy, Finland). Variables, including their definitions, are presented in Table 1. Data were collected for each individual from one month prior to the index case (i.e. from October 2010) up until the first positive MRSP finding (cases) or the latest date the patient was screened negative for MRSP (controls). Dates refer to

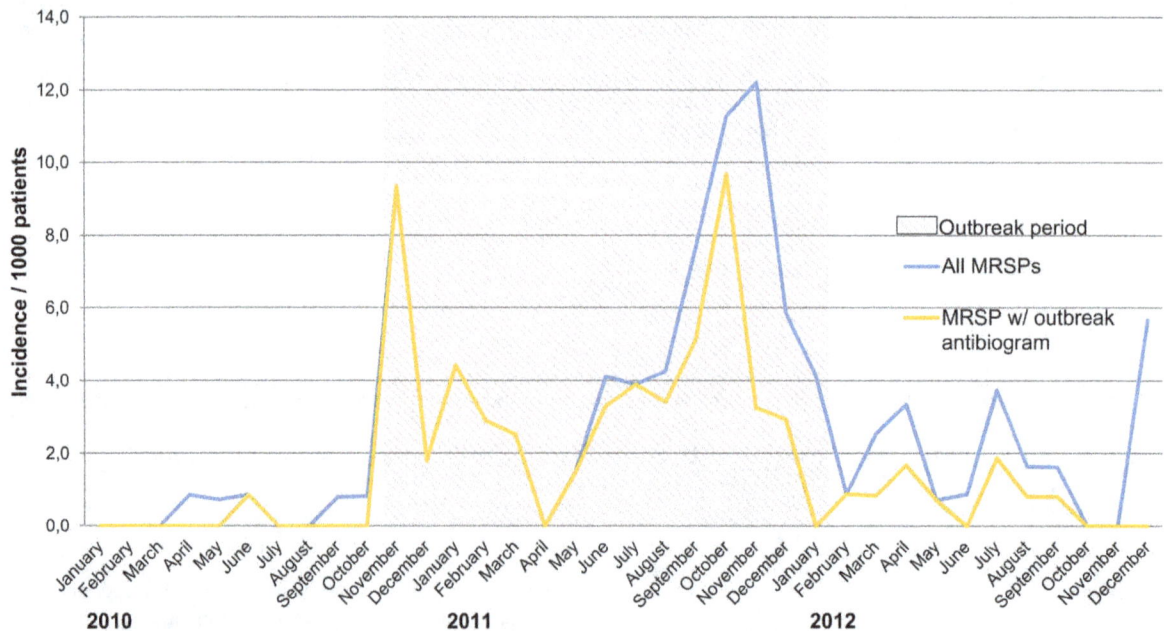

Figure 1. The monthly cumulative incidence of all MRSPs and MRSPs displaying the outbreak antibiogram (MRSP ST71) among patients of the Small Animal Hospital of Helsinki University from January 2010 to December 2012. In late 2011 a small cluster of ST45 among hospitalized patients contributed to an increase in incidence. From January 2012 onwards the great majority of new MRSP findings have been detected in screening targeted to risk patients on admission. In December 2012 the increase was not due to a cluster, but was due to the detection of different types of MRSPs mainly in patients belonging to risk groups.

when the specimen was taken. In addition, data on the cumulative incidence of MRSP before, during and after the outbreak was collected and presented as total incidence (all new MRSP findings) and as incidence of the outbreak MRSP. This data were extracted from the laboratory information system (connected to the patient registry software). Since one patient with the defined MRSP had been observed in July 2010, a trace-back analysis was performed to evaluate any relationship of that patient to the current outbreak.

This study did not require separate ethical approval since outbreaks are routinely investigated according to the hospital ethical guidelines to ensure patient safety. The owners of the animals were informed about the outbreak and study. They agreed to the investigation as well as any attempts to control the outbreak. Owners also gave permission to take the necessary specimens. The hospital covered the costs of screening specimens of exposed patients and specimens to monitor the efficacy of the control measures. Data was handled anonymously.

Data analysis and statistical methods

Descriptive analysis of cases was done by presenting the number of new cases per week over the outbreak and follow-up periods in the epidemic curve along with the implemented control measures. The number of colonized and infected patients was recorded. The attack rate was determined by using the number of hospitalized patients as the denominator. The risk factors (Table 1) for acquiring MRSP were assessed with logistic regression. For the risk factor study data were available for 55 cases and 213 controls. Each factor was first modeled using a univariable logistic regression models. To control for confounders, a stepwise multivariable logistic regression analysis was conducted for the risk factors with a P value ≤ 0.05 in the univariate analyses. In the stepwise selection process, a significance level of 0.15 was required to allow a variable into the multivariable model, and a significance level of 0.20 was required for a variable to stay in the multivariable model. Odds ratios (OR) with 95% confidence intervals (CI) were calculated. P values (Wald) ≤ 0.05 were considered statistically significant. All statistical analyses were done using SAS System for Windows, version 9.3 (SAS Institute Inc., USA).

Microbiological investigation

Specimens for bacterial cultures were taken from infection sites of all patients as soon as signs of infection were noticed. To screen for MRSP colonization (screening specimens), specimens were taken from the mucous membranes of patients with or without infection. For this, three sites were swabbed in patient; the nares and oral mucous membranes with one swab, and the perineum with another. If the patient had a wound or skin sore, that was also swabbed. Screening specimens were taken frequently from contact patients and regularly from all hospitalized patients (Figure 2) in order to monitor the extension of the outbreak and efficacy of control measures. Patients were screened repeatedly if they had long term hospitalization or several treatment periods. In the autumn 2011 there was a two month period of enhanced surveillance when every hospitalized patient (n = 72) was screened both on admission and on discharge. In addition, environmental swabs (n = 65) were taken to evaluate efficacy of daily cleaning and disinfection routines and the role of the environment as the source of MRSP on three occasions.

Specimens from superficial infection sites and urine were cultured aerobically, whereas specimens from deep lesions, aspirates and blood were also cultured anaerobically. Both non-selective and selective plates were used for primary cultures according to the laboratory protocol. The protocol also included direct plating onto MRSA selective agar (MRSA Select, Bio Rad Laboratories, France) and enrichment culture for MRSP (see below). Screening specimens from the patient were cultured by pooling the swabs into an enrichment broth (Brain Heart Infusion broth with 6.5% NaCl, Tammer-Tutkan Maljat Oy, Finland) and incubated for 16–22 h at +35.0°C (±0.2°C). The enrichment broth was then plated onto MRSA-selective agar and incubated up to 48 h at +35.0°C (±0.2°C), and were interpreted once a day. The limit of detection for enrichment culture method had been determined to be ≥ 10 CFU for MRSP with oxacillin minimum inhibitory concentration (MIC) of ≥ 4 µg/ml in internal valida-tion. Suspected MRSP colonies (pale pink to pink colonies) were subcultured onto tryptic soy agar with 5% sheep blood (Oxoid Ltd., UK). Presumptive identification of S. pseudintermedius was based on typical colony morphology, positive tube coagulation test (BBL Coagulase Plasma, Becton Dickinson, USA) and suscepti-bility to polymyxin B (300 U, Oxoid Ltd, UK) (sensitive ≥ 10 mm, resistant <10 mm). If identification was doubtful, sugar fermen-tation tests (Diatabs, Rosco Diagnostica A/S, Denmark) or API Staph ID 32 (bioMérieux SA, France) were used. Antimicrobial susceptibility testing was done in accordance with Clinical and Laboratory Standards Institute guidelines [10] by using the disk-diffusion method (Oxoid Ltd., UK). Breakpoints for oxacillin

Table 1. Variables analyzed from cases and controls during the MRSP outbreak in the Small Animal Hospital of Helsinki University between 2010 and 2011.

Species (dog/cat)	Emergency surgery (during weekend/evening/night)	Aminopenicillin medication given
Age (years)	Length of anesthesia (min)	[b]Days of aminopenicillin therapy
Gender	[b]Days in hospital	Cephalosporin medication given
Breed	[b]Days in surgery ward	[b]Days of cephalosporin therapy
Weight (kg)	[b]Days in intensive care unit	[c]Enrofloxacin medication given
[a]Severity of condition	[b]Days in other wards	[b]Days of enrofloxacin therapy
Skin lesions of any cause	Antimicrobial medication given	Proton pump inhibitor (PPI) given
Surgical procedure	[b]Days of any antimicrobial therapy	[b]Days of PPI therapy

[a]Severity was judged by the author (TG) on a scale of 1 to 5 after reviewing the patient record on admission and was based on the guidelines provided by the American Society of Anesthesiologists.
[b]The same patient might have had several visits or courses of medication, therefore the cumulative number of days for these variables was recorded until the first positive MRSP specimen (cases), or latest negative MRSP specimen (controls), see text for details.
[c]Enrofloxacin was the only fluoroquinolone used for these patients.

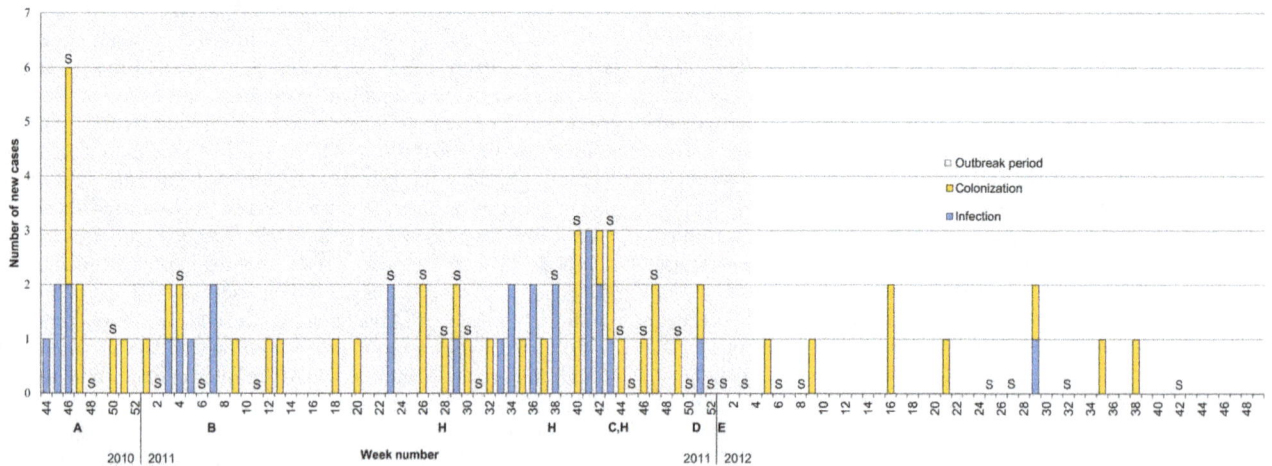

Figure 2. An epidemic curve showing new MRSP ST71 cases during the outbreak in 2010–2012 at the Small Animal Hospital of Helsinki University. The outbreak period was between November 2010 and January 2012, after which the follow-up period was started. A: hospital closed for 2 days for cleaning and disinfection, B: establishment of cohort ward, C: nurse responsible for hospital hygiene appointed, D: hospital closed for 5 days for cleaning and disinfection, E: veterinarian appointed as infection control officer. S: Screening of hospitalized patients, H: environmental swabs taken.

susceptibility presented by Bemis et al. [11] were used. Oxacillin MIC was determined by E-test (Oxoid Ltd., UK). MRSP isolates were sent to the Finnish Food Safety Authority (Evira) for verification of the presence of *mec*A [12].

Isolate characterization

Forty-seven isolates were available for pulsed field gel electrophoresis (PFGE) typing. A modified version of the HARMONY protocol as described by Murchan et al. [13] was used. Approximately 4×10^8 colony forming units per strain were suspended into 200 µl of EC-buffer (1 M sodium chloride, 0,5% Polyoxyethylene 20 cetyl ether, 0,2% w/v sodium deoxycholate, 0,5% w/v N-lauroyl-sarcosine sodium salt, 0,1 M EDTA, 6 mM 1,0 M Tris-HCl). The plugs were made by mixing the bacteria and EC-buffer suspension with 20 µl of lysostaphin (1 mg/ml, Sigma-Aldrich, USA), and 200 µl of 2% SeaPlaque GTG agarose (Lonza Inc., USA). The digestion was done using a 10% NEBuffer 4 and 20 U SmaI (New England BioLabs Inc., USA) for 4–18 hours. The pulse field electrophoresis was done in 1% SeaKem agar (Lonza Inc., USA) on the CHEF-DR III system (Bio-Rad Laboratories, USA). Gels were stained with SYBR Safe DNA gel stain (Life technologies, USA) and analyzed using GelCompar II v. 6.5 software (Applied Maths NV, Belgium), and cluster analysis was performed by UPGMA based on the Dice similarity coefficient, with optimization and position tolerance both set at 1%. Isolates were clustered using an 85% similarity cut-off. The strains were considered to be closely related (≤3 band differences) or subtypes of the same clone (4–6 band differences) according to Tenover *et al.* [14]. Based on PFGE, three strains representing subtypes of the clone (Figure 3) were further characterized by SCC*mec* [15] and multilocus sequence typing (MLST) [16], and confirmed to be *S. pseudintermedius* by species specific *nuc* PCR [17]. MLST type was determined by comparing sequences of the housekeeping genes to the *S. pseudintermedius* MLST database (http://pubmlst.org/spseudintermedius/).

Results

Description of the outbreak

During the outbreak period 63 cases were identified; 27 (43%) of these were infections, while 36 (57%) were colonized patients. Of the infected patients, three developed MRSP infection several weeks after colonization was detected. The types of the MRSP-infections are summarized in Table 2. The attack rate of MRSP among hospitalized patients was 2.1% (63/2969) and among patients discharged from the ICU 3.8% (43/1121). MRSP was the cause of a surgical wound infection in 0.9% of surgical procedures (17/1864). Fifty-eight of the cases (92%) were dogs and five (8%) were cats; dogs represented more than 40 different breeds, all five cats were domestic short haired. The epidemic curve indicating the number of new cases per week is presented in Figure 2; and the cumulative incidences both for the outbreak MRSP and all new MRSP findings before, during and after the outbreak in Figure 1.

The index patient was a 3 year-old dachshund that was referred to the Small Animal Hospital emergency care unit at the end of October 2010. The dog had systemic inflammatory response syndrome with disseminated intravascular coagulation due to necrotizing mastitis and a postoperative complication after cesarean section and ovariohysterectomy performed at two different private practices. The dog required surgery again at the Small Animal Hospital to remove necrotized tissue and was treated in the intensive care unit (ICU) for 1 week. The tissue specimen yielded pure growth of *Escherichia coli*. However, two days after discharge, in the beginning of November 2010, a surgical site infection was noted. The bacteriological culture revealed MRSP with the aforementioned multi-drug resistance antibiogram. The finding was extraordinary and therefore an outbreak investigation was initiated. This involved active case finding by culturing all infection sites and screening of patients potentially exposed to MRSP.

Trace-back analysis to the case in June 2010 did not reveal any apparent relationship to the outbreak. Subsequently the index case, active case finding revealed many new cases (Figure 2). After control measures in late 2010, and early 2011 the incidence of MRSP decreased for a while. The situation worsened again in the

MRSP SmaI Dice (Opt: 1.00%, Tol: 1.00%)

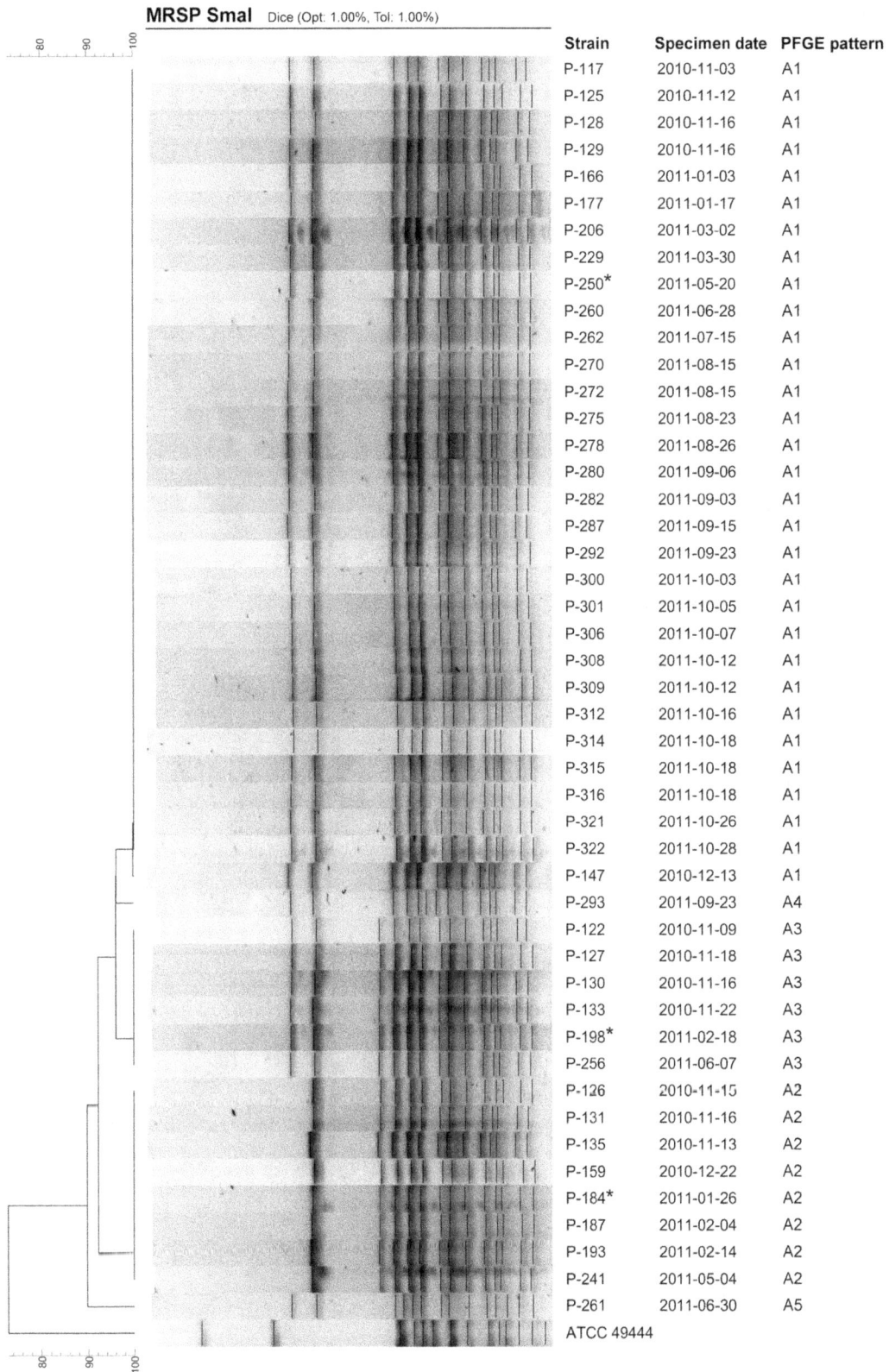

Strain	Specimen date	PFGE pattern
P-117	2010-11-03	A1
P-125	2010-11-12	A1
P-128	2010-11-16	A1
P-129	2010-11-16	A1
P-166	2011-01-03	A1
P-177	2011-01-17	A1
P-206	2011-03-02	A1
P-229	2011-03-30	A1
P-250*	2011-05-20	A1
P-260	2011-06-28	A1
P-262	2011-07-15	A1
P-270	2011-08-15	A1
P-272	2011-08-15	A1
P-275	2011-08-23	A1
P-278	2011-08-26	A1
P-280	2011-09-06	A1
P-282	2011-09-03	A1
P-287	2011-09-15	A1
P-292	2011-09-23	A1
P-300	2011-10-03	A1
P-301	2011-10-05	A1
P-306	2011-10-07	A1
P-308	2011-10-12	A1
P-309	2011-10-12	A1
P-312	2011-10-16	A1
P-314	2011-10-18	A1
P-315	2011-10-18	A1
P-316	2011-10-18	A1
P-321	2011-10-26	A1
P-322	2011-10-28	A1
P-147	2010-12-13	A1
P-293	2011-09-23	A4
P-122	2010-11-09	A3
P-127	2010-11-18	A3
P-130	2010-11-16	A3
P-133	2010-11-22	A3
P-198*	2011-02-18	A3
P-256	2011-06-07	A3
P-126	2010-11-15	A2
P-131	2010-11-16	A2
P-135	2010-11-13	A2
P-159	2010-12-22	A2
P-184*	2011-01-26	A2
P-187	2011-02-04	A2
P-193	2011-02-14	A2
P-241	2011-05-04	A2
P-261	2011-06-30	A5
ATCC 49444		

Figure 3. Dendrogram of 47 MRSP isolates with the outbreak antibiogram (see text). *Staphylococcus pseudintermedius* ATCC 49444 is displayed as a control. *Further characterized by multilocus sequence typing and SCC*mec*-typing.

Table 2. Nosocomial infections (n = 27) caused by the MRSP outbreak strain (ST71, SCC*mec* II–III) in the Small Animal Hospital of Helsinki University between 2010 and 2011.

Infection type	Number of infections
Surgical site infections (total)	19
Required surgical revision	3
Involved orthopedic devices[1]	7
Others (uncomplicated)	9
Other wound infections	3
Otitis[2]	1
Bite wound[3]	2
Dermatitis[4]	1
Cystitis complicated by uroliths[5]	1

[1]Some cases required removal of surgical devices and revision.
[2]Patient had orthopedic surgery and several visits to the hospital, otitis was subsequently diagnosed.
[3]Both patients presented with severe bite wounds; after prolonged hospital stay MRSP was cultured from the wound.
[4]Patient presented with pneumonia, autoimmune myositis and dermal vasculitis; later developed MRSP infection on the skin lesion.
[5]Colonization with MRSP preceded the cystitis.

summer and fall of 2011, leading to extensive control measures after which control was achieved. However, the investigation was interfered by a small cluster of MRSP ST45 detected in late 2011(Figure 1, File S2). The outbreak was considered to be over in January of 2012, when no new MRSP findings were revealed in three consecutive MRSP screenings of all hospitalized patients. After this the follow-up period was started. During the follow up period nine new MRSP findings with the outbreak antibiogram were detected. Of these, seven were explained by previous exposure due to hospitalization during the outbreak. Thus the total toll of cases connected to the outbreak was 70. The other two were not spatially or temporally connected to the outbreak. In the follow-up period all MRSP cases with the outbreak antibiogram were identified on admission using the risk patient classification criteria (Table 3). Regardless of this, all hospitalized patients were screened for MRSP on seven occasions, but no new cases were detected among these (Figure 2).

Risk factor analysis

Several risk factors were significant by univariable analyses (Table 4, Table S1). However, after controlling for confounders, the logistic regression model revealed only four significant risk factors; skin lesions of any origin (including surgical incisions) (OR 6.24, $CI_{95\%}$ 2.30–16.97), antimicrobial therapy regardless of duration (OR 3.80, $CI_{95\%}$ 1.04–13.92), cumulative number of days spent in the ICU (OR 1.33, $CI_{95\%}$ 1.13–1.57) or in the surgery ward (OR 1.13, $CI_{95\%}$ 1.01–1.27). The results of the univariable and multivariable analyses are presented in detail in Table 4.

Table 3. The current risk based classification of patients at the Small Animal Hospital of Helsinki University and resulting measures.

Classification	Criteria (any of the following)	Example of measures
High risk patients	MRSP-positive	Treated in cohort ward
	Has been hospitalized >24 hours and has signs of a hospital acquired	Barrier nursing
	infection	Surgery at the end of the day
		Disinfection of facilities
		Infection sites cultured
		Standard precautions*
Medium risk patients	Has a history of recurrent ear or skin infection	Screened for MRSP
	Has a history of prolonged or numerous hospital visits or visits at	Treated in separate rooms
	other veterinary clinics	reserved for medium risk
	Has a history of prolonged or numerous antimicrobial treatments	patients
	Has been exposed to a patient with MRSP	Surgery at the end of the day
	Has had surgery elsewhere and has a surgical site infection	Standard precautions
	Has a suppurative wound infection	Infection sites cultured
Low risk patients	All other patients	All other rooms
		Standard precautions

*Includes hand disinfection, hygienic work routine, and use of protective clothing in case of dirty procedures.

Table 4. Risk factors associated with acquisition of MRSP during the outbreak in the Small Animal Hospital of Helsinki University between 2010 and 2011.

Binary variables	MRSP-pos (n=55) n	%	MRSP-neg (n=213) n	%	Univariable logistic regression Unadjusted OR (95% CI)	Wald P	Multivariable logistic regression Adjusted OR (95% CI)	Wald P
Demographics								
Gender: M vs. F	30	54.5	96	45.1	1.46 (0.80–2.66)	0.212		
Species: dog vs. cat	50	90.9	192	90.1	1.09 (0.39–3.06)	0.864		
Epidemiological data								
Skin lesion	49	89.1	85	39.9	12.40 (5.06–30.37)	<0.001	6.24 (2.30–16.97)	0.0003
Antimicrobial treatment	52	94.6	130	61.0	11.07 (3.33–36.79)	<0.001	3.80 (1.04–13.92)	0.0442
Surgical procedure	45	81.8	67	31.5	9.81 (4.65–20.70)	<0.001		
Cephalosporin treatment	21	38.2	24	11.3	5.10 (2.54–10.26)	<0.001		
Enrofloxacin treatment	18	32.7	33	15.5	2.70 (1.3–5.2)	0.005		
Severity (1 vs. others)	46	85.5	8	14.5	2.84 (1.3–6.4)	0.012		
Aminopenicillin treatment	34	61.8	93	43.7	2.09 (1.14–3.85)	0.018		
Treatment in ICU	41	74.6	126	59.2	2.02 (1.03–3.95)	0.039		
Proton pump inhibitor treatment	36	65.5	114	53.5	1.65 (0.89–3.06)	0.115		
Orthopedic vs. soft tissue surgery	20	44.4	20	30.3	1.84 (0.83–4.08)	0.132		
Other antimicrobial treatment	12	21.8	32	15.0	1.58 (0.75–3.33)	0.229		
Emergency surgery	6	13.6	9	13.4	1.02 (0.33–3.13)	0.976		

Continuous variables	MRSP-pos (n=55) n	mean	MRSP-neg (n=213) n	mean	Unadjusted OR (95% CI)	Univariate P	Adjusted OR (95% CI)	Multiple regression P
Demographics								
Bodyweight	55	20.7	201	19.2	1.01 (0.99–1.03)	0.493		
Age	55	4.8	212	4.9	1.01 (0.92–1.10)	0.791		
Epidemiological data								
Cum. days in ICU	55	2.9	213	1.5	1.39 (1.20–1.61)	<0.001	1.3 (1.1–1.6)	0.0007
Cum. days in surgery ward	55	3.4	213	1.1	1.28 (1.15–1.42)	<0.001	1.1 (1.0–1.3)	0.0401
Cum. days in hospital (all wards)	55	7.2	213	4.5	1.15 (1.08–1.24)	<0.001		
Cum. days of proton pump inhibitors	36	5.5	114	2.9	1.08 (1.01–1.17)	0.037		
Length of surgical procedure (10 min change)	41	203.2	57	170.9	1.04 (0.99–1.10)	0.080		
Cum. days in other wards	55	2.0	213	2.6	0.92 (0.81–1.05)	0.210		
Cum. days antimic. given	55	12.0	213	5.4	1.01 (0.99–1.02)	0.364		

Table 4. Cont.

Continuous variables	MRSP-pos (n=55)		MRSP-neg (n=213)		Unadjusted OR (95% CI)	Univariate P	Adjusted OR (95% CI)	Multiple regression P
	n	mean	n	mean				
Cum. days of enroflox.	18	6.5	33	4.7	1.03 (0.96–1.11)	0.459		
Cum. days of aminopen.	34	13.9	93	10.1	1.00 (0.99–1.02)	0.481		
Cum. days of cephalosp.	21	5.3	23	4.1	1.03 (0.93–1.15)	0.518		
Cum. days of other antimic.	12	4.7	32	6.7	0.98 (0.91–1.06)	0.614		

OR = Odds Ratio, CI = Confidence Interval.

Characterization of the outbreak strain

PFGE analysis supported that the outbreak was due to clonal spread of MRSP. Isolates clustered to one dominant pulsotype, A1 (n = 31), and four subtypes; A2 (n = 8), A3 (n = 6), A4 (n = 1) with a one band difference and A5 (n = 1) with a four band difference (Figure 3). On the basis of the typing results of the three isolates, the strain responsible for the outbreak belonged to ST71 (File S1) and harbored SCC*mec* II–III.

Outbreak control measures

The staff and students were informed by e-mail about the situation on numerous occasions and training sessions were organized. The use of alcohol-based hand rubs before and after every patient contact was emphasised, and the use of protective gear (gloves and gowns) was required during dirty procedures (i.e. treatment of wounds, performing ear flushing, dental procedures or administering enemas), or when handling MRSP patients. The compliance to follow hygienic work order (i.e. performing clean procedures prior to dirty ones and examining healthy patients before diseased) was enhanced and immediate disinfection of secretions with 1% Virkon S (Antec International, UK) was demanded. The efficacy of the control measures were surveyed by frequent screening of hospitalized patients (Figure 2). Sixty-five environmental swabs from high-touch surfaces were collected. MRSP with the outbreak antibiogram was detected in only one environmental specimen, and originated from the cohort ward where MRSP patients were treated since February 2011. This ward was established to house MRSP-positive and high-risk patients (Table 3). Extensive cleaning and disinfection of all hospital surfaces were undertaken a few weeks after the first case (Figure 2). The ICU was closed during this time. Surface disinfection with a 1% Virkon S solution was increased.

In November 2011, a nurse responsible for hospital hygiene was appointed allowing a more effective tracking of discharged patients exposed to MRSP. These patients received a "MRSP exposed" tag in the electronic patient record. The tag was a sign for staff to screen the patient for MRSP and classify it as a medium-risk patient upon returning to the hospital (Table 3). Prior to the end of 2011 the hospital, excluding the emergency policlinic, was closed for five days for large scale cleaning and disinfection. All staff participated in the cleaning. From the beginning of 2012 a veterinarian was appointed as infection control officer to enforce prudent use of antimicrobials and consult in hospital hygiene and patients involving infections. After these measures control of the outbreak was finally achieved (Figure 2).

A "search-and-isolate" policy was launched in early 2012 to prevent further outbreaks and the spread of MRSP within the hospital and to the community. In addition to standard precautions (hand disinfection, hygienic work routine, and use of protective clothing in case of dirty procedures) this includes (1) the risk based classification of all patients (Table 3), (2) screening of patients at risk (at the expense of the owner), (3) isolation of high risk and MRSP positive patients, (4) screening of contact patients of new cases either in the hospital or upon revisit (at the expense of the hospital), (5) early initiation of the outbreak investigation, (6) surveillance and bacteriological sampling of treatment associated infections and (7) prudent use of antimicrobials.

Discussion

The MRSP outbreak spanned over a period of 14 months, during which 63 patients were found to be infected (n = 27) or colonized (n = 36). Additionally, seven more temporally and spatially connected cases were detected during the follow up period. There are several factors which suggest that this was a nosocomial outbreak: (i) the cases were spatially and temporally connected, (ii) the patients had no evidence of MRSP on admission and (iii) molecular characterization supported clonal spread. Also, all infections were related to hospital care as they were surgical site infections or other infections which appeared after prolonged hospital treatment. It was likewise considered very unlikely, that MRSPs of colonized patients were community acquired since this MRSP type was very rare prior to the outbreak and no similar type of MRSP was observed among outpatients or specimens submitted from private clinics during the outbreak. In addition, many of our cases (n = 30) had given a negative MRSP result in former bacteriological specimens taken on or soon after the first admission.

This is the first report of MRSP in Finland. The outbreak strain was the multi-drug resistant global MRSP clone ST71-SCCmec II–III [3]. This clone has also been found in other Nordic countries such as Denmark [3], Sweden [18] and Norway [19]. For our patients the strain caused a number of nosocomial infections ranging from dermatitis to osteomyelitis, with the majority being surgical site infections after non-elective procedures. In one case the colonization was followed by a urinary tract infection, complicated by urolith formation leading to surgery. In another case an MRSP infection was the most likely cause for euthanasia, but this could not be confirmed since no autopsy was done.

Many patients required prolonged hospital treatment or surgical procedure to combat the infection. Majority of infections were treated without systemic antimicrobials, but if considered necessary, amikacin was used. The exception was a case with urinary tract infection which was treated with nitrofurantoin. The fact that MRSP infections were manageable without systemic antimicrobials is encouraging. This approach could even be considered in infections caused by susceptible bacteria, provided that no systemic signs are present.

The risk factors for MRSP according to the multivariable analysis were skin lesions of any origin, antimicrobial therapy – regardless of duration, and cumulative number of days treated in the ICU or in the surgery unit. The length of antimicrobial therapy was not a significant risk factor in the final model. This indicates that any antimicrobial treatment may increase the risk for the acquisition of MRSP in an outbreak, possibly due to the high infection pressure. The result may not be generalized to the outpatient population, in which the cumulative use of antimicrobials could be the more important factor. Multiple factors operating in an intricate fashion lead to the elimination of many of the studied variables in the final model, suggesting the presence of confounders, such as surgery and skin lesions, and surgery and the use of antimicrobials.

In hospital outbreaks caused by multidrug resistant bacteria, it is often expected to have more colonized than infected patients, as were also the case in this outbreak. While infection is more harmful to the individual patient and more expensive to the hospital, failure to recognize colonized patients would likely have led to an underestimation of the extent of the outbreak, or even the unrecognition of the outbreak. Colonized and infected patients were pooled as cases for the risk factor analysis. If handled separately in the risk factor analysis one would not possibly reach the power to identify a common source or relevant factors associated with emergence of the pathogen. We think it is reasonable to assume that there is no biological difference in the acquisition of MRSP in colonized and infected patients. Colonization can precede the infection, as was the case also in our study in three of the patients, or colonization and infection may develop

simultaneously depending on where the pathogen enters the body as well as on the characteristics of the individual's immune status. In many cases infection never occurs. Also, exact differentiation between colonization and infection especially in mild cases can be difficult, since signs of inflammation can be very similar to infection.

Studies evaluating risk factors for MRSP have previously been done by comparing patients diagnosed with MRSP infection with patients with methicillin susceptible S. pseudintermedius (MSSP) infection [6,7], or comparing MRSP positive patients with MRSP negatives on admission to a hospital [5]. Antimicrobial treatment [5,6] as well as treatment duration [4] has been associated with an increased risk for MRSP. Interestingly, Lehner et al. [7] did not observe antimicrobial treatment as a risk factor for MRSP infection, but linked glucocorticoid therapy to an increased risk for MRSP infection. However, glucocorticoid therapy may also be associated with other factors, such as atopy or allergy [5]. Risk factors regarding MRSP in cats are poorly documented, but there is evidence that colonization rates of S. pseudintermedius [20] and MRSP are lower in cats compared to dogs [21]. Conversely, Lehner et al. [7] concluded that cats were at an increased risk of MRSP infection compared to dogs, although the result may have been due to bias caused by the sampling strategy. In our study the species was not a risk factor for MRSP. Cats were not separately analyzed in our study due to their low number. Still, species specific risk factors warrant further study.

Previous hospitalization has been shown to be a risk factor for MRSP [5,7], suggesting that MRSP is an important hospital associated pathogen. The epidemiology of MRSP appears to be comparable to that of MRSA in humans or animals, as also MRSA originally emerged in hospitals [1,22]. Other groups at risk for MRSP are patients with chronic dermatological disorders [4], most likely due to long-term antimicrobial pressure, frequent veterinary visits [7] and properties of the diseased skin [23], all of which favor the acquisition of MRSP. In light of these facts MRSP can currently be considered more a hospital associated than a community associated pathogen. In animals it may be challenging to differentiate between hospital and community acquired infections. Firstly, there is a lack of common definitions for these in veterinary medicine. Additionally, the majority of hospital acquired infections (such as surgical site infections) appear at home because the duration of hospitalization is usually short and many elective procedures are performed as outpatient surgery (day surgery). Therefore it is uncertain whether infections related to treatment are correctly classified as hospital acquired or veterinary care associated infections. If the spread is not controlled in the veterinary premises, it is inevitable that MRSP will become more prevalent in the community. This increases the likelihood of community acquired MRSP even in animals with no apparent risk factors. Similar development has already been observed in MRSA in humans [2,24].

There are limitations in this study. The quality of the data is dependent on how well information has been recorded in the patient management software, but this type of bias is expected to be equally distributed among cases and controls. In this study the data were not systematically available on underlying disorders such as allergies or metabolic diseases. In addition, information on variables related to patient care, such as the number of times the animal was handled or the exact placing of the patient (e.g. cage number), was not available. This sort of information could be helpful in order to understand the dynamics of the outbreak. Some degree of misclassification may have occurred due to the imperfect sensitivity of the MRSP screening method. Studies have reported the sensitivity of similar methods for MRSA in humans or livestock to be up to 98% [25–28]. Comparable methods have been used for MRSP detection in at least two studies [29,30], but currently no reference standard for the screening of MRSP exists. Many commercial MRSA selective agars contain cefoxitin as the selective antimicrobial which might impair the growth of MRSP. However, the outbreak strain was highly resistant to oxacillin (MIC >256 μg/ml) and based on our internal evaluation MRSP isolates with oxacillin MIC ≥4 μg/ml are detected even if the bacterial count in the specimen is low. Therefore it is unlikely that a significant amount of misclassification would have occurred. It can be considered a limitation that not all patients could be screened for MRSP upon admission. Consequently, it cannot be ruled out that some of the patients had MRSP already on admission. However, in outbreak situations it is not realistic, nor necessary to screen every patient to determine the admission status. As discussed above, the likelihood of a community acquired MRSP ST71 was very low when all evidence was considered.

In this outbreak no common source for MRSP was identified. Nevertheless, based on the epidemic curve (Figure 2), nosocomial patient-to-patient transmission was likely. It is widely accepted that contaminated hands favor the spread of nosocomial pathogens [31]. In humans the increased use of alcohol based hand rubs has been associated with a decrease in MRSA incidence in hospitals [32,33]. Barrier nursing has also been shown effective in reducing healthcare-associated MRSA infections [34]. Many hospital pathogens are likely transmitted by fomites, emphasizing the necessity of a clean environment and clothing [35–37]. However, the very high number (64 out of 65) of environmental specimens negative for MRSP suggests that the contaminated hospital environment was not the reason for maintenance of the outbreak. The control measures of our outbreak, including cohorting, patient flow planning, emphasis on hand hygiene, barrier nursing, prudent antimicrobial use and environmental cleaning are probably important [31]. Interestingly, Wilson et al. [38] found that while the use of enhanced cleaning procedures did reduce the amount of MRSA on hospital surfaces and the hands of healthcare staff, it did not reduce the number of new patients colonized with MRSA, although the authors thought that this may have been a result of a small sample size.

There could be numerous reasons for the long duration of the outbreak. There is evidence that ST71 is capable of efficient dissemination [3], perhaps due to multidrug resistance and a strong ability to form biofilm [19]. While the initial control measures seemed effective at first, it became clear that more rigorous efforts were needed. Initially the lack of resources allocated for infection control was likely to have contributed to the increased number of cases. New employees not familiar with the hygiene practices during the summer of 2011, combined with the lack of personnel due to holidays, may have influenced the increase in incidence. Also, the absence of effective tracking of patients exposed to MRSP until a hygiene nurse was appointed in late 2011 was probably an important factor, since after this the number of new MRSP cases decreased. The cleaning and disinfection at the end of 2011 likely favored the cessation of the outbreak.

In the literature concerning infection control in veterinary hospitals, the importance to recognize patients colonized with multidrug resistant organisms has not been properly acknowledged. Failure to recognize patients with multidrug resistant pathogens – regardless whether infected or colonized – will eventually lead to dissemination of resistant bacteria in hospitals and to the community. The search-and-isolate policy implemented in the Small Animal Hospital is similar to the search-and-destroy policy that has been used to control MRSA in some countries [24,39]. It does not, however, include the decolonization of patients as no research about the efficacy of decolonization therapy for MRSP has been published. Also, the veterinary use of some antimicrobials used for decolonization of MRSA in humans, such as mupirocin, rifampicin or linezolid, is legally prohibited in Finland. Currently only sporadic cases of MRSP displaying the outbreak antibiogram are identified, mainly among acknowledged risk patients, which indicates the success of present policy.

Conclusions

We show that multidrug resistant MRSP is capable of causing a large hospital outbreak difficult to control. Our findings suggest that skin lesions of any origin, antimicrobial treatment and prolonged hospital stay increase the probability of acquiring MRSP. We demonstrate that rigorous control measures are needed to control an outbreak and recommend the implementation of a search-and-isolate policy to reduce the burden of MRSP. However, standard precautions (hand disinfection, hygienic work routine, and use of protective clothing in unclean procedures) still remain the core in preventing the transmission of pathogens between patients.

Acknowledgments

The authors wish to thank laboratory technicians Mari Hyvönen, Marja Matikka, Taina Lehto and Tatjana Kristensen for their invaluable technical assistance. Special thanks go to the personnel of the University of Helsinki Veterinary Teaching Hospital, especially hygiene nurse Hanna Aaltonen. The outbreak was quenched due to their vital efforts. We also acknowledge Professor Outi Lyytikäinen for commenting on the manuscript.

Author Contributions

Conceived and designed the experiments: MR TG KT. Performed the experiments: TG MR LG AM SN. Analyzed the data: TG JJ MR. Contributed reagents/materials/analysis tools: AM JJ LG. Wrote the paper: TG AM SN JJ LG KT MR. Molecular analysis: AM SN LG MR TG. Statistical analysis: JJ. Drafted the manuscript: TG.

References

1. van Duijkeren E, Catry B, Greko C, Moreno MA, Pomba MC, et al. (2011) Review on methicillin-resistant *Staphylococcus pseudintermedius*. J Antimicrob Chemoth 66: 2705–2714.
2. Woodford N, Livermore DM (2009) Infections caused by Gram-positive bacteria: a review of the global challenge. J Infection 59 Suppl 1: S4–16.
3. Perreten V, Kadlec K, Schwarz S, Gronlund Andersson U, Finn M, et al. (2010) Clonal spread of methicillin-resistant *Staphylococcus pseudintermedius* in Europe and North America: an international multicentre study. J Antimicrob Chemoth 65: 1145–1154.

4. Huerta B, Maldonado A, Ginel PJ, Tarradas C, Gomez-Gascon L, et al. (2011) Risk factors associated with the antimicrobial resistance of staphylococci in canine pyoderma. Vet Microbiol 150: 302–308.

5. Nienhoff U, Kadlec K, Chaberny IF, Verspohl J, Gerlach GF, et al. (2011) Methicillin-resistant Staphylococcus pseudintermedius among dogs admitted to a small animal hospital. Vet Microbiol 150: 191–197.

6. Weese JS, Faires MC, Frank LA, Reynolds LM, Battisti A (2012) Factors associated with methicillin-resistant versus methicillin-susceptible Staphylococcus pseudintermedius infection in dogs. J Am Vet Med Assoc 240: 1450–1455.

7. Lehner G, Linek M, Bond R, Lloyd DH, Prenger-Berninghoff E, et al. (2014) Case-control risk factor study of methicillin-resistant Staphylococcus pseudintermedius (MRSP) infection in dogs and cats in Germany. Vet Microbiol 168: 154–160.

8. Zubeir IE, Kanbar T, Alber J, Lammler C, Akineden O, et al. (2007) Phenotypic and genotypic characteristics of methicillin/oxacillin-resistant Staphylococcus intermedius isolated from clinical specimens during routine veterinary microbiological examinations. Vet Microbiol 121: 170–176.

9. van Duijkeren E, Houwers DJ, Schoormans A, Broekhuizen-Stins MJ, Ikawaty R, et al. (2008) Transmission of methicillin-resistant Staphylococcus intermedius between humans and animals. Vet Microbiol 128: 213–215.

10. Clinical and Laboratory Standards Institute (2008) Performance standards for antimicrobial disk and dilution susceptibility tests for bacteria isolated from animals; Approved Standard – 3rd ed. CLSI, Wayne, PA, M31-A3.

11. Bemis DA, Jones RD, Frank LA, Kania SA (2009) Evaluation of susceptibility test breakpoints used to predict mecA-mediated resistance in Staphylococcus pseudintermedius isolated from dogs. J Vet Diagn Invest 21: 53–58.

12. Murakami K, Minamide W, Wada K, Nakamura E, Teraoka H, et al. (1991) Identification of methicillin-resistant strains of staphylococci by polymerase chain reaction. J Clin Microbiol 29: 2240–2244.

13. Murchan S, Kaufmann ME, Deplano A, de Ryck R, Struelens M, et al. (2003) Harmonization of pulsed-field gel electrophoresis protocols for epidemiological typing of strains of methicillin-resistant Staphylococcus aureus: a single approach developed by consensus in 10 European laboratories and its application for tracing the spread of related strains. J Clin Microbiol 41: 1574–1585.

14. Tenover FC, Arbeit RD, Goering RV, Mickelsen PA, Murray BE, et al. (1995) Interpreting chromosomal DNA restriction patterns produced by pulsed-field gel electrophoresis: criteria for bacterial strain typing. J Clin Microbiol 33: 2233–2239.

15. Kondo Y, Ito T, Ma XX, Watanabe S, Kreiswirth BN, et al. (2007) Combination of multiplex PCRs for staphylococcal cassette chromosome mec type assignment: rapid identification system for mec, ccr, and major differences in junkyard regions. Antimicr Agents Ch 51: 264–274.

16. Solyman SM, Black CC, Duim B, Perreten V, van Duijkeren E, et al. (2013) Multilocus sequence typing for characterization of Staphylococcus pseudintermedius. J Clin Microbiol 51: 306–310.

17. Sasaki T, Tsubakishita S, Tanaka Y, Sakusabe A, Ohtsuka M, et al. (2010) Multiplex-PCR method for species identification of coagulase-positive staphylococci. J Clin Microbiol 48: 765–769.

18. Borjesson S, Landen A, Bergstrom M, Andersson UG (2012) Methicillin-Resistant Staphylococcus pseudintermedius in Sweden. Microb Drug Resist 18: 597–603.

19. Osland AM, Vestby LK, Fanuelsen H, Slettemeas JS, Sunde M (2012) Clonal diversity and biofilm-forming ability of methicillin-resistant Staphylococcus pseudintermedius. J Antimicrob Chemoth 67: 841–848.

20. Lilenbaum W, Nunes EL, Azeredo MA (1998) Prevalence and antimicrobial susceptibility of staphylococci isolated from the skin surface of clinically normal cats. Lett Appl Microbiol 27: 224–228.

21. Nienhoff U, Kadlec K, Chaberny IF, Verspohl J, Gerlach G-F, et al. (2011) Methicillin-resistant Staphylococcus pseudintermedius among cats admitted to a veterinary teaching hospital. Vet Microbiol 153: 414–416.

22. Weese JS (2010) Methicillin-resistant Staphylococcus aureus in animals. ILAR J 51: 233–244.

23. Simou C, Thoday KL, Forsythe PJ, Hill PB (2005) Adherence of Staphylococcus intermedius to corneocytes of healthy and atopic dogs: effect of pyoderma, pruritus score, treatment and gender. Vet Dermatol 16: 385–391.

24. Holzknecht BJ, Hardardottir H, Haraldsson G, Westh H, Valsdottir F, et al. (2010) Changing epidemiology of methicillin-resistant Staphylococcus aureus in Iceland from 2000 to 2008: a challenge to current guidelines. J Clin Microbiol 48: 4221–4227.

25. Verkade E, Ferket M, Kluytmans J (2011) Clinical evaluation of Oxoid Brilliance MRSA Agar in comparison with bioMerieux MRSA ID medium for detection of livestock-associated meticillin-resistant Staphylococcus aureus. J Med Microbiol 60: 905–908.

26. Verkade E, Verhulst C, van Cleef B, Kluytmans J (2011) Clinical evaluation of Bio-Rad MRSASelect medium for the detection of livestock-associated methicillin-resistant Staphylococcus aureus. Eur Journal Clin Microbiol 30: 109–112.

27. Pletinckx LJ, De Bleecker Y, Dewulf J, Rasschaert G, Goddeeris BM, et al. (2012) Evaluation of salt concentrations, chromogenic media and anatomical sampling sites for detection of methicillin-resistant Staphylococcus aureus in pigs. Vet Microbiol 154: 363–368.

28. Veenemans J, Verhulst C, Punselie R, van Keulen PH, Kluytmans JA (2013) Evaluation of brilliance MRSA 2 agar for detection of methicillin-resistant Staphylococcus aureus in clinical samples. J Clin Microbiol 51: 1026–1027.

29. Gomez-Sanz E, Torres C, Lozano C, Saenz Y, Zarazaga M (2011) Detection and characterization of methicillin-resistant Staphylococcus pseudintermedius in healthy dogs in La Rioja, Spain. Comp Immunol Microb 34: 447–453.

30. Paul NC, Moodley A, Ghibaudo G, Guardabassi L (2011) Carriage of Methicillin-Resistant Staphylococcus pseudintermedius in Small Animal Veterinarians: Indirect Evidence of Zoonotic Transmission. Zoonoses Public Health 58: 533–539.

31. Weese JS (2012) Staphylococcal control in the veterinary hospital. Vet Dermatol 23: 292–298.

32. Lederer JW Jr, Best D, Hendrix V (2009) A comprehensive hand hygiene approach to reducing MRSA health care-associated infections. Jt Comm J Qual Patient Saf 35: 180–185.

33. Sakamoto F, Yamada H, Suzuki C, Sugiura H, Tokuda Y (2010) Increased use of alcohol-based hand sanitizers and successful eradication of methicillin-resistant Staphylococcus aureus from a neonatal intensive care unit: a multivariate time series analysis. Am J Infect Control 38: 529–534.

34. Perlin JB, Hickok JD, Septimus EJ, Moody JA, Englebright JD, et al. (2013) A bundled approach to reduce methicillin-resistant Staphylococcus aureus infections in a system of community hospitals. J Healthc Qual 35: 57–68.

35. Kramer A, Schwebke I, Kampf G (2006) How long do nosocomial pathogens persist on inanimate surfaces? A systematic review. BMC Infect Dis 6: 130.

36. Boyce JM (2007) Environmental contamination makes an important contribution to hospital infection. J Hosp Infect 65 Suppl 2: 50–54.

37. Singh A, Walker M, Rousseau J, Monteith GJ, Weese JS (2013) Methicillin-resistant staphylococcal contamination of clothing worn by personnel in a veterinary teaching hospital. Vet Surg 42: 643–648.

38. Wilson AP, Smyth D, Moore G, Singleton J, Jackson R, et al. (2011) The impact of enhanced cleaning within the intensive care unit on contamination of the near-patient environment with hospital pathogens: a randomized crossover study in critical care units in two hospitals. Crit Care Med 39: 651–658.

39. van Trijp MJ, Melles DC, Hendriks WD, Parlevliet GA, Gommans M, et al. (2007) Successful control of widespread methicillin-resistant Staphylococcus aureus colonization and infection in a large teaching hospital in the Netherlands. Infect Cont Hosp Ep 28: 970–975.

23

TCM Database@Taiwan: The World's Largest Traditional Chinese Medicine Database for Drug Screening *In Silico*

Calvin Yu-Chian Chen[1,2,3]*

1 School of Chinese Medicine, China Medical University, Taichung, Taiwan, **2** Department of Bioinformatics, Asia University, Taichung, Taiwan, **3** Department of Computational and Systems Biology, Massachusetts Institute of Technology, Cambridge, Massachusetts, United States of America

Abstract

Rapid advancing computational technologies have greatly speeded up the development of computer-aided drug design (CADD). Recently, pharmaceutical companies have increasingly shifted their attentions toward traditional Chinese medicine (TCM) for novel lead compounds. Despite the growing number of studies on TCM, there is no free 3D small molecular structure database of TCM available for virtual screening or molecular simulation. To address this shortcoming, we have constructed TCM Database@Taiwan (http://tcm.cmu.edu.tw/) based on information collected from Chinese medical texts and scientific publications. TCM Database@Taiwan is currently the world's largest non-commercial TCM database. This web-based database contains more than 20,000 pure compounds isolated from 453 TCM ingredients. Both cdx (2D) and Tripos mol2 (3D) formats of each pure compound in the database are available for download and virtual screening. The TCM database includes both simple and advanced web-based query options that can specify search clauses, such as molecular properties, substructures, TCM ingredients, and TCM classification, based on intended drug actions. The TCM database can be easily accessed by all researchers conducting CADD. Over the last eight years, numerous volunteers have devoted their time to analyze TCM ingredients from Chinese medical texts as well as to construct structure files for each isolated compound. We believe that TCM Database@Taiwan will be a milestone on the path towards modernizing traditional Chinese medicine.

Editor: Andreas Hofmann, Griffith University, Australia

Funding: The research was supported by grants from the National Science Council of Taiwan (NSC 99-2221-E-039-013-), China Medical University (CMU99-S-02) and Asia University (CMU98-ASIA-09). This study is also supported in part by Taiwan Department of Health Clinical Trial and Research Center of Excellence (DOH99-TD-B-111-004) and Taiwan Department of Health Cancer Research Center of Excellence (DOH99-TD-C-111-005). The funders had no role in study design, data collection and analysis, decision to publish, or preparation of the manuscript.

Competing Interests: The author has declared that no competing interests exist.

* E-mail: ycc@mail.cmu.edu.tw; ycc929@MIT.EDU

Introduction

For thousands of years, traditional Chinese medicine (TCM) holds an important role in medical diagnosis and treatments in Eastern Asia. However, due to lack of systematic investigation and poor understanding of TCM regimens, TCM is less recognized in the Western society. Recently, increasing effort has been devoted to study TCM, from which a large number of bioactive compounds have been isolated and studied. Hence, there is a need to establish a database to organize the enormous amounts of TCM data and make the virtual screening of TCM ingredients easily accessible.

Although there are many websites detailing information for TCM sources, traditional usage from ancient material medica texts, and processing and storage procedures, these databases, such as The Chinese medicine sampler (http://www.chinesemedicine sampler.com) and Dictionary of Chinese Herbs (http://alternati vehealing.org), contain little information of TCM ingredients at molecular level. The TCMGeneDIT database [1] is an effective search engine for TCM-related literature, but the information on the TCM constituents is not well organized. Other databases, including TCMD [2], Chinese Traditional Medicinal Herbs Database [3], and TCM-ID [4], provide general TCM information and 3D structures of TCM ingredients. However, these databases are either inaccessible or highly restricted for information sharing. To date, the ZINC database [5] is currently the

largest free 3D molecule database. However, there is no TCM related database similar to the scale of ZINC yet. In the hope of building a complete TCM ingredient library, we construct the TCM Database@Taiwan (http://tcm.cmu.edu.tw/).

In the past, our laboratory has performed screening for multiple TCM components and has successfully discovered novel lead compounds, such as anti-viral, anti-inflammation, anti-cancer, stroke prevention compounds, and hypnotic medications [6–17]. By constructing TCM Database@Taiwan, we can further facilitate the virtual screening process in the experiment design for the TCM lead drug discovery. We firmly believe that the constituents from TCM are the sources to derive novel pharmaceutical compounds.

Results and Discussion

TCM Database@Taiwan (http://tcm.cmu.edu.tw) is currently the largest non-commercial TCM database available for download. This web database is designed in both English and traditional Chinese languages. All 3D structures are constructed in mol2 format and are readily used for virtual screening.

TCM organization

Right now, the database contains 20,000 ingredients from 453 different herbs, animal products, and minerals TCM regimens. In the near future, the database will further record folk herb ingredients. The

TCM database is organized by proposed actions of Chinese medicines (Table S1). There are a total of twenty-two different drug classes and some are further divided into subclasses based on clinical applications recorded in TCM monographs. It should be noted that our TCM classification is based on traditional Chinese theories including the Yin-yang, the human Meridan/Channel system, the Five Elements theory, and the Zang Fu organ theory. It should also be noted that TCM listed under certain classes, such as parasites elimination, dampness reduction and itchiness relief medicinal, and topical application medicinal, contain toxic ingredients and are no longer prescribed in clinics. These ingredients are present in the TCM database for the completeness of TCM records. These data do not imply endorsement for any clinical or private use of the toxic TCM compounds nor for any animal products present in the database.

Search and Display

An overview of available search options and download options is shown in Figure 1. TCM Database@Taiwan can be browsed by simple and advanced search options. The simple search option enables users to browse the website either by TCM medicine or by TCM ingredients (Figure 2). The search-by-TCM-medicine option allows users to select the intended drug action group and then the desired TCM medicine. The search-by-TCM-chemical-composition option allows users to find possible TCM sources of the given molecule. This search result is directly linked to the TCM compound webpage without the need to specifying TCM action group.

For each search options, the result is organized in a "TCM profile" that provides the identified TCM compound(s) and the associated references. Clicking on a TCM compound in the profile will display the compound's 2D and 3D structures, as well as its molecular properties in a new page. Users can download the structure of the molecule in cdx (2D) or mol2 (3D) format at the bottom of the TCM compound webpage. In addition, users can also click on the links to browse other Chinese medicines that contains the selected TCM compound.

The advanced search option incorporates a molecular drawing interface (ChemAxon) for structure search (Figure 3). Users can also specify structure types, including exact search and substructure search, whichever best describes users' needs. Moreover, users can perform searches by specifying the molecular properties, such as molecular weight and ALogP. Both of the advanced search options can be used alone or in conjunction. The result will return molecule(s) that satisfy the input specification in a tabular format with name and 2D representation. For users who prefer search by Chinese medicine names and other TCM information, a website search engine is available at top of every page.

Download Interface

The TCM ingredients are organized by their drug action classes and their original sources. Users can download a specific drug class or a specific TCM or the whole TCM database on Download page.

Sharing TCM Constituents

As technology advances, new TCM ingredients have been isolated and studied each day. Therefore, we implemented an upload function for scientists who are interested in sharing their findings on Chinese medicines. Users may upload their own molecules to the TCM database server in mol2 format. The uploaded molecules will be reviewed and incorporated into the TCM database.

Overall, TCM Database@Taiwan is constructed in the hope to create the most complete TCM library and to strengthen the TCM research network to date. In addition, this web-based database is implemented with virtual screening and molecular simulation functions. For both biochemists studying TCM and medicinal chemists designing novel lead compounds, this database serves as a useful resource for virtual screening as well as for the references in biochemical assays. In the future, we will incorporate genetic algorithm (GA) and support vector machine (SVM) for further TCM classifications based on molecular properties. We

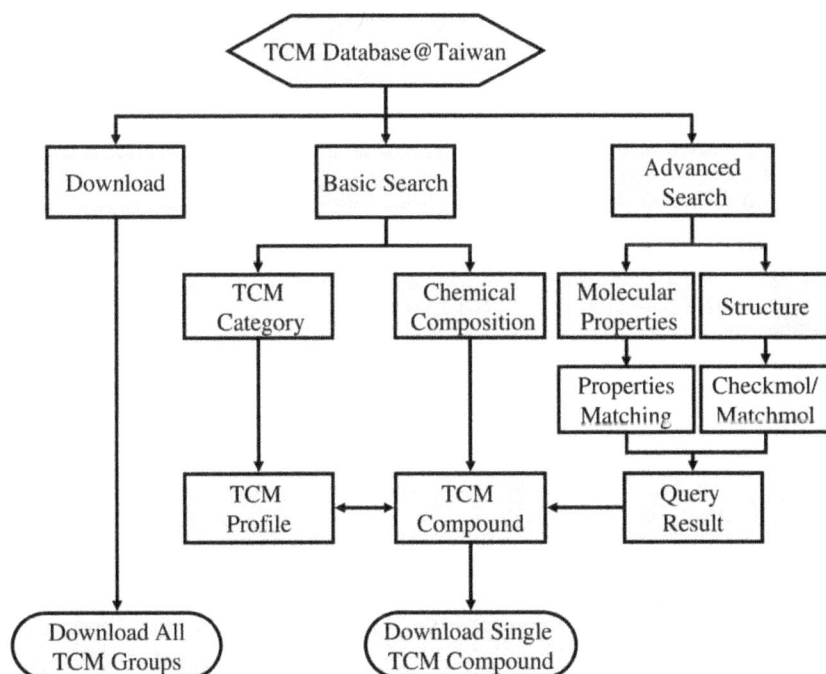

Figure 1. Search flowchart and available download options in TCM database.

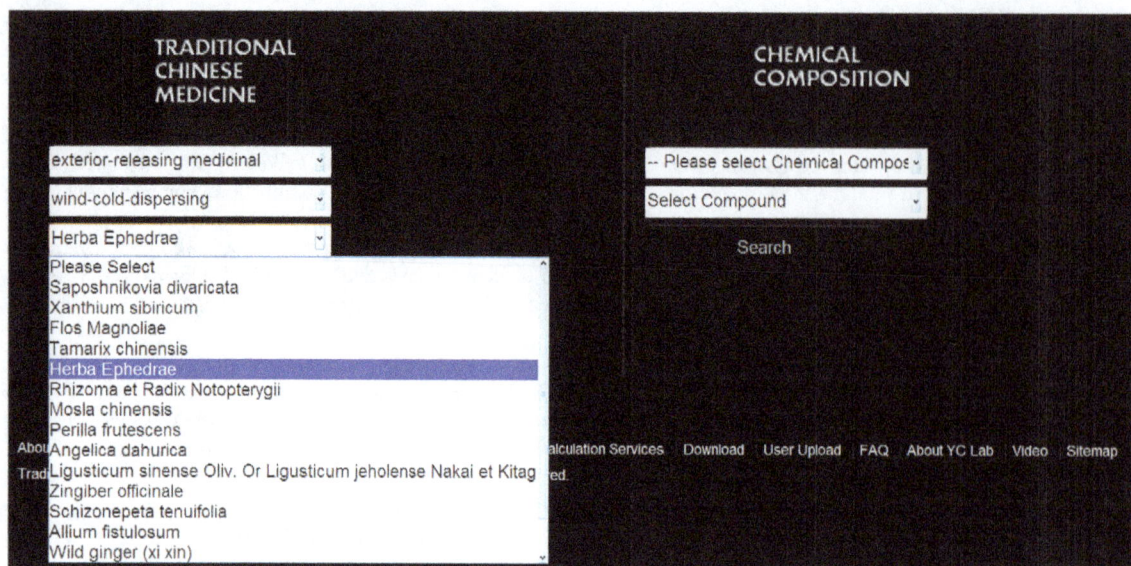

Figure 2. The search tool available in the TCM database. (a) search by TCM category and (b) search by chemical composition.

expect the construction of TCM Database@Taiwan to become a milestone for modern TCM researches.

Methods

The TCM herbs, animal products and minerals listed in the TCM Database @Taiwan were originated from Chinese medical texts and dictionaries [18–22]. In addition, the TCM constituents were collected manually from published results available on Medline [23] and ISI Web of Knowledge (http://apps.isiknowledge.com). The data were organized into twenty-two major classes based on their proposed therapeutic actions recorded in Chinese medical texts [24–26]. The 2D and 3D structures of TCM constituents were built by ChemBioOffice 2008 (CambridgeSoft, Cambridge, MA). The 3D structures were energy minimized in MM2 force field. Physicochemical properties,

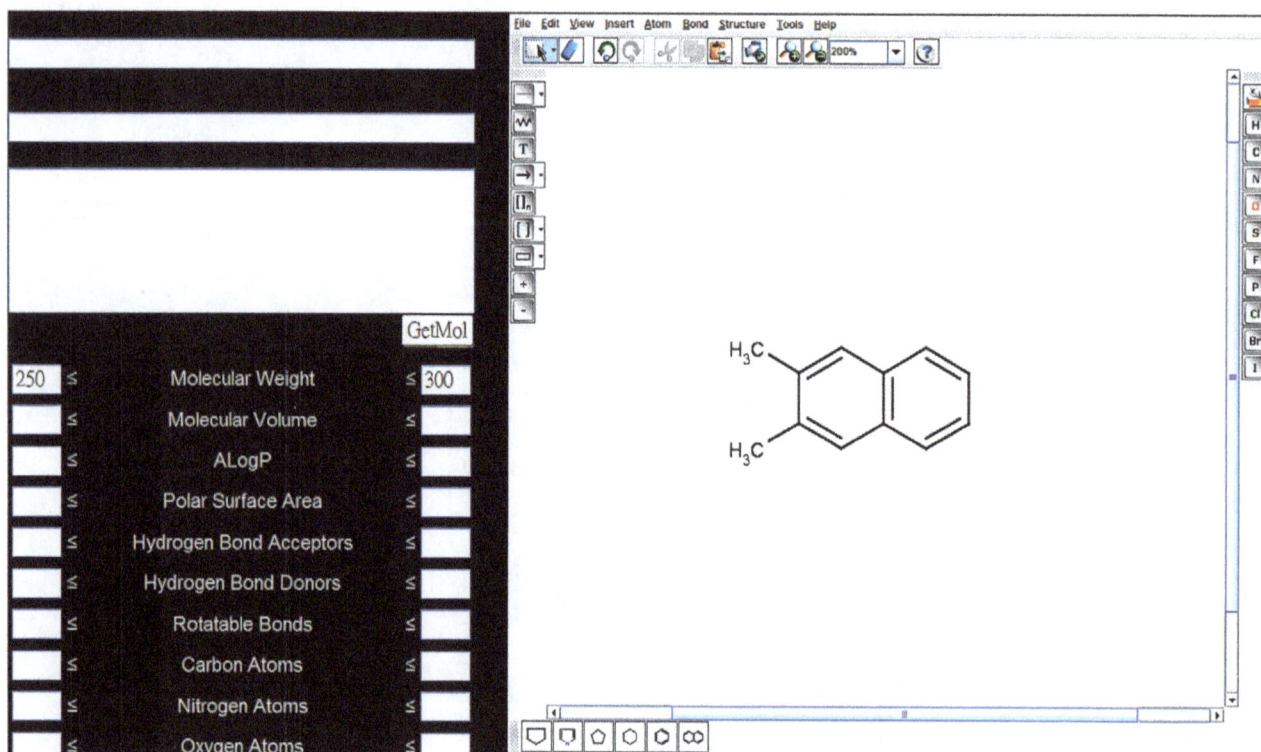

Figure 3. The advance search interface.

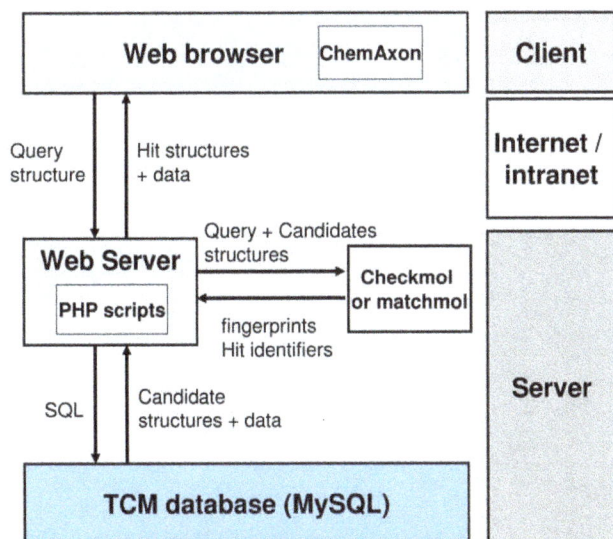

Figure 4. The infrastructure of the TCM database. The design is adapted from Norbert Haider's MolDB5R.

including ALogP and polar surface area, were calculated using ChemBioOffice.

With efficiency and stability as our main concern, we implemented our database on a Linux server, then use MySQL5.0, Apache, and hypertext preprocessor (PHP) for database and web server development. For friendly user interfaces, we used ChemAxon MarvinView applet (https://www.chemaxon.com) for 2D and 3D representation. In addition, we applied MarvinSketch tool from ChemAxon for structure drawing in the advanced search option.

In the advanced search section, the search engine was developed based on the Norbert Haider's MolDB5R package [27]. The infrastructure of the advanced search engine is shown in

Figure 4. For search-by-specifying-molecular-properties, a search script written in PHP is used to search and retrieve TCM compounds that satisfied all the input properties. Two programs, checkmol and matchmol, are used to perform the background structure searching and matching process. The queried structure is read by the checkmol program to generate molecular descriptors, which is then used in the preliminary search in the TCM database. The matchmol program is responsible for full structure comparison of the input structures from checkmol. For additional structure search options, such as substructure search, the matchmol program treat one compound as "needle" and other molecule(s) as "haystack" to determine the best-fit substructure of another structure. All the search options in the advanced search section can be used in conjunction. By specifying both molecular properties and query structure scaffold, an additional data screening process is performed to ensure that all the input criteria are met.

Supporting Information

Table S1 Summary of medicines present in each TCM class. The English translation of each class is taken from WHO publication.

Acknowledgments

I am grateful to hundreds of student volunteers who devoted their time checking the TCM compounds from the references and drawing these compounds for more than eight years and National Center of High-performance Computing for computer time and facilities. I also thank the professional suggestion by Drs. Chung Y Hsu, Kun-Lung Chang, Fuu-Jen Tsai of China Medical University, Nobel Laureate Ferid Murad, and professor Marc of Harvard University.

Author Contributions

Conceived and designed the experiments: CYCC. Performed the experiments: CYCC. Analyzed the data: CYCC. Contributed reagents/materials/analysis tools: CYCC. Wrote the paper: CYCC.

References

1. Fang YC, Huang HC, Chen HH, Juan HF (2008) TCMGeneDIT: a database for associated traditional Chinese medicine, gene and disease information using text mining. BMC Complement Altern Med 8: 58.

2. He M, Yan XJ, Zhou JJ, Xie GR (2001) Traditional Chinese medicine database and application on the Web. J Chem Inf Comput Sci 41: 273–277.

3. Qiao XB, Hou TJ, Zhang W, Guo SL, Xu SJ (2002) A 3D structure database of components from Chinese traditional medicinal herbs. J Chem Inf Comput Sci 42: 481–489.

4. Chen X, Zhou H, Liu YB, Wang JF, Li H, et al. (2006) Database of traditional Chinese medicine and its application to studies of mechanism and to prescription validation. Br J Pharmacol 149: 1092–1103.

5. Irwin JJ, Shoichet BK (2005) ZINC - A free database of commercially available compounds for virtual screening. J Chem Inf Model 45: 177–182.

6. Huang HJ, Lee KJ, Yu HW, Chen CY, Hsu CH, et al. (2010) Structure-Based and Ligand-Based Drug Design for HER 2 Receptor. J Biomol Struct Dyn 28: 23–37.

7. Chen CY, Chen CYC (2010) Insights into designing the dual-targeted HER2/HSP90 inhibitors. J Mol Graph Model 29: 21–31.

8. Huang HJ, Chen CY, Chen HY, Tsai FJ, Chen CYC (2010) Computational screening and QSAR analysis for design of AMP-activated protein kinase agonist. J Taiwan Inst Chem Eng 41: 352–359.

9. Chen CYC (2010) Virtual Screening and Drug Design for PDE-5 Receptor from Traditional Chinese Medicine Database. J Biomol Struct Dyn 27: 627–640.

10. Chen CYC (2010) Bioinformatics, chemoinformatics, and pharmainformatics analysis of HER2/HSP90 dual-targeted inhibitors. J Taiwan Inst Chem Eng 41: 143–149.

11. Chen CY, Huang HJ, Tsai FJ, Chen CYC (2010) Drug design for Influenza A virus subtype H1N1. J Taiwan Inst Chem Eng 41: 8–15.

12. Chen CYC (2009) Computational screening and design of traditional Chinese medicine (TCM) to block phosphodiesterase-5. J Mol Graph Model 28: 261–269.

13. Chen CY, Chang YH, Bau DT, Huang HJ, Tsai FJ, et al. (2009) Ligand-Based Dual Target Drug Design for H1N1: Swine Flu- A Preliminary First Study. J Biomol Struct Dyn 27: 171–178.

14. Huang HJ, Yu HW, Chen CY, Hsu CH, Chen HY, et al. (2010) Current developments of computer-aided drug design. J Taiwan Inst Chem Eng 41: 623–635.

15. Chen CYC (2009) Pharmacoinformatics approach for mPGES-1 in anti-inflammation by 3D-QSAR pharmacophore mapping. J Taiwan Inst Chem Eng 40: 155–161.

16. Chen CYC (2009) De novo design of novel selective COX-2 inhibitors: From virtual screening to pharmacophore analysis. J Taiwan Inst Chem Eng 40: 55–69.

17. Chen CYC (2009) Chemoinformatics and pharmacoinformatics approach for exploring the GABA-A agonist from Chinese herb suanzaoren. J Taiwan Inst Chem Eng 40: 36–47.

18. Chen G, Li S (1992) Ben cao gang mu tong shi = General explanation of Compendium of materia medica. Beijing Shi: Xue yuan chu ban she. 2 v. (10, 18, 13, 2323 p.), 2342, 2369 p. of plates) p.

19. Zhong N, Zhao G, Dai S, Chen R (2006) Zhong yao da ci dian. Shanghai: Shanghai ke xue ji shu chu ban she. 2 v. (2, 2, 15, 3875 p.) p.

20. Miao X, Zheng J (2002) Shennong ben cao jing shu. Beijing: Zhong yi gu ji chu ban she. 777 p.

21. Lü X (2002) Zhong yao jian bie da quan. Changsha Shi: Hunan ke xue ji shu chu ban she. pp 2, 3, 658.

22. Fang Y, Zhang Z, Miao X (1991) Shang han lun tiao bian. Shanghai: Shanghai gu ji chu ban she: Xin hua shu dian Shanghai fa xing suo fa xing. pp 2, 858.

23. Sayers EW, Barrett T, Benson DA, Bolton E, Bryant SH, et al. (2010) Database resources of the National Center for Biotechnology Information. Nucleic Acids Res 38: D5–D16.

24. Shen L, Li S (1998) Ben cao gang mu cai se tu pu. Beijing Shi: Hua xia chu ban she. pp 4, 21, 471.

25. Yang S (1998) The divine farmer's materia medica: a translation of the Shen Nong Ben Cao Jing. Boulder, CO: Blue Poppy Press. pp xvi, 198.

26. Yao D, Zhang J, Zhonghua RG. Guangzhou Shi: Guangdong ke ji chu ban she: Jing xiao Guangdong sheng xin hua shu dian. pp 3, 519.

27. Haider N (2010) Functionality Pattern Matching as an Efficient Complementary Structure/Reaction Search Tool: an Open-Source Approach. Molecules 15: 5079–5092.

24

From Traditional Medicine to Witchcraft: Why Medical Treatments Are Not Always Efficacious

Mark M. Tanaka[1]*, **Jeremy R. Kendal**[2], **Kevin N. Laland**[3]

1 Evolution & Ecology Research Centre, School of Biotechnology & Biomolecular Sciences, University of New South Wales, Sydney, New South Wales, Australia, **2** Department of Anthropology, University of Durham, Durham, United Kingdom, **3** School of Biology, University of St Andrews, Fife, United Kingdom

Abstract

Complementary medicines, traditional remedies and home cures for medical ailments are used extensively world-wide, representing more than US$60 billion sales in the global market. With serious doubts about the efficacy and safety of many treatments, the industry remains steeped in controversy. Little is known about factors affecting the prevalence of efficacious and non-efficacious self-medicative treatments. Here we develop mathematical models which reveal that the most efficacious treatments are not necessarily those most likely to spread. Indeed, purely superstitious remedies, or even maladaptive practices, spread more readily than efficacious treatments under specified circumstances. Low-efficacy practices sometimes spread because their very ineffectiveness results in longer, more salient demonstration and a larger number of converts, which more than compensates for greater rates of abandonment. These models also illuminate a broader range of phenomena, including the spread of innovations, medical treatment of animals, foraging behaviour, and self-medication in non-human primates.

Editor: James Holland Jones, Stanford University, United States of America

Funding: The work was supported by the Australian Academy of Sciences, the Research Councils UK, Biotechnology and Biological Sciences Research Council UK and the European Union. The funders had no role in study design, data collection and analysis, decision to publish, or preparation of the manuscript.

Competing Interests: The authors have declared that no competing interests exist.

* E-mail: m.tanaka@unsw.edu.au

Introduction

Traditional remedies, utilising medicinal plant and animal products, have been used as treatments for human diseases and medical conditions for millennia [1]. In recent years, 60–80% of the world's population, mainly from developing countries, depended primarily on traditional medicines, folk remedies and home cures, as well as treatment from witchdoctors and other 'supernatural practices', for their health-care needs [1]. In western societies, complementary and alternative medicine is garnering increasing interest and acceptance. At current growth rates, two-thirds of Americans are projected to be using alternative medicine by 2010 [2]. Asian governments are pouring billions of dollars into screening Traditional Chinese medicines in the hope that clinical trials will spawn lucrative drugs [3]. Traditional medicine has become big business.

While scientific studies have validated some traditional remedies, for instance, by confirming the biological activity of plant extracts [4,5], the use of complementary and traditional medicines remains contentious, and doubts about the efficacy and safety of many treatments remain [1,6,7,8]. Reservations over safety and efficacy underpin controversy over USA and UK universities' attempts to bring alternative medicines into medical school curricula [9]. The active ingredients used in many traditional medicines are potentially toxic, often containing dangerous elements, including heavy metals [5,10]. Even the use of ineffective non-toxic remedies can be harmful if it delays effective treatment. For instance, fears have been expressed that, in Nigeria, witchcraft and traditional remedies of unknown efficacy are widely employed as treatments for malaria, instead of, or delaying access to, modern medicines of proven effectiveness [11]. In sub-Saharan Africa there is a concern that the use of traditional remedies for mastitis, a condition often attributed to sorcery, may inadvertently be contributing to the spread of HIV [12].

In 2002 the WHO [1] launched a global plan to make the use of traditional medicine safer by encouraging evidence-based research on the safety, efficacy and quality of traditional practices. Accordingly, traditional medicines are currently undergoing scrutiny to evaluate their effectiveness and monitor adverse events [3,13]. Such analyses have often failed to confirm the efficacy of traditional remedies: for instance, of nearly 25,000 applications for registration of traditional medicines received by Malaysian authorities, 37.3% were rejected, either on grounds of safety or ineffectiveness [14]. However, there is currently no compelling explanation for the prevalence of low-efficacy treatments.

Here we develop mathematical models of the spread of self-medicative treatments for medical conditions to explore the factors that lead to treatments becoming widespread, and how a treatment's efficacy affects its rate of spread. A treatment is acquired through social learning, but its spread depends on a variety of factors, including its efficacy, and the rates of conversion, death, recovery from illness and abandonment of the treatment. The approach is to derive expressions for the cultural fitness (mean number of converts to the treatment resulting directly from observation of a given demonstrator), ϕ, and the probability of spread of new treatments. We show that the treatments that spread are not necessarily those that are most efficacious at curing the ailment, and explain how 'superstitious treatments' with little efficacy and even maladaptive practices can spread under broad conditions. The models draw from two bodies of theory, cultural evolution modeling [15,16,17,18] and stochastic (branching) processes [19], to develop theory applicable to investigating the spread of treatments of disease. Our analyses can also be viewed as contributing to the developing field of Darwinian medicine [20]. Although branching process models were developed to address the extinction of surnames [15], they have been more widely employed within biological evolution [21], and have yet to make further impact on the study of cultural evolution, despite extensive theory borrowing by the latter from the former [15,16,17,18].

Methods

Basic assumptions

The general structure of the model is illustrated in Figure 1 and the symbols used are summarised in Table 1. We assume that individuals are either in a diseased state or in a healthy state. We model the spread of a behavioural trait expressed in treatment of disease. The behavioural trait in question is any innovation, practice or treatment that could potentially affect the outcome of this disease. To model the spread of a behavioural trait, we make the following assumptions. A new behavioural trait arises in (or is invented by) an ill individual who may then *demonstrate* this practice; others who are ill may adopt the practice upon being exposed to it, and then become demonstrators themselves. In other words, demonstrators *convert* observers. There is empirical support for the assumption that self-medicative treatments spread through social learning [22]. Observers adopt the trait at a constant rate per demonstrator per unit time. This rate is α_1 when the demonstrator is ill and α_2 when the demonstrator is healthy. Allowing for different rates of cultural transmission from sick and well individuals is important, since treatments for many ailments, ranging from snake bites to the common cold, are primarily applied when sick, and discontinued, or practiced at a less frequent rate, when the sufferer has recovered. As our models are concerned with the initial spread of a treatment, we assume a constant supply of observers. As the dynamics of the spread of the

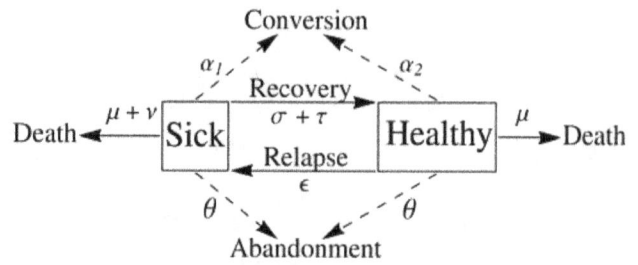

Figure 1. General structure of the model. This figure illustrates the processes through which demonstrators of a treatment can change health state. The parameters are defined in Methods.

trait are much faster than demographic changes, there are no explicit births in this model. Death, however, occurs at rate μ per individual per unit time; there is an additional death rate v for individuals with the disease.

Our assumption that observers adopt the trait in an unbiased fashion, and at a constant rate per demonstrator per unit time, may need further explanation. We do not assume that observers adopt self-medicative practices according to their efficacy in treating others, since we regard this to be difficult for an individual reliably to gauge. For instance, observers would be required to make a series of judgments: *Has the demonstrator the same condition as me? Is the demonstrator's judgment of its effectiveness reliable? Will the treatment work as well for me? Would the demonstrator have recovered anyway? Etc.* Rather, we leave judgments about the efficacy of treatments to self (i.e. the demonstrator), by allowing individuals to abandon the treatment, or revert to an alternative, based on their own evaluation of the treatment's effectiveness in curing themselves. Note, it does not follow from our assumption of unbiased copying that observers would be equally likely to adopt otherwise equivalent efficacious and ineffective practices, since demonstrators would be more likely to abandon the latter, as discussed below.

Table 1. Summary of symbols used in the model.

Symbol	Meaning
α_1	Rate of conversion of observers to the treatment practice when demonstrator is ill.
α_2	Rate of conversion of observers to the treatment practice when demonstrator is well.
τ	Efficacy of treatment; $\tau=0$ when treatment is ineffective.
σ	Rate of natural recovery from disease.
θ	Rate of abandoning the treatment. We set $\theta=\rho e^{-a(\sigma+\tau)}$.
ρ	Maximum rate of treatment abandonment.
a	Decay in abandonment rate as efficacy increases.
ϵ	Rate of relapse to disease. We set $\epsilon=\epsilon_0 e^{-b\tau}$.
ϵ_0	Maximum relapse rate.
b	Decay in relapse rate as efficacy increases.
μ	Background death rate.
v	Death rate due to the disease.
ϕ	Cultural fitness of the practice (function of the parameters).
N	Number of observers converted by a demonstrator.
U	Time spent by a demonstrator being ill.
W	Time spent by a demonstrator being well.

We are interested in both efficacious traits – those that hasten the recovery of the diseased individual – as well as those that are ineffective or even maladaptive (in that they retard or prevent recovery). The background rate of recovery is σ per individual per unit time, with an additional rate τ describing the efficacy of the treatment or practice ($\tau \geq -\sigma$). When $\tau = 0$ the treatment/practice is ineffective and the trait can be regarded as a superstition. When $\tau = -\sigma$ the trait is completely maladaptive because it prevents recovery, while if $\tau > 0$ the treatment is beneficial.

Further assume that an individual who adopts the trait may abandon it or revert to a previous practice. The rate of abandonment is a decreasing function of the rate of recovery from the disease. This response is based on the assumption that sick individuals will become increasingly dissatisfied with their treatment as the time to recovery increases, and will abandon treatments that are perceived to be ineffective. Let this function be

$$\theta(\rho,\sigma,\tau,a) = \rho e^{-a(\sigma+\tau)} \qquad (1)$$

where ρ is the maximum rate of abandonment, occurring when the trait is completely maladaptive ($\tau = -\sigma$), and a determines how strongly recovery influences abandonment (see Figure 2). While $\theta(\rho,\sigma,\tau,a)$ is a function of four parameters, we will write it simply as θ for convenience. Although we set this function to be an exponential decay, exploration of alternative forms of the relationship between abandonment and efficacy (e.g. hyperbolic function) showed they do not influence the qualitative outcomes of the analysis.

By letting recovered individuals relapse into the diseased state at rate ϵ per unit time we allow for multiple episodes of illness. This dynamic is suitable for describing recurring conditions. When $\epsilon = 0$ there is only a single bout of illness, a scenario we consider first in developing the models below. The rate ϵ itself can be set as a function of τ, where the treatment practiced in a well state has a

prophylactic effect. For example, the rate of relapse to disease might decrease exponentially at rate b with respect to efficacy τ. In other words, the probability that sick individuals will relapse to the diseased state decreases with increasing effectiveness of the treatment they utilise (τ).

Constructing the model

We consider a set of special cases of the general model. In the simplest case, recovery is permanent so that there is only a single episode of illness ($\epsilon = 0$), and demonstration of the treatment is restricted to the period of illness – that is, demonstration ceases upon recovery ($\alpha_2 = 0$). The second model generalises this situation by allowing demonstration to continue after recovery ($\alpha_2 > 0$), but there is still only a single episode of illness ($\epsilon = 0$). We also consider a model in which there can be multiple episodes of illness ($\epsilon > 0$) and where demonstration is restricted to sick individuals ($\alpha_2 = 0$). In the general case $\epsilon > 0$ and $\alpha_2 > 0$.

In each model, we focus on a single demonstrator and track the total number of individuals he or she converts. This is achieved by accounting for the conversion rates α_1, α_2 and the length of each period spent by the demonstrator being ill and well (U and W respectively). The time spent being an ill demonstrator within a given episode of illness is distributed exponentially with parameter

$$\lambda = \mu + v + \theta + \tau + \sigma.$$

When the demonstrator is well, the time until death, abandonment or becoming ill again is distributed exponentially with parameter

$$\zeta = \mu + \theta + \epsilon.$$

The cultural fitness of the treatment ϕ is given by the mean number of converts produced by the demonstrator. We report below the formulas for cultural fitness and provide derivations in Appendix S1. The appendix also considers the probability of spread of the treatment from the innovator, which can be derived analytically for the first model (Section A.1.1) and otherwise studied through computer simulation (Section A.2.3).

In the first model, where there is a single episode of illness and demonstration only occurs during illness, the cultural fitness is given by

$$\phi - \frac{\alpha_1}{\lambda}. \qquad (2)$$

Under the second model, where there is a single episode of illness and demonstration is continued after recovery,

$$\phi = \frac{\alpha_1}{\lambda} + \frac{\alpha_2(\tau+\sigma)}{\lambda\zeta}. \qquad (3)$$

Under the most general model, where there can be multiple episodes of illness and continuous demonstration of the treatment,

$$\phi = \frac{1}{\psi}\frac{\alpha_1}{\lambda} + \left(\frac{1}{\psi} - 1 + \frac{\tau+\sigma}{\lambda}\right)\frac{\alpha_2}{\zeta}, \qquad (4)$$

where $1/\psi$ is the mean number of episodes before abandonment of treatment or death and $\psi = 1 - \epsilon(\tau+\sigma)/(\zeta\lambda)$. The case where

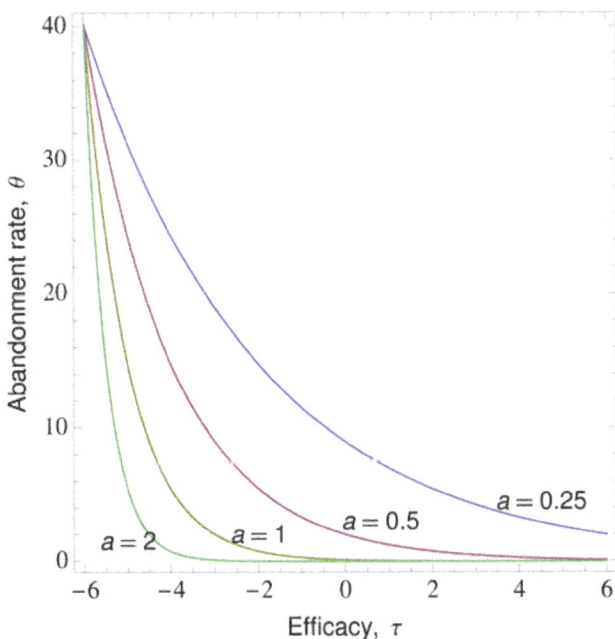

Figure 2. The relationship between rate of abandonment and efficacy. Here we show several curves by varying the parameter a and setting $\sigma = 6$ and $\rho = 40.1711$ (see Methods for interpretation of parameter values).

there are multiple episodes but restricted demonstration is specified by setting $\alpha_2 = 0$ in Equation 4, giving $\phi = \alpha_1/(\psi\lambda)$.

Parameter values

Unless otherwise specified, parameters in the numerical analysis take the following values. We assume $\mu = 0.016$ and $\nu = 0.008$ per individual per year, corresponding to a 62.5 year lifespan without disease and an illness-related death rate which is half that of natural causes. We set $\sigma = 6$, corresponding to an average episode of illness lasting 2 months. The number of converts per year per sick individual α_1 was set to 12, and that per healthy individual to $\alpha_2 = 1.2$. Other parameter values are: $\rho = 40.1711$, corresponding to an average time of around 0.3 months before abandonment when $\tau = -\sigma$ and gives a maximum cultural fitness ϕ when the treatment efficacy $\tau = 0$; $a = 0.5$, corresponding to an average time of 6 months before abandonment when $\tau = 0$ and $\rho = 40.1711$; and $\epsilon_0 = 2$, corresponding to an average time of 6 months of being healthy before relapse to disease when $b = 0$.

Results

We study our general model through subclasses, considering cases in which individuals experience either a single or multiple episodes of illness, and demonstration of the practice is either restricted to sick individuals, or continues after recovery.

First consider cases with a single bout of illness and treatment demonstration restricted to sick individuals (Equation (2), Figure 3). Across a broad range of conditions, the most efficacious treatments are not necessarily those most likely to spread, and superstitious treatments with no efficacy ($\tau \approx 0$), or even maladaptive practices ($\tau < 0$), frequently have the highest cultural fitness (ϕ). Superstitious treatments and maladaptive practices can spread because their very ineffectiveness results in sick individuals demonstrating the practice for longer than efficacious treatments, leading to more salient demonstration and more converts. This outcome occurs in spite of the fact that we assume that the less effective the treatment, the more likely a sick individual will abandon it, resulting in n-shaped functions for cultural fitness (Figure 3a–c) and probability of spread of the treatment (Figure 3d–f) The observed relationships represent a trade-off between duration of illness which is associated with demonstration of the treatment on one hand and retention of the treatment due to its efficacy on the other hand. That is, persistent illness leads to prolonged demonstration of the practice, yet an increased rate of abandonment of an ineffective treatment. In contrast, increased retention of an effective treatment is also associated with reduced demonstration of the practice.

The quality of treatments that successfully spread depends critically on the rates of recovery from illness and abandonment of the treatment, with high-recovery/low-abandonment favouring superstitious/maladaptive treatments, and low-recovery/high-

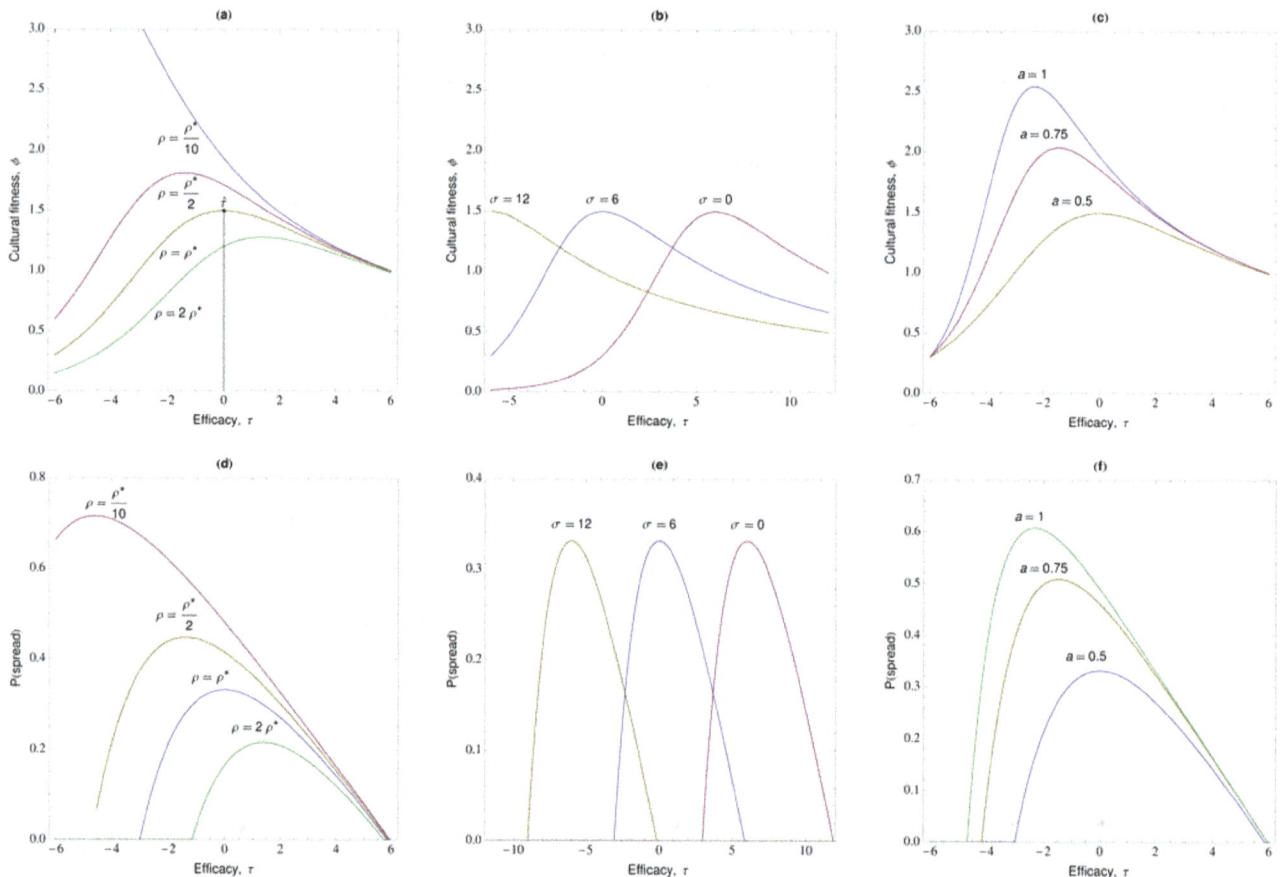

Figure 3. A single episode of illness and demonstration only during illness. The cultural fitness (a–c) and probability of spread (d–f) of self-medicative treatments, plotted as a function of treatment efficacy, τ, when there is a single episode of illness and demonstration occurs only during illness. Left (a and d), effect of varying maximum rate of abandonment, ρ. Middle (b and e), effect of varying rate of recovery, σ. Right (c and f), effect of varying rate of decay in treatment abandonment. Unless otherwise stated $a = 0.5$, $b = 0$, $\epsilon_0 = 0$, $\alpha_1 = 12$, $\alpha_2 = 0$, $\mu = 0.016$, $\nu = 0.008$, $\rho = \rho^* = 40.1711$ and $\sigma = 6$ (see also Methods and Table 1).

abandonment favouring efficacious treatments (Figure 3). From an evolutionary perspective, suppose the treatment or practice evolves through competition between alternative forms, each with its specific efficacy. Assuming treatments of higher cultural fitness always displace those of lower cultural fitness, the evolutionarily stable strategy in this system may well be a maladaptive treatment that hinders recovery. This scenario occurs when the abandonment parameter ρ is sufficiently low relative to the recovery rate σ. Intuitively, this case describes a situation where individuals are very persistent in using a treatment, resulting in the spread of poor practices in the long term. Factors that precipitate low abandonment, such as social norms favouring traditional remedies, or treatments that are costly to learn, potentially facilitate the spread of superstitions/maladaptive traits, particularly in chronic cases. This analysis can explain the ineffectiveness of many prominent complementary and traditional medicines.

Continued demonstration after recovery (α_2 positive) typically increases the probability that efficacious treatments will spread, by weakening the aforementioned trade-off between retention of treatment and duration of illness, because a fast recovery does not prevent subsequent recruitment of others to the practice (Figure 4). If the conversion rate after recovery is sufficiently high relative to that in sickness, efficacious treatments are more likely to spread than maladaptive/superstitious treatments. Numerical analysis leads to the general prediction that, other factors being equal, treatments solely demonstrated in sickness are typically less effective than treatments also demonstrated in wellness.

Multiple episodes of sickness typically favour efficacious treatments, and make it more likely in general that treatments will spread compared to single episodes (Equation (4), Figure 5a). Multiple episodes allow demonstrators of efficacious treatments repeated opportunities to convert others to the practice. High

efficacy, by enhancing recovery, increases the number of cycles of demonstration, weakening the trade-off between retention of treatment and duration of illness. Even with demonstration restricted to sick individuals, the efficacy of the treatment with the highest cultural fitness (or probability of spread) is typically high in cases where there is a high rate of relapse into sickness (i.e. large ϵ).

Prophylactic treatments ($b > 0$) disproportionately reduce the relapse rate of efficacious traits over maladaptive treatments, thereby decreasing their opportunity to acquire new converts (for $\alpha_2 \ll \alpha_1$). It follows that prophylactic self-medicative treatments should spread less readily than non-prophylactic treatments (Figure 5b). Figure 5c shows that the ultimate probability of spread across τ exhibits a similar pattern to that of the cultural fitness (Figure 5a,b) and that naturally, the probability of initially spreading from the inventor is always higher than the ultimate probability of spread.

Generally, highly efficacious treatments have higher cultural fitness than superstitious/maladaptive traits in multiple-episode cases, but nonetheless superstitious treatments (τ close to 0) can spread. Superstitious and maladaptive practices are most likely to spread where treatments are primarily demonstrated in sickness (i.e. a low ratio of α_2/α_1) and low abandonment (ρ), particularly where relapse is unlikely (ϵ small). Figure 6 illustrates this principle through a density plot of the τ with highest probability of spread as a function of ρ and the relative rate of conversion during healthy and sick periods (α_2/α_1).

Discussion

This study offers a simple, novel and counter-intuitive hypothesis for the prevalence of ineffective medical treatments: unbiased copying of new treatments can frequently lead to the prevalence of ineffective practices because such treatments are demonstrated more persistently than efficacious alternatives, even when there is enhanced abandonment of ineffective cures. By unbiased copying, we mean copying in direct proportion to the rate at which the alternative variants are demonstrated. Here, in simple terms, treatment frequency dynamics are typically dominated by two processes, representing the rates of acquisition and loss of remedies. Maladaptive and superstitious treatments can become prevalent because their ineffectiveness prolongs illness, enhancing their rate of demonstration relative to efficacious cures, and leading to elevated rates of acquisition that may compensate for greater loss.

Our finding that superstitious treatments can easily spread is supported by reports of extraordinary treatments for conditions such as leprosy (treated with a drink made of rotting snakes) and syphilis (treated by eating a vulture), and by similar myths for poisonous snake bites (apply 'guaco' leaves, poisonous lizard skin or snake's bile), dog bites (drink tea made from the dog's tail) and scorpion stings (tie a scorpion against the stung finger) [23]. The analysis also helps explain the persistence of medical treatments of animals, such as 'firing' (cautery) of working horses, employed for millennia as treatment for lameness, where recovery is rare, and still widely practiced in many countries in spite of trials establishing its ineffectiveness [24]. In such cases, of course, the treatment belief is acquired by the owner, rather than by the diseased individual.

Even when highly effective treatments have higher cultural fitness values than ineffective treatments, our analysis shows that such highly functional innovations can easily be lost due to stochasticity. This has not been apparent to researchers studying the diffusion of foraging innovations in animals, for whom the

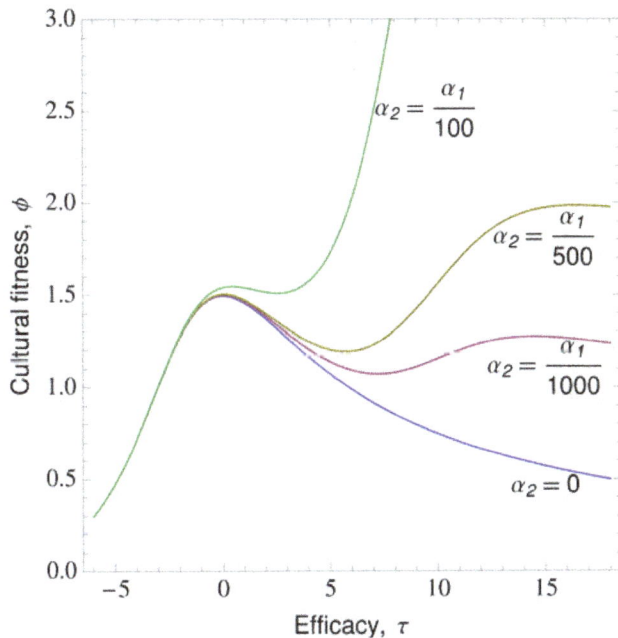

Figure 4. A single episode of illness and continued demonstration. The cultural fitness of self-medicative treatments (ϕ) plotted as a function of treatment efficacy, τ, when there is a single episode of illness ($\epsilon = 0$) and demonstration continues after recovery ($\alpha_2 > 0$). Parameter values are $a = 0.5$, $b = 0$, $\epsilon_0 = 0$, $\alpha_1 = 12$, $\mu = 0.016$, $v = 0.008$, $\rho = \rho^* = 40.1711$ and $\sigma = 6$ (see Methods for interpretation of parameter values).

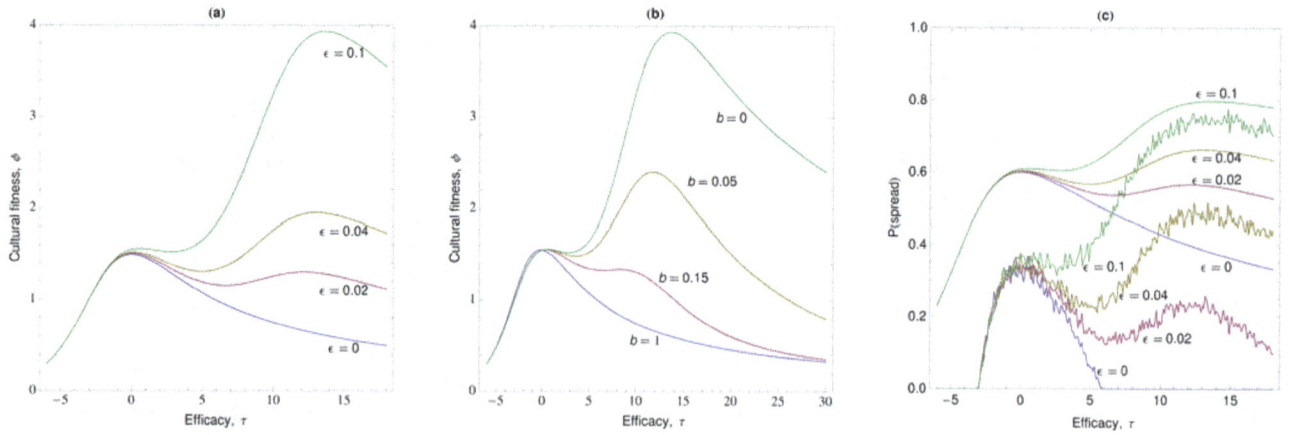

Figure 5. Multiple episodes of illness and demonstration restricted to sick individuals. The cultural fitness of self-medicative treatments ϕ, (left and middle), and probability of spread of treatments (right) plotted as a function of treatment efficacy, τ. Left (a): cultural fitness ϕ; we set $b=0$ so that $\epsilon = \epsilon_0$. Middle (b): cultural fitness ϕ; when treatment is prophylactic ($b>0$). Right (c): The ultimate probability of spread (rugged lines) and the probability of spread from an innovator (smooth lines) for various rates of relapse ϵ (indicated by colour). Unless stated otherwise, parameter values are $a=0.5$, $\alpha_1 = 12$, $\alpha_2 = 0$, $\epsilon_0 = 0.1$, $\mu = 0.016$, $v = 0.008$, $\rho = \rho^* = 40.1711$ and $\sigma = 6$ (see Methods for interpretation of parameter values).

failure of most innovations to spread, particularly those beneficial to the inventor, has been regarded as a mystery [25]. In fact, the observation that the majority of beneficial innovations are frequently lost is exactly what our model predicts.

The analyses presented here could usefully be extended to model disease frequencies explicitly, and to incorporate the costs of treatment. It is well-established that human life-history decision making is affected by costs [26], and this is also likely to be true of

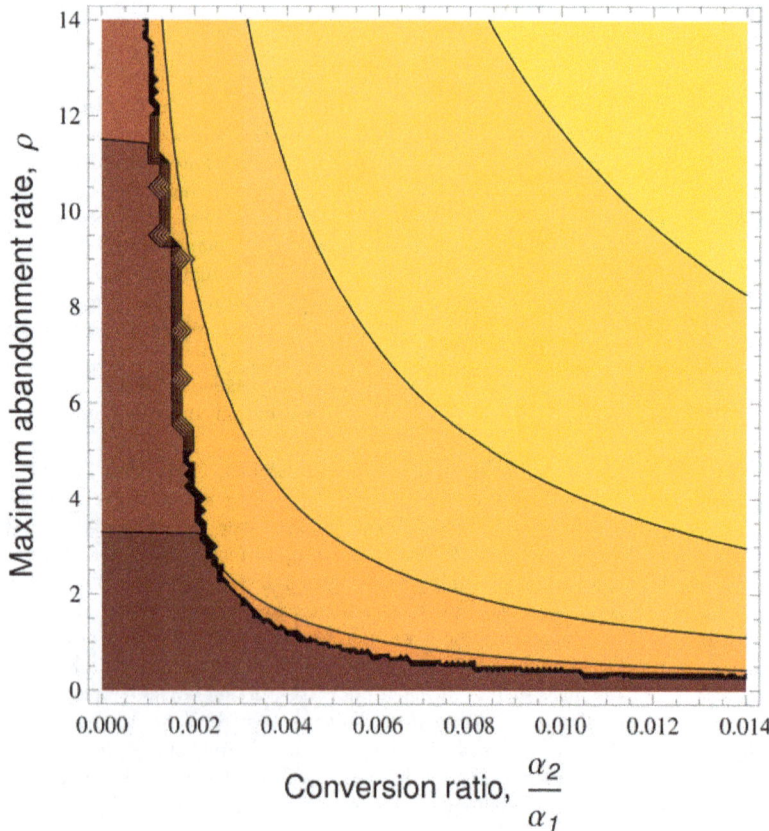

Figure 6. The effect of abandonment and conversion rates on the probability of spread. A density plot showing the treatment with the highest probability of spreading $\hat{\tau}$ as a function of ρ and the relative rate of conversion during healthy and sick periods (α_2/α_1), colour boundary range $\{-5, 17.5; \pm 2.5\}$ (low values, dark). Unless otherwise stated $a=0.5$, $b=0$, $\epsilon_0 = 0$, $\alpha_1 = 12$, $\alpha_2 = 0$, $\mu = 0.016$, $v = 0.008$, $\rho = \rho^* = 40.1711$ and $\sigma = 6$ (see Methods for interpretation of parameter values).

medical-treatment decisions. Nonetheless, our models make sense of a surprisingly broad set of phenomena.

Applications of the model

The primary application of our models is to the spread of self-medicative treatments in humans. The models are potentially relevant to any socially learned practice that is thought by the user to affect (that is, treat) their medical condition, through aiding recovery, reducing suffering, or reducing the probability of relapse, *irrespective of whether or not the treatment actually does bring about the improvements in condition assumed by the user*. The treatments include modern/established medical practices, complementary medicines, traditional medicines and alternative medicines. The models also potentially apply to instances of witchcraft, shamanism and magic in which the 'treatment' is believed to combat perceived underlying 'supernatural' causes of disease (e.g. the curse of a jealous neighbour, or a haunting by the ghost of an ancestor), so long as there exists a physical ailment in the user, and the treatment propagates through cultural transmission. While the use of modern medicines and well-documented and established complementary treatments is ontologically distinct from witchcraft and shamanism (they are not substitutes for each other, and their effectiveness is likely to be gauged by different criteria), nonetheless, all of these treatments share the fact that their use spreads through social learning and transmission, and uptake therefore is potentially a function of the rate of practice demonstration. Relevant medical conditions include physical and psychological disease, injuries and accidents. While the model can be applied to treatment of some infectious disease, we note that a satisfactory analysis of medical conditions that propagate rapidly relative to the rate of spread of treatments would require an extension of these models to track disease spread explicitly.

While the models assume treatments spread through social learning, the precise nature of the psychological mechanism is unspecified, and any of a range of established processes could be operating [27,28]. Nor do the models require the *conscious* imitation or observational learning of a practice. Accordingly, while the models are developed with humans in mind, they potentially are relevant to the spread of self-medicative treatments in other animals, particularly nonhuman primates. There is now good evidence for self-medicating behaviour in nonhuman primates, particularly African apes [29,30]. Chimpanzees, bonobos and gorillas are known to swallow whole and defecate intact leaves, traditional behaviour thought to be a means of purging intestinal parasites [29,30]. Experimental evidence reveals that this can spread through social transmission, leading to the suggestion that self-medicative practices in apes are maintained as behavioural traditions [29,30,31]. As intestinal parasites are likely to inflict multiple episodes ($\epsilon \gg 0$), circumstances that should favour the spread of efficacious treatments, our analysis supports claims of effective self-medication in apes.

The models are also potentially applicable to veterinary practices, although here the sick/treated animal is a different individual to the individual practicing the treatment (its owner). The models are not applicable to the activities of a veterinarian, but rather to animal owners who apply socially transmitted knowledge to treat their animal's condition.

The models apply broadly to any case where there are two states associated with higher and lower mortality, with the behavioural practice affecting the transition from the former to the latter. For instance, the model could be used to investigate the diffusion of foraging innovations, where hunger equates to sickness and satiation to wellness. With 'multiple episodes' of hunger ($\epsilon \gg 0$), a high rate of abandonment of poor foraging techniques or low

profitability foods ($\rho \gg 0$), and no 'recovery' without feeding ($\sigma = 0$), our model predicts that efficacious traits are most likely to spread, and that the frequency of maladaptive or superstitious foraging innovations should be low. This conclusion holds even if alternative foraging strategies were available ($\sigma \gg 0$), as would be the case where animals can feed without requiring social information. This may help to explain why there is not the same controversy over the spread of alternative foods and food-processing techniques as there is for treatments of disease: the latter are significantly more likely to be ineffective.

Remarks on unbiased copying

Our choice to set copying to be unbiased is a simple and parsimonious assumption. We also believe it is close to reality. Indeed, in recent years, considerable evidence has accumulated for such unbiased copying in the transmission of a broad range of cultural traits, from pottery designs, to baby names, to the popularity of dog breeds [32,33,34], but our analysis extends these findings to cultural traits that potentially affect Darwinian fitness. While individuals may seek to acquire effective remedies, they typically fail to do so in practice. In many circumstances, making judgments about the effectiveness of treatments deployed by others is challenging. For most ailments and practices, the decision to adopt a treatment is based on weak circumstantial evidence, cultural preconceptions and perceived efficacy, which may not reflect actual efficacy. Cultural mileux that frame natural phenomena in terms of supernatural causes would further weaken the connection between efficacy and the rate of adoption. Moreover, it is likely that people frequently recover irrespective of treatment (i.e. $\sigma > 0$), are poor at making judgments about what led to recovery, and different people offer conflicting advice. Our model therefore makes the simple assumption that sick people are willing to try new remedies – through unbiased copying – and drop them if they do not appear to work, and this suffices to explain superstitious and maladaptive treatments. We note that if copying were strongly biased so that individuals adopt effective treatments preferentially over ineffective ones, both acquisition and loss processes would favour effective remedies, leading to the spread of only efficacious treatments. At best, such a scenario could account for the presence of adaptive remedies, and could not by itself explain the existence of maladaptive or superstitious treatments. Yet, as described above, there is strong evidence that ineffective treatments are commonplace [1,6,7,8,11,12,13,14].

Unbiased copying should be distinguished from another notion – that sick people, in desperation, are willing to try any available treatment. Such a practice would not bring about unbiased copying (acquisition in proportion to observed frequency), but rather frequency independent copying, since all treatments would be equally likely to be adopted, irrespective of their frequency or efficacy. With no acquisition bias, treatment frequency dynamics would be dominated by the loss-process, which favours effective cures due to the abandonment of ineffective treatments. While the 'desperate flailing' process would preserve variation in treatments at low level, it could not explain how maladaptive or superstitious treatments could reach high frequencies. Moreover, this hypothesis runs counter to the strong empirical evidence that social learning increases with the frequency of demonstration [35,36,37,38,39]

Conceivably, in humans, the trade-off between trait efficacy and probability of spread predicted by our models will sometimes be negated through language. Individuals can simply sample others' evaluations, for instance, through conversation. However there is theoretical and empirical support for the hypothesis that individuals preferentially evaluate appropriate behaviour based on direct cues (e.g. self-evaluation), rather than observed behavioural decisions of others (e.g. evaluating others' treatments) [40,41,42]. Here, the contrast between technological/foraging innovations and medical treatments may be instructive. For technological/foraging innovations, the productivity of the innovation when employed by others is likely, in many situations, to be relatively straightforward to gauge, since observers can directly see the returns (higher yield, a better product etc) and make reliable judgments. This will mitigate against the spread of arbitrary of maladaptive practices, since observers would no longer be copying at random, but according to the efficacy of the trait. Individuals could equally inform others of effective self-medicative treatments, but with lower reliability, since the aforementioned factors (the difficulties of determining similarity of condition, demonstrator reliability, equivalence of treatment and the fact that individuals may have recovered independent of treatment), together with cultural norms about how medical conditions should be treated (e.g. the local convention in sub-Saharan Africa is to treat mastitis with witchcraft [12]) and placebo effects that accelerate recovery even when biologically inactive treatments have been adopted, render impartial evaluation of efficacy difficult.

Alternative hypotheses

While several established cultural evolution models explain the persistence of maladaptive traits, none are credible alternative explanations for the existence of ineffective or maladaptive self-medicative treatments on the scale observed. Selfish cultural variants, or memes [43], can lead to maladaptive traits spreading if the rate of imitation exceeds that of competing adaptive variants and overwhelms opposing selection [15,16]. To explain maladaptive treatments, however, this hypothesis would require people to prefer treatments that do not work over treatments that do, which is implausible. Conformist biases are known sometimes to lead to maladaptive outcomes, where environmental change renders a once adaptive solution no longer adaptive, or if conformity favours

group-beneficial traits [16,38]. Yet for many complementary medicines (e.g. the 'healing' power of crystals) there is no evidence that these treatments ever worked, nor any suggestion that they are group beneficial. Sexual selection, operating at genetic, cultural, or gene-cultural levels, is also known to be capable of propagating maladaptive variants [44,16,45] but people typically do not adopt medical treatments to render themselves attractive to the opposite sex. Prestige biases [16,46] are more credible, particularly in small scale pre-industrial societies, but in modern western societies where there is considerable prestige associated with doctors and the medical establishment, these institutions have typically lobbied against the use of complementary medicines and traditional treatments. These treatments appear to have spread in spite of a counteracting prestige bias, rather than because of one. In contrast to the above, the unbiased copying explanation that we favour is both simple and plausible.

Acknowledgments

We are grateful to Alex Bentley, Gillian Brown, Lewis Dean, Anne Kandler, Rachel Kendal, Luke Rendell and Jamie Tehrani for valuable comments on earlier drafts of this article, to Christine Broster, Charlotte Burn and Richard Byrne for drawing our attention to further potential applications of the models, and to Andrew Whiten for helpful discussion of self-medication in nonhuman primates.

Author Contributions

Conceived and designed the experiments: MMT JK KNL. Analyzed the data: MMT JK KNL. Contributed reagents/materials/analysis tools: MMT JK KNL. Wrote the paper: MMT JK KNL.

References

1. WHO (2002) WHO Traditional Medicine Strategy 2002–2005. World Health Organization Geneva.
2. Patwardhan B, Warude D, Pushpangadan P, Bhatt N (2005) Ayurveda and traditional Chinese medicine: a comparative overview. eCAM 2: 465–473.
3. Normile D (2003) The new face of traditional Chinese medicine. Science 299: 188–190.
4. Fiot J, Sanon S, Azas N, Mahiou V, Jansen O, et al. (2006) Phytochemical and pharmacological study of roots and leaves of *Guiera senegalensis* JF Gmel (*combretaceae*). Ethnopharmacol 106: 173–178.
5. Palombo EA (2006) Phytochemicals from traditional medicinal plants used in the treatment of diarrhoea: Modes of action and effects on intestinal function. Phytother Res 20: 717–724.
6. Abbott A (2005) Survey questions safety of alternative medicine. Nature 436: 898–898.
7. Abbott NC, White AR, Ernst E (1996) Complementary medicine. Nature 381: 361.
8. Shang A, Huwiler-Müntener K, Nartey L, Jüni P, Dörig S, et al. (2005) Are the clinical effects of homoeopathy placebo effects? Comparative study of placebo-controlled trials of homoeopathy and allopathy. Lancet 366: 726–732.
9. Giles J (2007) Degrees in homeopathy slated as unscientific. Nature 446: 352–353.
10. Garnier R, Poupon J (2006) Lead poisoning from traditional Indian medicines. Presse Med 35: 1177–1180.
11. Okeke TA, Okafor HU, Uzochukwu BSC (2006) Traditional healers in Nigeria: Perception of cause, treatment and referral practices for severe malaria. J Biosoc Sci 38: 491–500.
12. De Allegri M, Sarker M, Hofmann J, Sanon M, Bohler T (2007) A qualitative investigation into knowledge, beliefs, and practices surrounding mastitis in sub-saharan Africa: what implications for vertical transmission of HIV? BMC Public Health 7: 22.
13. Hsieh SC, Lai JN, Chen PC, Chen HJ, Wang JD (2006) Development of activesafety surveillance system for traditional Chinese medicine: an empirical

study in treating climacteric women. Pharmacoepid and Drug Safety 15: 889–899.
14. Ang HH, Lee KL (2006) Contamination of mercury in tongkat Ali hitam herbal preparations. Food Chem Toxicol 44: 1245–1259.
15. Cavalli-Sforza LL, Feldman MW (1981) Cultural transmission and evolution: a quantitative approach. Princeton University Press.
16. Boyd R, Richerson PJ (1985) Culture and the evolutionary process. Chicago University Press.
17. Tanaka MM, Kumm J, Feldman MW (2002) Coevolution of pathogens and cultural practices: a new look at behavioral heterogeneity in epidemics. Theor Popul Biol 62: 111–119.
18. Pagel M, Mace R (2004) The cultural wealth of nations. Nature 428: 275–278.
19. Karlin S, Taylor H (1975) A first course in stochastic processes. New York: Academic Press.
20. Nesse RM, Williams GC (1994) Why we get sick: The new science of Darwinian Medicine. New York: Vintage.
21. Ewens WJ (1979) Mathematical population genetics, volume 9 of *Biomathematics*. New York: Springer-Verlag.
22. Losada M, Ladio A, Weigant M (2006) Cultural transmission of ethnobotanical knowledge in a rural community of northwest Patagonia, Argentina. Econ Bot 60: 374–385.
23. Werner D (1983) Where there is no doctor. London: Macmillan Press.
24. Silver IA, Brown PN, Goodship AE, Lanyon LE, McCullagh KG, et al. (1983) A clinical and experimental study of tendon injury, healing and treatment in the horse. Equine Vet J Suppl 1: 1–42.
25. Reader SM, Laland KN, eds (2003) Animal Innovation. Oxford University Press.
26. Mace R (2000) Evolutionary ecology of human life history. Anim Behav 59: 1–10.
27. Whiten A, Ham R (1992) On the nature and evolution of imitation in the animal kingdom: reappraisal of a century of research. Adv Study Beh 21: 239–283.
28. Heyes CM (1994) Social learning in animals: categories and mechanisms. Biol Rev 69: 207–131.

29. Huffman MA (2003) Animal self-medication and ethno-medicine: exploration and exploitation of the medicinal properties of plants. Proc Nut Soc 62: 113–118.

30. Huffman MA, Hirata S (2004) An experimental study of leaf swallowing in captive chimpanzees: insights into the origin of a self-medicative behavior and the role of social learning. Primates 45: 113–118.

31. Whiten A, Goodall J, McGrew W, Nishida T, Reynolds V, et al. (1999) Cultures in chimpanzees. Nature 399: 682–685.

32. Bentley RA, Hahn MW, Shennan SJ (2004) Random drift and culture change. Proc Roy Soc Lond B 271: 1443–1450.

33. Bentley RA, Hahn MW (2003) Drift as a mechanism for cultural change: An example from baby names. Proc Roy Soc Lond B 270: S120–S123.

34. Bentley RA, Lipo C, Herzog M, Hahn MW (2006) Regular rates of popular culture change reect random copying. Evol Hum Behav 28: 151–158.

35. Laland KN, Williams K (1997) Shoaling generates social learning of foraging information in guppies. Anim Behav 53: 1161–1169.

36. Beck M, Galef Jr BG (1989) Social inuences on the selection of a protein-sufficient diet by Norway rats (*Rattus norvegicus*). J Comp Psychol 103: 132–139.

37. Lefebvre L, Giraldeau LA (1994) Cultural transmission in pigeons is affected by the number of tutors and bystanders present. Anim Behav 47: 331–337.

38. Henrich J, Boyd R (1998) The evolution of conformist transmission and the emergence of between-group differences. Evol Hum Behav 19: 215–241.

39. Coultas JC (2004) When in Rome… An evolutionary perspective on conformity. Group Proc and Intergroup Relat 7: 317.

40. Giraldeau LA, Valone TJ, Templeton JJ (2002) Potential disadvantages of using socially acquired information. Philos Trans R Soc Lond B Biol Sci 357: 1559–1566.

41. Bikhchandani S, Hirshleifer D, Welsh I (1992) A theory of fads, fashion, custom and cultural changes as informational cascades. J Polit Econ 100: 992–1026.

42. Bikhchandani S, Hirshleifer D, Welsh I (1998) Learning from the behavior of others: Conformity, fads and informational cascades. J Econ Perspect 12: 151–170.

43. Dawkins R (1976) The Selfish Gene. Oxford University Press.

44. Kirkpatrick M (1982) Sexual selection and the evolution of female choice. Evolution 36: 1–12.

45. Laland KN (1994) Sexual selection with a culturally transmitted mating preference. Theor Popul Biol 45: 1–15.

46. Henrich J, Gil-White FJ (2001) The evolution of prestige: freely conferred deference as a mechanism for enhancing the benefits of cultural transmission. Evol Hum Behav 22: 165–196.

PERMISSIONS

LIST OF CONTRIBUTORS

Taryn Roberts and Paul McGreevy
Faculty of Veterinary Science, University of Sydney, Sydney, New South Wales, Australia

Michael Valenzuela
School of Psychiatry, University of New South Wales, Sydney, New South Wales, Australia
Brain and Ageing Research Program, Faculty of Medicine, University of New South Wales, Sydney, New South Wales, Australia

Zhining Wen
National Center for Toxicological Research, U.S. Food and Drug Administration, Jefferson, Arkansas, United States of America
College of Chemistry, Sichuan University, Chengdu, Sichuan, China

Lun Yang and Leming Shi
National Center for Toxicological Research, U.S. Food and Drug Administration, Jefferson, Arkansas, United States of America
Department of Clinical Pharmacy and Center for Pharmacogenomics, School of Pharmacy, Fudan University, Shanghai, China

Zhijun Wang, Steven Wang, Ranadheer Ravula, Moses S. S. Chow and Ying Huang
Department of Pharmaceutical Sciences and Center for Advancement of Drug Research and Evaluation, College of Pharmacy, Western University of Health Sciences, Pomona, California, United States of America

Jun Xu
Clinical Transcriptional Genomics Core, Medical Genetics Institute, Cedars-Sinai Medical Center, David Geffen School of Medicine at UCLA, Los Angeles, California, United States of America

Charles Wang
Functional Genomics Core, Beckman Research Institute, City of Hope Comprehensive Cancer Center, Duarte, California, United States of America

Zhong Zuo
School of Pharmacy, Faculty of Medicine, The Chinese University of Hong Kong, Hong Kong, China

Pascale Rialland, Martin Guillot, Jérôme R. E. del Castillo, Daphnée Veilleux-Lemieux , Dominique Gauvin and Eric Troncy
1 Groupe de Recherche en Pharmacologie Animale du Québec (GREPAQ), Department of Biomedical Sciences, Faculty of veterinary medicine, Université de Montréal, Saint-Hyacinthe, Quebec, Canada

Simon Authier
Groupe de Recherche en Pharmacologie Animale du Québec (GREPAQ), Department of Biomedical Sciences, Faculty of veterinary medicine, Université de Montréal, Saint-Hyacinthe, Quebec, Canada
CiToxLAB North America, Laval, Quebec, Canada

Diane Frank
Department of Clinical Sciences; Faculty of veterinary medicine, Université de Montréal, Saint-Hyacinthe, Quebec, Canada

Johanna Judge, Neil Walker and Richard J. Delahay
The Food & Environment Research Agency, Sand Hutton, York, Yorkshire, United Kingdom

Robbie A. McDonald
The Food & Environment Research Agency, Sand Hutton, York, Yorkshire, United Kingdom
Environment and Sustainability Institute, University of Exeter, Cornwall Campus, Penryn, Cornwall, United Kingdom

Subhra Subhadra, Mohanraj Karthik and Muthusamy Raman
Department of Veterinary Parasitology, Madras Veterinary College, Tamil Nadu Veterinary and Animal Sciences University, Chennai, Tamil Nadu, India

Sebastian J. Padayatty, Andrew Y. Sun, Michael Graham Espey and Mark Levine
Molecular and Clinical Nutrition Section, National Institute of Diabetes and Digestive and Kidney Diseases, National Institutes of Health, Bethesda, Maryland, United States of America

Qi Chen and Jeanne Drisko
Program in Integrative Medicine, University of Kansas Medical Center, Kansas City, Kansas, United States of America

Katerina Karolemeas, James L. N. Wood, Trevelyan J. McKinley and Andrew J. K. Conlan
Disease Dynamics Unit, Department of Veterinary Medicine. University of Cambridge, Cambridge, United Kingdom

Christl A. Donnelly
MRC Centre for Outbreak Analysis and Modelling, Department of Infectious Disease Epidemiology, Imperial College, London, United Kingdom

Andrew P. Mitchell, Richard S. Clifton- Hadley and Paul Upton
Animal Health and Veterinary Laboratories Agency, Weybridge, Surrey, United Kingdom

Barbara Lamagna, Anna Guardascione, Luigi Navas and Manuela Ragozzino
Department of Veterinary Clinical Sciences, Unit of Surgery, University of Naples Federico II, Naples, Italy

Adelaide Greco and Arturo Brunetti
Department of Biomorphological and Functional Science, University of Naples Federico II, Naples, Italy
Ceinge, Biotecnologie Avanzate, scarl, Naples, Italy
Institute of Biostructure and Bioimaging, CNR, Naples, Italy

Orlando Paciello
Department of Pathology and Animal Health, Unit of Pathology, University of Naples Federico II, Naples, Italy

Leonardo Meomartino
Interdepartmental Veterinary Radiology Centre, University of Naples Federico II, Naples, Italy

Helen M. Higgins, Martin J. Green and Jasmeet Kaler
School of Veterinary Medicine and Science, University of Nottingham, Sutton Bonington, Leicestershire, United Kingdom

Laura E. Green
School of Life Sciences, University of Warwick, Coventry, West Midlands, United Kingdom

Sebastian Guenther, Katja Aschenbrenner, Astrid Bethe, Torsten Semmler and Lothar H. Wieler
Institute of Microbiology and Epizootics, Veterinary Faculty, Freie Universität Berlin, Berlin, Germany

Christa Ewers
Institute of Microbiology and Epizootics, Veterinary Faculty, Freie Universität Berlin, Berlin, Germany
Institute of Hygiene and Infectious Diseases of Animals, Veterinary Faculty, Justus-Liebig-Universität Giessen, Giessen, Germany

Ivonne Stamm
Vet Med Labor GmbH, Ludwigsburg, Germany

Annegret Stubbe and Michael Stubbe
Department of Zoology, Institute of Biology, Martin Luther Universität Halle-Wittenberg, Halle, Germany

Nyamsuren Batsajkhan
Department of Zoology, National University of Mongolia, Ulan-Bator, Mongolia

Youri Glupczynski
National Reference Laboratory for Antimicrobial Resistance in Gram-negative bacteria, Centre Hospitalier Universitaire de Mont-Godinne, Université Catholique de Louvain, Yvoir, Belgium

Kerstin E. Müller
Clinic for Ruminants and Swine, Faculty of Veterinary Medicine, Freie Universität Berlin, Berlin, Germany

Julia Klein
Clinic for Ruminants and Swine, Faculty of Veterinary Medicine, Freie Universität Berlin, Berlin, Germany
Center of Experimental and Applied Cutaneous Physiology, Department of Dermatology, Venerology and Allergology, Charité – Universitätsmedizin Berlin, Berlin, Germany

Maxim E. Darvin and Juergen Lademann
Center of Experimental and Applied Cutaneous Physiology, Department of Dermatology, Venerology and Allergology, Charité – Universitätsmedizin Berlin, Berlin, Germany

Kerstin M. Ahlgren, Nils Landegren, Anna Lobell and Olle Kämpe
Department of Medical Sciences, Science for Life Laboratory, Uppsala University, Uppsala, Sweden

Tove Fall
Department of Medical Sciences, Molecular Epidemiology and Science for Life Laboratory, Uppsala University, Uppsala, Sweden

Lars Grimelius
Department of Immunology, Genetics and Pathology, Uppsala University, Sweden

Henrik von Euler, Helene Hansson-Hamlin and Åke Hedhammar
Department of Clinical Sciences, Swedish University of Agricultural Sciences, Uppsala, Sweden

Katarina Sundberg and Göran Andersson
Department of Animal Breeding and Genetics, Swedish University of Agricultural Sciences, Uppsala, Sweden

Kerstin Lindblad-Toh
Broad Institute of Harvard and MIT, Cambridge, Massachusetts, United States of America
Science for Life Laboratory, Department of Medical Biochemistry and Microbiology, Uppsala University, Uppsala, Sweden

Åke Lernmark
Diabetes and Celiac Disease Unit, Department of Clinical Sciences, Lund University, Malmö, Sweden

Bamidele O. Tayo, Liping Tong and Richard S. Cooper
Department of Preventive Medicine and Epidemiology, Loyola University Chicago Stritch School of Medicine, Maywood, Illinois, United States of America

Marie Teil, Gregory Khitrov, Weijia Zhang, Quinbin Song, Omri Gottesman and Erwin P. Bottinger
Charles R. Bronfman Institute for Personalized Medicine, Mount Sinai School of Medicine, New York, New York, United States of America

Huaizhen Qin and Xiaofeng Zhu
Department of Biostatistics and Epidemiology, Case Western University, Cleveland, Ohio, United States of America

Alexandre C. Pereira
University of Sao Paulo Medical School, Sao Paulo, Brazil

Kate Sawford
Farm Animal & Veterinary Public Health, Faculty of Veterinary Science, University of Sydney, Camden, New South Wales, Australia
Department of Ecosystem and Public Health, Faculty of Veterinary Medicine, University of Calgary, Calgary, Alberta, Canada
Department of Medical Sciences, Faculty of Medicine, University of Calgary, Calgary, Alberta, Canada

Craig Stephen
Department of Ecosystem and Public Health, Faculty of Veterinary Medicine, University of Calgary, Calgary, Alberta, Canada

Ardene Robinson Vollman
Department of Community Health Sciences, Faculty of Medicine, University of Calgary, Calgary, Alberta, Canada

Ikram Guizani and Souheila Guerbouj
Laboratory of Molecular Epidemiology and Experimental Pathology, Pasteur Institute of Tunis, Université de Tunis el Manar, Tunis, Tunisia
Laboratory of Epidemiology and Ecology of Parasitic Diseases, Pasteur Institute of Tunis, Tunis, Tunisia

Fattouma Djilani
Laboratory of Epidemiology and Ecology of Parasitic Diseases, Pasteur Institute of Tunis, Tunis, Tunisia

Riadh Ben Ismail
Laboratory of Epidemiology and Ecology of Parasitic Diseases, Pasteur Institute of Tunis, Tunis, Tunisia
World Health Organization – Eastern Mediterranean Regional Office (WHO – EMRO), Cairo, Egypt

Mohamed Fethi Diouani
Laboratory of Epidemiology and Ecology of Parasitic Diseases, Pasteur Institute of Tunis, Tunis, Tunisia
Laboratory of Veterinary Epidemiology and Microbiology, Pasteur Institute of Tunis, Tunis, Tunisia

Afif Ben Salah and Jihene Bettaieb
Laboratory of Medical Epidemiology, Pasteur Institute of Tunis, Tunis, Tunisia

Bronwen Lambson
Molteno Institute for Parasitology, Department of Pathology, University of Cambridge, Cambridge, United Kingdom
Centre for HIV and STI, National Institute for Communicable Diseases of the National Health Laboratory Service, Johannesburg, South Africa

John D. Lippolis, Timothy A. Reinhardt, Randy A. Sacco and Brian J. Nonnecke
Ruminant Diseases and Immunology Research Unit, National Animal Disease Center, Agricultural Research Service (ARS), United States Department of Agriculture (USDA), Ames, Iowa, United States of America

Corwin D. Nelson
Department of Biochemistry, University of Wisconsin-Madison, Madison, Wisconsin, United States of America

Anna H. Le, Luis A. Bonachea and Shelley L. Cargill
Department of Biological Sciences, San José State University, San José , California, United States of America

Connie Chuang, Megan A. Ramaker, Sirjaut Kaur, Rebecca A. Csomos, Kevin T. Kroner, Jason A. Bleedorn, Susan L. Schaefer and Peter Muir
Comparative Orthopaedic Research Laboratory, and the Department of Surgical Sciences, School of Veterinary Medicine, University of Wisconsin-Madison, Madison, Wisconsin, United States of America

Julien Guevar, Jacques Penderis, Kiterie Faller, Carmen Yeamans, Catherine Stalin and Rodrigo Gutierrez-Quintana
School of Veterinary Medicine, College of Medical, Veterinary and Life Sciences, University of Glasgow, Glasgow, United Kingdom

Rowena M. A. Packer and Holger A. Volk
Department of Clinical Science and Services, Royal Veterinary College, Hatfield, Hertfordshire, United Kingdom

Nadia K. Shihab
Department of Clinical Science and Services, Royal Veterinary College, Hatfield, Hertfordshire, United Kingdom

Department of Neurology/Neurosurgery, Southern Counties Veterinary Specialists, Ringwood, Hampshire, United Kingdom

Bruno B. J. Torres
Department of Veterinary Medicine and Surgery, Federal University of Minas Gerais, Belo Horizonte, Minas Gerais, Brazil

Dipti W. Pitta, Nagaraju Indugu and Sanjay Kumar
Center for Animal Health and Productivity, School of Veterinary Medicine, University of Pennsylvania, Philadelphia, Pennsylvania, United States of America

Nidhi Parmar, Amrut K. Patel, Anand B. Patel, Bhaskar Reddy and Chaitanya Joshi
Ome Research Facility, Department of Animal Biotechnology, Anand Agricultural University, Anand, Gujarat, India

Karsanbhai B. Prajapathi
Livestock Production and Management Department, College of Veterinary Science and Animal Husbandry, Sardar Krushi Nagar Dantiwada Agricultural University, Sardar Krushi Nagar, Gujarat, India

Thomas Grönthal and Merja Rantala
Central Laboratory, Department of Equine and Small Animal Medicine, University of Helsinki, Helsinki, Finland

Arshnee Moodley and Luca Guardabassi
Department of Veterinary Disease Biology, Faculty of Health and Medical Sciences, University of Copenhagen, Copenhagen, Denmark

Suvi Nykäsenoja
3 Food and Feed Microbiology Research Unit, Finnish Food Safety Authority Evira, Helsinki, Finland

Jouni Junnila
4Pharma Ltd., Espoo, Finland

Katariina Thomson
Veterinary Teaching Hospital, University of Helsinki, Helsinki, Finland

Calvin Yu-Chian Chen
School of Chinese Medicine, China Medical University, Taichung, Taiwan

Department of Bioinformatics, Asia University, Taichung, Taiwan
Department of Computational and Systems Biology, Massachusetts Institute of Technology, Cambridge, Massachusetts, United States of America

Mark M. Tanaka
Evolution & Ecology Research Centre, School of Biotechnology & Biomolecular Sciences, University of New South Wales, Sydney, New South Wales, Australia

Jeremy R. Kendal
Department of Anthropology, University of Durham, Durham, United Kingdom

Kevin N. Laland
School of Biology, University of St Andrews, Fife, United Kingdom

Index